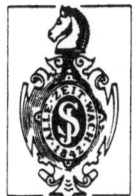

Clinical Medicine and the Nervous System

Series Editors: John P. Conomy and Michael Swash

Imaging of the Nervous System

Edited by Paul Butler

With 334 Figures

Springer-Verlag
London Berlin Heidelberg New York
Paris Tokyo Hong Kong

Paul Butler, MRCP, FRCR
Consultant Neuroradiologist, The London Hospital,
Whitechapel, London E1 1BB, UK

Series Editors:

John P. Conomy, MD, Head, Department of Neurology,
The Cleveland Clinic Foundation, Cleveland, Ohio, USA

Michael Swash, MD, FRCP, MRCPath, Consultant Neurologist,
The London Hospital, Whitechapel, London, UK

Front Cover Illustrations:
Cranial CT with intravenous contrast. Multiple tuberculomata.
Vertebral arterial DSA. Aneurysm of the posterior inferior cerebellar artery.
Cranial MRI (sagittal section) – T1 weighted image. Pituitary tumour.

ISBN-13:978-1-4471-1639-4   e-ISBN-13:978-1-4471-1637-0
DOI: 10.1007/978-1-4471-1637-0

British Library Cataloguing in Publication Data
Imaging of the nervous system.
  1. Man. Nervous system. Diagnosis. Imaging
  I. Butler, Paul, *1952–* II. Series
  616.8'047575
  ISBN-13:978-1-4471-1639-4

Library of Congress Cataloging-in-Publication Data
Imaging of the nervous system/Paul Butler (ed.).
     p. cm. — (Clinical medicine and the nervous system)
     ISBN-13:978-1-4471-1639-4 (alk. paper)
1. Nervous system — Imaging. 2. Nervous system — Diseases — Diagnosis. I. Butler, Paul, 1952 June 4–
II. Series. [DNLM: 1. Magnetic Resonance Imaging. 2. Nervous System Diseases — diagnosis. 3. Tomography, X-ray Computed. WL 141 1315]
     RC349.D52143 1990
     616.8'0475 — dc20
     DNLM/DLC.   89-26083
     for Library of Congress   CIP

2128/3916–543210. Printed on acid-free paper

Series Editors' Foreword

Traditionally, investigation of the nervous system has been primarily a clinical matter. The great era of clinical assessment of patients with neurological disease in the first half of the century was determined by the necessity both to understand the phenomena of neurological disease in relation to structure and function and to localise lesions, in order to facilitate the twin processes of diagnosis and management. Over the years diverse techniques have been applied to clinical practice in order to improve the accuracy of diagnosis. These have comprised extensions of clinical method, for example clinical neuropsychology, electro-encephalography, radiography of the skull and spine, angiography and other contrast procedures, including the now abandoned technique of air encephalography, and myel-ography, perhaps itself soon to be little used. Isotope studies of the brain have possibly not realised their full potential in clinical neurology. All these different investigations found an integrated place in clinical management, enhancing the classical clinical database and its associated information, derived from biochemical, immunological and haematological studies.

The advent of computerised tomographic X-ray scanning changed all this. The quality of the images derived from CT scanning was so much superior to that obtainable by conventional X-ray methods, and the method was so non-invasive in its conception, that clinical practice in both medical and surgical neurology changed profoundly. An image of the affected part of the nervous system was now available that could be used to study the location and X-ray absorbence characteristics of a lesion in the brain, and that could be applied to medical treatment or used to direct the surgical approach with hitherto undreamt of accuracy. The development of magnetic resonance imaging, digital angiography, and also of positron emission tomography and SPECT imaging, has further refined the role of imaging in clinical neurology. Some long-cherished beliefs about lesion location and size in relation to certain clinical phenomena have been abandoned, the diagnosis of many previously difficult disorders has been simplified, and otherwise unrecognisable lesions have come to be seen as important. Nonetheless, the image is not yet everything in clinical neurology and neurosurgery. Indeed, although clinical problem solving has been greatly enhanced by modern imaging, and has changed its emphasis, some of the commonest clinical problems, for example headache and epilepsy, are relatively unlikely to yield information to the imager.

In this book Paul Butler has set out to provide a review of most of what matters to clinicians about neuro-imaging within a relatively short volume commensurate with the aims of the Clinical Medicine and the Nervous System series. We trust that the book will find its way onto the bookshelves of neurologists and neurosurgeons everywhere, and that they will find it useful and informative in their everyday clinical practice and, in the case of younger physicians and surgeons, in their training. The format of the book is such that it should also be useful to general physicians and surgeons, and to general radiologists, as a source of information about the nervous system.

London, UK   Michael Swash
Cleveland, Ohio   John P. Conomy
March 1990

Preface

The introduction of computed tomographic (CT) scanning in the late 1970s brought with it the prospect of less-invasive neuroimaging and soon led to the welcome demise of air encephalography (a rare example of one radiological technique truly replacing another). This trend has been continued with magnetic resonance imaging (MRI) which provides quite remarkable displays of the neuraxis without the use of ionising radiation. How the two techniques are best used is still emerging but each has its own peculiar advantages and in many instances they are complementary. Their relative simplicity also allows repeated examinations to follow the progress of disease and monitor therapeutic response.

Conversely cerebrovascular imaging remains largely invasive although screening for degenerative cervical arterial disease is now undertaken in many centres using real time "B" mode ultrasound in combination with Doppler studies (duplex sonography). Digital subtraction techniques have gone some way to make angiography both safer and less unpleasant for the patient, but early enthusiasm has been dampened by problems with spatial resolution.

CT and MRI have made a great contribution to spinal imaging. CT obviates myelography in many cases of lumbar degenerative disease and complements it elsewhere in the spine, but in many centres MRI has led to the near total abandonment of myelography. Paradoxically MRI may lead to a renaissance of the plain radiograph, which has been rather neglected in the age of CT. There is increasing interest in functional radioisotope studies of the central nervous system and, coupled with the development of more "user friendly" radiopharmaceuticals, nuclear medicine has also experienced something of a revival in recent years.

This text provides an overview of current neuroradiological practice and demonstrates the appearances of a wide range of craniospinal pathology using modern techniques. It is intended primarily for residents in neurology, neurosurgery and radiology, but it is hoped that their senior colleagues and those in related specialties will also find it relevant. A detailed account of MRI technology is considered beyond the scope of this book, but the interested reader is referred to the excellent and concise account "Magnetic Resonance Imaging" by Sigal, Doyon, Ph Halimi and Atlan (Springer-Verlag, 1988).

A number of illustrations have been inserted by the editor (denoted by P.B. in the legends) in chapters other than his own; for these and many of the other illustrations I would like to express my thanks to the Department of Medical Illustration at The London Hospital. I am also grateful to the series editor, Michael Swash and the publisher, Michael Jackson, for their patient advice and to the contributors for their tolerance.

London　　　　　　　　　　　　　　　　　　　　　　　　　　　　　　　Paul Butler
September 1989

Contents

Contributors

Philip L. Anslow, MA, FRCR
Consultant Neuroradiologist, Radcliffe Infirmary, Oxford OX2 6HE, UK

Nagui M. Antoun, MRCP, FRCR
Consultant Neuroradiologist, Addenbrooke's Hospital, Cambridge CB2 2QQ, UK

Paul Butler, MRCP, FRCR
Consultant Neuroradiologist, The London Hospital, Whitechapel, London E1 1BB

Peter Dawson, PhD, MRCP, FRCR
Senior Lecturer and Honorary Consultant Radiologist, The Royal Postgraduate Medical School, Hammersmith Hospital, London W12 0HS

W. St Clair Forbes, MA, MB, BCh, DMRD, FRCR
Consultant Neuroradiologist, Hope Hospital, Salford M6 8HD, UK

Charles E. L. Freer, MRCP, FRCR
Consultant Neuroradiologist, Addenbrooke's Hospital, Cambridge CB2 2QQ, UK

Neil W. Garvie, MA, MSc, MRCP, FRCR
Consultant in Radiology and Nuclear Medicine, The London Hospital, Whitechapel, London E1 1BB

Margaret D. Hourihan, MRCP, FRCR
Consultant Neuroradiologist, University Hospital of Wales, Heath Park, Cardiff CF4 4XW, UK

Glyn A. S. Lloyd, DM, FRCR
Consultant Radiologist, The Royal National Throat, Nose and Ear Hospital, London WC1X 8DA

John M. Stevens, DRACR, FRCR
Consultant Radiologist, St Mary's Hospital and The Hospital for Nervous Diseases, Maida Vale, London W9 1TO

Michael Swash, MD, FRCP, MRCPath
Consultant Neurologist, The London Hospital, Whitechapel, London E1 1BB

Evelyn Teasdale, BSc, MRCP, FRCR
Consultant Radiologist, Institute of Neurological Sciences, Southern General Hospital, Glasgow GS1 4TF, UK

Chandra H. Thakkar, MD, FRCR
Consultant Neuroradiologist, The London Hospital, Whitechapel, London E1 1BB

Ian W. Turnbull, FRCR
Consultant Neuroradiologist, North Manchester General Hospital, Manchester M8 6RB,
UK

Chapter 1

Cerebrovascular Disease

Paul Butler

CEREBRAL ISCHAEMIA

Arterial Disease

Pathogenesis of Stroke

The Harvard Stroke Registry Group found that the most common cause of stroke was cerebral arteriosclerosis with thrombotic or thromboembolic occlusion (Mohr et al. 1978).

In the craniocervical arterial tree the sites of predilection for arteriosclerosis include the carotid bifurcation (Fig. 1.1), the carotid siphons and the basal intracranial arteries, particularly the middle cerebral. Rarely the process can be diffuse. The early changes of intimal and subintimal infiltration cause minor irregularity of the opacified vessel lumen at angiography. Stenosis then develops which may be smooth and regular but which is more often irregular and ulcerated. Platelet aggregation can be provoked causing local thrombus formation which may lead ultimately to arterial occlusion or embolism.

The consequence of any vascular occlusion will depend on its site and the adequacy of the collateral circulation. Thrombotic occlusion of the internal carotid artery can lead to major cerebral infarction and death but if the occlusion is gradual and collateral pathways are available, neurological deficit need not be severe. Anastomoses exist between the internal and external carotid arteries – notably via the maxillary and ophthalmic arteries – and between the external carotid and vertebral arteries. Intracranially the Circle of Willis links the internal carotid arteries and the basilar artery. Surface cortical anastomoses are seen between anterior, middle and posterior cerebral arteries and transdural connections occur especially in children between cortical and meningeal arteries.

Embolisation from carotid bifurcation disease may cause distal cerebral arterial occlusion either of a permanent or a temporary nature. Barnett (1980) states that stenotic or ulcerative lesions of the extracranial carotid arteries are the principal

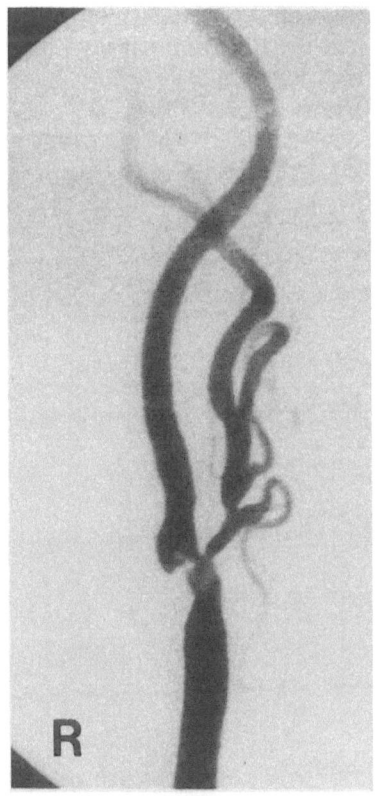

Fig. 1.1. Carotid arterial DSA with atheromatous disease of the cervical carotid bifurcation.

sources of non-cardiac cerebral emboli. It is also possible that some patients with severe arterial stenoses experience cerebral ischaemia due to a failure to maintain adequate cerebral perfusion.

Cerebral angiography in the first few days after cerebral infarction may show a blush in the infarcted region due to "luxury perfusion" consequent upon ischaemic small vessel dilatation. Early venous filling due to local arteriovenous shunting may also occur.

The heart is recognised as an important source of cerebral emboli with disorders of cardiac rhythm the most frequent cause – particularly atrial fibrillation (Salgado et al. 1987; Grosgogeat 1985).

Cerebral embolism may follow a myocardial infarction or cardiomyopathy and is related to the abnormal movement of the damaged ventricle. Intracardiac tumours, notably atrial myxomas, are uncommon but well recognised to cause cerebral embolism – perhaps as a presenting feature.

Lacunes are small, deeply situated ischaemic lesions with diameters between 0.5 and 15 mm (Fisher 1965). They are thought to result from occlusions of small perforating arteries and are often multiple. There is a strong association with hypertensive disease. The thalami, basal ganglia and pons are typically affected but lacunes also occur in the white matter of internal capsule, the corona radiata and centrum semiovale (Fig. 1.2).

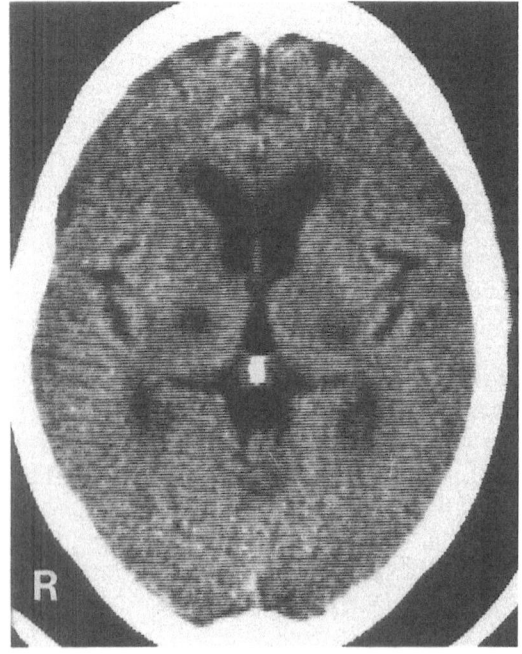

Fig. 1.2. Cranial CT. Lacunar infarcts involving both internal capsules.

It is apparent that a number of mechanisms for stroke exist in patients with degenerative vascular disease. Emboli can arise from the heart or from arteriosclerotic extracranial arteries and in the latter case, thrombosis in situ can also lead to stroke.

A similar arteriosclerotic process may affect the proximal portions of the major cerebral arteries – especially the middle cerebral artery and small vessel occlusion with lacune formation additionally emphasises the importance of intrinsic cerebral vascular disease. If an extracranial arterial stenosis is severe and the collateral circulation poorly developed then cerebral ischaemia may result from inadequate perfusion.

In the elderly hypertensive patient with myocardial ischaemia any of these causes may be responsible and the actual cause of stroke may prove difficult to determine.

The causes of cerebral ischaemia are listed in Table 1.1.

Table 1.1. Causes of cerebral ischaemia

Arteriosclerosis
Embolism
Arteritis
Fibrodysplasia
Dissection
Moya moya disease
Trauma
Hypotension
Arterial spasm
Blood dyscrasia
Migraine
Venous infarction

Computed Tomography in Cerebral Infarction

A mature cerebral infarct appears as a zone of hypodensity conforming to a vascular territory with shrinkage leading to dilatation of adjacent cerebrospinal fluid (CSF) spaces. The vascular territories are summarised in Figs 1.3–1.6. It is important to realise that the cerebral arterial tree is subject to normal anatomical variations and that there is some overlap between vascular territories particularly in the posterior circulation. The majority of cerebral infarcts occur in the territory of the middle cerebral artery followed by the posterior cerebral and anterior cerebral artery territories.

During maturation the infarct evolves through a number of acute changes. The cessation of oxidative metabolism following cerebral infarction leads to failure of membrane transport mechanisms with the development of intracellular (cytotoxic) oedema. Similar mechanisms lead to increased vascular permeability and the occurrence of vasogenic oedema which is dependent on the reperfusion of ischaemic brain. Such vascular damage also leads to the breakdown of the blood–brain barrier (Brant Zawadzki et al. 1987).

A CT scan undertaken within 24 hours of an ischaemic stroke may be ostensibly normal or show only subtle changes. Such early scans may reveal increased density of an occluded middle cerebral artery due to thrombus or embolus (Pressman et al. 1987; Schuierer and Huk 1988) (Fig. 1.7). The main purpose of an early CT scan in stroke is to exclude cerebral haemorrhage.

Mass Effect

Mass effect may precede the appearance of hypodensity. It occurs in only a minority of patients and accompanies the more extensive infarcts, regressing after about one week. Its existence is an adverse prognostic factor.

Hypodensity

Hypodensity in infarction usually becomes visible at 24 hours and the margins become clearer over the next few days. In some patients this hypodensity diminishes at 2–3 weeks leaving an apparently normal scan. This "fogging effect" was found in 54% of cases studied by Skriver and Olsen (1981). To exclude an infarct reliably at this time it may be necessary to resort to intravenous contrast administration.

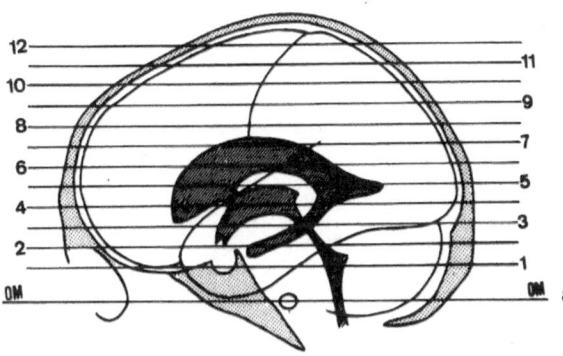

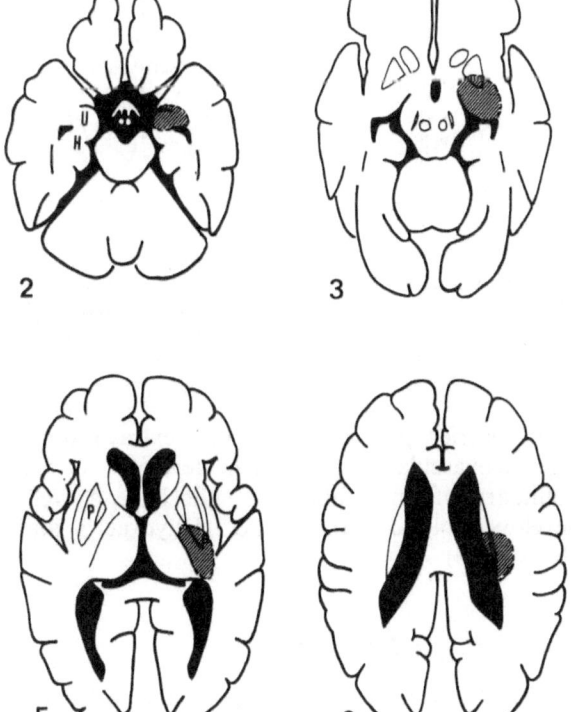

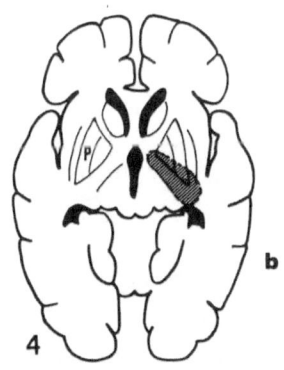

Fig. 1.3. a System of 12 cuts parallel to the orbito- or cantho-meatal line (OM). **b** Anterior choroidal artery (using only cuts 2 to 6). H, para-hippocampal gyrus; U, uncus; P, putamen. (From Bories et al. 1985.)

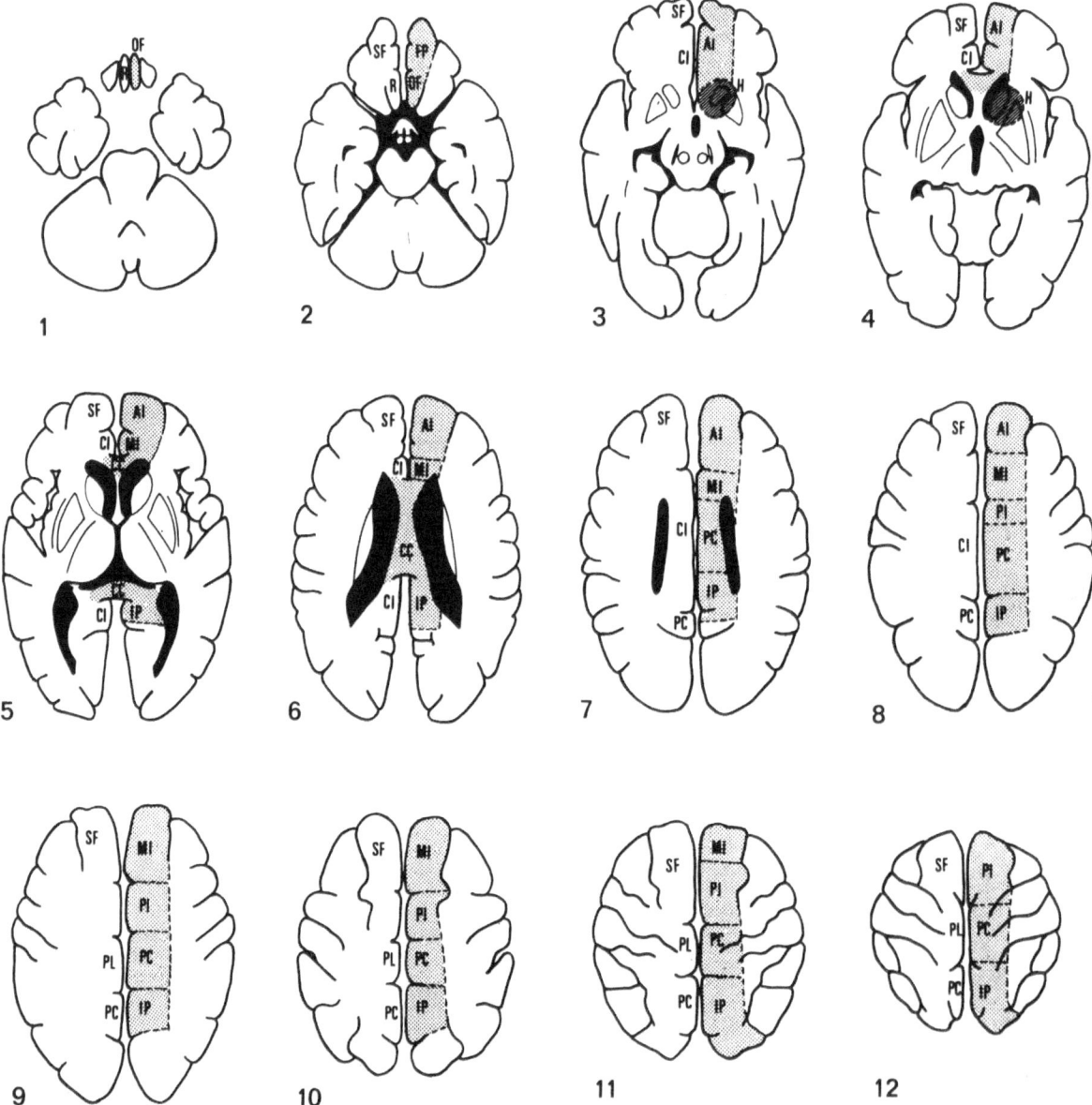

Fig. 1.4. Anterior cerebral artery (ACA) territory. (The numbers refer to the cuts in Fig. 1.3(a).) Gyri (G) and other structures: R, rectal G; SF, superior frontal G; CI, cingulate G; PC, precuneus; PL, paracentral lobule. Arteries (A): OF, orbito-frontal A; FP, fronto-polar A; AI, anterior frontal A; MI, middle internal frontal A; PI, posterior interior frontal A; H, Heubner A; IP, internal parietal A (superior and inferior branches); CC, pericallosal arteries; PC, paracentral A. (From Bories et al. 1985.)

Enhancement

It is likely that the majority of infarcts enhance with intravenous contrast at some stage in their time course (Fig. 1.8) but enhancement is infrequent before day 7 and rare after 6 weeks. Enhancement in a lesion after this time should alert the radiologist to the possibility of alternative pathology.

The pattern of enhancement is variable. It can be ring-like (typical of deep infarcts), total or gyriform and is thought to be due to a disordered blood–brain barrier permitting contrast extravasation. The neovascularisation which develops at the boundary of an infarct may not have a well-developed blood–brain barrier (Duyckaerts and Hauw 1985).

Haemorrhagic Infarction

Cerebral infarcts can be haemorrhagic with restoration of blood flow into the vascular bed of the

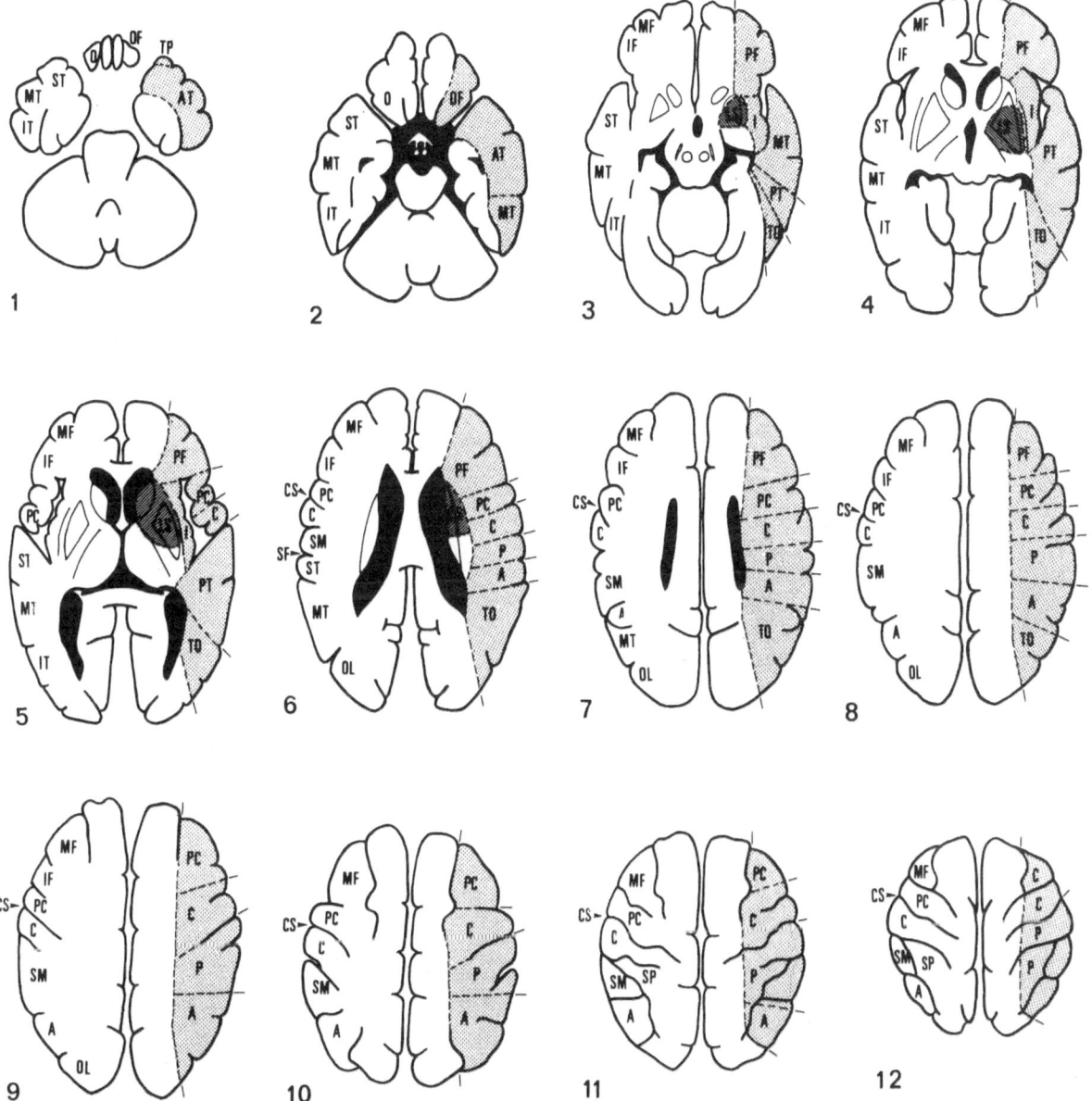

Fig. 1.5. Middle cerebral artery (MCA) territory. (The numbers refer to the cuts in Fig. 1.3(a).) Gyri (G) and other structures: O, orbital G; ST, superior temporal G; MT, middle temporal G; IT, inferior temporal G; MF, middle frontal G, IF, inferior frontal G; PC, precentral G; C, post-central G; SM, supramarginal G; A, angular G; OL, occipital lobe; SP, superior parietal lobule; CS, central sulcus; SF, sylvian fissure. Arteries (A): OF, orbito-frontal A; TP, temporo-polar A; AT, anterior temporal A; MT, middle temporal A; PT, posterior temporal A; TO, temporo-occipital A; PF, prefrontal A; I, insular arteries; LS, lenticulo-striate arteries; PC, precentral A; C, central A; P, parietal A (anterior and posterior branches); A, angular A. (From Bories et al. 1985.)

infarcted zone, consequent upon dislodgement of an embolus (Fisher and Adams 1987). It has been shown that up to 40% of infarcts show petechial haemorrhage (Horning et al. 1986), the most frequent sites for haemorrhagic infarcts being within the territories of the middle cerebral artery and the posterior circulation (Bonafe et al. 1985).

Differential Diagnosis

Differentiation of haemorrhagic infarction from a spontaneous intracerebral haemorrhage may be difficult but the latter is usually surrounded by a relatively modest halo of hypodensity and may extend beyond the bounds of vascular territories.

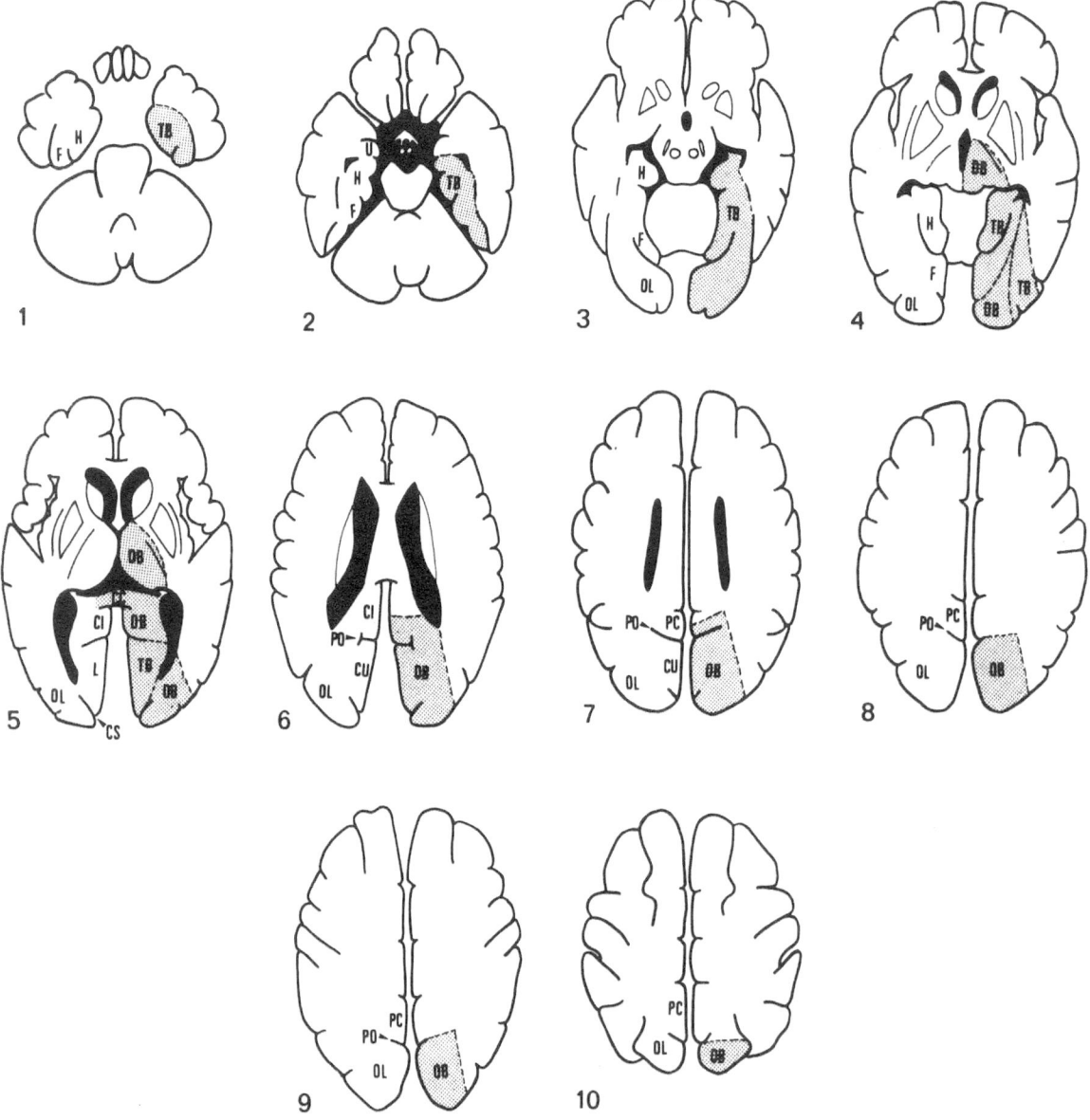

Fig. 1.6. Posterior cerebral (PCA) territory (using only cuts 1 to 10, see Fig. 1.3). Gyri (G) and other structures: H, para-hippocampal G; F, fusiform G; U, uncus; OL, occipital lobe; CI, cingulate G; L, lingual G; CU, cuneus; PC, precuneus; CS, calcarine sulcus; PO, parieto-occipital fissure. Arteries (A): TB, temporal and occipito-temporal branches; OB, occipital and parieto-occipital branches; CC, posterior pericallosal A; DB, deep branches (thalamostriate, thalamogeniculate and posterior choroidal arteries). (From Bories et al. 1985.)

Haemorrhagic contusion may need to be considered when it is uncertain whether head injury could have been a consequence of a primary intracerebral event. In contusion there may be considerable low density but it is not confined within vascular boundaries and there may be associated features of an adjacent vault fracture, extracerebral haemorrhage or evidence of contre-coup damage.

Patients with cerebral venous infarction present clinically in a rather different fashion from those with arterial occlusion and CT findings of bilateral enhancing lesions in the subcortical parasagittal white matter perhaps with haemorrhage are important clues to the diagnosis of venous infarction.

Cerebral ischaemia may present in a stepwise or even progressive manner raising the possibility of a cerebral tumour. The CT appearance of hypodense, infiltrative neoplasms can, on occasion, closely resemble infarcts. The hypodensity of infarction involves both grey and white matter and does not

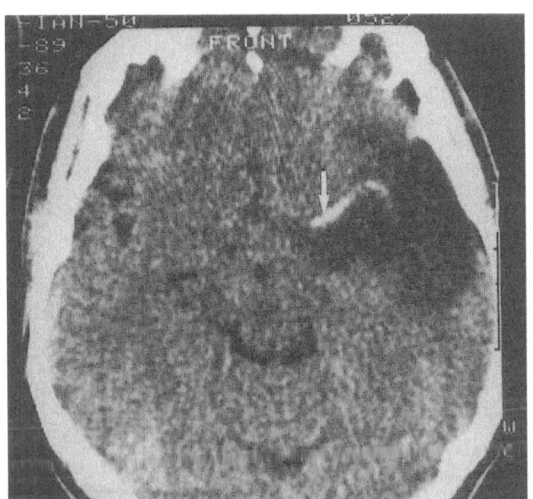

Fig. 1.7. Cranial CT. Hyperdense thrombosed middle cerebral artery (*arrow*). (By courtesy of Dr. A. D. Platts.)

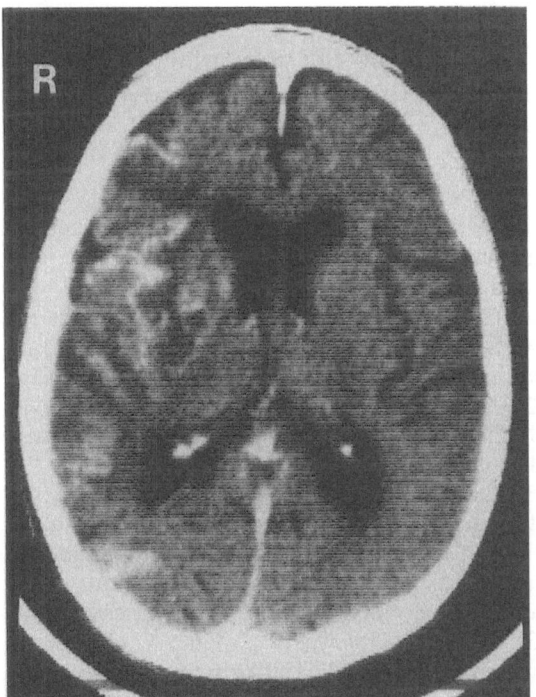

Fig. 1.8. Cranial CT: Right middle cerebral artery territory infarct with gyriform enhancement after intravenous contrast.

extend beyond the bounds of the involved vascular territory. According to Masdeu (1983), regarding lesions affecting the supratentorial compartment, grey matter enhancement with contrast and sparing of the thalamus favour infarction; oedema and ring enhancement in white matter characterise

neoplasm. Oedema associated with tumour affects mainly white matter and extends along definable tracts, especially the internal and external capsules and corpus callosum. Arcuate fibres in the subcortical white matter serve to connect adjacent gyri and their involvement in oedema results in the typical finger-like processes of tumoral oedema.

A cerebral infarct undergoes a process of evolution leading to maturation in which contrast enhancement and mass effect are transient but in tumour these persist and may become more marked as the mass grows. Low-grade hypodense malignancies which show no enhancement may prove the most problematic and it may be necessary to resort to surgical biopsy or, at the very least, sequential CT scanning to resolve the issue.

Deep Hemisphere Infarction

The internal capsule is a V-shaped white matter tract where even small lesions may result in severe neurological impairment. Its arterial supply is derived from three sources – the artery of Heubner from the anterior cerebral artery, the lenticulostriate arteries of the middle cerebral artery and the anterior choroidal artery arising from the internal carotid artery. As might be expected a degree of overlap exists between these territories particularly in the region of the genu.

Manelfe et al. (1981) investigated capsular ischaemic lesions using CT. The commonest lesion in this series involved the putamen, the body of the caudate and the superior internal capsule. Sterbini et al. (1987) described 28 cases of infarction in the territory of the anterior choroidal artery which includes the genu and posterior limb of the internal capsule. These infarcts constituted only 2.9% of their material and, along with isolated anterior and posterior limb lesions, are rare. Since the anterior choroidal artery arises directly from the internal carotid artery, infarcts in its territory are associated with carotid arterial degenerative disease.

The study by Cobb et al. (1987) of subinsular infarction suggests that at least a proportion of such lesions involving the putamen, caudate nucleus and internal capsule is the result of haemorrhage. It is often not clear with CT which process was responsible for low-density lesions in this region, but magnetic resonance imaging (MRI) will indicate the presence of chronic haemorrhage and permit a distinction (Brant Zawadzki et al. 1987). Cole and Yates (1967) found microaneurysms in the thalamus, basal ganglia, pons and cerebellum and postulated that small deep "cystic cavities" were often the consequence of haemorrhage.

Watershed Infarctions

Watershed infarcts occurring in the border zones
between vascular territories are rare and characteristically occur when there has been a failure of
cerebral perfusion, for instance, during a severe
hypotensive episode. The usual border zone
involved is that of the middle cerebral artery territory and bilateral and symmetrical wedge-shaped
lesions may be found (Fig. 1.9).

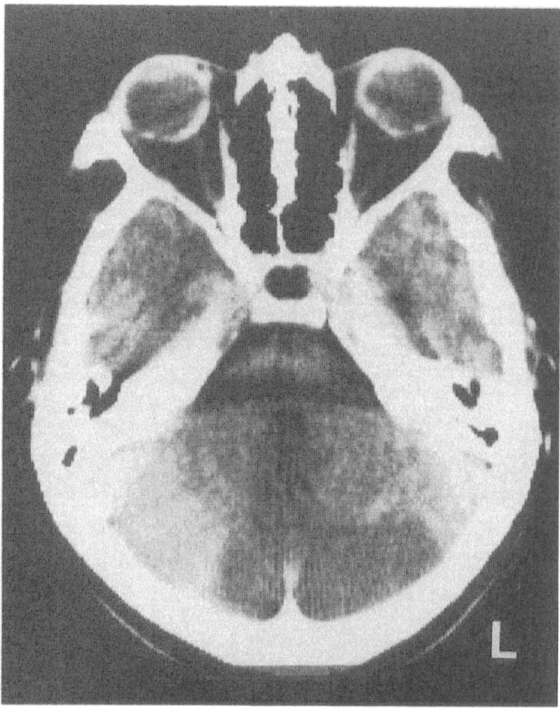

Fig. 1.10. Cranial CT. Posterior inferior cerebellar artery territory infarct.

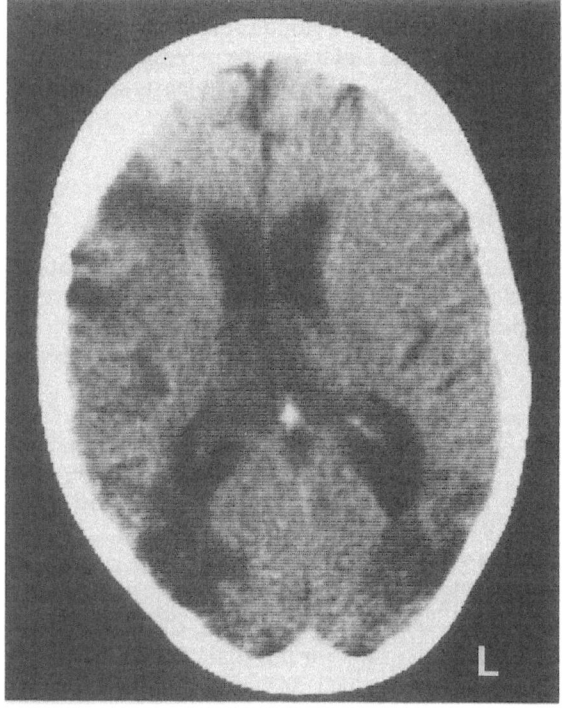

Fig. 1.9. Cranial CT. Bilateral watershed infarcts between middle
and posterior cerebal artery territories.

Infarcts in the Vertebrobasilar Territory

The vascular territories of the cerebellum and brainstem are inconstant and subject to frequent variation but it is often possible to ascribe a posterior
fossa ischaemic lesion seen on CT reliably to a
vascular territory (Savoiardo et al. 1987). The posterior inferior cerebellar artery (PICA), a branch of
the vertebral artery, supplies the postero-inferior
surface of the cerebellum and the ipsilateral inferior
vermis and the majority of cerebellar infarcts
involve the territory of this artery (Fig. 1.10). The
anterior petrosal surface of the cerebellum is supplied by the anterior inferior cerebellar artery and
the superior cerebellar artery, the most constant
branch, supplies the superior surface of the cerebellum and ipsilateral superior vermis (Fig. 1.11).

The medulla and pons are supplied mainly by
small perforating branches from the vertebral arteries and PICA. The pons is also supplied by per-
forators from the dorsum of the basilar artery.
Infarcts at these levels are limited by the midline
because the penetrating arteries do not cross it (Fig.
1.12). Midline lesions can occur at midbrain level
with thalamoperforate artery occlusions which may
additionally involve both thalami.

Hinshaw et al. (1980) in a CT study of 49 patients
with posterior fossa infarcts concluded that most
brainstem lesions were associated with cerebellar
lesions and that most branch occlusions were
related to vertebrobasilar arterial disease (Fig.
1.13).

Massive cerebellar infarction may result in swelling sufficient to cause obstructive hydrocephalus,
which may necessitate ventricular drainage. A diagnosis of cerebellar haemorrhage by CT should be
made after careful consideration since it is asserted
that 25% of cerebellar infarctions are haemorrhagic
(Bonafe et al. 1985).

Occlusion of the basilar artery usually involves
the proximal portion and is due to arteriosclerosis.
Distal occlusion is usually embolic either from
atheroma in the proximal vertebral arteries or from
a cardiac source (Castaigne et al. 1973).

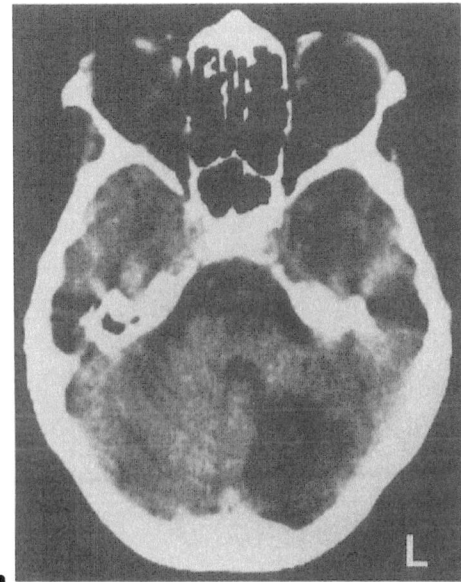

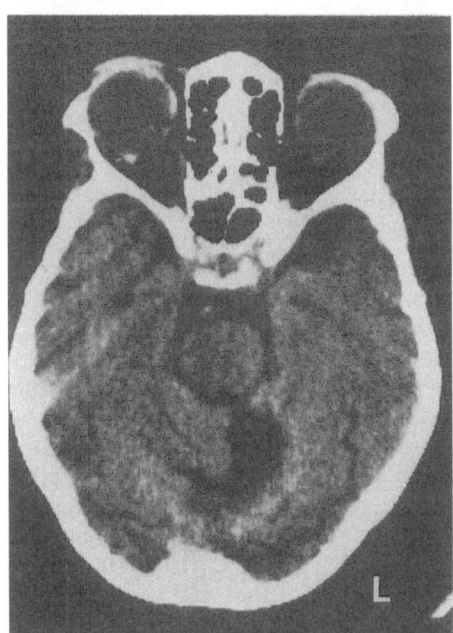

Fig. 1.11. Cranial CT. Superior cerebellar artery territory infarct involving the superior cerebellar hemisphere (**a**) and superior vermis (**b**).

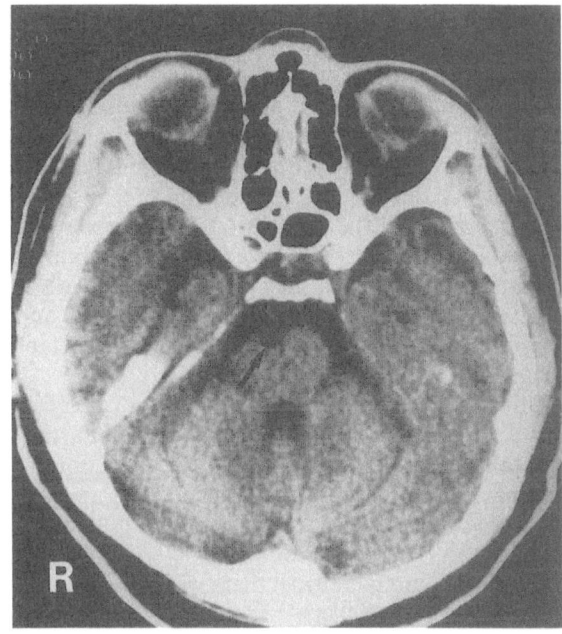

Fig. 1.12. Cranial CT. Right pontine infarct (*arrow*).

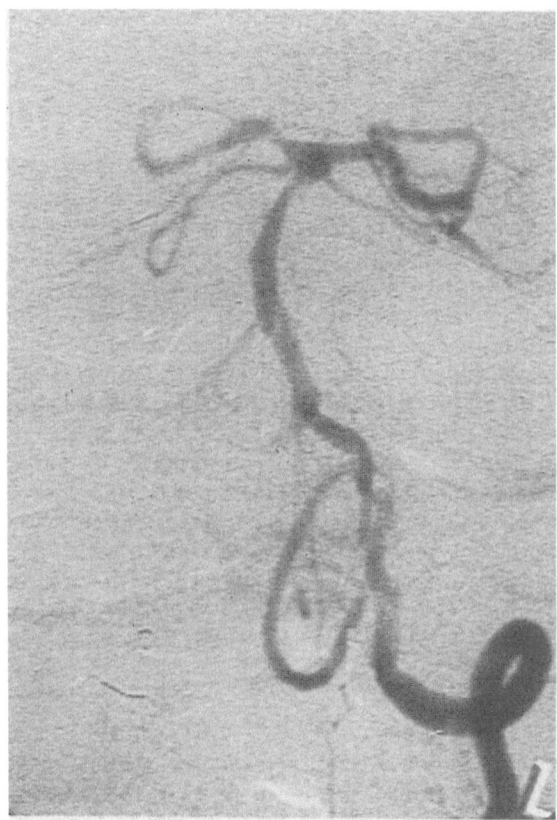

Fig. 1.13. Vertebral arterial DSA (frontal projection) showing atheromatous irregularity of the vertebral and basilar arteries.

Sato et al. (1987) conducted sequential angiography on patients with posterior circulation infarcts and showed recanalisation in some cases which strongly supported an embolic cause. There may be propagation of thrombus within the basilar artery in a craniad or caudad direction and clinical features will depend not only on the site of occlusion but also on the sufficiency of the collateral circulation. Because of this, the CT scan after basilar artery occlusion may demonstrate a variety of lesions in brainstem cerebellum, thalami and occipital lobes. Bilateral lesions are an important feature.

Direct evidence of vascular occlusion on CT is unusual but on occasion the occluded basilar artery may fail to enhance following intravenous contrast administration. The occluded basilar artery appears hyperdense on a plain scan with an attenuation value greater than that of whole blood and following intravenous contrast there will be no change (Vonofakos et al. 1983a).

The principles of detection and the evolution of infarcts of the posterior circulation are similar to those occurring in the carotid territories. A notable difference is in the appearance of the cortical enhancement following intravenous contrast. Parallel stripes of enhancement are seen because of the arrangement of the cerebellar folia.

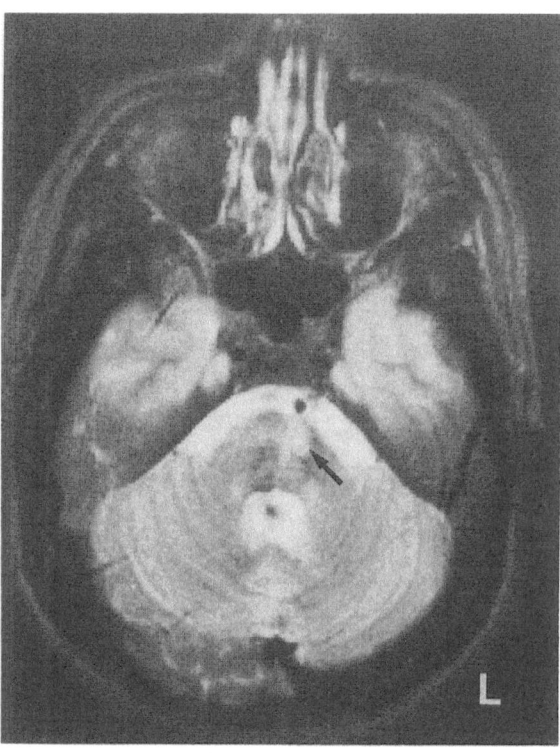

Fig. 1.14. Cranial MRI scan (T2 weighted image). Left pontine infarct (*arrow*).

MRI of Cerebral Ischaemia

The early radiological investigation of acute stroke is directed towards differentiating cerebral haemorrhage from infarction and in this role CT is more reliable than MRI. MRI has nevertheless proved very sensitive in the detection and extent of cerebral ischaemia and is superior to CT especially in the posterior fossa where CT interpretation is often made difficult by bony artefacts (Fig. 1.14) (Heiss et al. 1986). Lacunar infarcts are also detected more readily with MRI (Brown JJ et al. 1988). In a study of acute infarction induced in monkeys by Unger et al. (1987), at 2–4 h post-embolisation, infarcts were visible on MRI but not with CT and lesions were always more clearly delineated with MRI showing a high signal intensity with T2 weighted images. Cerebral infarction results in a prolongation of both T1 and T2 relaxation times with the T2 weighted sequences showing infarction more sensitively.

Despite the drawbacks of MRI regarding early discrimination of cerebral haemorrhage and infarction, the existence of subacute haemorrhage within an infarct is well shown by MRI due to the paramagnetic effect of methaemoglobin (Brant Zawadzki et al. 1987).

Gadolinium DTPA (diethylenetriamine pentaacetic acid) is an intravenous contrast for MRI. Like conventional iodinated CT contrast media it extravasates through a disordered blood–brain barrier but unlike the CT media it does not appear within the arterial vasculature since flowing blood creates a signal void on MRI scans. Imakita et al. (1987) investigated gadolinium DTPA in cerebral infarction and found that the enhancement was more obvious than that with CT, perhaps indicating an increased sensitivity of the MRI contrast agent to blood–brain barrier breakdown.

Cerebral Vasculitis

There are many causes of cerebral vasculitis (Table 1.2) but the range of angiographic findings is fairly restricted no matter what the underlying disease process. These changes consist of occlusions and irregular stenoses of affected arteries and small fusiform aneurysms may also be found. If small vessels are involved there may be no demonstrable angiographic abnormality and the changes may be reversible. Systemic lupus erythematosus (SLE) is one such microvasculitis where cerebral infarcts may result from either cerebral arterial disease or from

Table 1.2. Causes of vasculitis

Drugs
Irradiation
Collagen diseases
  Systemic lupus erythematosus
  Polyarteritis nodosa
  Rheumatoid arthritis
  Scleroderma
  Dermatomyositis
Inherited connective tissue disorder
  Pseudoxanthoma elasticum
  Ehlers–Danlos syndrome
  Marfan's syndrome
Infection
  Tuberculosis
  Syphilis
Haematological disorders
  e.g. Sickle cell disease
Temporal arteritis
Takayasu's disease
Sarcoid
Amyloid
Moya moya disease
Behçet's disease
Metabolic conditions
  Diabetes mellitus
  Hyperlipidaemia

cardiac emboli. Vasculitis is a rare accompaniment in other collagen diseases and in polyarteritis nodosa, in contradistinction to the renal arteriographic findings, cerebral arterial microaneurysms are infrequent.

Behçet's syndrome and SLE enter into the differential diagnosis of multiple sclerosis and whereas systemic features may point to the former, neurological disturbance may occasionally be seen in isolation.

Miller et al. (1987) have identified several features on MRI scanning which may help to distinguish a vasculitis from multiple sclerosis. In vasculitis, periventricular lesions are milder than those seen in multiple sclerosis and in some cases of vasculitis hemisphere lesions were found in the absence of periventricular lesions. The occurrence of large infarcts, cortical lesions or cortical atrophy favoured vasculitis.

Cerebral amyloid angiopathy results from amyloid deposition in the arteries of the cerebral cortex and leptomeninges. It is often associated with dementia and should be considered when repeated, multiple and bilateral intracerebral haemorrhages occur in the elderly patient (Sobel et al. 1985).

Moya Moya Disease

Moya moya disease is a rare, chronic cerebrovascular occlusive disorder with characteristic angiographic findings of stenosis of the distal inter-

nal carotid artery and its branches and enlargement of perforating vessels at the base of the brain (Fig. 1.15). As occlusion proceeds so the number of collaterals increases but ultimately both the internal carotid branches and the collaterals disappear, leaving the external carotid arteries and the vertebrobasilar system to supply the brain. Collateral arterial connections develop between the anterior and posterior choroidal arteries and between the anterior and posterior pericallosal arteries. Vessels may "bridge" a proximal middle cerebral artery occlusion and ethmoidal and transdural collaterals connect the external and internal carotid arteries. These small moya moya vessels are particularly numerous in children.

There are two peaks of incidence: in the first and in the fourth decades. Children present with repeated episodes of cerebral ischaemia. The course is progressive but can ultimately "arrest" and stabilise. Adults with moya moya disease usually present with subarachnoid haemorrhage.

The diagnosis is primarily angiographic and besides an idiopathic form occurring typically in Japanese females below the age of 20, there are associations with cerebral arteriovenous malformations (3% in the series of Mawad et al. 1984), cerebral aneurysms, sickle cell disease and neurofibromatosis. A slowly growing basal skull tumour such as meningioma may also result in progressive

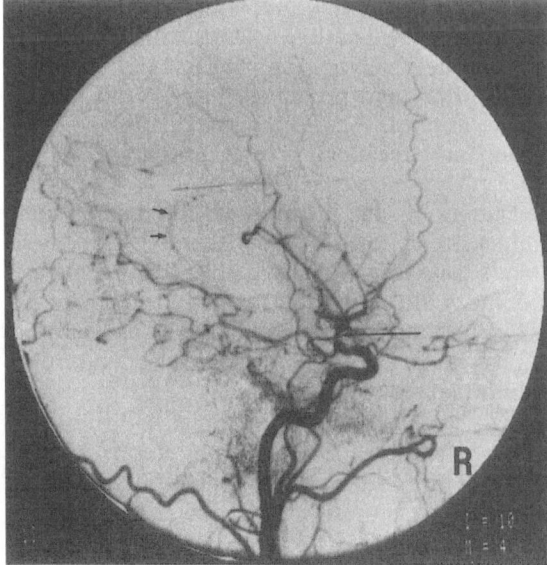

Fig. 1.15. Carotid arterial DSA (lateral projection). Moya moya disease. There is extensive occlusion involving the supraclinoid portion of the internal carotid artery and its major branches. Bridging collaterals can be seen (*arrows*). The posterior communicating and posterior cerebral arteries are well preserved..

vascular occlusion. The angiographic findings in moya moya disease have been described by Takahashi (1980).

The existence of cerebral aneurysms in some cases is interesting. Almost half develop in the posterior cerebral circulation, especially in the posterior choroidal vessels. It was postulated by Kodama and Suzuki (1978) that some of these were pseudo-aneurysms resulting from rupture of collateral vessels and their disappearance on sequential angiography was noted. True berry aneurysms, presumably related to the altered haemodynamic stresses on the posterior circulation, also occur.

High quality CT may also show moya moya vessels (Takahashi et al. 1980; Takeuchi et al. 1982). Multiple low-density areas and cerebral atrophy may also be encountered. Contrast administration reveals basal ganglial enhancement due to collateral vessels which may be shown best by coronal CT scans (Asari et al. 1982).

MRI can demonstrate arterial occlusion and show the collateral vessels particularly within the basal ganglia as punctate regions of "signal void" due to flowing blood (Fujisawa et al. 1987).

Sickle Cell Disease

Cerebral infarction is a serious neurological complication of sickle cell disease and occurs most often in children. Although the sickling process may be responsible for the arterial occlusion it is probable that cerebral ischaemic events are also related to an occlusive angiopathy of the forebrain. Intimal hyperplasia involves the intracranial internal carotid artery and proximal anterior and middle cerebral arteries. The posterior circulation is rarely affected and the angiographic appearances may conform to a moya moya pattern.

Angiography and intravenous contrast medium administration for CT are hazardous for these patients especially when hyperosmolar agents are used. Strict attention must be paid to the patient's state of hydration and blood transfusion is carried out prior to angiography to reduce the proportion of abnormal red cells.

El-Gammel et al. (1986) correlated CT and MRI findings in sickle cell patients with cerebrovascular disease. Their discovery of asymptomatic white matter lesions in those without stroke underscores the sensitivity of MRI in cerebral ischaemia and may provide a non-invasive method whereby "at risk" groups can be identified and early measures taken.

Pulseless Disease

The first case of pulseless disease was reported by Takayasu in 1908 and the accepted clinical triad consists of absence of radial pulsation, a hypersensitive carotid sinus reflex and ophthalmoangiopathy.

The aortic arch, its major branches and the pulmonary arteries are involved in this chronic non-specific arteritis which typically affects young females between the second and third decades. Systemic upset also occurs. Fibrosis and thickening of arterial walls results in stenosis or occlusion of the vessel lumina. Masuzawa et al. (1986) have described an association with intracranial aneurysms and postulate that their development may be due to the altered circulatory dynamics of the Circle of Willis.

Arterial Dissection and Fibromuscular Dysplasia

Spontaneous dissection of the internal carotid or vertebral arteries is becoming increasingly recognised as a cause of cerebral ischaemia in relatively young patients. Cervical pain accompanying cerebral ischaemia is an important clinical pointer to the diagnosis.

In a retrospective review of 42 cases by Houser et al. (1984) dissection was revealed angiographically by an eccentric tapered stenosis in 47%, stenosis and aneurysm formation in 28%, occlusion in 18% and aneurysm alone in 7%. Petro et al. (1986) have stressed that pseudoaneurysm formation following internal carotid artery dissection is more likely when the artery is coiled.

In 25% of the patients, more than one vessel was involved and where a single carotid artery had dissected, the right was more frequently involved than the left. Intradural extension of dissection of both internal carotid and vertebral arteries was described. The outlook in these cases was generally favourable with a regression of angiographic abnormalities in the majority. Recurrence was rare.

The appearance of an internal carotid artery occluded by dissection may differ from atheromatous occlusion. In the former, the internal carotid artery may be occluded just distal to its origin, its terminal portion appearing flame – or radish-shaped. The cervical carotid bifurcation appears normal. The termination of an internal carotid artery occluded due to arteriosclerotic thrombosis typically has a rounded shape and the bifurcation is often involved in the same disease process. Despite these differences, dissection may be difficult to distinguish at angiography from a tapering thromboembolic occlusion of the internal carotid artery.

Fibromuscular dysplasia (Fig. 1.16) is the commonest predisposing factor but is seen in only a minority of dissections, occurring in six of Houser's 42 patients. Of those with cervical disease 50% will have co-existing fibrodysplasia of the renal arteries (Osborn and Anderson 1977). Fibrodysplasia is commoner in females but the female preponderance in dissection is less marked. Of 20 cases of vertebral artery dissection described by Chiras et al. (1985), 30% had underlying fibromuscular dysplasia. In 30% both vertebral arteries were involved and cervical pain preceding a vertebrobasilar stroke was a prominent symptom. The vertebral artery segments at the level of the first and second cervical vertebrae were mainly involved.

Axial MRI in arterial dissection has shown a hyperintense signal in both T1 and T2 weighted images expanding the wall and narrowing the arterial lumen. These are the appearances of subacute mural haematoma with short T1 and long T2 relaxation times.

Follow-up of cases in the study by Goldberg et al. (1986) showed resolution in both cases examined which is in agreement with the findings of Houser et al. (1984) that, in the absence of occlusion, there is a return to normal after several months.

Cerebral Artery Ectasia

Arteriosclerosis of the basilar artery (Fig. 1.17) may result in ectasia which may be so marked as to cause brainstem compression and obstructive hydrocephalus. Typically, the patients are elderly, hypertensive males and there is often evidence of preexisting cerebral ischaemic change such as lacunar infarction or generalised white matter low density in the pattern of Binswanger disease (Moseley and Holland 1979). In the series of Goldstein et al. (1983) the intracranial carotid and vertebrobasilar arteries were most affected followed by the proximal anterior and middle cerebral arteries (Fig. 1.18). Of their 15 patients, 11 were male and cerebral ischaemia was the main presenting complaint. In the younger age groups connective tissue disorders may be responsible, e.g. Ehlers–Danlos syndrome, pseudoxanthoma elasticum and Marfan's syndrome.

Hypertensive Encephalopathy

Weingarten et al. (1985) reported the CT findings in 11 patients with hypertensive encephalopathy. White matter oedema affecting the supratentorial compartment was found in all their cases and in the infratentorial compartment in eight. The changes

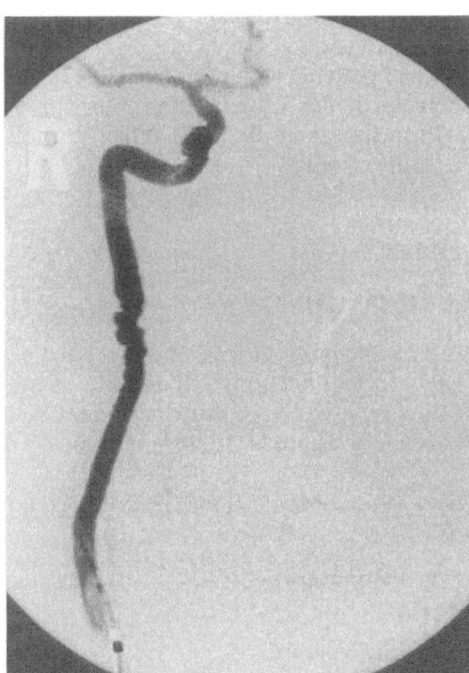

Fig. 1.16. Internal carotid arterial DSA (frontal projection). Fibromuscular dysplasia showing the typical beaded luminal contour.

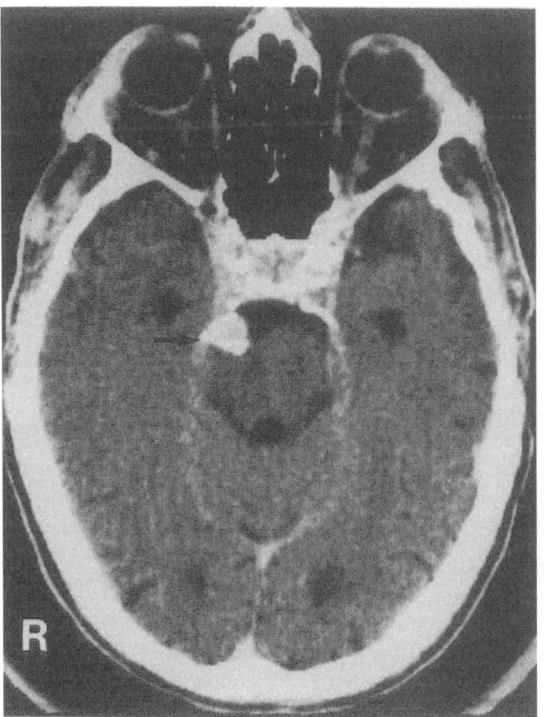

Fig. 1.17. Cranial CT after IV contrast. Basilar artery ectasia (arrow).

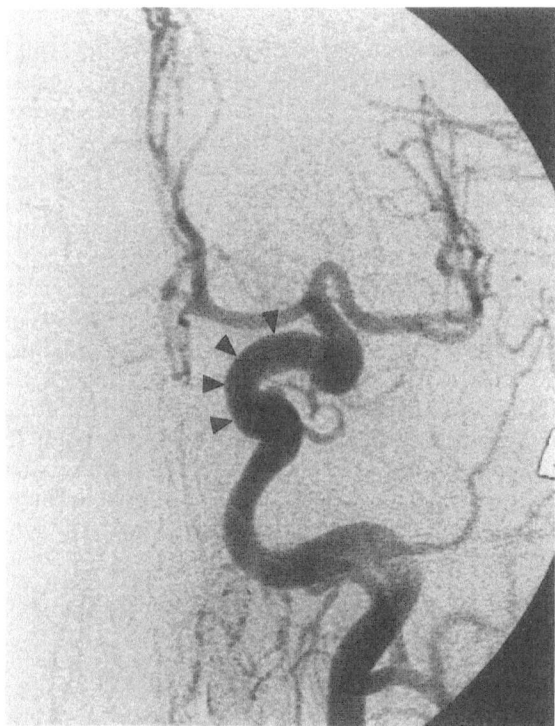

Fig. 1.18. Carotid arterial DSA. Ectasia of the supraclinoid portion of the left internal carotid artery (*arrowheads*).

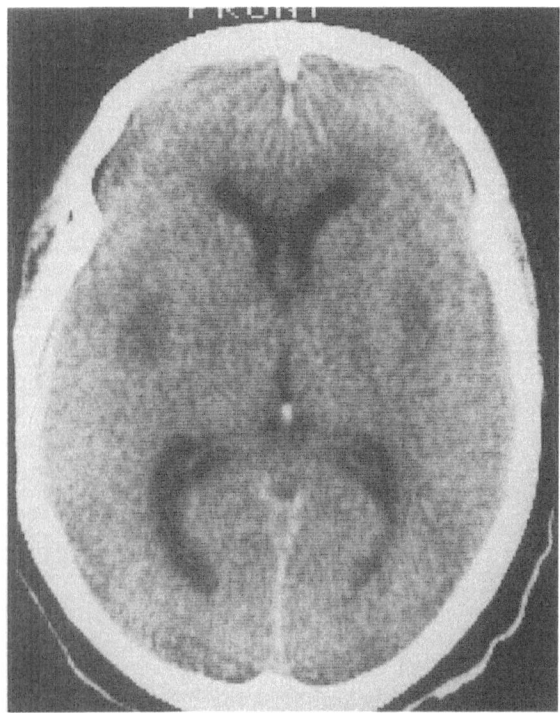

Fig. 1.19. Cranial CT. Global hypoperfusion with symmetrical basal ganglial low density lesions.

were mostly reversible but three patients went on to develop frank infarction.

Eclampsia

Colosimo et al. (1985) found CT changes consistent with cerebral oedema in patients with eclampsia which subsequently regressed. Cerebral haemorrhage may also occur.

CT in Global Hypoperfusion

Kjos et al. (1983) studied 10 patients with global hypoperfusion and found diffuse mass effect, loss of grey–white matter differentiation and low density lesions in both basal ganglia (Fig. 1.19) and watershed territories. With intravenous contrast, enhancement of the cerebral cortex and basal ganglia was found emphasising the vulnerability of those structures to such an insult.

Bilateral hypodense lesions in the basal ganglia also occur in carbon monoxide poisoning, hypoglycaemia, cyanide and barbiturate poisoning.

CT in Migraine

Although the mechanism is incompletely understood, cerebral infarcts may follow severe migraine (Bousser et al. 1985). Du Boulay et al. (1983) found an association between cerebral atrophy and migraine of greater than five years' duration which was probably more severe in men.

MRI studies of patients with migraine have demonstrated periventricular white matter lesions in a large proportion (Soges et al. 1988). Their pathological basis is uncertain.

Venous Disease

Sinovenous Occlusion

Dural sinus thrombosis was formerly an important complication of facial infections and of mastoiditis. Frequently now no underlying cause is evident but recognised associations are listed in Table 1.3.

Table 1.3. Causes of superior sagittal sinus thrombosis (Fig. 1.20)

Pregnancy and the puerperium
Oral contraceptives
Infection
Dehydration (especially in infants)
Trauma (including postoperative)
Haematological disorders (especially leukaemias)
Tumours adjacent to the sagittal sinus (e.g. calvarial metastases)
Behçet's syndrome

Cerebrovascular Disease 15

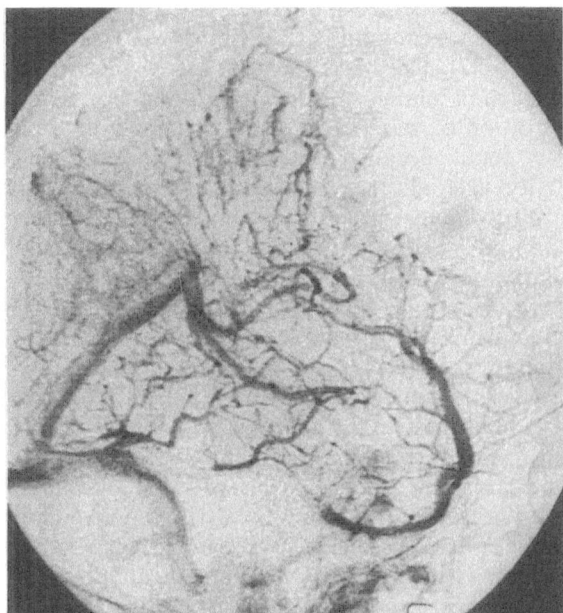

Fig. 1.20. Carotid arterial DSA (lateral projection) late venous phase. Superior sagittal sinus thrombosis. The occlusion is evidenced by non-opacification of the sinus.

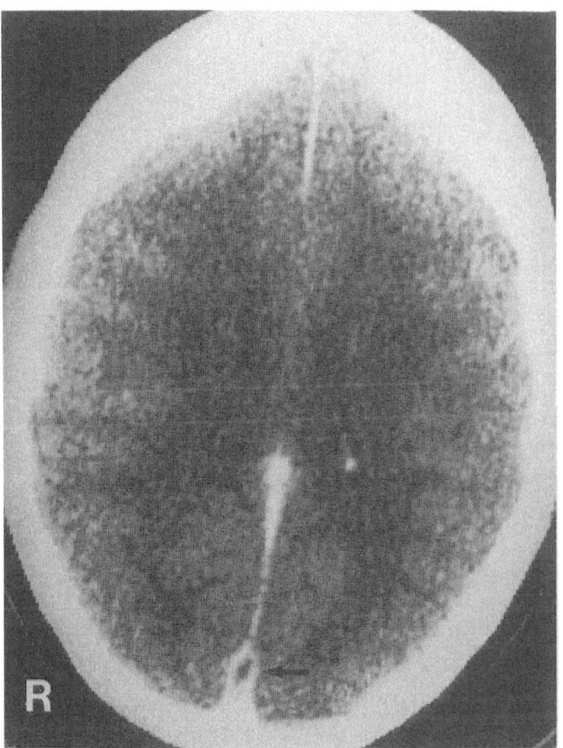

Fig. 1.21. Cranial CT after IV contrast. The empty triangle sign (*arrow*).

Dural sinus thrombosis also enters into the differential diagnosis of "idiopathic intracranial hypertension" (benign intracranial hypertension or pseudotumour cerebri). In this latter condition both CT and MRI are characteristically normal (Silbergleit et al. 1989).

Contrast enhanced CT may demonstrate the empty delta or empty triangle sign (Fig. 1.21). Originally described by Buonanno et al. (1978), it consists of enhancement of the sinus wall with a relatively lucent lumen and is explained by a rich dural venous collateral circulation of lateral lacunae, dural cavernous spaces and meningeal venous tributaries. A study by Virapongse et al. (1987) of 76 cases of superior sagittal sinus thrombosis showed that the empty delta sign occurred in 28%.

An empty triangle sign and haemorrhagic venous infarction are unfavourable prognostic features in those with superior sagittal sinus thrombosis and in any case, the diagnosis carries a poor outlook in children.

Unenhanced cranial CT may show hyperdensity indicating thrombus within the dural venous sinus which may extend laterally into adjacent cortical veins. MRI may also reveal thrombosis as a high signal within the sinus (McMurdo et al. 1986).

Venous infarction is much less common than the arterial counterpart. The CT appearances are somewhat variable but hypodensity occurs typically in parasagittal subcortical white matter. Contrast enhancement is usually cortical but may also involve the subcortical white matter. Mass effect is usually not pronounced.

Venous infarcts are not uncommonly haemorrhagic (Fig. 1.22) when they are almost invariably asssociated with superior sagittal sinus involvement. Conversely superior sagittal sinus thrombosis can occur in the absence of haemorrhagic infarction and indeed with an apparently normal cranial CT scan.

The haematomas of venous infarction are often multiple, of varying size and with irregular edges in contrast to the normally smooth margins of spontaneous intracerebral haemorrhage. It is also important to realise that the CT changes are reversible (unlike arterial infarction) and within about two months the scan may return to normal.

The causes of venous infarction and dural sinus thrombosis are in the main similar but cerebral venous occlusion can occur without dural sinus thrombosis (Gabrielsen et al. 1981). Venous infarction can also result from the presence of a dural arteriovenous fistula leading to stagnation of the blood in the cortical veins.

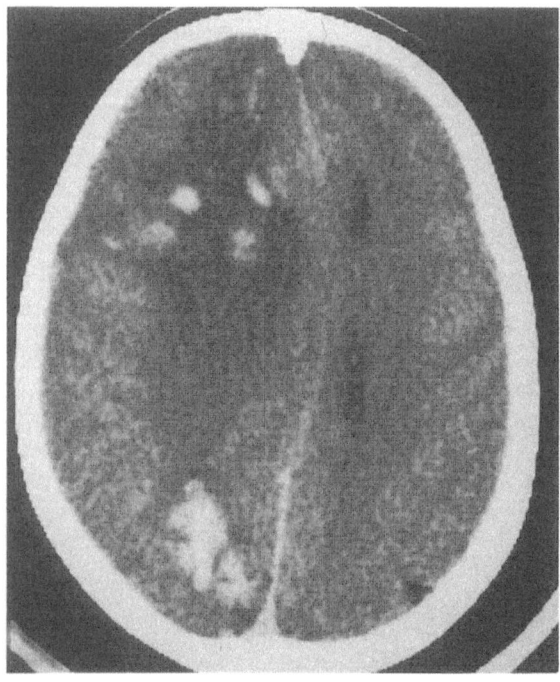

Fig. 1.22. Cranial CT. Haemorrhagic venous infarction.

niques have emerged as alternatives to conventional film/screen angiography (Butler 1986, 1987; Butler et al. 1987). DSA is a means whereby electronic subtraction allows the near instantaneous demonstration of vascular anatomy essentially free of bony detail. Because of its exquisite contrast sensitivity, arterial images can be produced following an intravenous injection of contrast (intravenous DSA) as well as following selective arterial cannulation (arterial DSA).

Intravenous DSA is a minimally invasive procedure which is both simple and safe and which can readily be performed on outpatients. There are, however, a number of drawbacks, mainly related to its inferior spatial resolution, which have called its value into question (Hoffman et al. 1984).

Several centres are now exploiting digital subtraction arch aortography in the investigation of craniocervical degenerative disease (McCreary et al. 1985; Gritter et al. 1987). Patients attend on a day-case or true outpatient basis and this approach appears to be a satisfactory compromise between intravenous DSA and full selective angiography.

Angiography in Cerebral Ischaemia

Although CT and MRI are the primary diagnostic tools in the investigation of cerebral ischaemia, angiography remains valuable in a number of circumstances. It will certainly be required prior to carotid endarterectomy or other surgical procedures designed to alleviate cerebral ischaemia. Angiography may be necessary if it is uncertain as to whether a lesion demonstrated by CT is a tumour or infarct. It may also be unclear whether primary cardiac disease or cervical arterial disease is responsible for cerebral ischaemic events and angiography may go some way to resolving the issue.

When angiography is performed and indeed whether it is performed are very much matters of individual clinical judgement since by no means all physicians are convinced of the efficacy of carotid artery surgery and the optimum treatment of arteriosclerotic craniocervical degenerative disease remains to be established.

Angiography is usually delayed following an acute infarct but in the presence of transient ischaemic episodes and a normal CT scan, early angiography is often performed. Both angiography and surgery may be deemed necessary at an early stage for a stroke in evolution in an attempt to limit the extent of the damage.

With the advent of digital subtraction angiography (DSA) two further angiographic tech-

INTRACRANIAL HAEMORRHAGE

Intracranial haemorrhage may be classified according to its location into intracerebral, intraventricular, subarachnoid, subdural and extradural. Haemorrhage in one compartment may of course come to involve the others. For instance the rupture of a berry aneurysm may cause intraventricular, intracerebral and subdural haemorrhage in addition to the primary subarachnoid haemorrhage.

Intracerebral haemorrhage

The causes of intracerebral haemorrhage are given in Table 1.4.

Table 1.4. Causes of intracerebral haemorrhage

1. "Spontaneous"
2. Aneurysm
3. Arteriovenous malformation
4. Haemorrhagic infarction (arterial and venous)
5. Trauma
6. Tumour
7. Arteritis e.g. Amyloid
              Moya moya

"Spontaneous" Intracerebral Haemorrhage

"Spontaneous" intracerebral haemorrhage is closely related to the existence of hypertensive disease and the majority are said to be due to the rupture of Charcot Bouchard micro-aneurysms located in the basal ganglia, thalamus, pons and the dentate nuclei of the cerebellum. They are of the order of 1–2 mm in diameter and are often multiple. Micro-aneurysms found in the posterior fossa in the study of Cole and Yates (1967) were always associated with hypertension. Rupture of a berry aneurysm with haematoma formation may closely resemble a spontaneous haemorrhage and the presence of an intracranial haematoma should alert the observer to the possibility of an underlying vascular anomaly. Haemorrhage within a neoplasm may precipitate a stroke syndrome.

CT of Intracerebral Haemorrhage

A fresh intracerebral haematoma appears as a region of hyperdensity which, depending on its size, may exert considerable mass effect (Fig. 1.23). There is usually little surrounding oedema since bleeding dissects through cerebral tissue but a hypo-intense "halo" is a frequent accompaniment. There is a linear relationship between the haematocrit and CT attenuation values. Fresh whole blood is readily discriminated and subsequent clot retraction leads to a further increase in attenuation since low density serum is extruded. This hyperdensity recedes with time and after about one to two weeks the haematoma may become isodense with adjacent brain. Ultimately the residuum may simply be a low density region.

The protein component of haemoglobin (globin) is the main determinant of attenuation, the iron in haemoglobin having little part to play. Should the patient be anaemic the CT detection of haemorrhage may be difficult (New 1976).

A ring enhancement pattern after intravenous contrast is not uncommon in spontaneous haematomas and need not necessarily imply tumour. It can persist for up to 6 months (Zimmerman et al. 1977). Enzmann et al. (1981) induced parietal lobe haematomas in dogs and found that the contrast enhancement resulted from the existence of an inflammatory infiltrate.

MRI of Intracerebral haemorrhage

Dooms et al. (1986) have assessed the value of MRI in the diagnosis of cerebral haemorrhage. Acute haematomas (less than 3 days old) yield rather non-

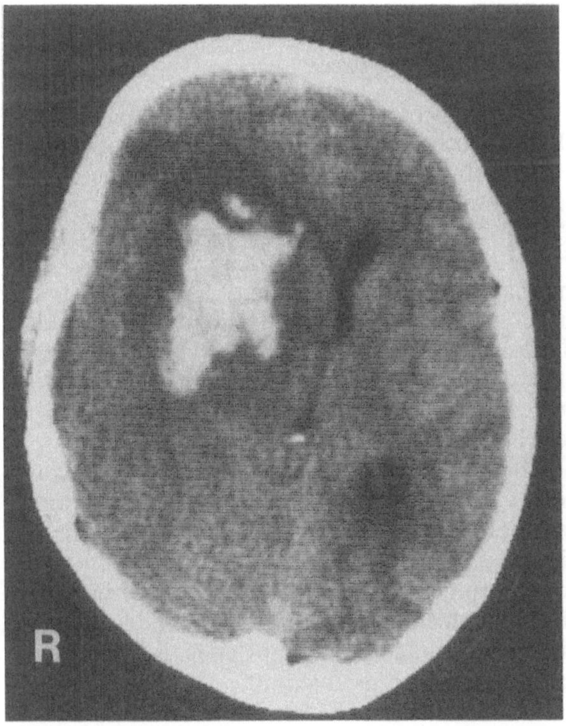

Fig. 1.23. Cranial CT. Spontaneous intracerebral haemorrhage. Note the surrounding halo of low density and the mass effect with right to left shift of midline structures.

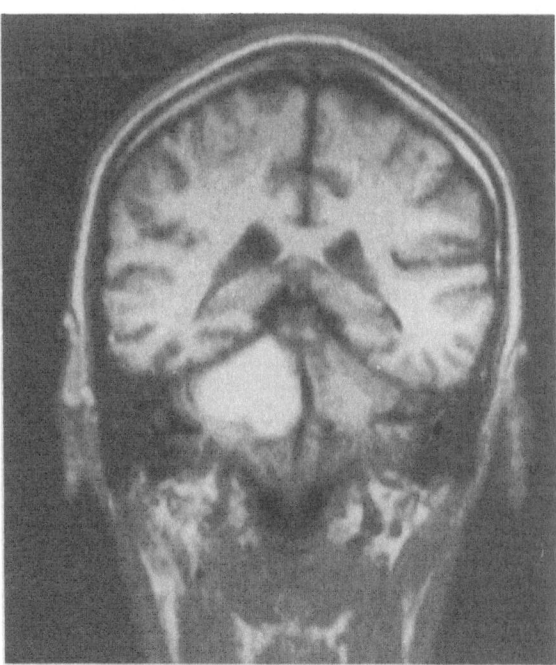

Fig. 1.24. Cranial MRI (T1 weighted image). Right cerebellar haematoma. (By courtesy of Dr. D. P. E. Kingsley.)

specific MRI features. The long T1 and T2 relaxation times of fresh blood are shared by infarct, tumour and oedema. After 3 days, the T1 time shortens and signal intensity increases. This is explained by the oxidation of haemoglobin to methaemoglobin – a paramagnetic substance – which influences T1 relaxation time. The long T2 relaxation time persists but this pattern of a short T1 and a long T2 relaxation time for chronic haematomas is more specific (Fig. 1.24). Gomori et al. (1985) examined the MRI characteristics of acute (less than 1 week), subacute (1–4 weeks) and chronic (greater than 1 month) haematomas. Acute haematomas were seen to have a central reduction in signal intensity on T2 weighted images due to deoxyhaemoglobin formation.

In subacute and chronic haematomas, an increase in the signal intensity in both T1 and T2 weighted images occurred initially as a peripheral rim before becoming uniform throughout the haematoma. Hypointensity was found around both subacute and chronic haematomas and was thought to be due to haemosiderin within macrophage lysosomes.

Subarachnoid Haemorrhage

The commonest cause of subarachnoid haemorrhage is rupture of a berry aneurysm, and a classification of intracranial aneurysms is given in Table 1.5.

Table 1.5. Classification of intracranial aneurysms

Berry aneurysm
Charcot Bouchard micro-aneurysms
Arteriosclerotic fusiform aneurysms (arterial ectasia)
Traumatic aneurysms
Mycotic aneurysms
Dissecting aneurysms
Pseudo aneurysms, e.g. moya moya disease

Berry Aneurysms

Berry aneurysms occur typically at arterial bifurcations and the majority arise on or near to the Circle of Willis. The location of aneurysms in 500 operated patients is given in Table 1.6. Aneurysmal subarachnoid haemorrhage has a peak age incidence of 50–54 years and is commoner in females in the ratio 3:2. Males predominate below the age of 40.

Internal carotid artery aneurysms are twice as common in females and middle cerebral artery aneurysms also have a female preponderance in the ratio 3:2. Conversely, 58% of anterior com-

Table 1.6. Distribution of aneurysm sites (500 operated patients)

	No.	%
Anterior cerebral artery	174	34.8
Anterior communicating	160	32.0
A$_1$ segment	4	0.8
Pericallosal	10	2.0
Middle cerebral artery	99	19.8
Internal carotid artery	197	39.4
Posterior communicating	116	23.2
Bifurcation	32	6.4
Carotid-ophthalmic	24	4.8
Anterior choroidal	10	2.0
Cavernous	3	0.6
Non-specific	12	2.4
Posterior circulation	30	6.0
Basilar bifurcation	14	2.8
PICA	10	2.0
Vertebrobasilar junction	2	0.4
Superior cerebellar	2	0.4
Posterior cerebral	2	0.4

From Sengupta RP, McAllister VL (1986) *Subarachnoid Haemorrhage*. Springer, Berlin, Heidelberg, New York, p. 120.

municating artery aneurysms occur in males (Locksley 1966).

Arterial aneurysms are rare in childhood. Meyer et al. (1989) found that there was a male preponderance in this age group and a relatively high percentage of giant aneurysms occurring in unusual locations.

Aneurysm Development

The aetiology of berry aneurysm formation is probably due to an interplay of acquired and congenital predisposing factors (Sahs 1966). At the points of bifurcation of the cerebral arteries there is a gap in the muscular layer (the medial defect). It is here that aneurysms arise but probably only when the internal elastic lamina is damaged. Arteriosclerosis and hypertension may have a role to play in the elastic lamina degeneration, particularly in the older patient. The sac of an aneurysm is thin-walled and continuous with the adventitia of the adjacent vessel.

Although berry aneurysms are very rare in children, a familial tendency for aneurysm formation has been found (see p. 25). Some inherited conditions such as the Ehlers–Danlos syndrome and neurofibromatosis are associated with intracranial aneurysms lending further weight to the likelihood of a genetic influence perhaps manifested through defective collagen production.

Mycotic Aneurysms

Intracranial aneurysms may develop as a consequence of infective emboli, most commonly in association with endocarditis. Those due to septic emboli are usually small and peripherally sited, mainly on branches of the middle cerebral artery. Their frequency is difficult to determine with the decline of rheumatic heart disease but a 5% incidence in endocarditis has been cited (Roach and Drake 1965).

Computed Tomography in Subarachnoid Haemorrhage

CT provides a non-invasive means of demonstrating blood in the subarachnoid space and may obviate the need for a, sometimes hazardous, diagnostic lumbar puncture. The CT appearances may reflect the severity of the initial bleed and the patient's subsequent pre- and postoperative course can be monitored for any complications.

It is important to bear in mind that *a normal cranial CT examination in a patient with suspected subarachnoid haemorrhage in no way excludes the diagnosis.*

The Aneurysm

Aneurysms as small as about 2–3 mm in diameter may be demonstrated using intravenous contrast enhanced thin section axial CT (Vonofakos et al. 1983b). Angiography normally shows only that part of an aneurysm in continuity with the circulation whereas CT will show both the patent lumen and any coexisting mural thrombus, so as to reflect the true size of the lesion more accurately. Mural ring calcification may also be present in the larger aneurysms. If subarachnoid blood is present on the plain scan there seems little point in repeating the scan after intravenous contrast since angiography is the definitive method of demonstrating intracranial aneurysms. Such a step may be valuable in patients with a suspicious history but with a normal unenhanced CT scan and in those with suspected cranial vascular malformations.

The hyperdensity of subarachnoid blood persists for about one week after which the cerebrospinal fluid becomes isodense with adjacent brain. At this stage the scan may appear near normal and it may be difficult to appreciate the loss of definition of the normal CSF spaces in the absence of scans prior to the ictus.

The distribution of intracranial bleeding, especially when intraparenchymal, following aneurysmal rupture can often point to the location of the aneurysm or at least lateralise it (Silver et al. 1981). Cerebral angiography will still be necessary prior to surgery but in the event of clinical deterio-

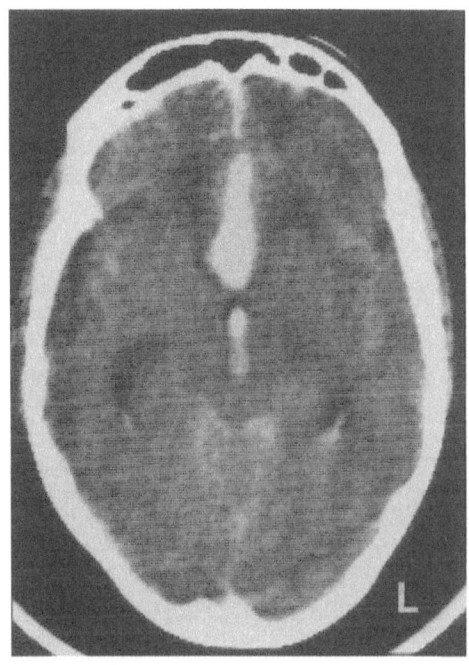

Fig. 1.25. Cranial CT. Rupture of an anterior communicating artery aneurysm with pellucidal haematoma.

ration necessitating urgent surgery a limited study may be possible directed by the CT findings. When a patient is found to have more than one intracranial aneurysm, CT may indicate which has ruptured.

Anterior communicating artery aneurysm rupture is probably the easiest to localise with CT (a 92% accuracy in Inouc ct al.'s (1981) series (Fig. 1.25). The densest subarachnoid blood will be in the interhemispheric fissure and haematoma formation may occur in the septum pellucidum and inferomedial frontal lobe – often in a flame-shaped distribution.

A pericallosal artery aneurysm may cause a corpus callosum haematoma.

Carotid tip aneurysm rupture results in subarachnoid blood in the ipsilateral Sylvian fissure and in the suprasellar cistern. Haematoma formation in frontal or temporal lobes may also occur. If, as can happen, the haematoma involves the thalamic and basal ganglial region, there may be difficulty in distinguishing it from a spontaneous hypertensive haemorrhage.

Haematoma formation is unusual following rupture of a *posterior communicating artery aneurysm* but if present it is found within the temporal lobe. The subarachnoid blood may be maximal in the ipsilateral Sylvian fissure but often it becomes generalised throughout the basal cisterns.

Middle cerebral artery aneurysm rupture (Fig. 1.26) causes the maximal blood density to occur in

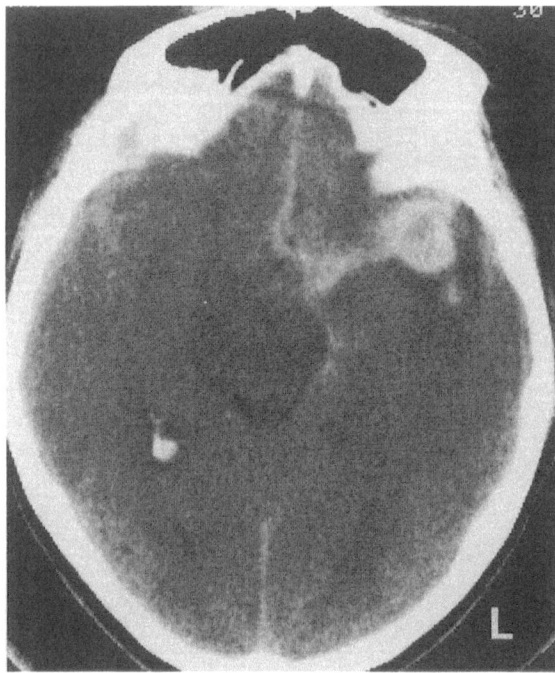

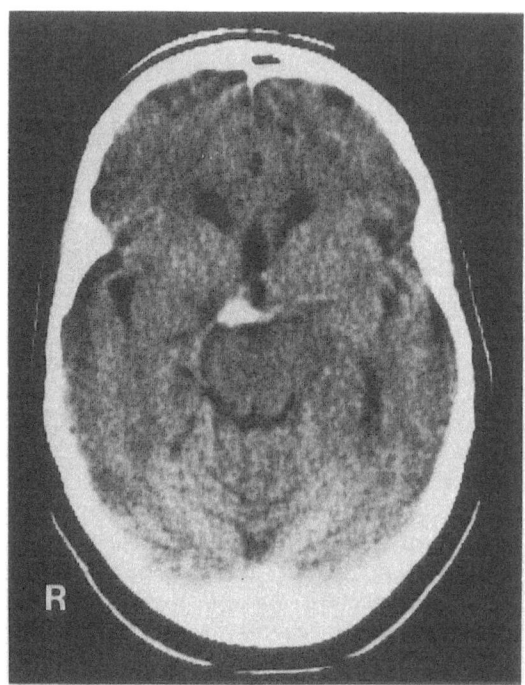

Fig. 1.26. Cranial CT. Rupture of a left middle cerebral artery aneurysm.

Fig. 1.27. Cranial CT after IV contrast. Basilar tip aneurysm.

the Sylvian fissure, often as a discrete haematoma which may involve the temporal lobe and which again may bear a close resemblance to a "spontaneous" haemorrhage.

Aneurysms of the posterior circulation rarely cause haematomas. Indeed following rupture of a posterior inferior cerebellar artery aneurysm it is common to see no evidence of subarachnoid blood on CT. Blood especially within the fourth ventricle can be an important clue to the presence of a posterior inferior cerebellar artery aneurysm (Silver et al. 1981).

With a *basilar tip aneurysm* it is not unusual to visualise the aneurysm itself as a hyperdense lesion which enhances following intravenous contrast medium (Fig. 1.27).

Basal cistern enhancement has been reported in 21 of 42 patients in the series by Sobel et al. (1981) and in 21 out of 27 patients in Inoue et al.'s (1981) series. This appears to represent an adverse prognostic feature being associated with the development of complications, notably hydrocephalus. The existence of basal cistern enhancement appears to bear no temporal relation to the initial bleed.

Complications

Intraventricular haemorrhage may follow aneurysmal rupture, particularly with aneurysms of the anterior communicating artery or of the carotid tip (Silver et al. 1981). The size of the intraventricular haemorrhage does not appear to affect the prognosis nor does it seem to presage the development of late hydrocephalus. Conversely, early hydrocephalus occurred in 35% of cases in the above authors' series.

Hydrocephalus can occur very soon after aneurysm rupture when it is due to the presence of basal cistern blood obstructing cerebrospinal fluid flow. It may also develop between 2 and 6 weeks after the subarachnoid haemorrhage when meningeal fibrosis causes either an obstruction to cerebrospinal fluid flow at the tentorial hiatus or creates an absorption block affecting the arachnoid granulations. Hydrocephalus occurs most commonly following rupture of anterior communicating artery aneurysm (Silver et al. 1981).

Angiographic vasospasm (see Fig. 1.32) correlates well with low density regions seen on CT scanning. Such change may be temporary or progress to frank infarction. Vasospasm of the cerebral vessels can be asymptomatic but there is a broad correlation between its severity and the neurological status of the patient. That there can also be neurological deficit without evident vasospasm emphasises the complexity of cerebral haemodynamics following subarachnoid haemorrhage and the importance of changes in small vessels which are not seen at angiography.

CT undertaken soon after subarachnoid haemorrhage will not normally be expected to show hypodensity since there is a delay of about 3 days between the bleed and the onset of vasospasm which becomes maximal at 6–9 days and then regresses. Its development is greatly influenced by the amount of subarachnoid blood present.

Subdural haematoma following subarachnoid haemorrhage occurs in 1%–2% of cases usually following internal carotid artery aneurysm rupture.

CT and Prognosis Following Subarachnoid Haemorrhage

Davis et al. (1980) found that the amount of bleeding, as judged by its anatomic extent on CT, correlated with both the clinical grade of the patient and with the severity of the pre-operative vasospasm. Turnbull (1980) in a study involving 93 patients found that a normal CT scan following haemorrhage pointed to a complete recovery but that low attenuation areas were an adverse prognostic factor showing a close correlation with demonstrable angiographic spasm. Of patients with an intracerebral haematoma of less than 2.5 cm diameter 80% made a complete recovery whereas only 20% recovered when the haematomas were larger.

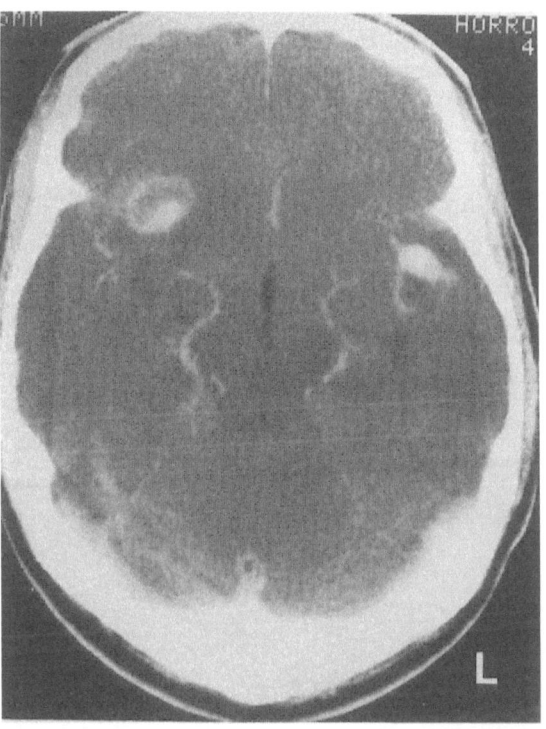

Fig. 1.28. Cranial CT after IV contrast. Bilateral middle cerebral artery aneurysms. That on the right is partially thrombosed. (Reproduced by kind permission of the *British Journal of Radiology*.)

MRI and Subarachnoid Haemorrhage

Acute subarachnoid haemorrhage is very difficult to diagnose with MRI but within one week, the signal is intensified on T1 weighted images due to methaemoglobin formation (Bradley and Schmidt 1985). As with spontaneous cerebral haemorrhage, CT appears better in the acute stage. MRI may nevertheless be of value when the CT is normal and seems to be more sensitive to the detection of an intracranial aneurysm (Satoh and Kadoya 1988).

Giant Intracranial Aneurysms

Giant intracranial aneurysms by convention exceed 25 mm in diameter and usually present due to compression of adjacent structures. They arise more commonly from the anterior circulation (Bull 1969). The CT appearances of large aneurysms have been described by Pinto et al. (1979). Patent, thin-walled aneurysms are hyperdense and enhance uniformly with intravenous contrast.

Partially thrombosed aneurysms present as ring-shaped hyperdensities often with calcification and an enhancing centre (a "target lesion") (Fig. 1.28). In a completely thrombosed aneurysm, there is no central enhancement. Adjacent ischaemic low density may be present. MRI has been used to study giant aneurysms (Olsen et al. 1987). Its ability to show flow within the lumen of the aneurysm as a signal void is an important advantage over CT which, in turn, shows calcification to better effect. The high signal characteristics on T1 and T2 weighted images of completely thrombosed aneurysms are also helpful since in these instances the diagnosis may remain unproven following angiography (Fig. 1.29).

Atlas et al. (1987) in an MRI study of partially thrombosed aneurysms showed that a high signal intensity rim due to methaemoglobin surrounds the lumen and peripherally there is a laminated appearance due to thrombus at different stages of organisation.

Parasellar Aneurysms

Intracavernous aneurysms or those arising from the supraclinoid segments of the internal carotid artery may project into the pituitary fossa and the clinical features of such aneurysms may suggest a pituitary tumour. If a trans-sphenoidal approach to such a "tumour" is planned, it is of vital importance to make the distinction.

Intravenous DSA can demonstrate patent aneurysms of a size sufficient to mimic a pituitary tumour in a quite simple manner. One can also envisage a useful role for MRI in these circumstances.

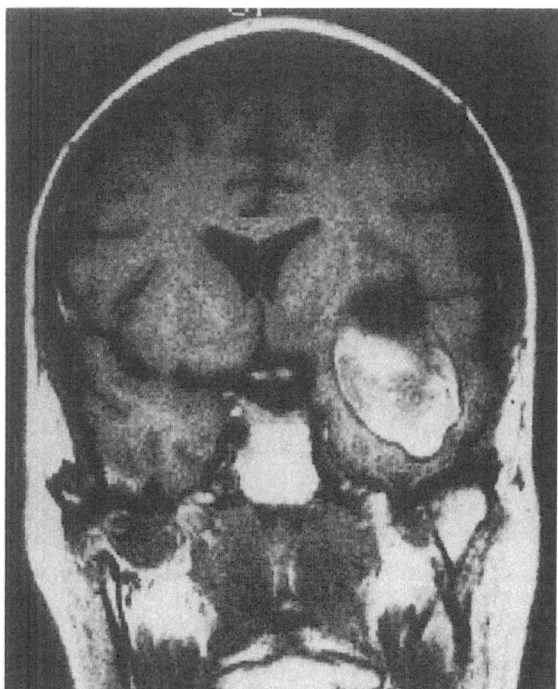

Fig. 1.29. Cranial MRI (T1 weighted image). Partially thrombosed middle cerebral artery aneurysm with a signal void superiorly due to blood flow in patent lumen.

Angiographic Findings

Anterior Cerebral Artery Aneurysms

The majority (90%) of anterior cerebral artery aneurysms arise at the junction of the horizontal portion of the anterior cerebral and the anterior communicating arteries (Fig. 1.30). It is important to undertake bilateral carotid angiography in such cases because an aneurysm may fill from one side only and this will influence the surgical approach. It may be necessary to perform a cross-compression study in order to demonstrate the anterior communicating artery complex adequately. In the absence of spontaneous cross flow, one cervical carotid artery is manually compressed whilst its fellow is injected.

Another favoured site for anterior cerebral artery aneurysms is at the junction of the pericallosal and calloso-marginal arteries (Fig. 1.31). These small pericallosal artery aneurysms are best seen in lateral projection. Berry aneurysms occurring at other sites are rare.

Middle Cerebral Artery Aneurysms

The usual site for middle cerebral artery aneurysms is at the terminal portion of the sphenoidal segment at its bifurcation or trifurcation (Fig. 1.32).

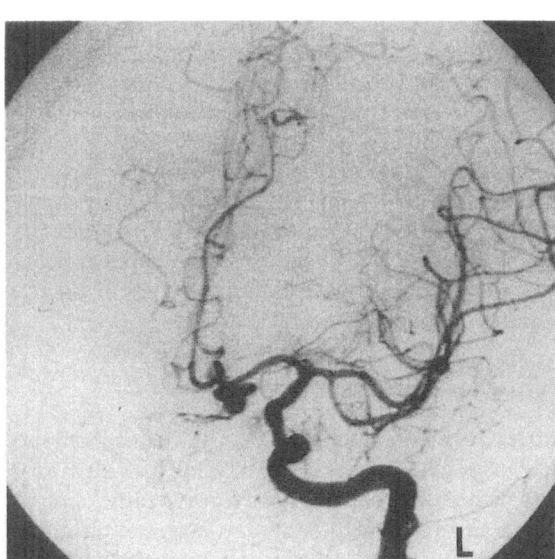

Fig. 1.30. Carotid arterial DSA (frontal oblique projection). Multiloculate anterior communicating artery aneurysm.

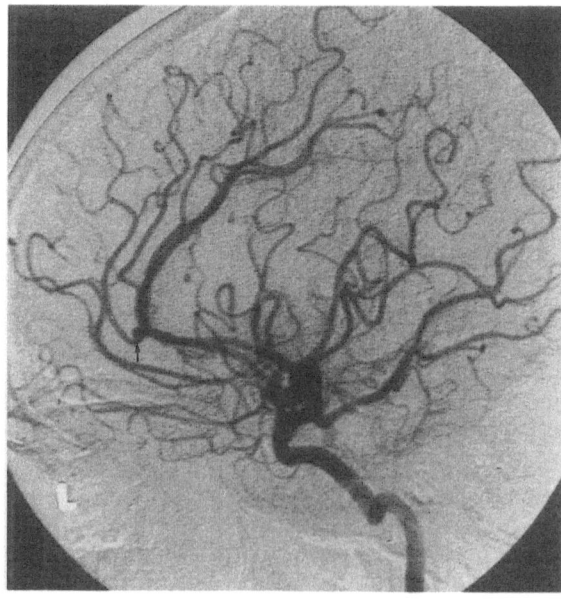

Fig. 1.31. Carotid arterial DSA (lateral projection). Pericallosal artery aneurysm (*arrow*).

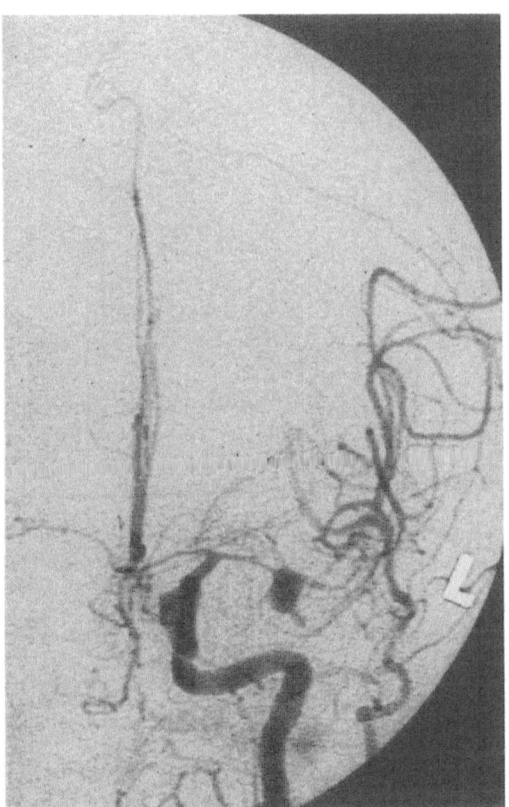

Fig. 1.32. Carotid arterial DSA. Middle cerebral artery aneurysm with spasm of the basal arteries.

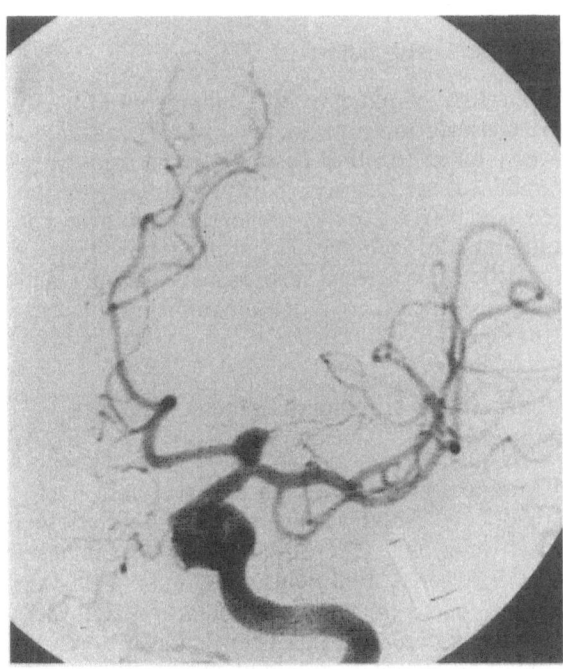

Fig. 1.33. Carotid arterial DSA (frontal oblique projection). Left carotid tip aneurysm.

Internal Carotid Artery Aneurysms

Internal carotid artery aneurysms comprise:

1. Posterior communicating artery aneurysms which arise at the junction of the internal carotid and the posterior communicating arteries (Fig. 1.36)
2. Anterior choroidal artery aneurysms which may be confused with (1)
3. Carotid tip aneurysms arising at the terminal carotid bifurcation (Fig. 1.33)
4. Ophthalmic artery aneurysms
5. Intracavernous aneurysms (Fig. 1.34)

Ophthalmic artery aneurysms usually project anteriorly and medially and if, in addition, they project upwards they can constitute a suprasellar mass. Intracavernous aneurysms need to be distinguished from the ophthalmic artery aneurysms. The latter arise more distally and project above the anterior clinoid process. An intracavernous artery aneurysm lies mainly below the anterior clinoid process at a level corresponding to the intracavernous portion of the internal carotid artery which it overlaps in the lateral projection.

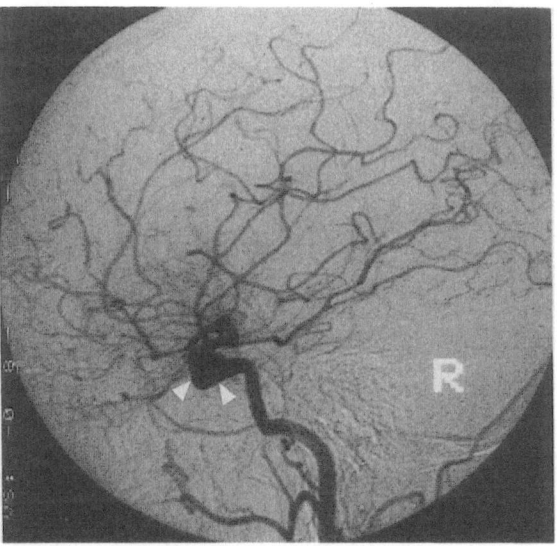

Fig. 1.34. Carotid arterial DSA (lateral projection). Cavernous aneurysm (*arrowheads*).

Vertebrobasilar Aneurysms

Vertebrobasilar aneurysms can arise from the basilar tip (Fig. 1.35) where a posteriorly directed sac can be intimately related to important perforating vessels. More distal posterior cerebral

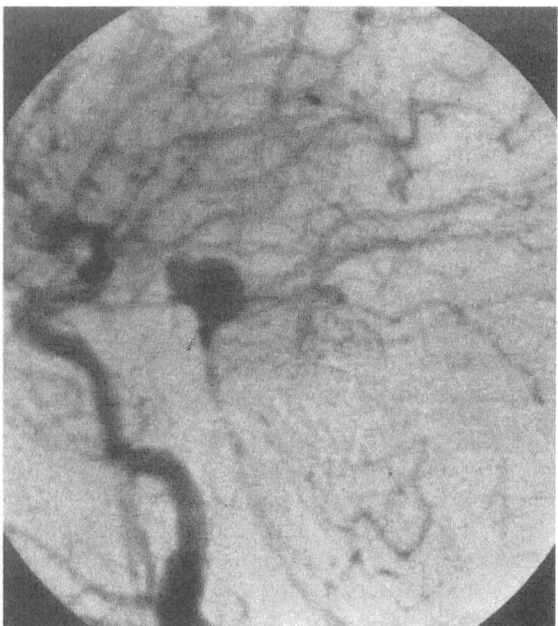

Fig. 1.35. Cranial intravenous DSA (lateral projection). Basilar tip aneurysm.

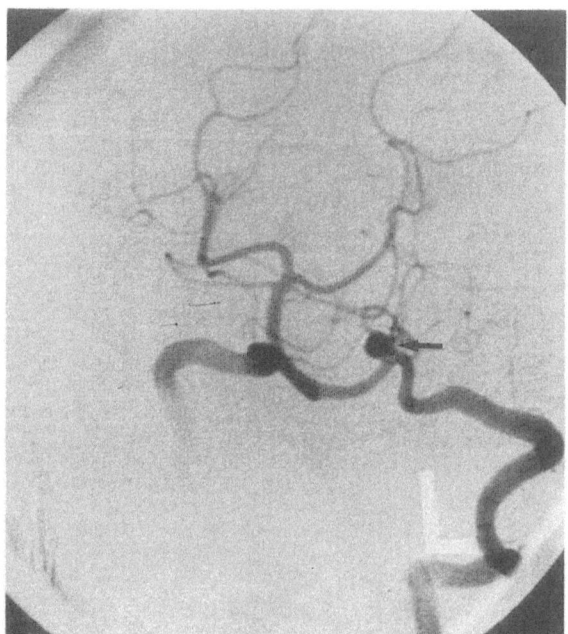

Fig. 1.37. Vertebral arterial DSA (frontal oblique projection). Aneurysm at the origin of the left posterior inferior cerebellar artery (*arrow*).

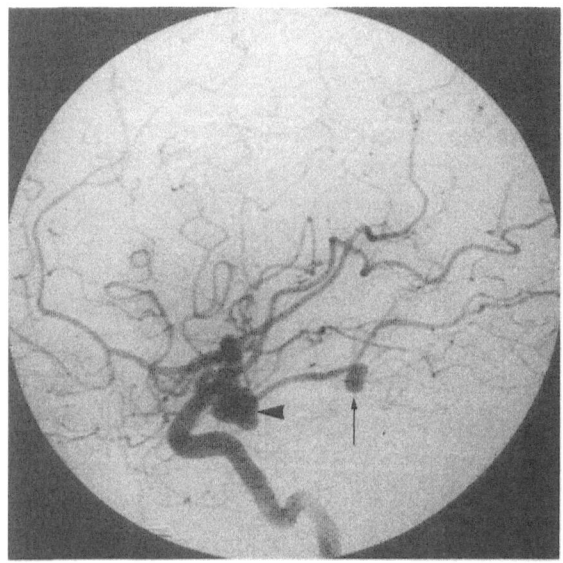

Fig. 1.36. Carotid arterial DSA. Left posterior cerebral artery (*arrow*) and posterior communicating artery (*arrowhead*) aneurysms.

artery aneurysms are also seen (Fig. 1.36). Berry aneurysms can also arise at the junction of the posterior inferior cerebellar (PICA) and the vertebral arteries (Fig. 1.37) and the demonstration of both PICA origins is a sine qua non of cerebral panangiography for intracranial aneurysms. Along

the basilar trunk, aneurysms can arise at the origins of the anterior inferior cerebellar and superior cerebellar arteries and at the vertebrobasilar confluence.

Multiple Aneurysms

About 20% of patients with subarachnoid haemorrhage have multiple aneurysms. CT and angiography taken together bestow a large measure of confidence in identifying which aneurysm has bled (see pp. 19–20). At angiography a large and multiloculate aneurysm is the most likely culprit especially when arterial vasospasm is maximal in its vicinity or when there is demonstrable intraluminal thrombus.

Subarachnoid Haemorrhage with Negative Angiography

In a minority of those with subarachnoid haemorrhage cerebral panangiography fails to disclose a causative lesion – 13% of patients in Alexander et al.'s (1986) series. Failure to visualise an aneurysm may be due to thrombotic obliteration following rupture or severe vasospasm which may prevent the filling of an otherwise patent aneurysm. In genuine angiogram-negative cases small vascular malformations around the brainstem have been incriminated which are either too small to be seen at angiography or which thrombose after rupture. The outlook for patients with normal angiography following subarachnoid haemorrhage is generally favourable although Hawkins et al. (1989) in a long-term follow-up have shown a reduced life expectancy because of supervening cardiovascular and cerebrovascular disease. The danger lies in overlooking small berry aneurysms and exposing the patient to the sometimes dire consequences of a further haemorrhage. To avoid such catastrophies a rational approach has to be devised. The CT and angiographic findings should be carefully reviewed. If vasospasm is present, angiography should be repeated when it is judged clinically to have regressed. If, even in the absence of vasospasm, the arterial anatomy of any region has been incompletely displayed then further angiography with additional views is warranted. Aneurysms of the anterior communicating complex and of the carotid tip can be overlooked. PICA aneurysms are especially likely to cause no CT abnormality following rupture. The origins of both PICAs must be adequately shown by injection of both vertebral arteries if necessary.

Forster et al. (1978) asserted that with a normal high quality angiogram following subarachnoid haemorrhage further angiography in the absence of a further bleed is seldom justified.

Familial Aneurysms and Infundibula

Patrick and Appleby (1983) presented details of a family with a high incidence of intracranial aneurysms and provided a review of the literature. They supported the view that a dominant mode of inheritance is operative and that familial aneurysms present at an earlier age than those in the general population.

Familial cases showed a lower incidence of anterior communicating artery aneurysms and an increased incidence of posterior communicating artery aneurysms. An infundibulum appears to be the precursor of a posterior communicating artery aneurysm and is a triangular or round dilatation at the junction of the posterior communicating and internal carotid arteries – by definition less than 3 mm in diameter. The posterior communicating artery should also enter at the apex of the infundibulum. The incidence in normal angiograms is 7% (Saltzmann 1959); in familial aneurysm cases 20%–40%. Trasi et al. (1981) documented the development of an aneurysm from an infundibulum of the posterior communicating artery in a young female.

Caroticocavernous Fistula

Caroticocavernous fistulae may arise spontaneously or may be acquired due to trauma, rupture of an intracavernous carotid aneurysm or arterial dissection. They are also associated with collagen deficiency syndromes (Halbach et al. 1987). Indirect fistulae are supplied by dural branches of the external carotid artery. CT may show proptosis and enlargement of the superior ophthalmic vein due to increased flow (Fig. 1.38) and angiography will demonstrate the fistulous connection (Fig. 1.39).

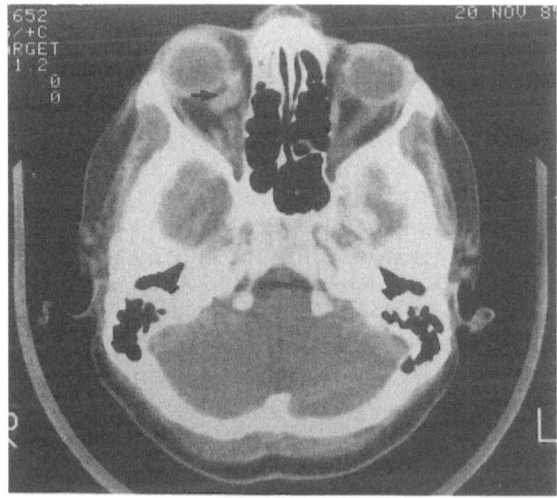

Fig. 1.38. Cranial CT after IV contrast. Caroticocavernous fistula. Note the right proptosis and enlarged superior ophthalmic vein (*arrow*).

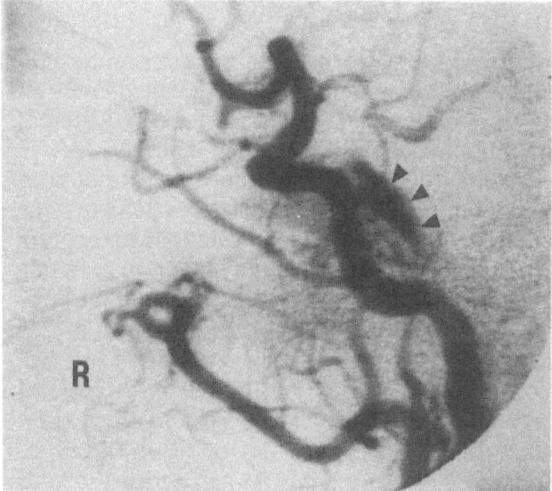

Fig. 1.39. Carotid arterial DSA (lateral projection), same patient as Fig. 1.38. *Arrowheads* outline contrast within the cavernous sinus.

Catastrophic haemorrhage may occur following rupture of a resultant cavernous sinus varix either as a subarachnoid haemorrhage or an epistaxis. With the interruption of normal drainage channels from the cavernous sinus, drainage into cortical veins may occur and this may also lead to intracerebral haemorrhage. Orbital venous hypertension and arterial insufficiency may each contribute to visual failure.

Vascular Malformations

McCormick (1966) has described a classification of vascular malformations. Arteriovenous malformations are the commonest type and are mostly found in the supratentorial compartment within the territory of the middle cerebral artery. Of 70 cases studied by Kelly et al. (1969) 57 were hemispheric, eight central (thalamus, basal ganglia, midbrain) and five were within the posterior fossa.

Venous angiomas, consisting entirely of veins, occur more commonly in spinal cord but are found intracranially.

Cavernous angiomas consist of large sinusoidal vascular spaces uninterrupted by parenchyma. They are particularly likely to calcify. A varix of one or several large veins may occur within the leptomeninges or parenchyma and occasionally gives rise to massive haemorrhage.

Telangiectases are small capillary angiomas usually found at autopsy but which may be encountered during life.

Arteriovenous Malformations

Arteriovenous malformations are congenital non-neoplastic lesions consisting of a coiled mass of arteries and veins. Affected individuals may present with intracranial haemorrhage or epilepsy.

The majority of arteriovenous malformations involve the cerebral hemispheres, particularly the frontal and parietal lobes. The lesions displace brain rather than invade it and supply by more than one major cerebral artery is common. Frontal arteriovenous malformations may be supplied by both the anterior and middle cerebral arteries. Temporal lesions may be supplied by the posterior cerebral artery as well as by the middle cerebral artery (Fig. 1.40). Saccular aneurysms may occur on the major arterial feeders presumably, in part at least, due to altered haemodynamics. Venous drainage depends on the site of the malformation but may be via the superficial or deep venous systems (Fig. 1.41).

Deep hemisphere arteriovenous malformations may rupture into the ventricular system leading ultimately to a communicating hydrocephalus. Obstructive hydrocephalus may result from pressure from enlarged cerebral vessels adjacent to the cerebral aqueduct.

Dural arteriovenous malformations arise near a major venous sinus and are supplied by extradural branches of the carotid and vertebral arteries. These can exist in isolation or accompany large intracerebral malformations.

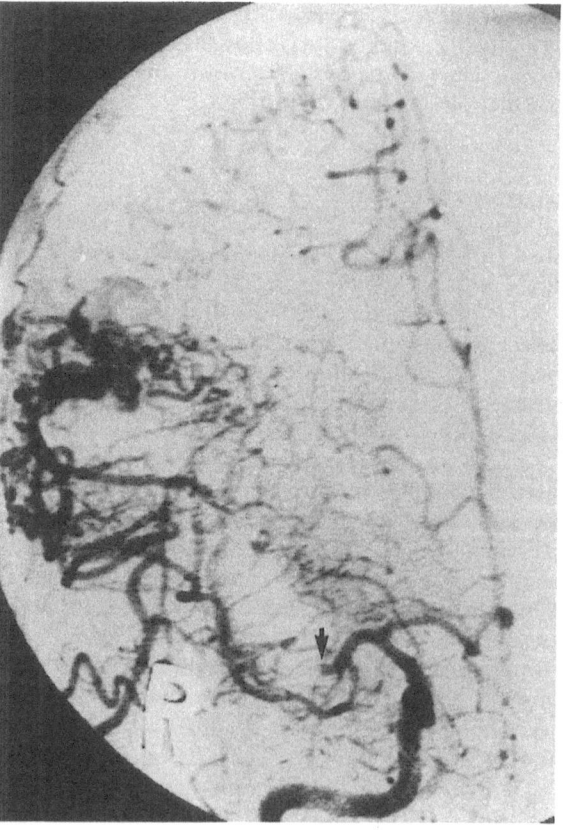

Fig. 1.40. Carotid arterial DSA (frontal projection). Right temporal arteriovenous malformation in association with middle cerebral artery occlusion (*arrow*) (moya moya variant).

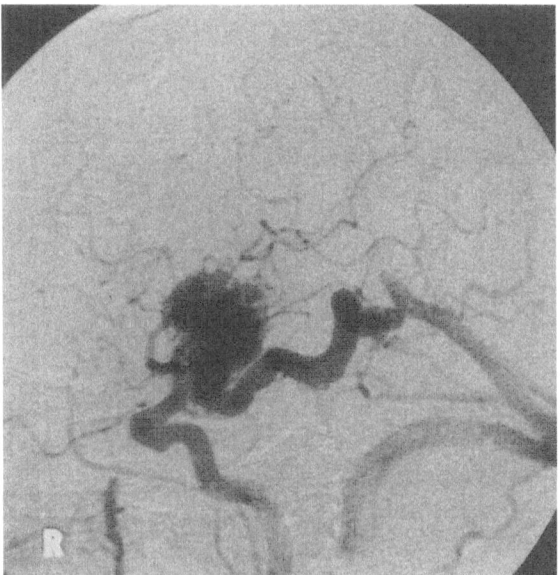

Fig. 1.41. Carotid arterial DSA (lateral projection). A deep hemisphere arteriovenous malformation with an enlarged basal draining vein and early opacification of the straight and lateral venous sinuses.

CT in Arteriovenous Malformations

On the plain CT scan the unruptured arteriovenous malformation will show serpiginous densities due mainly to prominent draining veins. There may be calcification which can be fleck-like or in the form of conglomerates (Figure 1.42). The basal cisterns adjacent to an arteriovenous malformation may be enlarged corresponding to the increased size of vessels coursing through them.

White matter hypodensity in relation to some arteriovenous malformations has been ascribed to oedema (Kumar et al. 1984), but may also be due to ischaemia – perhaps involving a local steal phenomenon. Kumar et al. (1984) also noted venous wall enhancement due to thickening and occasional local gyral effacement and enhancement. In their series, 44 of 48 patients with supratentorial arteriovenous formations had abnormal precontrast scans as had six out of 12 with malformations in the infratentorial compartment.

Prior to CT, the demonstration of mass effect at angiography was taken as evidence that a vascular malformation had bled. Kumar et al. (1985) studied 60 patients with unruptured malformations and showed mass effect to be exerted in 33 (55.9% of cases). The degree correlated grossly with the size of the lesion, particularly with the size of the venous channels.

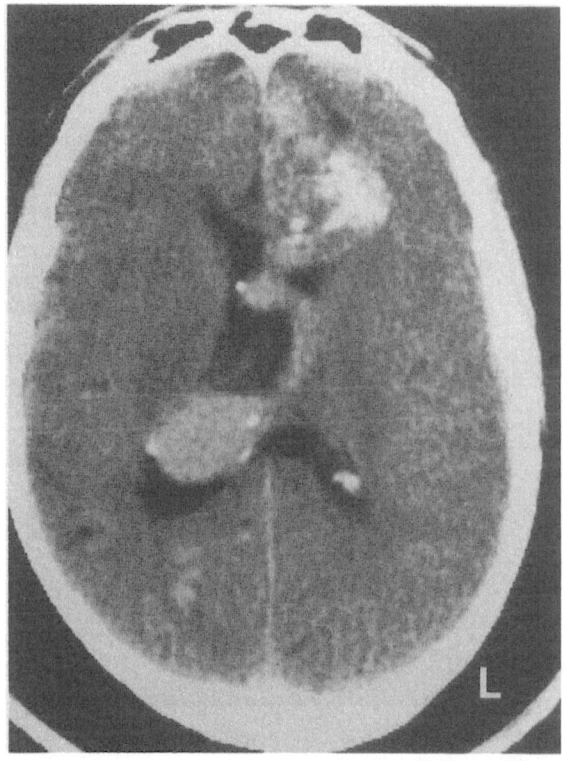

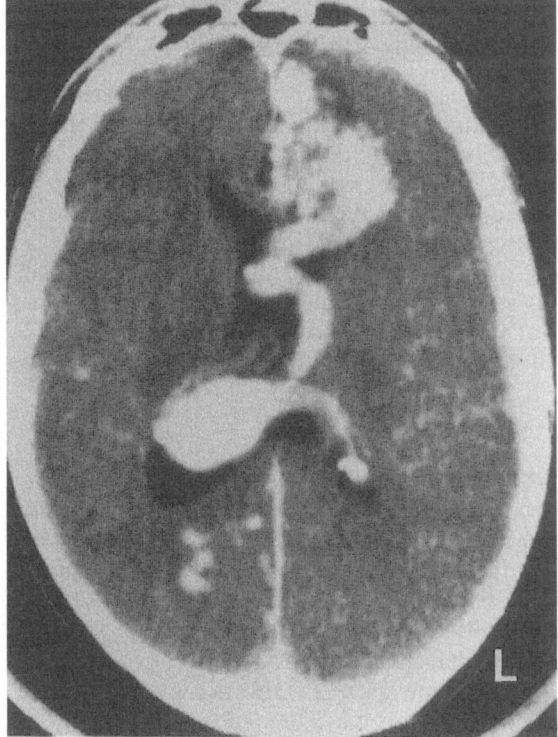

Fig. 1.42. Cranial CT before (**a**) and after (**b**) IV contrast. Calcified frontal arteriovenous malformation showing a large distended posteriorly coursing draining vein leading to an aneurysmal vein of Galen.

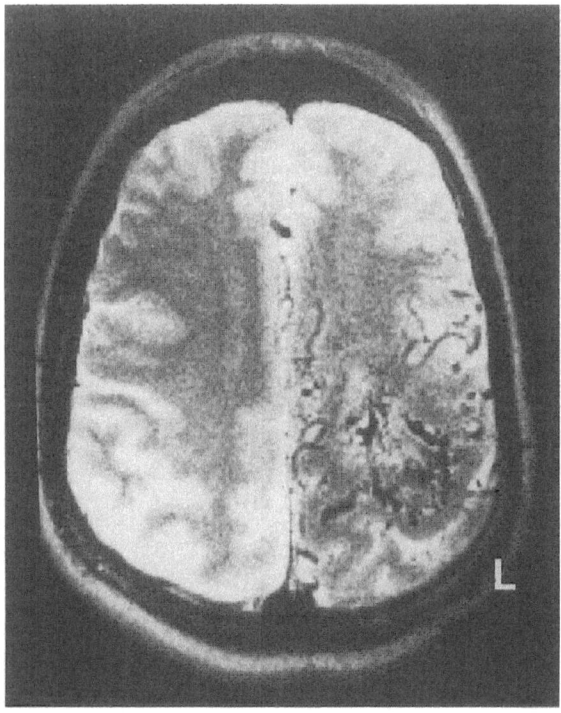

Fig. 1.43. Cranial MRI scan (T2 weighted image). Left parietal arteriovenous malformation.

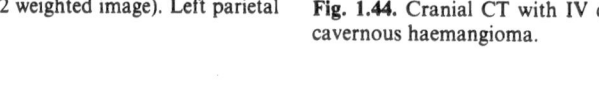

Fig. 1.44. Cranial CT with IV contrast. Left medial temporal cavernous haemangioma.

MRI in Vascular Malformations

MRI has been shown to be of value in vascular malformations (Fig. 1.43) and is particularly useful in those lesions close to the midline where the relationship to adjacent structures can be accurately assessed. Those in the infratentorial compartment are also well shown. Flowing blood contributes a poor signal since stimulated protons are carried away from the scan plane to be substituted by non-stimulated protons leaving a "signal void" (Schorner et al. 1986).

Cavernous Haemangiomas

CT studies may show a well-demarcated hyperdense lesion which enhances – often poorly – and which may contain flecks of calcification (Fig. 1.44). There is no appreciable mass effect but there may be associated haemorrhage. Ahmadi et al. (1985) studied 10 patients with histologically verified cavernous haemangiomas and in four, two or more distinct types of vascular malformation were identified.

The CT findings are thus not specific and in addition cavernous angiomas often fall within the category of "occult" vascular malformations (see below).

Venous Angiomas

At angiography, venous angiomas consist of a radiating collection of medullary veins with a large central draining vein, appearing first in the early venous phase and then persisting into the late venous phase. There is no increase in the size or number of arterial feeding vessels. Olsen et al. (1984) showed that CT demonstrated the large draining vein as the most consistent feature. They are usually found within anterior or middle cerebral artery territories but Pelz et al. (1983) described a brainstem location. They may also be found within a cerebellar hemisphere.

Augustyn et al. (1985), studying MRI in this pathology, identified the enlarged transcerebral vein and obtained positive findings in all seven angiographically verified patients studied.

Occult Vascular Malformations

Occult or "cryptic" vascular malformations are lesions which fail to show abnormal vessels at angiography. All histological varieties are represented by this definition. Their appearance is rather non-specific and may resemble tumours. Yeates and Enzmann (1983) suggested that important clues to the diagnosis on CT were hyperdense lesions perhaps with some calcification, little or no mass effect and little or no contrast enhancement. Particularly in the brainstem, glioma is the main differential diagnosis but these are usually iso- or hyperdense on the plain scan and do not normally enhance.

MRI is a sensitive means of characterising chronic haematomas and has been shown to be valuable in the diagnosis of cryptic malformations (Fig. 1.45) (Lemme Plaghos et al. 1986; New et al. 1986). In the series of Gomori et al. (1986) the co-existence of different types of vascular malformation again posed the question as to how distinct the pathological types are. Sze et al. (1987) have cautioned that occult vascular malformations with haemorrhage may be indistinguishable from haemorrhagic neoplasms but that multiplicity and oedema favour the latter.

Angiography in Aneurysms and Vascular Malformations

Angiography is usually undertaken just prior to surgery, the timing of which depends on the patient's clinical condition. Surgery on intracranial aneurysms is directed towards the prevention of recurrent haemorrhage which is most frequent in the second week after the initial bleed. Against this

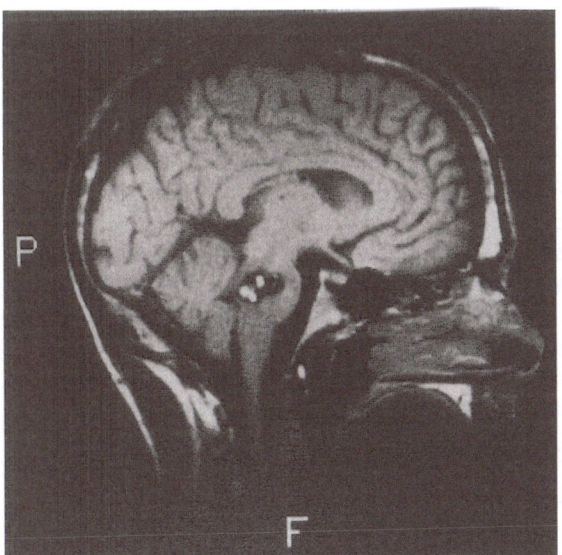

Fig. 1.45. Cranial MRI scan (T1 weighted image). Cavernous haemangioma of the brainstem. (By courtesy of Dr. C. E. L. Freer.)

has to be balanced the evidence which suggests that operation in the presence of vasospasm affects the prognosis adversely (Allcock and Drake 1965). Accordingly many neurosurgeons favour early surgery in relatively well patients before the onset of vasospasm, although the optimum time for surgery is by no means universally agreed.

The risks of recurrent bleeding from an arteriovenous malformation are rather different from those of berry aneurysms. Haemorrhage occurs mostly in the second, third and fourth decades and beyond the age of 40 years the likelihood of bleeding rapidly diminishes. The time interval between bleeds is in any case irregular and the risk of recurrent haemorrhage is estimated at 6% in the first year and 2% per year thereafter (Graf et al. 1983). In the series of Brown RD et al. (1988) the risk of death from rupture was 29%.

Emergency angiography and surgery may be required to evacuate an intracerebral haematoma but since the risk of rebleeding is lower the timing of intervention is less problematic than in the case of berry aneurysms. In addition since the haemorrhage is predominantly intraparenchymal, vasospasm may not be encountered.

DUPLEX SONOGRAPHY OF CAROTID ARTERIES

Margaret D. Hourihan

The management of extracranial carotid degenerative disease has depended to a large extent on estimates of the degree of stenosis of the vessels. This anatomical approach is flawed by the limitations of the angiography and particularly by the absence of functional information. To overcome these problems, the range of diagnostic modalities used to study the extracranial carotid tree has increased in recent years. The principal developments have been in the application of ultrasound techniques to provide anatomical and functional information about the arteries and flow within them. Most good vascular laboratories and departments of diagnostic vascular imaging now utilise the duplex ultrasound system to gather this information. The role of duplex ultrasound is established, if not precisely defined. The role of intravenous digital subtraction angiography (DSA) is less certain as it provides little functional information.

Sound and Ultrasound

Sound waves audible to the normal human ear are transmitted through air at frequencies in the range 20–20 000 Hz. Ultrasound waves are inaudible with frequencies in the range 1–15 MHz for medical application and require a solid or liquid medium for transmission.

Ultrasound waves are generated by the application of an electric field which causes realignment of electrically charged molecules within a piezoelectric crystal which creates a mechanical response in the form of a sound wave. Excitation of the piezoelectric crystal by an alternating voltage produces ultrasonic waves, the frequency of which is determined by the frequency of the applied voltage.

Ultrasound waves travel at similar velocities in all soft tissues without refraction of the incident beam. At tissue boundaries, however, the incident beam is partly reflected and partly transmitted. The amount reflected is determined by the acoustic impedance of the tissues at either side of the tissue interface. A similar partition occurs at each tissue interface with partial reflection and partial transmission of the incident beam. Reflected ultrasound waves returning from the tissue to the piezoelectric crystal cause a potential difference between the front and rear faces of the crystal which can be measured and displayed.

Ultrasound Techniques

Ultrasound techniques are described as indirect or direct according to the way they provide information about the blood vessels. The principal indirect techniques used to assess the carotid vessels are oculoplethysmography and supraorbital doppler analysis (Keller et al. 1976; Thiele et al. 1980). Each can provide information about the carotids by examination of distal vessels, but apart from screening for high-grade stenosis or occlusion, the techniques are relatively insensitive.

Other methods examine the structure or function of the carotid arteries directly. The early continuous wave Doppler and pulsed Doppler (Mavis-C) imaging methods have now been largely superseded by B-mode ultrasound imaging to provide direct structural information. In B-mode imaging, pulsed ultrasound waves enter the tissue to be examined and are reflected from the interface between tissues of different acoustic impedance. This provides range and amplitude data which can be displayed visually so that the brightness of the image increases with increasing amplitude of the reflected wave.

Structural detail of the vessel, its walls, lumen and atheromatous plaque (if present) is provided. The static B scanner is rarely used in carotid imaging, which is the domain of high resolution real time B-mode scanners.

The second direct method involves haemodynamic assessment. The ability of ultrasound to detect the flow of blood was first described in 1959 by Satomura. He based his calculations on the principle formulated by 1842 by Christian Doppler to describe the change apparent in the wavelength of light emitted from moving stars when measured by a fixed observer. Doppler's principle applies equally to sound and additionally whether there is a moving sound source or, as in the case of cellular elements of blood, a moving sound reflector. The Doppler shift principle can be used to detect movement of the cellular elements of blood; the movement being detected and recorded from the change in frequency of the reflected ultrasound waves.

Continuous Wave Doppler

Continuous wave Doppler (CWD) utilises two piezoelectric crystal transducers, one emitting and the other receiving ultrasound waves. When directed at a blood vessel the CWD can detect the movement of cellular elements because their movement towards the probe causes an increase in the frequency of the reflected ultrasound waves, whereas flow away from the probe causes a decrease in that frequency. This is the Doppler Principle and the Doppler shift frequency can be described mathematically as a function of the velocity of ultrasound in tissue, the velocity of the cellular elements in the blood, the angle between the incident ultrasound beam and the direction of blood flow. Whether blood flow is laminar or turbulent, there will be a range of velocities of the cellular elements in the flowing blood. Moreover, blood flow is dynamic, so velocities will vary throughout the cardiac cycle, being higher in systole than in diastole. In some cases the diastolic flow will be reversed. These CWD systems detect blood flowing at all points within the ultrasound beam so that signals can be confused by reflection from adjacent vessels.

Pulsed Doppler

Pulsed Doppler (PD) has one piezoelectric transducer which acts as both transmitter and receiver, with the reflected signals received and processed during gaps in transmission. Such systems are range-gated. The time taken for the incident ultrasound to reach and return from reflectors allows determination of the distance between these reflectors and the ultrasound source. Varying the time between transmission and reception allows alteration of the distance of the sampling site from the probe. In this way the PD can "focus" on a particular vessel, overcoming the possible confusion of multiple signals detected by CWD.

Direct Imaging

Continuous Wave Systems

The imaging system comprises a continuous wave transducer, a probe position resolver and a storage monitor. A bright spot is generated on an oscilloscope each time the CWD probe detects a Doppler shift signal so that movement back and forth in the neck can generate an image of the sources of the Doppler shift signals. These images are uniplanar and of low quality and difficulties encountered with continuous wave Doppler in defining the source of flow signal led to the development of two-dimensional imaging of the carotid vessels.

Pulsed Doppler Systems

Pulsed Doppler can provide much greater morphological detail than CWD systems. The introduction of multigated systems allows analysis of variations of blood velocity throughout the cardiac cycle in all gates simultaneously. Moreover the probe can be positioned to allow the generation of images in different planes, e.g. anteroposterior, lateral and transverse.

In addition to the anatomical image, PD systems allow Doppler shift analysis to provide information concerning the velocity and volume of blood flow in the vessel.

B-Mode Imaging

Systems in current use show real-time images by employing arrays of transducers or mechanical, rotating transducers. The frame rate of these systems is typically 20–30/s.

Ultrasound frequencies of 7.5–10 MHz which can image vessel walls at depths of 3–6 cm are appropriate to examine the cervical carotid arteries. The lower frequency (7.5 MHz) has better penetration but the image quality is superior with the higher (10 MHz) frequency of the incident ultrasound signal. The reflected ultrasound waves are converted into grey scale images by either digital or analogue signal processing.

Anatomical images of the carotid vessels are usually made in both transverse and sagittal planes. The normal anatomy of the vessel wall is seen contrasted against the echolucent, blood-filled lumen. Additionally, the dynamic nature and high resolution of B-mode ultrasound allows assessment in all phases of the cardiac cycle and alterations in the luminal diameter are seen easily. Abnormalities of the vessel wall such as intimal ulceration, irregularity, plaque, or smooth stenosis can be identified. The composition of mural lesions can be assessed. Fibrotic and calcified plaques can be distinguished and intraplaque haemorrhage identified (Fig. 1.46).

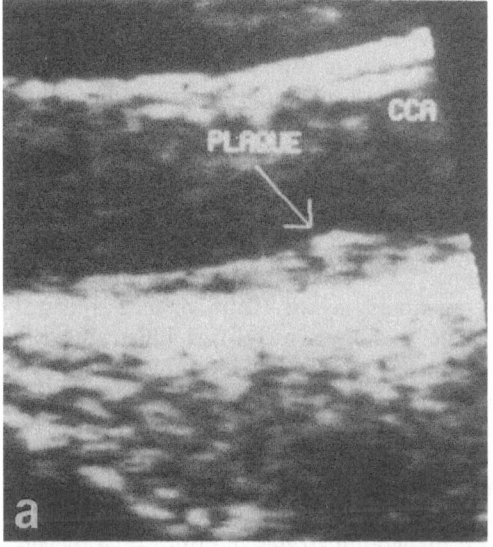

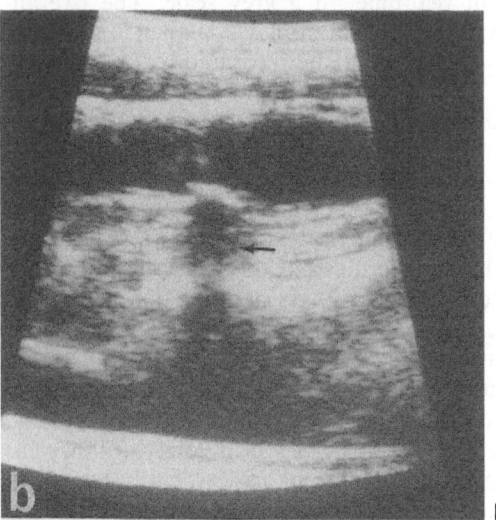

Fig. 1.46. B-mode images: cervical carotid artery. **a** Homogeneous echo pattern from a fibrous plaque; **b** calcified plaque with acoustic shadowing (*arrow*).

These assessments are probably important if cerebral ischaemic episodes are the result of embolisation by cholesterol crystals and atheromatous debris following intraplaque haemorrhage, or if the emboli derive from the platelet and fibrin thrombi which form on the diseased intima.

There are a number of limitations if carotid morphology is assessed by B-mode imaging alone. The study may be flawed if the bifurcation is particularly deep or high in the neck. Luminal lesions may not be differentiated from blood if they are hypoechoic (sonolucent), or if they are in the acoustic shadow of hyperechoic tissue, e.g. calcified plaque. The precise luminal area and diameter cannot always be determined and a particular difficulty is the differentiation of tight stenosis from vessel occlusion. In general, however, the morphological information about the vessel wall from the B-mode may allow the clinician to assess the relative risk of plaque breakdown, ulceration, and embolisation leading to cerebral ischaemic episodes or stroke.

Doppler Signal Analysis

Doppler analysis of blood flow may be represented as either an analogue waveform or as a spectral display. The analogue waveform illustrates the weighted average velocity of blood as an instantaneous function of time. It has two major limitations in that it is susceptible to distortion by extraneous signals and it provides no information regarding the range or spectrum of velocities within the vessel.

Spectral display illustrates the full range of velocities in real-time on a grey scale. The overall pattern of the spectral display is similar to the analogue waveform but the informational content is greater.

In normal blood vessels the movement of cellular elements is laminar – more rapid centrally with lower velocities adjacent to the vessel walls. This range of velocities is smaller in systole when the cellular elements move at a rapid and more uniform speed than it is in diastole; though peak and mean velocities are higher in systole than in diastole. In systole, the spectral display (Fig. 1.47) reveals a rapid rise in velocity with narrowing of the vertical bandwidth (range of velocities), and a spectral window which indicates the absence of slowly moving cells. A lowering of velocity follows in diastole, with widening of the vertical bandwidth, seen on grey scale as a broader distribution of brightness.

In the normal internal carotid artery (ICA) antegrade blood flow is continuous throughout the

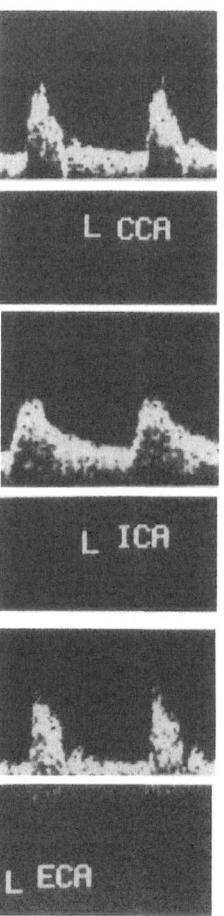

Fig. 1.47. Spectral display of frequency (y axis) against time (x axis) from the common (CCA) internal (ICA) and external (ECA) carotid arteries, showing two cardiac cycles. Each shows a rapid rise in systole. The spectral window is seen in both the CCA and the ICA, but is less obvious in the ECA. The ICA display is all above the base line, indicating forward flow but an element of reversed flow is seen below the line for the ECA. The rapid decrease in frequencies in diastole indicate a high peripheral resistance in the ECA, in contrast to the fairly continuous flow in the low resistance ICA.

cardiac cycle so that all elements of the spectral display are above the base line. In the normal external carotid artery (ECA) antegrade flow predominates but the higher peripheral resistance may cause cessation or reversal of flow in diastole, shown as a return to or below the zero baseline in the spectral display. The Doppler profile for the ECA and ICA are so characteristic that, in combination with realtime B-mode imaging, accurate vessel identification is possible.

Doppler analysis is not perfect but a sensitivity and specificity of about 95% has been reported (Blackshear 1980; Dreisbach et al. 1983). Difficulty may arise when calcified plaques distort or absorb the ultrasound beam, or when blood flow in a dis-

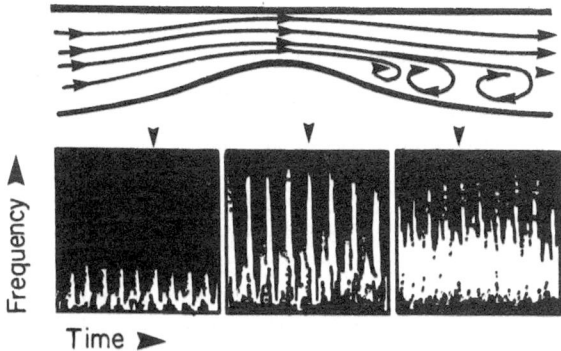

Fig. 1.48. Redrawn spectral displays from a carotid artery proximal to, at and downstream from, a stenosis as illustrated diagrammatically. At the stenosis, peak frequency increases markedly. Downstream from the stenosis there is filling of the spectral window and a decrease in peak frequency.

eased ECA is mistaken for flow in an ICA which is, in reality, occluded. Alterations in the velocity and pattern of blood flow may occur when the vessels are diseased. Changes in the spectral display are seen proximal to, at and distal to an arterial stenosis (Fig. 1.48). Proximally, the slowing of blood flow causes a decrease in peak frequency. At the stenosis peak frequency is increased and distal to the stenosis broadening of the vertical bandwidth occurs, i.e. an increasing range of velocities is

encountered as the vortices produced by the stenosis rotate in the ultrasound field. Turbulence and flow disturbance occur irrespective of whether the cause is a simple smooth stenosis, a plaque, an ulcer or some other form of irregularity of the vessel wall. This turbulence produces a marked broadening of the vertical bandwidth as red cells are moving in many directions simultaneously (Fig. 1.49).

The patterns of spectral display which may occur are endlessly variable but some characterisation has been undertaken on the basis of peak frequency and vertical bandwidth. Many workers try to match the spectral display from an individual patient with one in the five categories (Table 1.7) which Fell et al. (1981) suggested correspond with angiographic findings.

Table 1.7. Characteristics of the spectral display in relation to varying degrees of arterial stenosis

Stenosis %	Peak frequency kHz	Spectral broadening
0	3.5	Nil
10%	3.5	Systolic deceleration
10%–49%		Pan systolic
50%	4	Whole cardiac cycle
100%	Nil	Nil

After Fell et al. (1981).

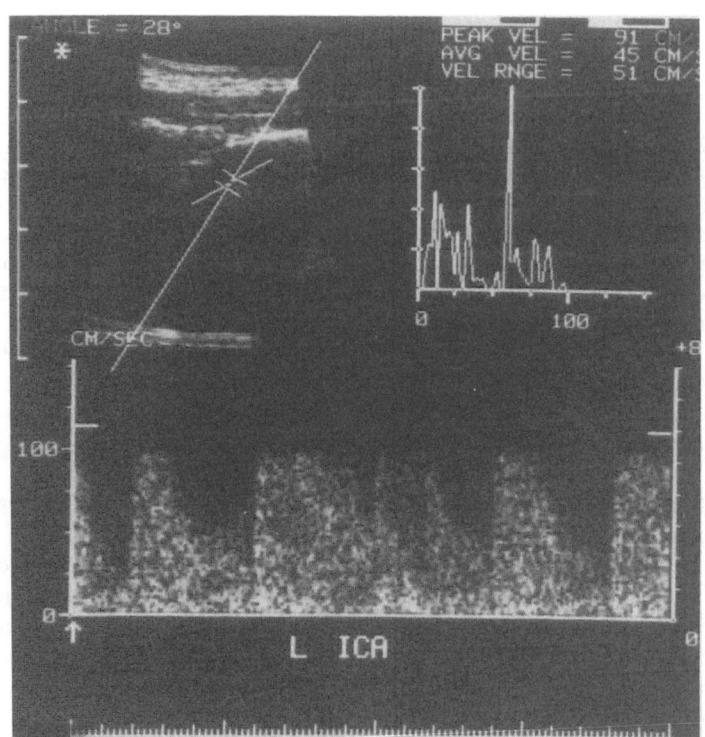

Fig. 1.49. Composite illustration showing the spectral display (*below*) in an internal carotid artery with a greater than 75% stenosis, the sampling site within the internal carotid (*above left*) and velocity data (*above right*).

In addition to the visual display, spectral data can be analysed in other ways. The Fourier transform is used to display spectral information at specific times in the cardiac cycle and is particularly useful for generating data on the velocity of blood flow. This Fourier analysis is displayed for any selected sampling site as amplitude versus frequency which, with knowledge of the angle of the incident beam, can allow computation of the velocity of blood flow.

Duplex Scanning

Duplex scanning refers to the concurrent assessment of structural and functional data about blood vessels by the use of high-resolution realtime. B-mode ultrasound and spectral analysis. Since the concept was introduced (Barber et al. 1974) hardware development and the quality of data generated have progressed rapidly. Modern systems allow the generation of a B-mode image from which the site for assessment of blood flow characteristics can be determined. Sample volumes for spectral analysis can be taken from any chosen site in the vessels. This is important because it allows sampling at a distance from the slower-moving cellular elements of blood adjacent to a vessel wall thus avoiding a spuriously broad spectrum. In addition, it allows sample volumes to be taken from each of the common carotid artery (CCA), carotid bulb, ICA and ECA; and sample volumes can be taken proximal to, at and downstream from any identified lesion in each of these sites. Spectral analysis is used to complement the structural B-mode assessment in determining the degree of stenosis by consideration of velocity patterns, for some stenoses, e.g. those due to soft plaque or recent thrombus do not show well on B-mode. This limitation of B-mode may be overcome with duplex scanning as, for instance, the Doppler sample volume may produce no signal thus demonstrating vessel occlusion.

Duplex scanning also overcomes some of the limitations of spectral analysis alone. A common practical problem usually encountered with spectral analysis made at the carotid bifurcation is a demonstration of a broadening of the spectral display which occurs because of an inappropriately steep angle of the incident beam to the longitudinal axis of the artery.

The ability of duplex scanning correctly to identify the presence of disease in up to 97% of carotid vessels irrespective of the degree of stenosis is not matched by its accuracy in estimating the precise degree of stenosis, though the accuracy is equivalent to angiography with stenoses above 50%. Just how accurate duplex scanning is in assessing the degree of stenosis depends on whether the yardstick is conventional angiography or operative findings, each of which is no less observer-dependent than duplex scanning (Croft et al. 1980; Chilcote et al. 1981; O'Donnell et al. 1985; Rubin et al. 1987). Three-way comparisons show duplex scanning to be marginally more accurate than angiography in detecting stenoses greater than 50% and significantly more accurate for ulceration, irregularity and plaque conformation (Goodson et al. 1987). Nonetheless duplex scanning and angiography should not be seen to be in competition but rather to be complementary (Table 1.8). Several comments are relevant to the comparison of duplex scanning with angiography.

Table 1.8. Advantages and limitations of duplex sonography

Advantages	Disadvantages
Non-invasive, inexpensive	User dependent
Multiplanar imaging	Field of view is fairly restricted
Mural detail is shown	
Enables qualitative evaluation of plaque	Acoustic shadowing from calcific plaque may obscure other major lesions
Physiological data are obtained	It may be difficult to differentiate a "near occlusion" from an occlusion (colour Doppler may make this easier)
Normal vessels are reliably identified	

There is considerable interobserver variation in assessing the severity of stenosis from angiograms and the minimal diameter cannot be measured with certainty within 0.5 mm. Duplex scanning tends to "overestimate" disease in patients shown to have normal or minimally diseased carotids. This may be a result of the static nature of angiography and its consequent inability to display luminal changes throughout the cardiac cycle or it may be due to the ability of ultrasound to show both the thickness of the vessel wall and changes in vessel distensibility with developing stenosis.

Investigative Strategy

How the vessels are imaged in patients with, or suspected of having, extracranial vascular disease varies according to the clinical presentation, the experience and personal preference of the physician and the imaging hardware available. This is a dynamic calculus and continues to evolve in many centres but ultrasonography is becoming established as the screening method of choice (Sandercock 1987).

Duplex scanning can be used to identify patients with significant disease at the carotid bifurcation which may warrant further investigation by angiography. Equally important for a screening tool, it can also demonstrate that carotid bifurcation regions are normal. This may be of value for instance in excluding carotid disease in patients prior to coronary artery surgery.

Intravenous DSA provides a more complete assessment of the extracranial carotid vasculature than duplex scanning, but the image quality is dependent on a number of factors including the ability of the patient to remain motionless, cardiac output and correct anatomical positioning to prevent superimposition of vessels (Connolly et al. 1985).

Duplex scanning is less expensive and involves no irradiation or contrast medium. It defines areas of stenosis and provides information on consequent haemodynamic alterations in carotid blood flow. Small plaques, intimal irregularity and ulceration are all better shown by duplex scanning than by DSA or conventional angiography (Rubin et al. 1987; Goodson et al. 1987). The technique does not depend on the patient's cardiac output or ability to remain motionless. It is, however, highly operator dependent and requires a high degree of expertise before quoted figures of 95% sensitivity are attained.

References

Ahmadi J, Teal JS, Segall HD, Zee CS, Hans JS, Becker TS (1983) Computed tomography of carotid-cavernous fistula. AJNR 4:131–136

Ahmadi J, Miller CA, Segall HD, Park SY, Zee GS, Becker RL (1985) CT patterns in histopathologically complex cavernous hemangiomas. AJNR 6:389–393

Alexander MSM, Dias PS, Uttley D (1986) Spontaneous subarachnoid haemorrhage and negative cerebral panangiography: Review of 140 cases. J Neurosurg 64:537–542

Allcock JM, Drake CG (1965) Ruptured intracranial aneurysms: The role of arterial spasm. J Neurosurg 22:21–29

Asari S, Satoh T, Sakurai M, Yamamoto Y, Sadamoto K (1982) The advantage of coronal scanning in cerebral computed angiotomography for diagnosis of Moyamoya disease. Radiology 145:709–711

Atlas SW, Grossman RI, Goldberg HI, Hackney DB, Bilaniuk LT, Zimmerman RA (1987) Partially thrombosed giant intracranial aneurysms: Correlation of MR and pathological findings. Radiology 162:111–114

Augustyn GT, Scott JA, Olsen E, Gilmor RL, Edwards MK (1985) Cerebral venous angiomas: MR imaging. Radiology 156:391–395

Barber FE, Baker DW, Nation AWC, Strandness DE, Reid JM (1974) Ultrasonic duplex echo-doppler scanner. IEEE Trans Biomed Eng 21:109–113

Barnett HJM (1980) Progress towards stroke prevention: Robert Wartenberg lecture. Neurology 30:1212–1225

Blackshear WM (1980) Comparative review of OPG – K + M,

OPPG – G and pulsed doppler ultrasound for carotid evaluation. Vascular Diagnosis and Treatment 1:43–52

Bonafe A, Manelfe C, Scotto B, Pradere MY, Pascol A (1985) Role of computed tomography in vertebrobasilar ischaemia. Neuroradiology 27:484–493

Bories J, Derhy S, Chiras J (1985) CT in hemispheric ischaemic attacks. Neuroradiology 27:468–483

Bousser MG, Baron JC, Chiras J (1985) Ischaemic strokes and migraine. Neuroradiology 27:583–587

Bradley WG, Schmidt PG (1985) Effect of methaemoglobin formation on the MR appearance of subarachnoid haemorrhage. Radiology 156:99–103

Brandt Zawadzki M, Weinstein P, Bartkowski H, Moseley M (1987) MR imaging and spectroscopy in clinical and experimental cerebral ischaemia: A review. AJNR 8:39–48

Brown JJ, Hesselink JR, Rothrock JF (1988) MR and CT of lacunar infarcts. AJNR 9:477–482

Brown RD, Wiebers DO, Forbes G et al. (1988) The natural history of unruptured intracranial arteriovenous malformation. J Neurosurg 68:352–357

Bull J (1969) Massive aneurysms at the base of the brain. Brain 92:535–570

Buonanno FS, Moody DM, Ball MR, Laster DW (1978) Computed cranial tomographic findings in cerebral sinovenous occlusion. J Comput Assist Tomogr 8:281–291

Butler P (1986) Intravenous digital subtraction angiography (review Article). Br J Hosp Med 35:30–36

Butler P (1987) Digital subtraction angiography (DSA): a neurosurgical perspective. Br J Neurosurg 1:323–333

Butler P, Freer CEL, Jha AN, Lye RH (1987) Intravenous digital subtraction angiography in intracranial aneurysms. Br J Radiol 60:323–326

Castaigne P, Lhermitte F, Gautier JC et al. (1973) Arterial occlusions in the vertebrobasilar system: A study of 44 patients with post-mortem data. Brain 96:133–154

Chilcote WA, Modic MT, Pavilicek WA et al. (1981) Digital subtraction angiography of the carotid arteries: a comparative study in 100 patients. Radiology 139:287–295

Chiras J, Marciano S, Vega Molina J, Touboul J, Poirier B, Bories J (1985) Spontaneous dissecting aneurysm of the extracranial vertebral artery (20 cases). Neuroradiology 27:288–292

Cobb SR, Mehringer CM, Itabashi HH, Pribram H (1987) CT of subinsular infarction and ischaemia. AJNR 8:221–227

Cole FM, Yates P (1967) Intracerebral microaneurysms and small cerebrovascular lesions. Brain 90:759–767

Colosimo C, Fileni Mushchini M, Guerrini P (1985) CT findings in eclampsia. Neuroradiology 27:313–317

Connelly JE, Brownell DA, Levine EF, McCart PM (1985) Accuracy and indications of diagnostic studies for extracranial carotid disease. Arch Surg 120:1229–1232

Croft RJ, Ellam LD, Harrison MJG (1980) Accuracy of carotid angiography in the assessment of atheroma of the internal carotid artery. Lancet i:997–1000

Davis JM, Davis KR, Crowell RM (1980) Subarachnoid haemorrhage secondary to ruptured intracranial aneurysms: Prognostic significance of cranial CT. AJNR 1:17–21

Dooms GC, Uske A, Brant Zawadzki M et al. (1986) Spin-echo MR imaging of intracranial haemorrhage. Neuroradiology 28:132–138

Dreisbach JN, Seibert CE, Smazal SF, Stavros AT, Daigle RJ (1983) Duplex sonography in the evaluation of carotid artery disease. AJNR 4:678–680

Du Boulay GH, Ruiz JS, Rose FC, Stevens JM, Zilkha KJ (1983) CT changes associated with migraine. AJNR 4:472–473

Duyckaerts C, Hauw JJ (1985) Pathology and pathophysiology of brain ischaemia. Neuroradiology 27:460–467

El-Gammel T, Adams RJ, Nichols FT et al. (1986) MR and CT investigations of cerebrovascular disease in sickle cell patients. AJNR 7:1043–1049

Enzmann DR, Britt RH, Lyons BE, Buxton JL, Wilson DA (1981) Natural history of experimental intracerebral hemorrhage sonography, computed tomography and neuropathology. AJNR 2:517–526

Fell G, Phillips DJ, Chikos PM, Harley JD, Thiele BL, Strandness DE (1981) Ultrasonic duplex scanning for disease of the carotid artery. Circulation 64: 1191–1195

Fisher CM (1965) Lacunes: Small, deep cerebral infarcts. Neurology 15:774–784

Fisher CM, Adams RD (1987) Observations on brain embolism with special reference to haemorrhage infarction. In: Furlan AJ (ed) The heart and stroke. Springer-Verlag, Berlin, Heidelberg, New York

Forster DMC, Steines L, Hakanson S, Bergvall V (1978) The value of repeat pan angiography in cases of unexplained subarachnoid hemorrhage. J Neurosurg 48:712–716

Fujisawa I, Asato R, Nishimara K et al. (1987) Moya moya disease: MR imaging. Radiology 164:103–105

Gabrielsen TO, Seeger JF, Knake JE, Stilwill EW (1981) Radiology of cerebral vein occlusion without dural sinus occlusion. Radiology 140:403–408

Goldberg HI, Grossman RI, Gomori JM, Asbury AK, Bilanuik LT, Zimmerman RA (1986) Cervical internal carotid artery dissecting hemorrhage: Diagnosis using MR. Radiology 158:157–161

Goldstein SJ, Sacks JG, Lee C, Tibbs PA, McCready RA (1983) Computed tomographic findings in cerebral arterial ectasia. AJNR 4:501–504

Gomori JM, Grossman RI, Goldberg HI, Zimmerman RA, Bilanuik LT (1985) Intracranial haematomas: Imaging by high field MR. Radiology 157:87–93

Gomori JM, Grossman RI, Goldberg HI, Hackney DB, Zimmerman AR, Bilanuik L (1986) Occult cerebral vascular malformations: High field MR imaging. Radiology 158:707–713

Goodson SF, Fanigan DP, Bishara RA, Schuler JJ, Kikta MJ, Meyer JP (1987) Can carotid duplex scanning supplant arteriography in patients with focal carotid territory symptoms? J Vasc Surg 5:551–557

Graf CJ, Perret GE, Torner JC (1983). Bleeding from cerebral arteriovenous malformations as part of their natural history. J Neurosurg 58:331–337

Gritter KJ, Laidlaw WW, Peterson NT (1987) Complications of out patient transbrachial intra-arterial digital subtraction angiography. Radiology 162:125–127

Grosgogeat Y (1985) Cerebral ischaemic accidents of cardiac origin. Neuroradiology 27:579–582

Halbach W, Hieshema GB, Higashida RT, Reicker M (1987) Carotid cavernous fistulae: Indications for urgent treatment. AJNR 8:725–802

Hawkins TD, Sims C, Hanka R (1989) Subarachnoid haemorrhage of unknown cause: a long term follow up. J Neurol Neurosurg Psychiatry 52:230–235

Heiss WD, Herholz K, Bocherswarz HG et al. (1986) PET, CT and MR imaging in cerebrovascular disease. J Comput Assist Tomogr 10:903–911

Hinshaw DB, Thompson JR, Hasso AN, Casselman ES (1980) Infarctions of the brainstem and cerebellum: A correlation of computerised tomography and angiography. Radiology 137:105–112

Hoffman M, Gomes AS, Pais SO (1984) Limitations in the interpretation of intravenous carotid digital subtraction angiography. AJR 142:261

Horning CR, Dorndorf W, Agnoli AL (1986) Hemorrhagic cerebral infarction: A progressive study. Stroke 17:172–184

Houser UW, Mokri B, Sundt TM, Baker HL, Reese DF (1984) Spontaneous cervical cephalic arterial dissection and its residuum angiographic spectrum. AJNR 5:27–34

Imakita S, Nishimura T, Naito H et al. (1987) Magnetic resonance imaging of human cerebral infarction: Enhancement with Gd DTVA. Neuroradiology 29:422–429

Inoue Y, Saiwai S, Migamoto T et al. (1981) Postcontrast computed tomography in subarachnoid hemorrhage from ruptured aneurysms. J Comput Assist Tomogr 5:341–344

Keller H, Meier W, Yonekawa Y, Kumpe D (1976) Noninvasive angiography for the diagnosis of carotid artery disease using doppler ultrasound (carotid artery doppler). Stroke 7: 354–363

Kelly DL, Alexander E, Davis CH, Maynard DC (1969) Intracranial arteriovenous malformations: Clinical review and evaluation of brain scans. J Neurosurg 31:422–428

Kjos BO, Brant Zawadzki M, Young RG (1983) Early CT findings of global central nervous system hypoperfusion. AJNR 4:1043–1048

Kodama N, Suzuki J (1978) Moyamoya disease associated with aneurysm. J Neurosurg 48:565–569

Kumar AJ, Fox AJ, Vinuela F, Rosenbaome AE (1984) Revisited old and new CT findings in unruptured large arteriovenous malformations of the brain. J Comput Assist Tomogr 8:648–655

Kumar AJ, Vinuela F, Fox AJ, Rosenberg AE (1985) Unruptured intracranial arteriovenous malformations do cause mass effect. AJNR 6:29–32

Lemme Plaghos L, Kucharczyk W, Brandt Zawadski M et al. (1986) MR imaging of angiographically occult vascular malformations. AJNR 7:217–222

Locksley HB (1966) Natural history of subarachnoid haemorrhage, intracranial aneurysms and arteriovenous malformations. J Neurosurg 25:219–237

Lutz PR, Bullinger WE, Auisling RG (1986) Subcortical arteriosclerotic encephalopathy CT spectrum and pathologic correlation. AJNR 7:817–822

Manelfe C, Clanet M, Gigand M, Bonafe A, Guirand B, Rascol A (1981) Internal capsule: Normal anatomy and ischaemic changes demonstrated by computed tomography. AJNR 2:149–155

Masdeu JC (1983) Infarct versus neoplasm on CT: Four helpful signs. AJNR 4:525–528

Masuzawa T, Kurokawa T, Oguro K et al. (1986) Pulseless disease associated with multiple intracranial aneurysms. Neuroradiology 28:17–22

Mawad ME, Hilal SK, Michelsen WJ, Stein B, Ganti SR (1984) Occlusive vascular disease associated with cerebral arteriovenous malformation. Radiology 153:401–440

McCormick WF (1966) The pathology of vascular ("arteriovenous") malformations. J Neurosurg 24:807–816

McCreary JA, Schellhas KP, Brant Zawadzki M, Norman D, Newton TH (1985) Outpatient DSA in cerebrovascular disease using transbrachial arch injections. AJNR 6:795–801

McMurdo SK, Brant Zawadski M, Bradley WG, Chang GY, Berg BO (1986) Dural sinus thrombosis: Study using intermediate field strength MR imaging. Radiology 161:83–86

Meyer FB, Sundt TM, Fode NC, Morgan MK, Forbes GS, Mellinger JF (1989) Cerebral aneurysms in childhood and adolescence. J Neurosurg 70:420–425

Miller DH, Ormerod IEC, Gibson A, du Boulay EPGH, Rudge P, McDonald WI (1987) MR Brain scanning in patients with Vasculitis: Differentiation from multiple sclerosis. Neuroradiology 29:226–231

Mohr JP, Caplan LR, Melski JW et al. (1978) The Harvard Cooperative Stroke Registry: A prospective registry. Neurology 28:754–762

Moseley IF, Holland IM (1979) Ectasia of the basilar artery:

The breadth of the clinical spectrum and the diagnostic value of computed tomography. Neuroradiology 18:83–91

New PF, Aronow S (1976) Attenuation measurements of whole blood and blood fractions in computed tomography. Radiology 121:635–640

New PF, Ojemann RG, Daris KR et al. (1986) MR and CT of occult vascular malformations of the brain. AJNR 7:771–779

O'Donnell TF, Erdoes L, Mackey WC et al. (1985) Correlation of B-mode ultrasound imaging and arteriography with pathologic findings at carotid endarterectomy. Arch Surg 120:443–449

Olsen E, Gimor RL, Richmond B (1984) Cerebral venous angiomas. Radiology 151:97–104

Olsen WL, Brant Zawadski M, Hodes J, Noman D (1987) Giant intracranial aneurysms: MR imaging. Radiology 163:431–435

Osborn AG, Anderson RE (1977) Angiographic spectrum of cervical and intracranial fibromuscular dysplasia. Stroke 8:617–626

Patrick D, Appleby A (1983) Familial intracranial aneurysm and infundibular widening. Neuroradiology 25:329–334

Pelz DM, Vinuela F, Fox AJ (1983) Unusual radiologic and clinical presentation of posterior fossa venous angiomas. AJNR 4:81–84

Petro GR, Witwer G, Cacayorin E et al. (1986) Spontaneous dissection of the cervical internal carotid artery: Correlation of arteriography, CT and pathology. AJNR 7:1053–1058

Pinto RS, Kricheff I, Butler AR, Murali R (1979) Correlation of computed tomographic, angiographic and neuropathological changes in giant cerebral aneurysms. Radiology 132:85–92

Pressman BD, Tourje RS, Thompson JR (1987) An early CT sign of ischaemic infarction: Increased density in a cerebral artery. AJNR 8:645–648

Roach MR, Drake CJ (1965) Ruptured cerebral aneurysms caused by micro-organisms. N Engl J Med 273:240–244

Rubin JR, Bondi JA, Rhodes RS (1987) Duplex scanning versus conventional arteriography for the evaluation of carotid artery plaque morphology. Surgery 102:749–755

Sahs AL (1966) Observations on the pathology of saccular aneurysms. J Neurosurg 14:792–806

Salgado ED, Furlan AJ, Conomy JP (1987) Cardioembolic sources of stroke. In: Furlan AJ (ed) The heart and stroke. Springer-Verlag, London, Berlin, Heidelberg

Saltzmann GF (1959) Infundibular widening of the posterior communicating artery studied by carotid angiography. Acta Radiol 51:415–421

Sandercock P (1987) A symptomatic carotid stenosis: spare the knife. Br Med J 294:1368–1369

Sato M, Tanaka S, Kohama T (1987) "Top of the basilar" syndrome: Clinico-radiological evaluation. Neuroradiology 29:354–359

Satoh S, Kadoya S (1988) Magnetic resonance imaging of subarachnoid haemorrhage. Neuroradiology 30:361–364

Satomura S (1959) A study of the flow patterns in peripheral arteries by ultrasonics. J Acoust Soc Jpn 15:151–158

Savoiardo M, Bracchi M, Passerini A, Visciani A (1987) The vascular territories in the cerebellum and brainstem: CT and MR study. AJNR 8:199–209

Schorner W, Bradac GB, Treisch J, Bender A, Felix R (1986) Magnetic resonance imaging (MRI) in the diagnosis of cerebral arteriovenous angiomas. Neuroradiology 28:313–318

Schuierer G, Huk W (1988) The unilateral hyperdense middle cerebral artery: An early CT sign of embolism or thrombosis. Neuroradiology 30:120–122

Silbergleit R, Junck L, Gebarski SS, Hatfield MK (1989) Idiopathic intracranial hypertension (pseudotumour cerebri): MR imaging. Radiology 170:207–209

Silver AJ, Pederson ME, Ganti SR, Hilal SK, Michelsen WJ (1981) CT of subarachnoid haemorrhage due to ruptured aneurysm. AJNR 2:13–22

Skriver EB, Olsen TS (1981) Transient disappearance of cerebral infarcts on CT scan: the so-called fogging effect. Neuroradiology 22:61–65

Sobel D, Li FC, Norman D, Newton TH (1981) Cisternal enhancement after subarachnoid haemorrhage. AJNR 2:549–552

Sobel DF, Baker E, Anderson B, Kretzschmar H (1985) Cerebral amyloid angiography associated with massive intracerebral haemorrhage. Neuroradiology 27:318–321

Soges LJ, Cacayorin ED, Petro GR, Ramachandran TS (1988) Migraine: Evaluation by MR. AJNR 9:425–429

Spencer MP (1987) Ultrasound diagnosis of cerebrovascular disease. Martinus Nijhoff, Dordrecht

Sterbini GLP, Agatiello LM, Stocchi A, Solivetti FM (1987) CT of ischaemic infarctions in the territory of the anterior choroidal artery: A review of 28 cases. AJNR 8:229–232

Sze G, Krol G, Olsen WL et al. (1987) Haemorrhagic neoplasms: MR mimics of occult vascular malformations. AJNR 8:795–802

Takahashi M, Miyauchi T, Kowada M (1980) Computed tomography of Moyamoya disease: Demonstration of occluded arteries and collateral vessels as important diagnostic signs. Radiology 134:671–676

Takahashi M, Bussaka H, Nakagawa N (1984) Evaluation of the cerebral vasculature by intra-arterial DSA – with emphasis on in vivo resolution. Neurology 9:253–260

Takahashi S (1980) Magnification angiography in Moyamoya disease. Radiology 136:379–386

Takeuchi S, Kobayasi K, Tsuchida T, Imamura H, Tanaka R, Ito J (1982) Computed tomography in Moyamoya disease. J Comput Assist Tomogr 6:24–32

Thiele BL, Young JV, Chikos PM, Hirsch JH, Strandness DE (1980) Correlation of arteriographic findings and symptoms in cerebrovascular disease. Neurology 30:1041–1046

Trasi S, Vincent LM, Zingesser LH (1981) Development of aneurysm from infundibulum of posterior communicating artery with documentation of prior haemorrhage. AJNR 2:368–370

Turnbull IW (1980) Computed tomographic pointers to the prognosis of subarachnoid haemorrhage. Br J Radiol 53:416–420

Unger EC, Gado MH, Fulling KF, Littlefield JL (1987) Acute cerebral infarction in monkeys: An experiment study using MR imaging. Radiology 162:789–795

Viraponge C, Cazenave C, Quisling R, Sarwar M, Hunk S (1987) The empty delta sign: Frequency and significance in 76 cases of dural sinus thrombosis. Radiology 162:779–785

Vonofakos D, Marcu H, Hacker H (1983a) CT diagnosis of basilar artery occlusion. AJNR 4:525–528

Vonofakos D, Hacker H, Grau H (1983b) Direct visualisation of intracranial aneurysms by multiplane dynamic CT. AJNR 4:425–428

Weingarten KL, Zimmerman RD, Pinto RS, Whelan MA (1985) Computed tomographic changes of hypertensive encephalopathy. AJNR 6:395–398

Yeates A, Enzmann D (1983) Cryptic vascular malformations involving the brainstem. Radiology 146:71–75

Yock DH (1981) CT demonstration of cerebral emboli. J Comput Assist Tomogr 5:190–196

Zimmerman RD, Leeds NE, Naidich TP (1977) Ring blush associated with intracranial hematoma. Radiology 122:707–711

Chapter 2

Intracranial Tumours

Charles E. L. Freer

Introduction

Computed tomography (CT) is the primary investigation for cerebral tumours. Plain radiography is reserved for further clarification of a CT abnormality in the calvarium, skull base or as part of surgical planning. Angiography has a similarly limited role and is mainly used to assess tumour vascularity, especially of meningiomas.

CT is highly efficient in detecting tumours in the supratentorial compartment, but the specificity of the diagnosis is less secure. Claveria et al. (1978) and Kendall et al. (1979) found that 9% and 5% respectively of the diagnoses were incorrect. Infarcts and radiation necrosis were the major causes of diagnostic confusion.

Magnetic resonance imaging (MRI) has advantages in terms of high contrast sensitivity, multiplanar imaging, and absence of ionising radiation – all of which are valuable in the diagnosis and management of intracranial tumours. MRI is superior in the detection and subsequent management of tumours in the brainstem, middle and posterior cranial fossae (Bydder et al. 1983; Johnson et al. 1983; Bradac et al. 1985; Flannigan et al. 1985) where CT interpretation is hindered by the presence of artefacts. Comparisons with CT have shown that MRI has a superior sensitivity (Bydder et al. 1985; Lee BCP et al. 1985) although tumours which do not show any substantial increase in T1 or T2 relaxation times (up to 12% in one series (Mackay et al. 1985)) can be difficult to detect. Fortunately the majority of these tumours are large and exert mass effect (Haughton et al. 1986). It is important to note that if only T1

weighted and proton density spin echo techniques are used substantial tumours can be missed (Brant-Zawadzki et al. 1984; Smith et al. 1985). Gadolinium-labelled diethylenetriamine pentaacetic acid (gadolinium DTPA), a stable chelate complex of a rare earth ion with strong paramagnetic properties, is an effective contrast agent for MRI and may be used in much the same way as the conventional iodinated contrast agents in CT.

Central nervous system tumours encompass a wide range of histological types and are listed in Table 2.1.

Radiotherapeutic and postoperative changes will be considered separately.

Table 2.1. A classification of intracranial tumours

Intra-axial
Glial and oligodendroglial series
 Low-grade astrocytomas
 Glioblastoma multiforme
 Cystic glioma
 Oligodendroglioma
Ependymoma
Lymphoma and leukaemia
Haemangioblastoma
Gangliocytoma
Metastasis

Intraventricular
Neuroepithelial cysts
Choroid plexus tumours

Extra-axial
Meningioma
Pituitary and associated tumours
Pineal region tumours
Dermoid, epidermoid and lipoma
Neuroma
Chordoma and tumours of cartilaginous origin

Intra-axial Tumours

Low-Grade Astrocytomas

The CT appearances are variable. Generally they appear as an area of ill-defined mixed attenuation surrounded by a zone of low attenuation which may have the typical appearance of white matter oedema, but which may nevertheless be tumour since the true tumour – oedema interface is often difficult to identify. Contrast medium enhancement is also variable; uncommon in the genuine low-grade tumour, but increasing in frequency as the tumour blends with the more aggressive histological types (Silverman and Marks 1981). Calcification is common but is not often marked. CT is a highly sensitive technique for the detection of calcification but there is a lack of specificity. An area of patchy calcification in a hemisphere detected on plain radiographs has a high likelihood of being a low-grade glioma or oligodendroglioma but on CT calcification is also seen in high-grade gliomas. The general principle of curvilinear calcification indicating a cyst or vascular anomaly is always valuable. Areas of calcification will not return a signal with MRI and appear as a "signal void". MRI is also less sensitive than CT in the detection of calcification.

With MRI low-grade astrocytomas appear as areas of increased signal intensity on T2 weighted images and variable low signal intensity on T1 weighted images. There is an increased sensitivity in the detection of low-grade gliomas but the problems relating to the definition of the tumour margin remain (Fig. 2.1).

Glioblastoma Multiforme

These tumours have usually attained a large size at presentation although there is a small subgroup with epilepsy, or other neurological symptoms (Bolender et al. 1983), whose scans are normal initially but 6–8 weeks later demonstrate typical appearances. CT shows a region of mixed attenuation usually with low attenuation centrally (Fig. 2.2). After IV contrast there is marked irregular enhancement of the tumour. An homogeneously enhancing mass which is round or lobular suggests a gliosarcoma (Lee Y-Y et al. 1985).

MRI will demonstrate these tumours as extensive areas of heterogeneous signal intensity, increased on T2 weighted images and decreased on T1 weighted images. As with low-grade astrocytomas there is difficulty in separating the tumour from surrounding secondary effects. Contrast enhancement with gadolinium DTPA will demonstrate local

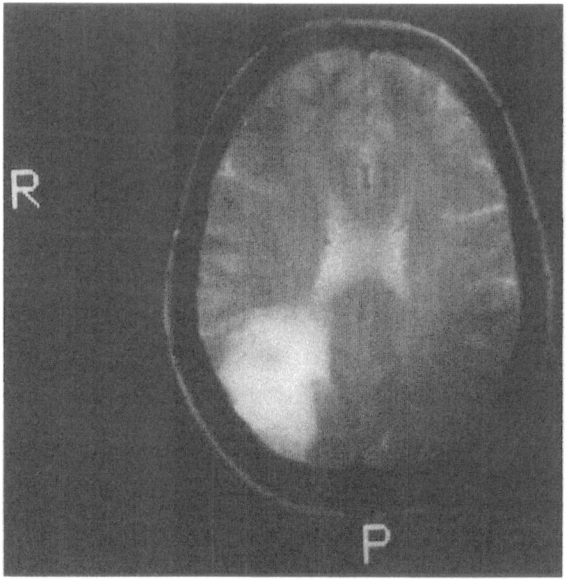

Fig. 2.1. Cranial MRI (T2 weighted image). Low-grade glioma. Tumour margins are indefinite.

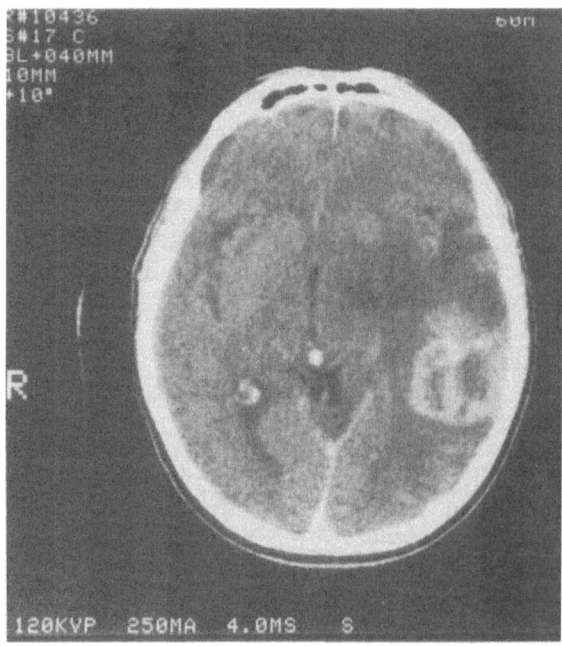

Fig. 2.2. Cranial CT after contrast. High-grade glioma.

breakdown of the blood–brain barrier but this will leave areas of indeterminate signal intensity which may represent tumour but might also be a reactive zone, old haemorrhage, or the margin of white matter oedema. With high field imagers there is often a peripheral low signal area from haemosiderin outlining the margin of the tumour – a phenomenon

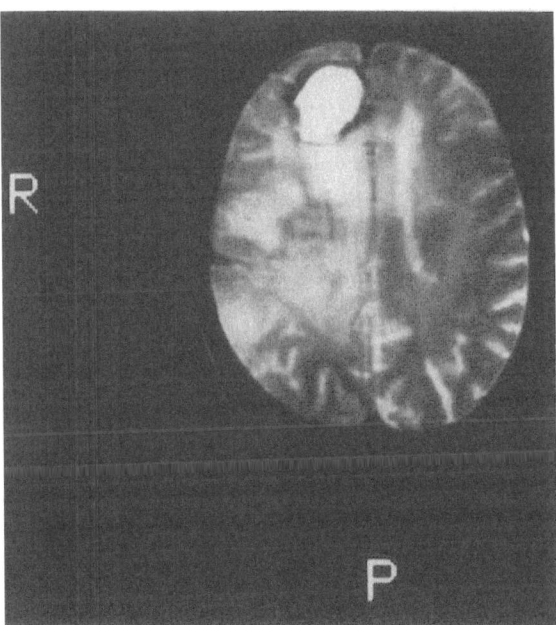

Fig. 2.3. Cranial MRI (T2 weighted image). High-grade glioma. There is a rim of low signal surrounding the tumour.

not visualised at medium field strengths (Fig. 2.3) (Weinstein et al. 1986). A number of authors (Claussen et al. 1985a, b; Felix et al. 1985; Graif et al. 1985) have suggested that differentiation between tumour and surrounding brain is possible but Earnest et al. (1988) with CT and MR enhancement followed by stereotactic biopsy were unable to confirm the location of the tumour margin in a small series. In any case the boundaries of a typical diffuse and infiltrating glioma may be difficult to define histologically with a continuum from frank tumour through reactive changes to unequivocal white matter oedema. The definition of tumour margins may be an unattainable goal though MRI often demonstrates a more extensive lesion than is evident from the CT especially where there is spread into the corpus callosum or where there is a multifocal component, which occurred in up to 7% on one histological study (Barnard and Geddes 1987).

Cystic Gliomas

This is a subgroup of low-grade pilocytic astrocytomas occurring predominantly in children which are usually found in the cerebellum or hypothalamus but also occasionally in the cerebrum and which have a favourable prognosis (Palma and Guidetti 1986). When a well-circumscribed area of low attenuation at or near that of cerebrospinal fluid (CSF), with or without peripheral enhance-

ment, is present a cyst is suspected although in reality this may represent either solid tumour or necrosis. The attenuation value per se is a poor indicator of content (Latchaw et al. 1977). The definitive sign of fluid content is a fluid level corroborated by a change in its direction with a change in the position of the head or rarely the demonstration of contrast fluid level after intravenous enhancement. A thin well-circumscribed wall visible before contrast is suggestive of a cyst rather than necrosis; a smooth inner border is further evidence whereas an irregular thick wall suggests necrosis. The differentiation of cyst from abscess on CT parameters alone is difficult since both have a thin wall, although with an abscess the wall may not be seen before contrast and occasionally will show local thinning when adjacent to a lateral ventricle. A cyst on a delayed scan may show a contrast fluid level whereas in an abscess there may be homogeneous enhancement where no true capsule is present.

As MRI images "water" it might be expected that the differentiation between solid and cystic lesions would be easier. Unequivocal cysts (Weiner et al. 1987) have appearances similar to cerebrospinal fluid on T1 and T2 weighted images but there is a spectrum through intermediate signal intensities to cysts with higher signal intensity than CSF on T1 and T2 weighted images (Kjos et al. 1985). The intermediate lesions were considered to be the result of increased protein concentration reducing the mobility of water but simple signal intensity observations are poor indicators of protein content (Hackney et al. 1987). The high signal intensity cysts are probably due to cellular debris and the residua of occult haemorrhage.

Oligodendroglioma

An irregular area of low attenuation with prominent calcification is typical of oligodendroglioma especially where this lesion is situated in the frontal lobe (Fig. 2.4).

With MRI there are areas of high and low signal intensity on T2 weighted image and T1 weighted image respectively with prominent "signal voids" corresponding to the calcifications.

Grading and Prognostic Factors in Gliomas

Kazner et al. (1982) analysed a large series of results. Grade 1 gliomas are low attenuation lesions on CT, with neither vasogenic oedema nor contrast enhancement. Conversely glioblastomas have a ring enhancement which is thick and irregular in 85% of cases. These findings are corroborated by other studies and in day to day practice. Attempts using

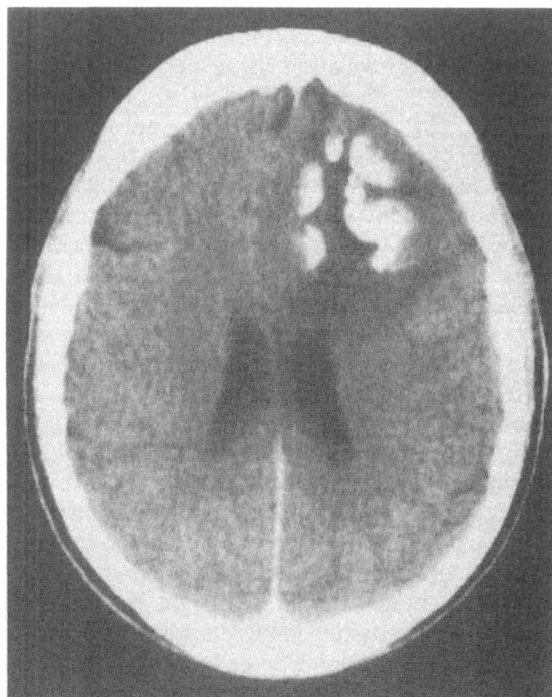

Fig. 2.4. Cranial CT. Oligodendroglioma showing prominent calcification.

both CT and MRI to distinguish intermediate grades of malignancy have been disappointing. Vonofakos et al. (1979) examining oligo-dendrogliomas showed that the development of cystic change was associated with progression to a higher, more aggressive grade. Levin et al. (1980) examined the prognosis with respect to shift, tumour size, oedema and degree of necrosis when an improved survival was noted with a small tumour and prominent oedema.

Differential Diagnosis of Gliomas

Virtually any pathological process in the brain especially where there is space occupancy and enhancement may be confused with a glioma. An abscess, a solitary metastasis and an area of infarction are common difficulties. The majority of infarcts and tumours present a typical appearance but there remains a small minority where the differentiation is difficult. They may be distinguished by their position, mass effect, enhancement pattern especially in relation to the clinical stage and their overall progress (see Chap. 1).

With primary intracranial haemorrhage, especially in the parietal lobe, the initial event may be clinically silent but the patient may present with epilepsy when the CT demonstration of an enhancing ring lesion can be a potential source of confusion (Clugston et al. 1988). The presence of a central high attenuation area with a thin peripheral enhancing ring is typical of a haematoma. Arteriovenous malformations with enlarged arteries and veins are unlikely to be confused. Cryptic vascular malformations, including cavernous haemangiomas which present with haemorrhage or cyst formation, may require follow-up scanning – particularly using MRI – for clarification.

Large multiple sclerosis plaques have irregular ring enhancement but the relative lack of oedema and mass effect in conjunction with the clinical findings are helpful diagnostic pointers (Reith et al. 1981).

Neurosarcoidosis usually presents with lepto-meningeal spread but high attenuation and enhancing focal intracranial masses with white matter oedema may be difficult to diagnose where pulmonary sarcoidosis is unsuspected (Kendall and Tatler 1978; Powers and Miller 1981). The MRI appearances are variable but it is a sensitive technique in detection of hypothalamic and peri-ventricular lesions though Hayes et al. (1987) failed to visualise two CT-positive cases probably due to the suppression of oedema by high doses of corticosteroids.

Exceptionally gliomas have an extra-axial origin from glial rests suggesting a more benign diagnosis (Shungshotti et al. 1984; Derrig et al. 1986) and the very rare diffuse leptomeningeal gliomatosis (Ho et al. 1981) is not visualised by CT or MRI in spite of extensive neurological symptoms and signs.

With status epilepticus there is occasionally a poorly defined area of low attenuation with faint peripheral enhancement (Rumack et al. 1980) which resolves with control of the focus although careful follow-up is required to ensure that this is not a tumour.

Ependymoma

Ependymomas are most frequently found in the posterior fossa, and then almost exclusively in childhood. In the supratentorial compartment they are usually intraparenchymal and adjacent to the trigone rather than being truly intraventricular. They have usually attained a considerable size at presentation with a variable degree of contrast enhancement and cyst formation (Armington et al. 1985) (Fig. 2.5). Ependymal spread may be rapid and extensive (Enzmann et al (1978b)).

Ependymoblastoma is a highly malignant form that grows with local infiltration and subarachnoid seeding.

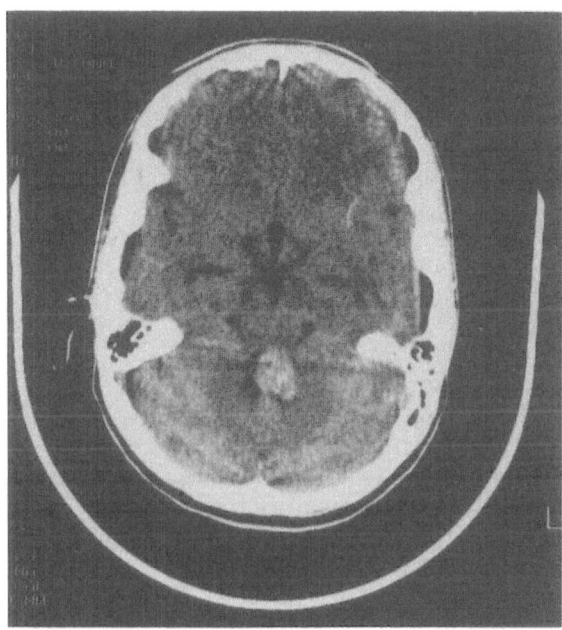

Fig. 2.5. Cranial CT. Ependymoma of the fourth ventricle.

Subependymoma is a variant of ependymoma which contains subependymal glial elements. They are most frequently found coincidentally at post mortem typically in the floor of the fourth ventricle but also in the lateral ventricle adjacent to the foramen of Monro and rarely at more distant sites. Symptomatic tumours are rare (Scheithaeur 1978; Vaquero et al. 1984) but a well-circumscribed mass (half of which are calcified) causing hydrocephalus is the usual appearance (Stevens et al. 1984). Up to 15% are more cellular tumours resembling true ependymomas and present in the first decade in the floor of the fourth ventricle (Scheithaeur 1978).

Lymphoma

Primary lymphoma is an uncommon tumour comprising less than 1% of primary central nervous system tumours though the incidence is rising due to the increase of immunocompromised patients, resulting both from organ transplantation and AIDS. The majority are large cell B-type lymphomas and only very rarely of the Hodgkins type (Ashby et al. 1988a, b). They may present with a solitary mass, typically in the frontal lobe – though no region is exempt including the corpus callosum. Multiple masses clustered around the ventricles may also be found (Enzmann et al. 1979; Paganii et al. 1981) (Fig. 2.6). The CT attenuation is slightly increased with marked homogeneous enhancement after contrast medium. Surrounding low attenu-

ation may be the typical pattern of oedema but non-enhancing tumour can be extensive. In spite of the often large size of the tumour central low attenuation areas are uncommon, only 9% in one series (Ashby et al. 1988b), which is surprising in view of the common occurrence of histological evidence of necrosis. These tumours are usually confused with high-grade gliomas when solitary though the high attentuation before contrast medium and the absence of necrosis is against this diagnosis. A peripherally situated tumour may mimic a meningioma – indeed on rare occasions they may arise from the dura (Ashby et al. 1988a). In the presence of multiple mass lesions and where there is typical periventricular clustering, especially with involvement of the corpus callosum, lymphoma can be diagnosed with some certainty. If corticosteroids have been administered following the incorrect assumption that the lesion is a glioma the tumour may disappear, albeit transiently (Vaquero et al. 1984). Secondary involvement of the central nervous system by lymphoma is usually meningeal (Fig. 2.7) or related to involvement from the calvarium.

It is anticipated that MRI will show increased signal intensity on T1 and T2 weighted image but there is limited experience with this rare group of tumours.

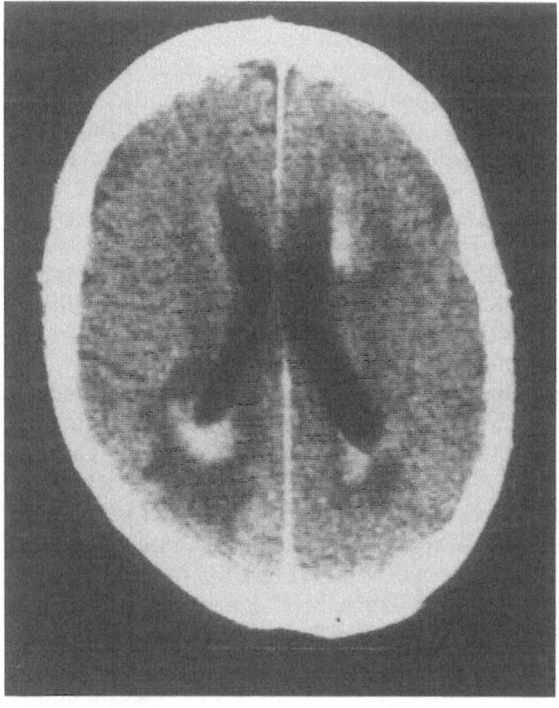

Fig. 2.6. Cranial CT after IV contrast. Lymphoma. The hyperdense periventricular lesions enhance uniformly.

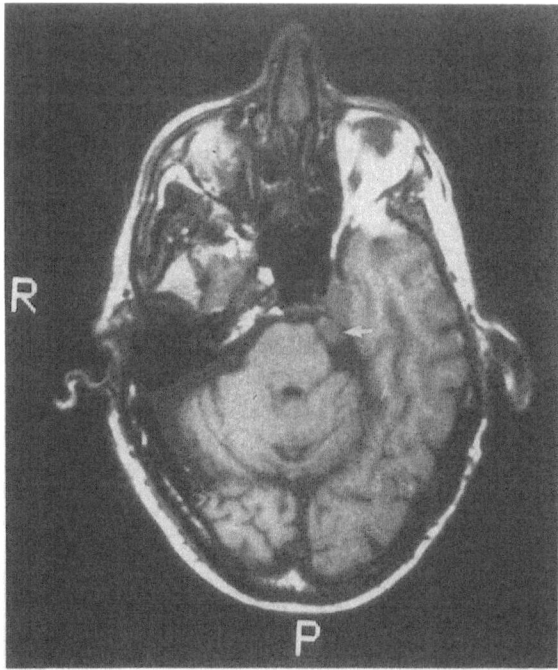

Fig. 2.7. Cranial MRI (T1 weighted image). Leptomeningeal deposit from lymphoma (*arrow*). The patient suffered trigeminal neuralgia.

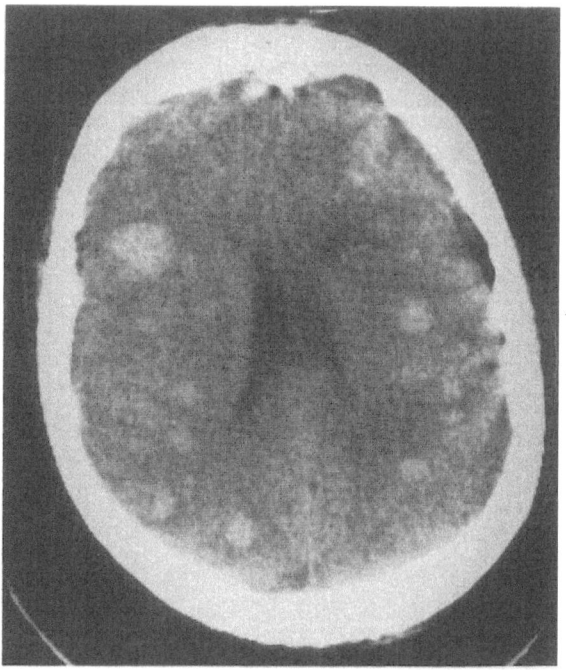

Fig. 2.8. Cranial CT. Multiple haemorrhagic leukaemic deposits.

Leukaemia

Leukaemic infiltration of the meninges is common though infrequently visualised on CT (meningeal enhancement with or without a communicating hydrocephalus) as cerebrospinal fluid analysis is the primary diagnostic procedure. Focal parenchymal masses are uncommon but when present they are iso- or hyperdense with a tendency to a periventricular site and a variable degree of enhancement (Kao et al. 1987). In myeloid leukaemia, focal intracranial masses – granulocytic sarcomas (or chloromas) – may occur when there is a large well-marginated mass with prominent enhancement. Granulocytic sarcomas are extra-axial in origin but may invade the parenchyma. When focal signs are present, haemorrhage is the usual cause which is commonly secondary to thrombocytopenia but multiple haemorrhagic leukaemic infiltrates can occur (Kelly et al. 1985) (Fig. 2.8).

As with lymphoma MRI experience in cerebral leukaemia is limited although there is a single case report of a chloroma which was iso-intense with adjacent brain (Kao et al. 1987). Gadolinium-enhanced MRI scanning appears promising in the diagnosis of meningeal disease.

Haemangioblastomas

These tumours most frequently present in the third and fourth decades associated with the Von Hippel–Lindau syndrome with sporadic cases occurring in later life (Horton et al. 1976). A cerebellar hemisphere is the almost invariable site (Fig. 2.9) although supratentorial lesions have been described (Miller et al. 1986).

The typical CT appearance is of a well-circumscribed low attenuation area, representing the cyst with a focal enhancement from the nodule, or nodules, which if small may not be visualised. Even if a vascular nodule is seen, angiography is helpful in detecting further small nodules (Fig. 2.10).

The symptomatic cysts are well demonstrated on MRI and in addition focal areas of high signal intensity on T2 weighted image may be seen separate from the main bulk of the mass. These are presumed to be additional lesions which are also seen in the supratentorial compartment though the significance of small high signal areas on T2 weighted image may only be clarified on long-term follow-up (Sato et al. 1988).

The appearance of a haemangioblastoma is usually typical especially in combination with angi-

its typical position and if there is a low attenuation area this will be small compared to the size of the mass as a whole.

Gangliocytomas

Gangliocytomas, which embrace gangliogliomas and ganglioneuromas, are uncommon tumours of childhood and young adults. They appear as low-grade gliomas, typically in the temporal, frontal and basal ganglial regions, with calcification, which may be marked, in 50% and little surrounding oedema (Nass and Whelan 1981).

A diffuse variant occurring in the cerebellum is gangliocytoma dysplasticum, or Lhermitte–Duclos syndrome, which is a mass with indeterminate margins with the affected side of the posterior fossa enlarged reflecting its origin in childhood or infancy. Pre-operative or even intra-operative diagnosis may prove difficult but a report by Wong et al. (1989) describes one case shown on MRI as a process primarily involving the cerebellar cortex.

Metastatic Disease

Metastases to the brain are the most common metastatic complication of systemic cancer and are present in up to 25% of patients who die of cancer of whom more than 75% have some neurological symptoms. These figures are higher than found in a neurosurgical unit with its selected population. A wide range of CT changes accompany metastatic disease reflecting the diverse histology, positions and rates of growth of the tumours (Pechora-Peterova and Kalvach 1986). Most metastases occur in the subcortical cerebrum especially in the middle cerebral artery distribution, with approximately 10% in the cerebellum. A typical lesion is about 1 cm in diameter, iso- or slightly hyperdense with respect to average brain, with a large amount of surrounding oedema – greater than that associated with a glioma. Contrast enhancement is the norm with a varying degree of central non-enhancement which is usually due to necrosis (Fig. 2.11).

The presence of multiple typical lesions in a patient with known cancer clearly poses no major diagnostic problems though multifocal glioma, primary lymphomas, infarcts, or infections may cause difficulties. The apparently separate components of a multifocal glioma may be shown to be connected especially via the corpus callosum. Lymphoma is infrequently necrotic and, when multiple, lesions tend to cluster around the third and lateral ventricles (Paganii et al. 1981; Kelly et al. 1985). Infarcts rarely have associated white matter oedema and a subcortical position would be very

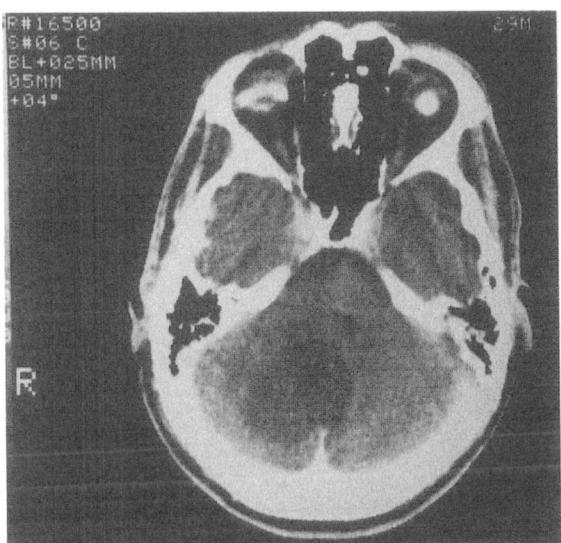

Fig. 2.9. Cranial CT after IV contrast. Cystic cerebellar haemangioblastoma. Note the ocular lesions in this patient with Von Hippel–Lindau disease.

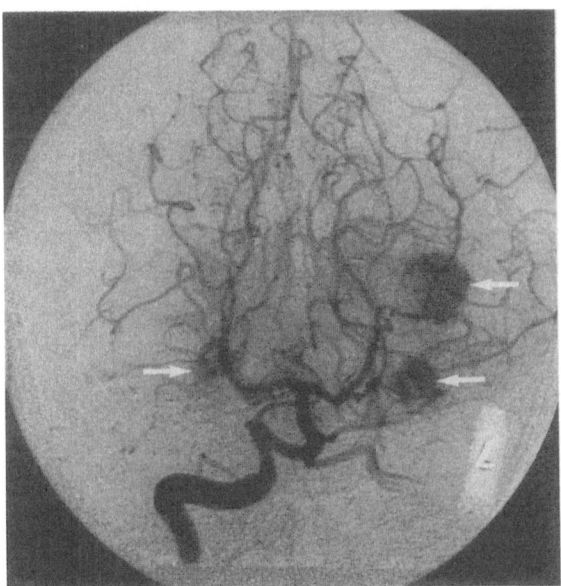

Fig. 2.10. Vertebral arterial DSA (frontal projection). Multiple cerebellar haemangioblastomata (*arrows*). (P.B.)

ography. Cystic pilocytic gliomas are uncommon in the age range of haemangioblastomas; the more anaplastic gliomas are infrequent occupants of the cerebellar hemispheres and a cystic appearance would be exceptional. A cystic secondary may be difficult to distinguish but an irregular margin and enhancement are usual. The rare adult medulloblastoma (Hughs 1984) can be distinguished by

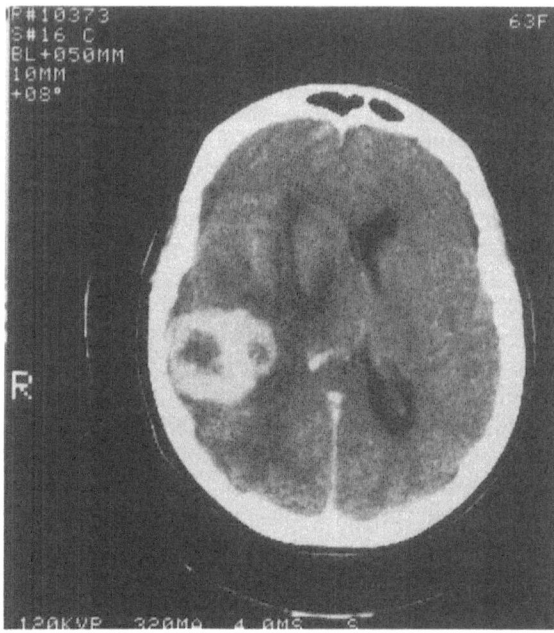

Fig. 2.11. Cranial CT after IV contrast. Necrotic metastasis from carcinoma of the breast (note similarity to Fig. 2.2).

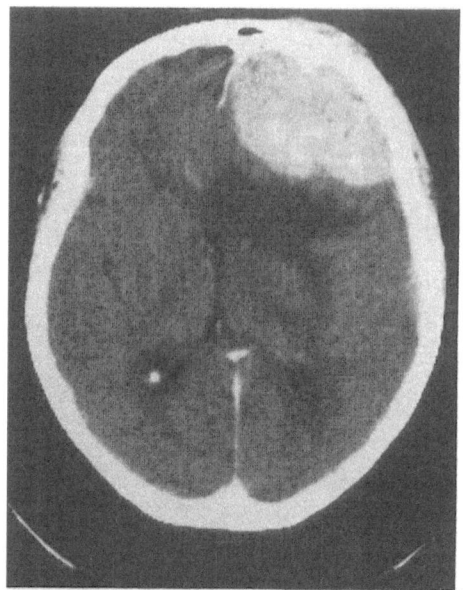

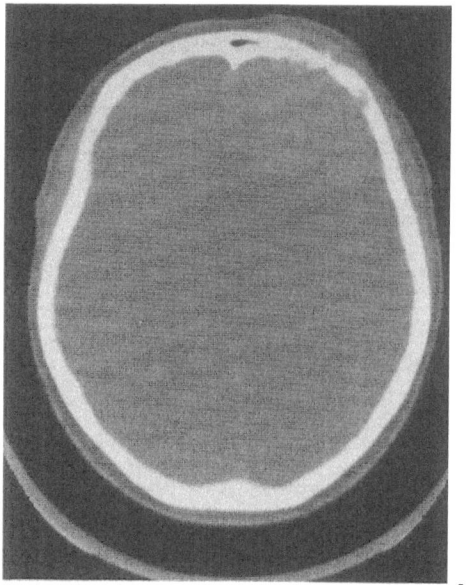

Fig. 2.12a and **b.** Cranial CT after IV contrast. Metastatic adenocarcinoma with calvarial involvement.

unusual (Masdeu 1983). Infections, especially when metastatic, occur in the middle cerebral artery distribution but oedema is generally more prominent with a greater neurological disability for a given size of lesion.

Atypical appearances of cerebral metastases include a single area of ring enhancement or generalised brain swelling but no discrete mass visualised due to multiple tiny tumour seedlings. Rarely, a metastasis adjacent to the dura will closely resemble a meningioma.

Sometimes the nature of the primary tumour can be hinted at, although no specific criteria exist. A large lesion with a very thin rim of enhancement and central low attenuation suggest a squamous cell origin. Calcification classically occurs with adenocarcinomas of gastrointestinal origin or very rarely from osteogenic sarcomas but breast and lung are the most usual causes on account of their frequency as primary tumours and propensity to metastasise to the central nervous system (Anand and Potts 1982). High attenuation lesions, especially those which contain haemorrhage, are typical of melanomas, hypernephromas and the rare chorioncarcinoma.

Cerebellar metastases frequently present before the primary tumour becomes apparent clinically and are usually single (Weisberg 1985) though this may reflect the insensitivity of CT in the posterior fossa. Primary tumours in the age group in which metastasis occurs are uncommon. Thus, a posterior fossa intra-axial lesion in the middle-aged or elderly patient is likely to be a metastasis especially in the vermis. Cranial nerve dysfunction is generally part of a more diffuse leptomeningeal spread. Secondary spread into the subdural space is most frequently due to extensive calvarial involvement (Fig. 2.12) but metastatic prostatic carcinoma may present de novo, presumably via the vertebral venous plexus (Castaldo et al. 1983).

Leptomeningeal Metastasis

Leptomeningeal metastasis is the widespread seeding of the leptomeninges by systemic cancer either by haematogenous spread or invasion from a pre-existing metastasis. Malignant cells disseminate throughout the subarachnoid spaces with especially heavy deposition in the basal cisterns, the Sylvian and hippocampal fissures (Fig. 2.13). Hydrocephalus, meningism and cranial nerve lesions may result. Leptomeningeal involvement occurs in 8%–10% of systemic cancers, especially the leukaemias, lymphoma (Fig. 2.7), breast and lung carcinomas (Erlich and Davis 1978; Wasserstrom et al. 1982). Germinomas, pinealomas, and medulloblastomas are also well known to seed throughout the CSF. In the rare meningeal gliomatosis (Bradley et al. 1984) CT remains normal.

CT in leptomeningeal metastasis may reveal communicating hydrocephalus, obliteration of the basal cisterns and enhancement of the cisterns, sulci, tentorium, ependyma or subependyma (Enzmann et al. 1978b; Lee et al. 1984). Focal peripheral nodules are occasionally seen. One or more of these signs were present in 22 of 75 in a series of patients studied sequentially (Ascherl et al. 1981) though no CT changes were diagnostic. Communicating

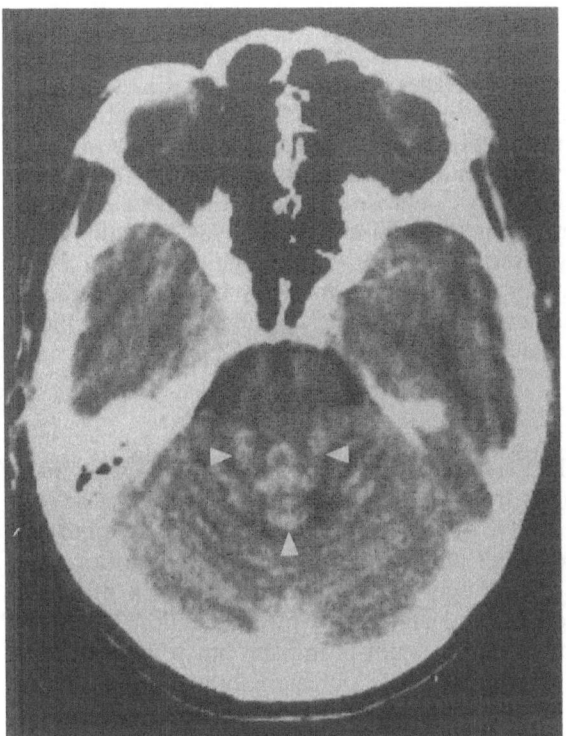

Fig. 2.13. Cranial CT after IV contrast. Leptomeningeal metastases (*arrowheads*) from carcinoma of the bronchus.

hydrocephalus is a non-specific sign but in a patient with systemic cancer or a known tumour abutting the ventricular or subarachnoid space should be considered to indicate leptomeningeal spread even in the absence of positive cytology. It has been emphasised that CSF abnormalities often post date CT changes (Jaeckle et al. 1985). Cisternal and tentorial enhancement may also be encountered in infectious meningitis especially TB and in sarcoidosis (see Chap. 5).

Incidental Vascular Disease

At autopsy about 15% of patients with systemic cancer have cerebrovascular disease though not all have symptoms or signs (Graus et al. 1985). However, with an increasingly aged population and prolonged survival, this possibility should be considered where the CT findings are atypical. Symptomatic infarction may also be due to non-bacterial thrombotic ("marasmic") endocarditis which is most often associated with the presence of an adenocarcinoma. Disseminated intravascular coagulation may cause venous infarctions which might be considered to be due to intratumoral haemorrhage (see Chap. 1). Occlusion of the venous sinuses is usually due to local invasion but may occur as a non-metastatic complication (Sigbee et al. 1979) or following treatment with L-asparaginase (Priest et al. 1980).

Magnetic Resonance Imaging in Metastatic Disease (Fig. 2.14)

The sensitivity of MRI often leads to the demonstration of multiple lesions when CT has shown only one (Claussen et al. 1985a, b; Healey et al. 1987; Russell et al. 1987). This may pose a number of problems:

1. The multifocal elements of a glioma are detected more frequently which may raise the possibility of metastasis.
2. High signal intensity lesions on T2 weighted image in the cerebrum are common in the aged patient.
3. The non-specific nature of the MR image does not aid advance diagnosis of the source.
4. In spite of the increased sensitivity of MRI without enhancement still further lesions are seen with gadolinium DTPA.

It might be argued that the increased sensitivity, with or without contrast agents, is not a problem, especially where the patient has a known cancer, but there is a tendency for aggressive surgeons to

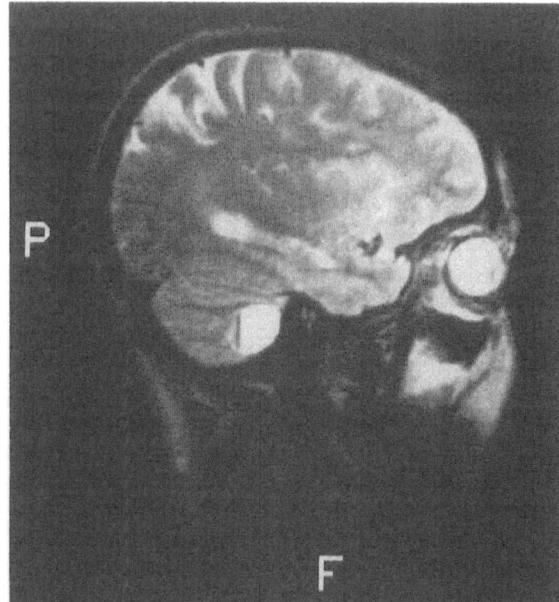

Fig. 2.14. Cranial MRI, sagittal section (T2 weighted image). Cystic cerebellar metastasis.

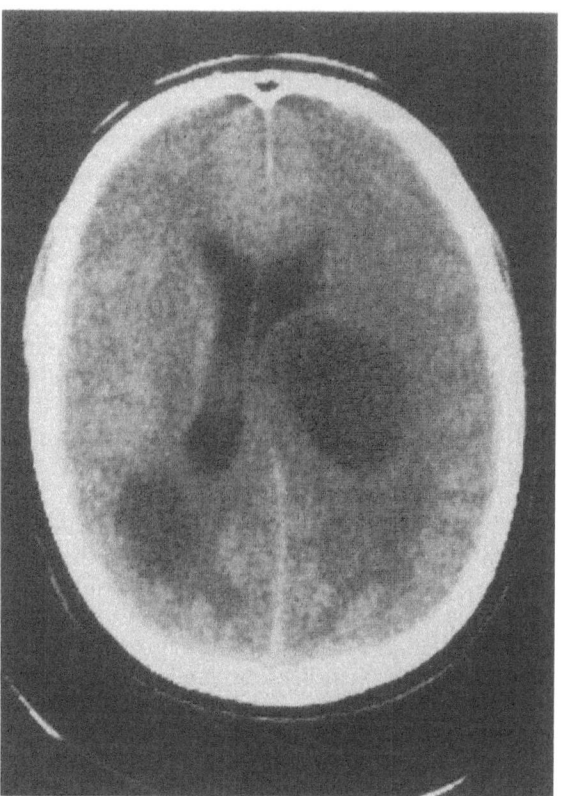

Fig. 2.15. Cranial CT. Neuroepithelial cysts.

remove one or several metastatic tumours. The apparent multiplicity of lesions might dissuade them from such an approach. Co-existing cerebro-vascular disease may prove difficult to distinguish. Sze et al. (1988) have suggested that punctate lesions in the centrum semi-ovale and basal ganglia should be considered as infarcts. It is interesting to note that MRI without gadolinium DTPA appears less sensitive than CT to leptomeningeal spread (Davis et al. 1987a).

Intraventricular Tumours

A wide range of tumours or tumorous conditions, for example astrocytoma, ependymoma medul-loblastoma, craniopharyngioma, dermoid, epi-dermoid, teratoma, arachnoid and ependymal cysts, may present within the ventricles (Morrison et al. 1984). The majority are discussed in their separate sections but neuroepithelial cyst and choroid plexus tumours will be considered here.

Neuroepithelial Cysts

Neuroepithelial cysts, i.e. cystic structures with fea-tures of primitive ependyma and/or choroid plexus with or without basement membrane, occur else-where in the brain, in both the supra- and infra-tentorial compartments (Fig. 2.15). The most common reported sites are adjacent to the third and

lateral ventricles (Borch et al. 1973; Czervionke et al. 1987; Numaguchi et al. 1987 where they are substantial well-circumscribed low density masses, without enhancement, with attenuation values similar to cerebrospinal fluid. Infratentorial sites are reported (Andrews et al. 1984), notably one example at the craniovertebral junction, extra-axial and of high attenuation without contrast medium enhancement – similar appearances to a typical colloid cyst (Romero et al. 1987).

Colloid Cyst

The most common form is the colloid cyst which arises from the roof of the third ventricle near the foramen of Monro. These are usually round or oval high attenuation lesions in which lobulation is exceedingly rare (Fig. 2.16). About a fifth are isodense and a few are of low attenuation. Contrast enhancement is not prominent but when it occurs is homogeneous or occasionally a ring pattern is seen. The septum pellucidum is generally thickened and the posterior aspect of the third ventricle is collapsed with a variable degree of dilatation of the lateral ventricles.

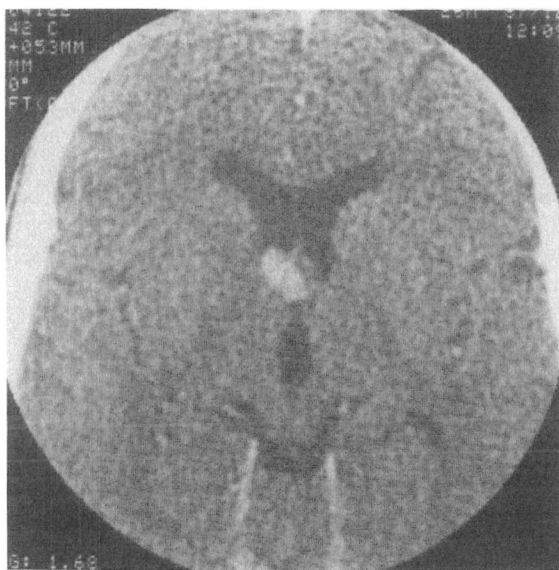

Fig. 2.16. Cranial CT. Colloid cyst of the third ventricle. The cyst has prolapsed through the foramen of Monro into the right lateral ventricle. (P.B.)

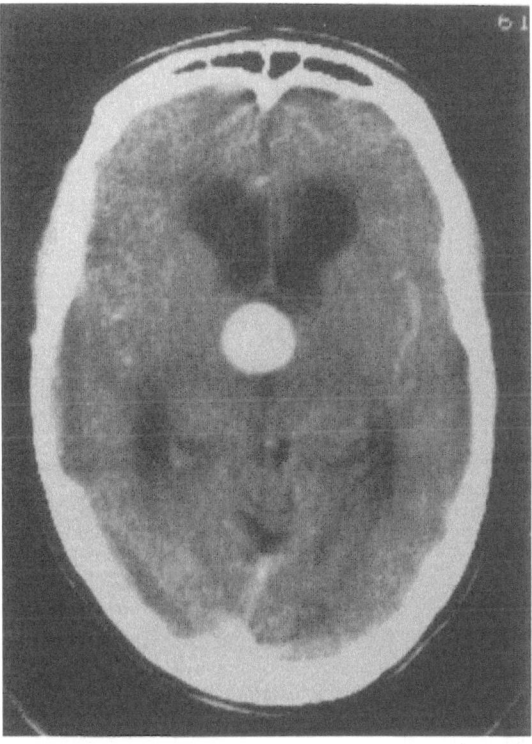

Fig. 2.17. Cranial CT after IV contrast. Ectatic basilar artery.

MRI demonstrates the position of a tumour at the foramen of Monro very clearly in axial, sagittal and coronal planes. Colloid cysts are well visualised with a high signal on T1 and T2 weighted image. Alternative diagnoses, such as the ectatic basilar artery, will be evident from the flow void and the communication between a pituitary tumour or craniopharyngioma can be clearly seen with sagittal or coronal imaging.

The appearances of a colloid cyst are generally typical but the differential diagnosis includes an ectatic basilar artery (Fig. 2.17), meningioma, choroid plexus papilloma, ependymoma, glioma (Fig. 2.18), craniopharyngioma, pituitary tumour and teratoma. A meningioma is a rare tumour in the third ventricle but occurs in childhood (Lee et al. 1979), when colloid cysts are rare.

The choroid plexus papilloma is lobular with marked enhancement. Ependymomas are rare occupants of the third ventricle and have an irregular contour. Gliomas are usually irregular with variable enhancement but smooth round, or oval varieties occur especially the giant cell glioma associated with tuberose sclerosis: tubers will be evident elsewhere. Pituitary tumours and craniopharyngiomas may extend superiorly to block the foramen of Monro but the slightly asymmetrical position and generally obvious connection with sellar/suprasellar region will not cause difficulties. A teratoma has typical heterogeneous attenuation and contains fat with foci of calcification.

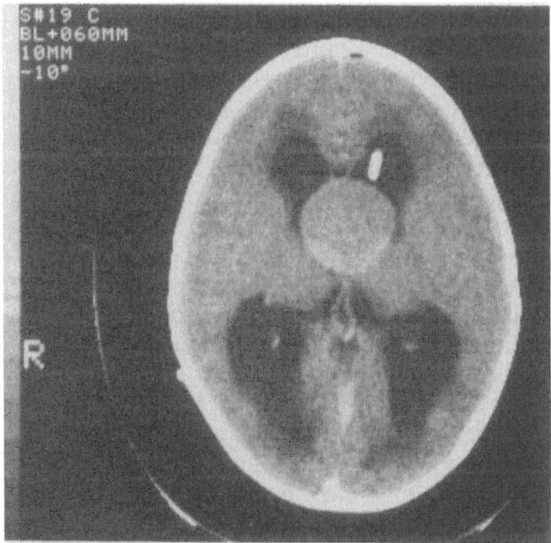

Fig. 2.18. Cranial CT after IV contrast. Intraventricular glioma.

Choroid Plexus Tumours

Choroid plexus tumours are uncommon and the histological spectrum includes papilloma, carcinoma, meningioma, metastasis and xanthogranuloma (Pearl 1984).

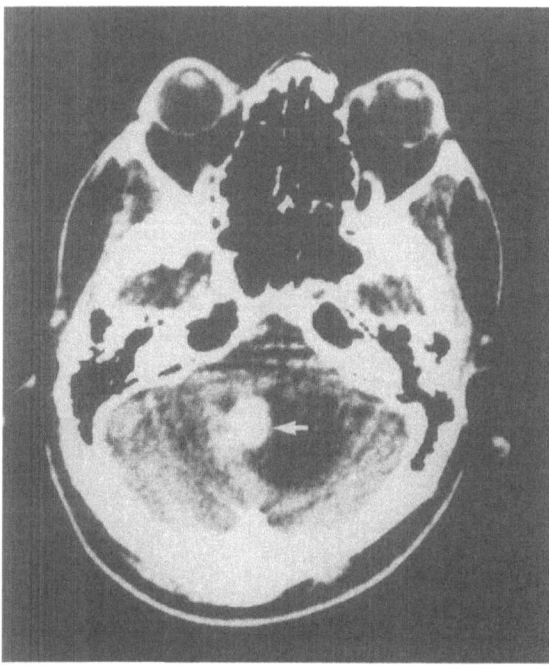

Fig. 2.19. Cranial CT after IV contrast. Choroid plexus papilloma. The tumour is seen within a dilated fourth ventricle (*arrow*).

Papillomas are most common in infancy within the lateral ventricle though when they occur in adults the fourth ventricle is the usual location (Fig. 2.19). They are generally of increased attenuation, displacing rather than engulfing the choroid, with patchy calcification and prominent enhancement after intravenous contrast. Hydrocephalus is a classic feature which may be due to an increased cerebrospinal fluid production though these tumours are fragile and hypervascular suggesting that the hydrocephalus may be communicating secondary to tumour debris, haemorrhage or a combination of both. If there is increased cerebrospinal fluid production this is secondary to the very large surface areas of these lobulated tumours.

Carcinoma, also frequent in children, is of increased attenuation with marked enhancement. Local invasion is an important distinguishing feature.

Meningiomas are the most common of the choroid plexus tumours and appear typically as hyperdense, perhaps calcified, lesions with uniform contrast enhancement. The most frequent intraventricular location is within the lateral ventricle.

Metastases are present in about 2% in autopsy series though few are seen ante mortem. Increased attenuation with enhancement and local invasion are usual CT features (Kart et al. 1986).

Xanthogranulomas are seen frequently on histological examination but are rarely of clinical relevance unless they are large and obstruct cerebrospinal pathways (Pearl 1984). They are low attenuation and non-enhancing masses.

Haemangiomas and arteriovenous malformations which also occur in the choroid plexus should be included in the differential diagnosis of a choroid plexus mass especially where there is haemorrhage. They may be bilateral and are associated with Sturge Weber and Wyburn Mason syndromes.

Magnetic resonance imaging has not been extensively reported in these rare tumours but the use of multiplanar imaging would be expected to aid in their localisation.

Extra-axial Tumours

Meningioma

The typical CT appearances, regardless of the site, are of a well circumscribed, high attenuation, enhancing mass with hyperostosis of the adjacent skull vault. The associated oedema is variable but may be far greater than the size of the primary lesions. Those lesions which are vascular, have a large surface area, and are situated in the anterior parasagittal region with dural sinus involvement tend to have prominent oedema (Stevens et al. 1983) though the mechanism remains obscure. If calcification is present transitional (especially if the calcification is homogeneous) or fibroblastic types are likely. Low attenuation areas or irregular margins suggest angioblastic or syncytial forms (Vassilouthis and Ambrose 1979).

The majority of meningiomas are easy to diagnose with typical features regardless of their position (Fig. 2.20). In a series of 130, 9 were incorrectly diagnosed (Russell et al. 1980) due to a variety of causes:

1. Adjacent focal low attenuation from oedema or a subarachnoid cyst far greater in size than the meningioma.

2. The true hypodense meningioma.

3. Focal non-enhancing low attenuation areas within the mass due to myxomatous degeneration, xanthomatous change, necrosis, old haemorrhage, true cyst formation and exceptionally a secondary within the tumour. (There is an increased incidence of meningiomas with carcinoma of the female breast (Shoenberg et al. 1975.)

4. Focal areas of increased attenuation due to haemorrhage which may be in the adjacent sub-

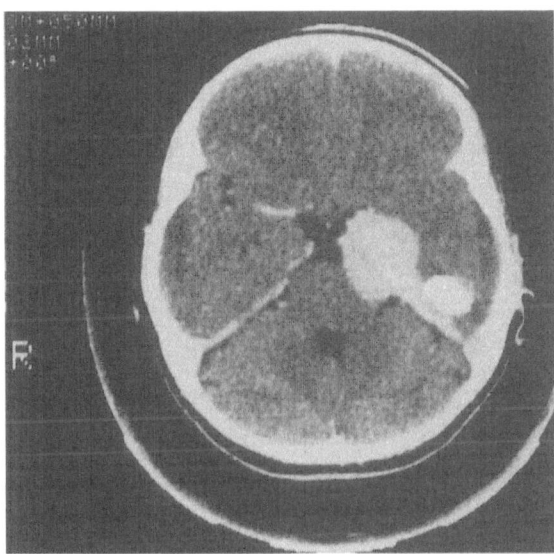

Fig. 2.20. Cranial CT after IV contrast. Meningioma.

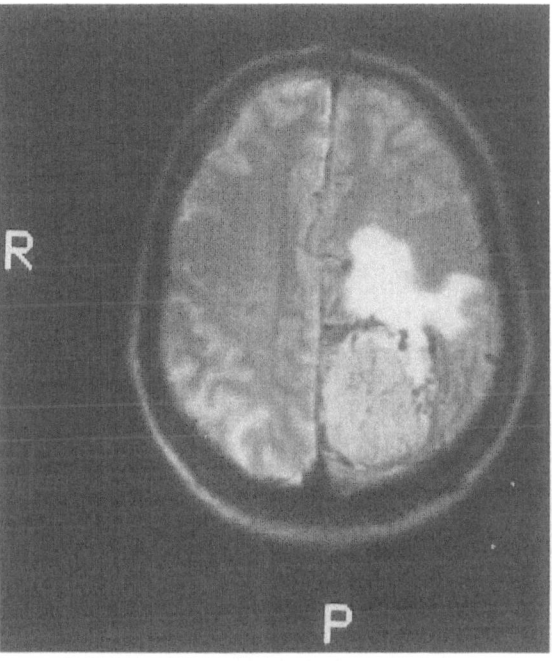

Fig. 2.21. Cranial MRI (T2 weighted image). Meningioma. Note the high signal oedema anterior to the tumour.

arachnoid or subdural space, intra- or peri-tumoral. Intraventricular tumours are the most likely to bleed (Helle and Conley 1980).

Purely cystic meningiomas presenting as areas of ring enhancement are difficult to diagnose partly due to their infrequency but also because the signs of an extra-axial mass are absent.

Malignant change in a meningioma is suggested on CT by a lobulated poorly defined margin, heterogeneous attenuation and enhancement with bony destructive changes and, rarely, a draining vein (Dieterman et al. 1982; New et al. 1982; Shadir et al. 1985).

Lymphoma, metastasis, extramedullary haematopoiesis, plasmacytoma and glioma should be included in the differential diagnosis of a meningioma.

CT is a highly effective imaging technique for the diagnosis of meningiomas and is unquestionably the superior technique for the demonstration of calcification and hyperostosis. MRI demonstrates the majority of meningiomas partly due to their size and in particular their extra-axial origin especially with multiplanar imaging around the tentorium and high vertex (Fig. 2.21). Meningiomas usually fail to exhibit major alterations in T1 or T2 relaxation times (Mackay et al. 1985; Spangoli et al. 1986) so that a small lesion may be overlooked. If the small meningioma is calcified MRI will probably fail to detect it unless there is a prominent signal void. However, in spite of the bulk of the tumour not having major change in relaxation parameters there is often a thin peripheral margin of low attenuation

(Zimmerman et al. 1985) which probably represents a CSF cleft. Haemorrhage within the tumour is detected far more frequently than on CT and there is marked enhancement with gadolinium DTPA which may be more dramatic than with CT enhancement (Bydder et al. 1985).

Pituitary Tumours

Pituitary tumours are conventionally divided into micro- and macroadenomas. Hardy (1973) suggested that a microadenoma is a "well localised nodule embedded in the pituitary parenchyma varying in size from 3 to 10 mm". A tumour with a 3 mm diameter has a volume of $14\,mm^3$ and one with a 10 mm diameter has a volume of $523\,mm^3$ which is approximately that of a normal pituitary gland! This distinction is not supported by clinical data and would seem to be artificial. Small tumours are not uncommon; 27% in one autopsy series (Burrows et al. 1981). Swartz et al. (1983), in a CT study of the pituitary gland in women of child-bearing age, found focal defects of varying size in 36% and Chambers et al. (1982) found 10 well-defined low attenuation areas greater than 3 mm in a series of 50 patients scanned for orbital disease.

A small pituitary tumour may be manifest on CT as a region of focal high or low density within the gland (Fig. 2.22). There may also be "indirect" signs which include a convex upper border to the gland,

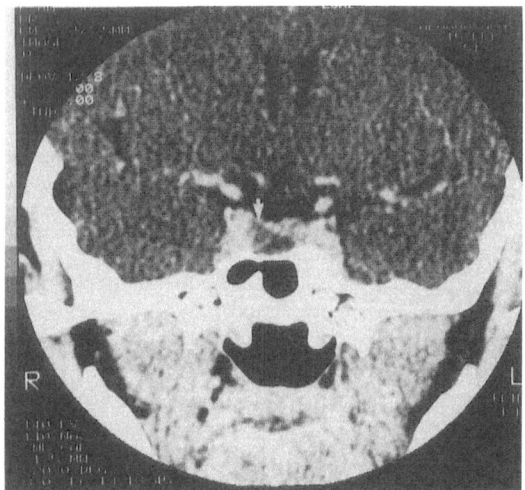

Fig. 2.22. Coronal CT after IV contrast. Prolactinoma (*arrow*). (P.B.)

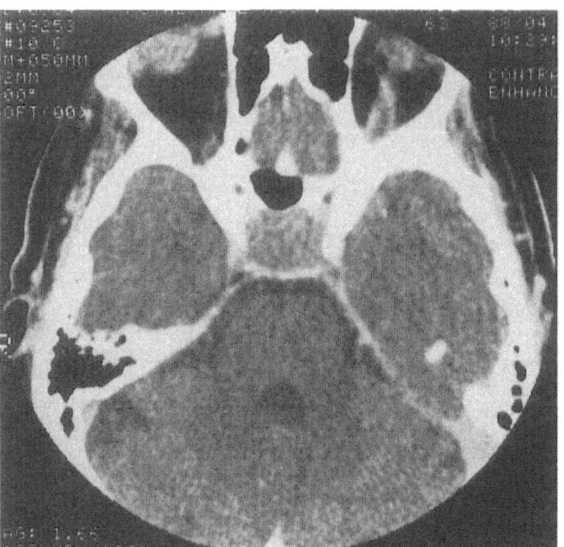

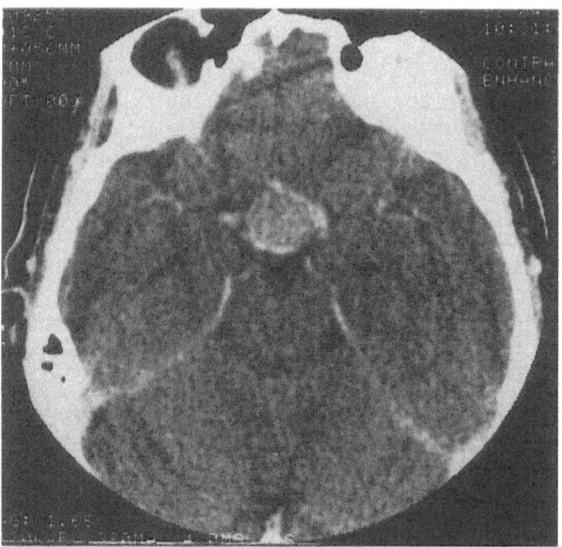

Fig. 2.23. Cranial CT after IV contrast. Pituitary adenoma. The pituitary fossa is occupied by a uniformly enhancing mass (**a**) which extends into the suprasellar cistern (**b**). (P.B.)

displacement of the infundibulum away from the tumour and focal thinning of the sellar floor.

It is important to realise that all of these signs have a considerable margin of error and that a normal scan does not exclude a tumour. In a study by Teasdale et al. (1986), of 34 patients who underwent high resolution CT and trans-sphenoidal hypophysectomy, 28 had abnormal pituitary glands but only 20 contained tumours. In nine patients with tumours no abnormality was seen on CT and a good correlation between the CT and the operative findings was present only when the tumour was greater than 6 mm in diameter. Apart from stalk deviation the indirect signs were unhelpful.

The very small ACTH-secreting tumour is a particular problem where petrosal sinus venous sampling may be valuable in the presence of normal CT (Doppman et al. 1984).

Substantial pituitary tumours do not present any great difficulty in their detection or in establishing their relationship to adjacent structures (Fig. 2.23). Lateral extension may be difficult to determine on CT though tumour generally enhances less than adjacent cavernous sinus or carotid artery (Ahmadi et al. 1985). The role of angiography has declined with high resolution CT but it may be required to assess the degree of lateral extension, to exclude an aneurysm and to assess the position of the carotid arteries prior to surgery if MRI is not available.

The majority of tumours of the pituitary arise from the anterior lobe cell series and occasionally glioma, pituicytoma and choristoma from the adenohypophysis occur but there are no specific CT features to suggest these diagnoses pre-operatively.

Metastases in the pituitary are not uncommon at autopsy usually associated with widespread disease typically from the female breast. They are infrequently symptomatic but diabetes insipidus is the most common presentation (71%) (Max et al. 1981).

Occasionally there may be diffuse enlargement of the gland from endocrine failure, typically hypothyroidism (Bilaniuk et al. 1985). Very rarely an enhancing mass in the pituitary may present in pregnancy or in the postpartum period – lymphocytic hypophysitis (Asa et al. 1981; Quencer 1980).

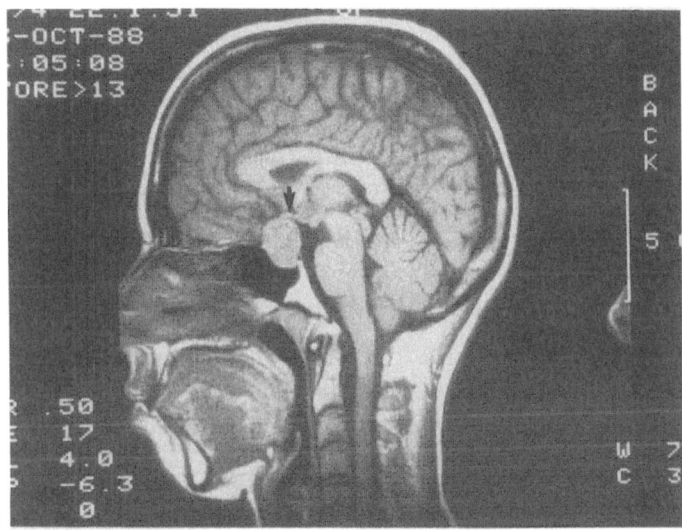

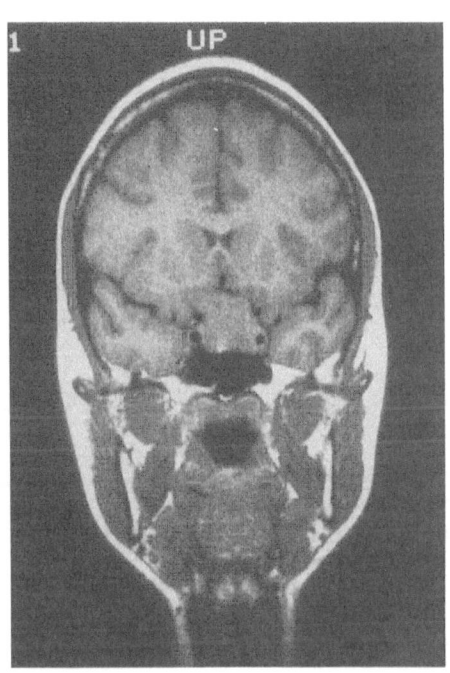

Fig. 2.24. Cranial MRI (T1 weighted image). Pituitary adenoma, sagittal (**a**) and coronal (**b**) views. Note the position of the optic chiasm (*arrow*) (P.B.)

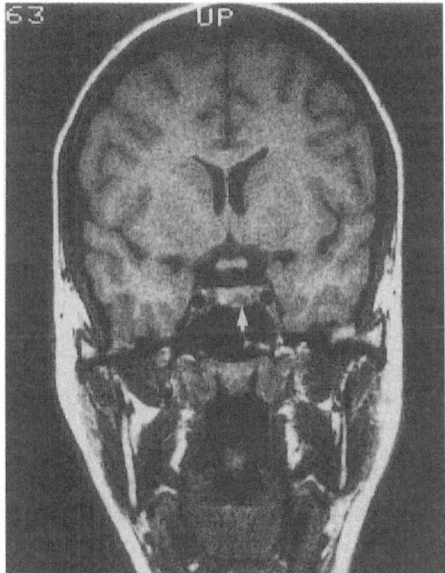

Fig. 2.25. Cranial MRI (T1 weighted image). Microadenoma (*arrow*). Note the clear delineation of the optic chiasm in this coronal image. (By courtesy of P. Kennedy.)

Magnetic Resonance Imaging and the Pituitary

MRI and high resolution CT have been shown to be of equal value in the examination of large pituitary tumours (Sartor et al. 1987) (Fig. 2.24). MRI also has the advantage of multiplanar imaging without the need for contrast agents and not only demonstrates the tumour but also the carotid arteries due to the signal flow void. Angiography may no longer be required when MRI is available.

The use of higher field strengths which allow greater definition have enabled a more detailed examination of the pituitary gland (Kucharczyk et al. 1987). It is now possible to image focal areas of abnormal signal intensity within the gland (Fig. 2.25), infundibular deviation and the superior margin of a normal-sized gland although the problems of specificity remain as with CT (Pojunas et al 1986; Davis et al. 1987b; Kulkarni et al. 1988). The empty sella is well shown (Fig. 2.26), the diagnosis of which depends on the pituitary stalk being identifiable as far as the base of the sella.

At high field strength the anterior lobe can be distinguished from the higher signal in the posterior lobe (Fujisawa et al. 1987a). Diabetes insipidus from any cause will reduce the signal from the posterior lobe so that it becomes iso-intense with the anterior lobe. Occasionally in diabetes insipidus "infundibulomas" with increased signal intensity develop in the stalk which should not be mistaken for primary tumours (Fujisawa et al. 1987b).

The role of gadolinium DTPA in pituitary tumours remains to be established but Dwyer et al. (1987) using delayed MRI scanning, demonstrated cystic ACTH-secreting microadenomas with good surgical correlation. Nakamura et al. (1988) found gadolinium DTPA particularly valuable in assessing cavernous sinus involvement by tumour in a study of 44 patients with macroadenomas.

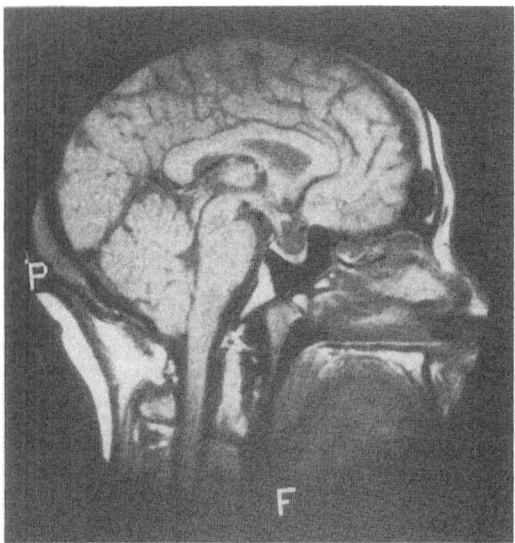

Fig. 2.26. Cranial MRI (T1 weighted image). Empty sella.

Craniopharyngiomas

The low attenuation, partially calcified sellar and suprasellar mass showing peripheral ring enhancement is the typical CT appearance of craniopharyngioma especially in a child or adolescent. Sometimes lesions are iso- or even hyperdense (Braun et al. 1982). Calcification is frequent in the young but is less common when the tumour presents in later years when there is also a tendency for craniopharyngiomas to occur in the posterior aspect of the third ventricle.

Magnetic resonance is effective in imaging these tumours although the difficulty in detecting anything other than large amounts of calcification is a relative disadvantage. There is increased signal intensity on the T2 weighted image reflecting the generally cystic nature of these tumours and a range of signal intensities may be encountered on T1 weighted image (Pusey et al. 1987; Freeman et al. 1987) (Fig. 2.27).

Rathke Cleft Cysts

Rathke cleft cysts, remnants of Rathke's pouch, are usually found between anterior and posterior lobes of the pituitary and occasionally in a suprasellar location. On CT there is a well-circumscribed area of low attenuation perhaps with peripheral enhancement (Okamata et al. 1985). The few cases studied by MRI have a heterogeneous signal intensity (Kucharczyk et al. 1987). Cysts may appear hyperintense on T1 weighted images and isointense on T2 weighted images reflecting their mucopolysaccharide content (Nemoto et al. 1988).

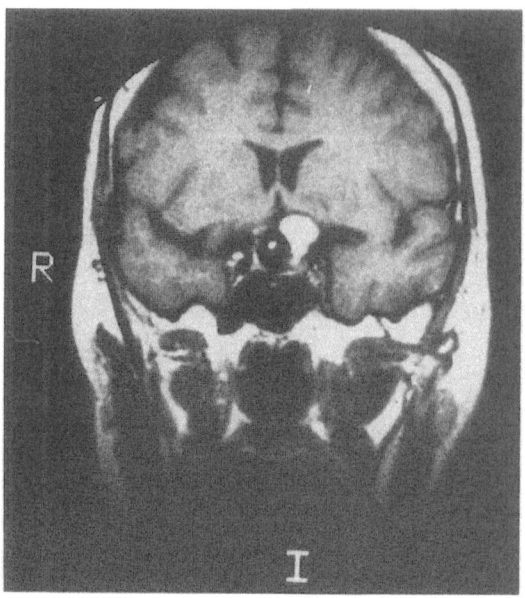

Fig. 2.27. Cranial MRI (T1 weighted image). Craniopharyngioma. High signal fat or haemorrhage is seen to the left of a signal void resulting from calcification.

Hypothalamic Tumours

Primary tumours such as gliomas and hamartomas are uncommon and the hypothalamus is more frequently involved as a part of a more diffuse process. Germinomas, metastases (Fig. 2.28), sarcoidosis, lymphoma, histiocytosis and tuberculomas may be encountered.

Microscopic hamartomatous malformations are frequent because of the complex embryological development of the hypothalamus (Sherwin et al. 1962) but tumours arising from the tuber cinereum which cause precocious puberty are rare. CT demonstrates an isodense mass without prominent enhancement. Calcification is said to be a major feature but this was not prominent in two large series (Diebler and Ponsot 1983; Hibi and Fujiwara 1987). MRI may find an important role here since Hibi and Fujiwara found three hamartomas, as shown by focal high signal intensity, with large cysts which previously had been considered to be arachnoid in origin.

Pineal Tumours

This group of tumours includes germinomas, teratomas, gliomas, pineocytomas, pineoblastomas and meningiomas. They are diagnosed on CT by their attenuation characteristics pre- and post-contrast medium administration and by the type of calcification, if any (Ganti et al. 1986).

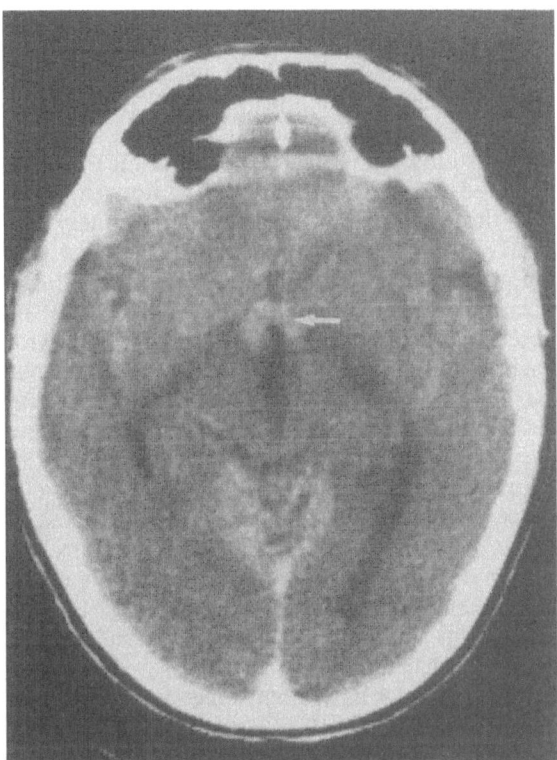

Fig. 2.28. Cranial CT after IV contrast. Hypothalamic secondary deposit (*arrow*).

Germinomas (the most common) are typically high attenuation lesions before contrast showing uniform enhancement and contain a variable amount of calcification. Synchronous or asynchronous development of a second lesion in the hypothalamus and suprasellar region is frequent. Rarely tuberculosis, metastases or sarcoidosis may give a similar pattern of a mass in the pineal and hypothalamus (Waal et al. 1985).

Teratomas have heterogeneous attenuation with little or no enhancement but marked calcification so that the normal pineal calcification is engulfed. *Gliomas* are hypo- or isodense with nodular or ring enhancement and the normal pineal calcification is displaced anteriorly and superiorly.

Pineocytomas are iso- or hyperdense with nodular enhancement but no accompanying alteration in the distribution of pineal calcification.

Pineoblastomas (Fig. 2.29) and *meningiomas* are similar with increased attenuation and marked homogeneous enhancement following intravenous contrast medium. The pineoblastoma may be associated with retinoblastoma(s) (Border 1980; Ehlers et al. 1983) and are rarely familial (Peyster et al. 1986).

These changes are the classic alterations but there is considerable overlap between histological types of pineal region tumours.

MRI is effective in demonstrating the pineal region and its tumours. There is the advantage of multiplanar imaging especially in the sagittal plane. Small areas of calcification will not be detected though the larger areas can be inferred by areas of signal void. One report (Kilgore et al. 1986) noted that MRI failed to detect a germinoma that was in a normal size gland and homogeneously calcified. In general these tumours give a signal similar to grey matter but there is good contrast from the adjacent posterior aspect of the third ventricle, CSF in the Galenic cistern and flow effects in the vein of Galen. Astrocytomas as elsewhere tend to have increased signal on T2 weighted image.

Pineal cysts are infrequent, occurring in 4%–5% of an unselected population (Mamourian and Towfight 1986; Lee et al. 1987). They are easily recognised by appearing larger than the usual pineal and having a cystic appearance with long T1 and T2 (Fig. 2.30). They are of no known significance and some degree of cystic change was seen in 40% of cases in an autopsy series (Tapp and Huxley 1972). Arachnoid cysts and cysticerci give similar appearances though arachnoid cysts are generally larger and with cysticercosis there is usually a multiplicity of lesions.

Small lipomatous deposits occasionally occur in the pineal region but are characterised by the typical

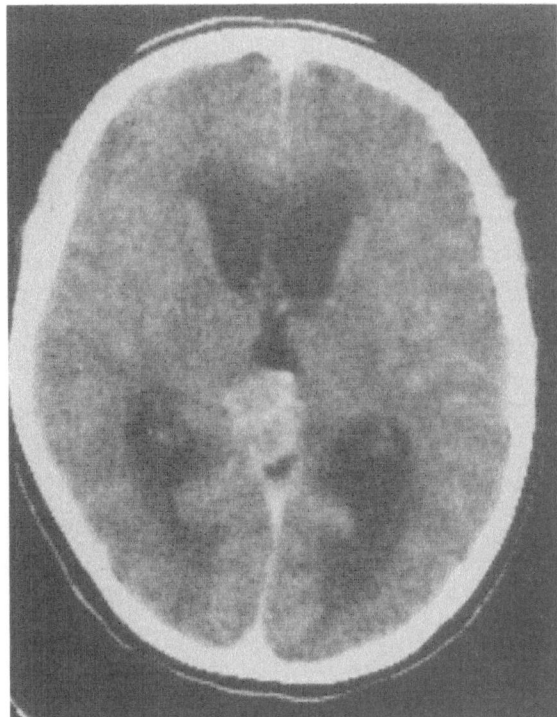

Fig. 2.29. Cranial CT after IV contrast. Pineoblastoma.

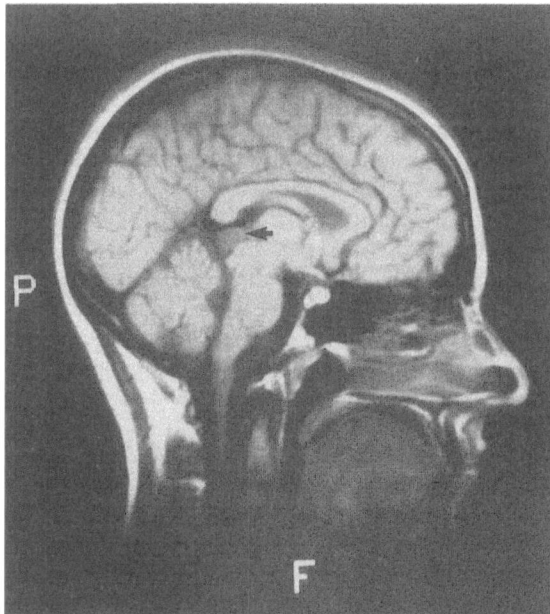

Fig. 2.30. Cranial MRI, sagittal section (T1 weighted image). Pineal cyst (*arrow*).

appearances of fat with high signal on T2 and T1 weighted image. Larger fat deposits in an enlarged pineal would suggest a teratoma.

Epidermoid, Dermoid and Lipoma

These tumours arise from the inclusion of epidermal tissue in the case of epidermoids with dermoids containing elements of ectoderm, mesoderm and endoderm.

Epidermoids are most common in the posterior fossa, especially within the cerebellopontine angle (Latack et al. 1985) (Fig. 2.31). Occasionally these tumours present as supratentorial hemispheric masses which usually arise in the Sylvian fissure or basal cisterns. A typical CT appearance is of a lobulated mass of low attenuation without enhancement though this may occur at the periphery secondary to local reactive changes rather than the tumour per se. A small amount of marginal calcification, either curvilinear or nodular, may be present. These tumours may be confused with arachnoid cysts where there is a smooth contour and homogeneous low attenuation corresponding to CSF or with a low-grade glioma where there is calcification. Although they are extra-axial in nature, this may be difficult to appreciate since epidermoids tend to invaginate into brain substance.

Dermoids are midline tumours found mainly in the posterior fossa. The combination of a very low attenuation mass of fat density and a variable degree of calcification are virtually diagnostic. Rarely they may have homogeneous high attenuation (Braun et al. 1977) or leak into the subarachnoid or ventricular system to cause an intense meningitis or ventriculitis (Fig. 2.32) which may

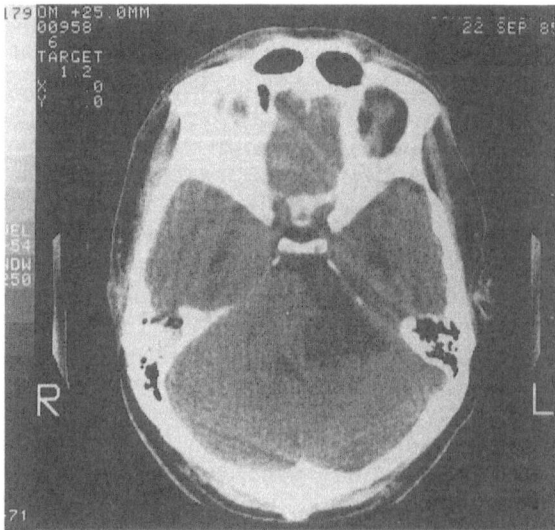

Fig. 2.31. Cranial CT. Cerebellopontine angle epidermoid. (P.B.)

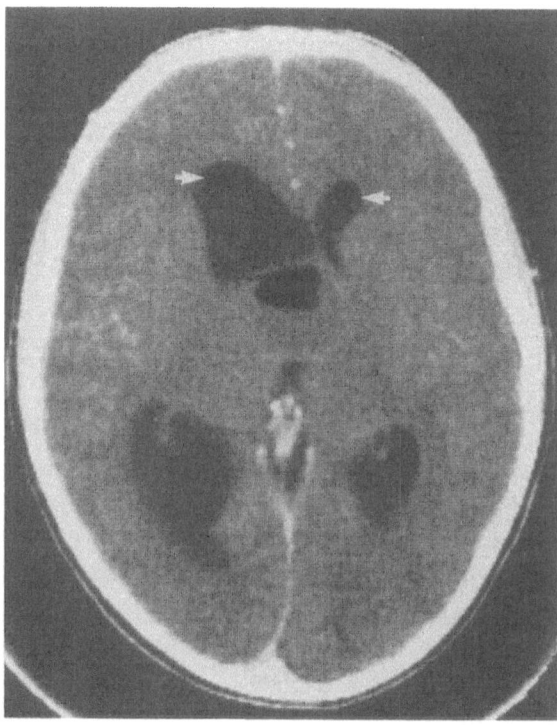

Fig. 2.32. Cranial CT after IV contrast. Suprasellar dermoid tumour with layering intraventricular fat (*arrows*).

cause hydrocephalus per se or exacerbate ventriculomegaly already present from mass effect.
This possibility should be considered in the differential diagnosis of recurrent sterile meningitis.

A lipoma as a symptomatic mass is uncommon
and small deposits of fat are now increasingly recognised in the region of the pineal, quadrigeminal
plate, suprasellar and cerebellopontine angle cisterns.

MRI demonstrates these tumours well with high
signal on T1WI and T2WI due to the fat content.
On CT the full extent of epidermoids may be difficult to assess when they are of a similar attenuation
to cerebrospinal fluid but it is most unlikely that
this is the case with MRI (Kortman et al. 1985).
There are also the general advantages of using MRI
in the posterior fossa (Latack et al. 1985), basal
cisterns and suprasellar region.

Neurinomas

The majority of these tumours arise from the VIIth
and VIIIth cranial nerves (see Chap. 9), but the
trigeminal nerve may be involved and rarely the
other cranial nerves.

Trigeminal neurinomas may be pre- or postganglionic in origin or arise within Meckel's cave
accounting for the variety of CT appearances. They
may be confined to the posterior or middle cranial
fossae and frequently straddle the petrous apex
which shows local erosion. They, like the more
familiar neurinomas, are isodense enhancing

masses on CT with MRI features of increased signal
intensity on T2 weighted image and iso- or
decreased signal intensity on T1 weighted image
(Gentry et al. 1987; Yuh et al. 1988). The demonstration of very low attenuation with CT or with
MRI, the signal intensities of fat, may represent
fatty degeneration but these findings are more likely
to represent a trigeminal lipoma (Yuh et al. 1987)
(Fig. 2.33).

Chordomas and Cartilage Tumours

Chordomas, rare tumours of the skull base, are
most frequently found near the spheno-occipital
synchondrosis but occasionally they present as a
sellar, foramen magnum, or nasopharyngeal mass.
They also occur in the sacral region. Bone destruction is common but sclerosis is present in about
5%. The substantial mass frequently contains calcification or ossification and exhibits a variable
degree of patchy contrast enhancement with CT
(Banna et al. 1980). With MRI the high signal of
the normal marrow cavity of the clivus is replaced
by tumour which is clearly separated from adjacent
bone (Fig. 2.34). Calcification will be evident as
signal voids. Sagittal and coronal images are valuable in assessing local extension (Han et al. 1984).

Cartilage tumours, chondromas and chondrosarcomas, also most frequently arise from the
sphenoid bone with the cerebellopontine angle the
next most commonly involved site. Exceptionally
the calvarium may be involved (Berkmann and
Blatt 1968). Calcification and bone erosions are
common.

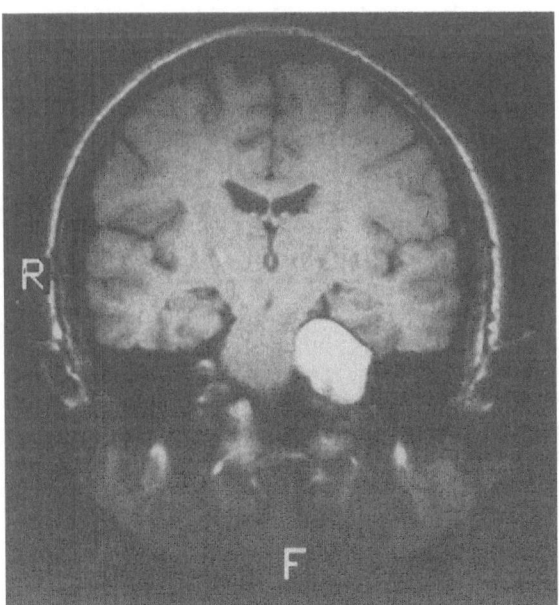

Fig. 2.33. Cranial MRI (T1 weighted image). Coronal section: trigeminal lipoma.

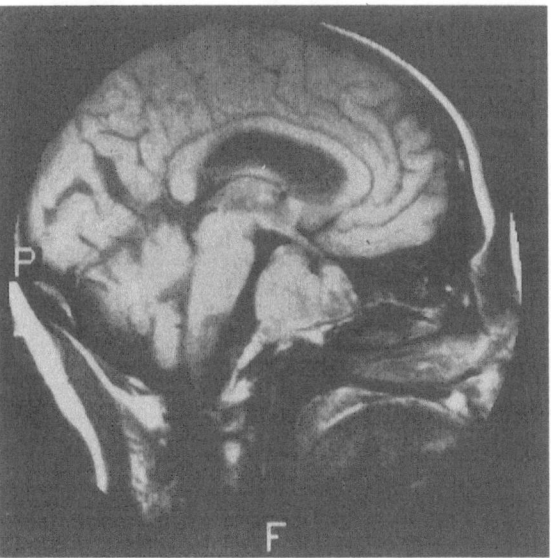

Fig. 2.34. Cranial MRI (T1 weighted image). Chordoma of the clivus.

There is, therefore, considerable similarity between chordomas and cartilaginous tumours. Hefelfinger et al. (1973) in a large series noted that, historically, chordomas had been considered to be chondromas or chondrosarcomas and that there was a subgroup in which, whilst unequivocal evidence of chordomatous tissue was present, there was also a substantial cartilaginous component, chondroid chordomas. This group pursued a slowly progressive course in comparison to the typical aggressive chordoma. There is therefore a spectrum from the true chordoma through chondroid chordoma to chondroma.

Effects of Radiation Therapy

Gliomas and other primary tumours of the brain are managed by a combination of surgery, radiotherapy and chemotherapy. Neuronal damage caused by radiotherapy may be exacerbated by the additional use of radiosensitisers and chemotherapy. Radiation damage may result in both early and late effects. The early changes at between one week and three months are due to glial cell damage with consequent vasogenic oedema. These self-limiting changes are effectively controlled by steroids and may be visualised on CT as increasing

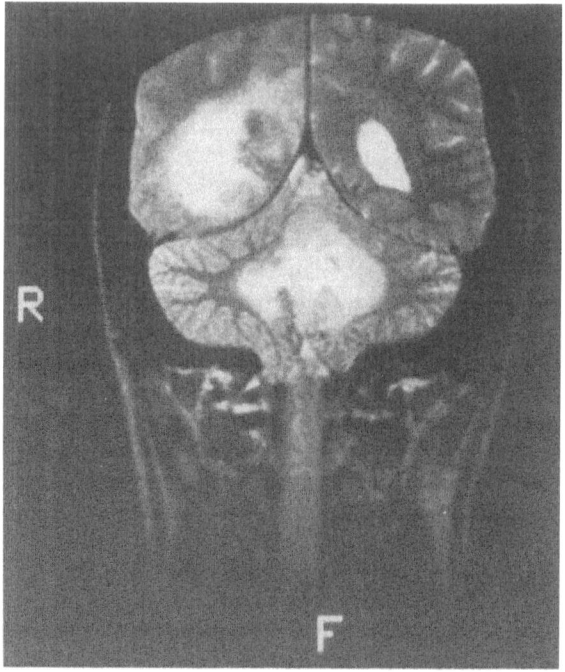

Fig. 2.36. Cranial MRI (T2 weighted image). Frontal glioma with cerebellar white matter demyelination due to irradiation.

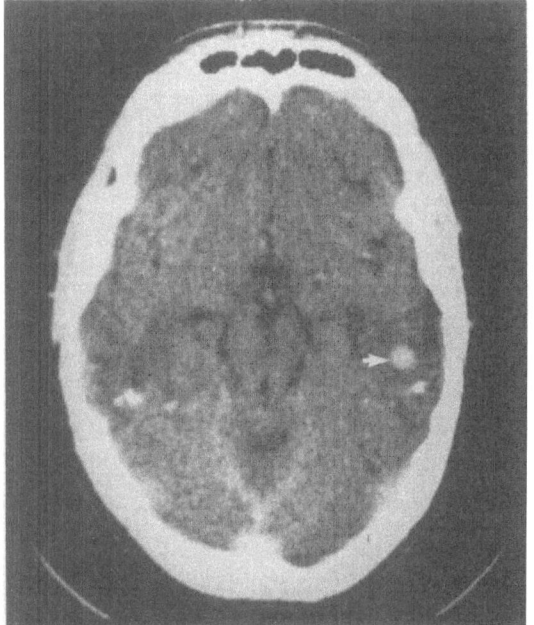

Fig. 2.35. Cranial CT after IV contrast. Radiation necrosis. The effects of cross field irradiation with bilateral low-density regions, calcification and a focus of enhancement (*arrow*).

degrees of contrast enhancement and adjacent low attenuation. The delayed effects, manifest from several months to several years after treatment, present a diagnostic challenge as the clinical signs closely resemble those of tumour recurrence. The mechanism is uncertain but may well be due to a vasculopathy which may be evident with angiography.

CT demonstrates an area of low attenuation, associated white matter oedema and a variable degree of mass effect. Contrast enhancement is invariable even if the tumour was initially non-enhancing. These are changes that are indistinguishable from tumour recurrence. However, Mikhael (1979) suggested that if the isodose curves are plotted and superimposed upon the subsequent CT there will be coincidence with the area of ring enhancement representing necrosis but where there is tumour regrowth the isodose boundaries will not be observed. A less formal approach may be adequate where crossed fields have been applied (Fig. 2.35). Exceptionally delayed radiation effects may resolve (Yanashita et al. 1980).

MRI has not provided specific appearances for radiation changes in the brain though the increased sensitivity of local and more generalised increased signal intensity on T2WI is noted (Curness et al. 1986; Dooms et al. 1986; Tsuruda et al. 1987) (Fig. 2.36). MR spectroscopy is of potential value for the detection of biochemical changes but spectra localisation is inadequate at present.

Positron emission tomography may be able to provide the answer. ^{18}F-labelled 2-fluorodeoxy-D-glucose (^{18}FDG) is a tracer of glucose metabolism which has been shown to have increased uptake in gliomas, most marked in the high grades. Deficient uptake in radiation necrosis was noted by Patronas et al. (1982) and confirmed by Doyle et al. (1987).

Postoperative Changes

Low attenuation is frequently seen at the sites of retraction especially in the frontal and temporal lobes. Grey and white matter are involved and patchy areas of haemorrhage are often present in the early stages. Gradual resolution over 24–36 hours is the usual course. Intravenous contrast medium will not show enhancement in this early period unless there is residual tumour but between days 5 and 14 postoperatively breakdown of the blood–brain barrier will be apparent. This phenomenon is not expected to be present, for example after lobectomy where there is good exposure, minimal trauma and excellent haemostasis, but where even a small cortical incision has been made with limited access and haemorrhage, postoperative enhancement is more marked and can rarely persist for months or even years (Cairncross et al. 1985).

Following craniectomy there is a single, smooth curvilinear enhancing membrane (meningogaleal complex) (Lanzieri et al. 1986) covering the brain. Its normal thickness should be no more than 6 mm and may be increased due to infection. Nodular changes may result from extra-axial tumour recurrence.

References

Ahmadi J, North CM, Segall HD, Zee C-S (1985) Cavernous sinus invasion by pituitary adenoma. AJNR 6:893–898

Anand AK, Potts DG (1982) Calcified brain metastases: Demonstration by CT. AJNR 3:527–530

Andrews BT, Halks-Miller M, Berger MS, Rosenblum ML, Wilson ML (1984) Neuroepithelial cysts of the posterior fossa: pathogenesis and report of two cases. Neurosurgery 15:91–95

Armington WG, Osborn AG, Cubberly DA et al. (1985) Supratentorial ependymoma: CT appearance. Radiology 157:367–372

Asa SL, Bilbao JM, Kovacs K, Josse RG, Krenes K (1981) Lymphocytic hypophysitis of pregnancy resulting in hypopituitarism: a distinct clinicopathological entity. Ann Intern Med 95:166–171

Ascherl GF, Hilal SK, Brisman R (1981) Computed tomography of disseminated meningeal and ependymal enoplasms. Neurology 31:567–574

Ashby MA, Barber PC, Homes AE, Freer CEL, Collins RD (1988a) Primary intracranial Hodgkin's disease. Am J Surg Pathol 124:294–299

Ashby MA, Bowen D, Bleehen NM, Barber PC, Freer CEL (1988b) Primary lymphoma of the central nervous system: Experience at Addenbrooke's Hospital, Cambridge. Clin Radiol 39:173–181

Banna M, Baker HL, Houser OW (1980) Pituitary and para-pituitary tumours on computed tomography: a review article based on 230 cases. Br J Radiol 53:1123–1143

Barnard RO, Geddes JF (1987) The incidence of multifocal gliomas: A histologic study of hemisphere sections. Cancer 60:1519–1531

Berkman YM and Blatt ES (1968) Cranial and extracranial cartilaginous tumours. Clin Radiol 19:327–333

Bilaniuk LT, Moshang T, Cara J et al. (1985) Pituitary enlargement mimicking pituitary tumour. J Neurosurg 63:39–42

Bolender NF, Cromwell LD, Graves V, Margolis MT, Kerber CW, Wendling L (1983) Interval appearance of glioma. J Comput Assist Tomogr 7:599–603

Borch DC, Mitchell I, Maloney AFJ (1973) Ependymal lined paraventricular cysts: a report of three cases. J Neurol Neurosurg Psychiatry 36:611–617

Border JL (1980) Trilateral retinoblastoma. Lancet ii:582–583

Bradac GB, Shcorner W, Bender A, Felix R (1985) MRI (NMR) in the diagnosis of brain stem tumours. Neuroradiology 27:208–213

Bradley WG, Waluch V, Yadley RA, Wycoff RR (1984) Comparison of CT and MR in 400 patients with suspected disease of the brain and cervical spinal cord. Radiology 152:695–702

Brant-Zawadzki M, Norman D, Newton H et al. (1984) Magnetic resonance of the brain: the optimal screening technique. Radiology 152:71–77

Braun IF, Naidich TP, Leeds NE, Koslow M, Zimmerman HM, Chase NE (1977) Dense intracranial epidermoid tumours. Radiology 122:717–719

Braun IF, Pinto RS, Epstein F (1982) Dense cystic craniopharyngiomas. AJNR 3:139–141

Burrows G, Wortzman G, Rewcastle N (1981) Microadenomas of the pituitary and abnormal sellar tomograms in an unselected autopsy series. N Engl J Med 304:156–158

Bydder GM, Steiner RE, Thomas DJ, Marshall J, Gilderdale DJ, Young IR (1983) Nuclear magnetic resonance imaging of the posterior fossa: 50 cases. Clin Radiol 34:173–188

Bydder GM, Kingsley DPE, Brown J, Niendorf HP, Young IR (1985) Meningiomas including studies with and without Gadolinium DTPA. J Comput Assist Tomogr 9:690–697

Cairncross JG, Pexman JWW, Rathbone MP, Del-Maestro RF (1985) Post operative contrast enhancement in patients with brain tumour. Ann Neurol 17:570–572

Castaldo JE, Bernat JL, Merer FA, Schned AR (1983) Intracranial metastases due to prostatic carcinoma. Cancer 52: 1739–1747

Chambers EF, Turski PA, LaMasters DC, Newton TH (1982) Regions of low density in the contrast enhanced pituitary gland: Normal and pathological processes. Radiology 144:109–113

Claussen C, Laniado M, Kazner E, Schorner W, Felix, R (1985a) Applications of contrast agents in CT and MRI (NMR): their potential in imaging of brain tumours. Neuroradiology 27:164–171

Claussen C, Laniado M, Schorner M et al. (1985b) Gadolinium–DTPA in MR imaging of glioblastoma and intracranial metastases. AJNR 6:669–674

Claveria LE, Du Boulay GH, Kendall BE (1978) The diagnostic limitations of computerised axial tomography in hemispheric tumours. In: Bories J (ed) The diagnostic limitations of computerised axial tomography. Springer, Berlin, Heidelberg, New York, pp 2–16

Clugston R, Wong G, Chakera TMH (1988) Intracerebral haematoma mimicking intracranial neoplasm at computed tomography. Med J Aust 148:92–94

Curness JT, Laster DW, Ball MR, Moody DM, Witcofski RL
(1986) MRI of radiation injury to the brain. AJR 147:119–
124

Czervionke LF, Daniels DL, Meger GA, Poujnas KW, Williams
AL, Houghton VM (1987) Neuroepithelial cysts of the lateral
ventricles: MR Appearance. AJNR 8:609–613

Davis PC, Friedman NC, Fry SM, Malko JA, Hoffman JC,
Braun IF (1987a) Leptomeningeal metastasis: MR imaging.
Radiology 163:449–454

Davis PC, Hoffman JC, Spencer T, Tindall GR, Braun IF
(1987b) M.R. imaging of pituitary adenomas: CT, clinical and
surgical correlation. AJNR 8:107–112

Derrig P, O'Connor L, Brammer HM, Meriwether M (1986)
Glioblastom multiforme masquerading as a more benign
process. AJNR 7:166–167

Diebler C, Ponsot G (1983) Hamartomas of the tuber cinereum.
Neuroradiology 25:93–101

Dieterman JF, Heldt N, Burguet JF, Medjek L, Maitrit D,
Wackenheim A (1982) CT findings in malignant meningiomas.
Neuroradiology 23:207–209

Dooms GC, Hecht S, Brant-Zawadski M, Berthiaume Y,
Norman D, Newton TH (1986) Brain radiation lesions: MR
imaging. Radiology 158:149–155

Doppman JL, Oldfield EH, Krudy AG, Chrousos GP, Schulte
HM, Schaff M, Loriaux DC (1984) Petrosal sinus sampling for
Cushing syndrome: Anatomical and technical considerations.
Radiology 150:99–103

Doyle WK, Budinger TF, Valk PE, Levin VA, Gutin PH (1987)
Differentiation of cerebral radiation necrosis from tumour
recurrence by [18F]FDG and 82Rb positron emission tomography. J Comput Assist Tomogr 11:563–570

Dwyer AJ, Frank JA, Doppman JL et al. (1987) Pituitary adenomas in patients with Cushing disease: Initial experience with
Gd-DTPA enhanced MR imaging. Radiology 163:421–426

Earnest F, Kelly PJ, Scheithauer BW et al. (1988) Cerebral
astrocytomas: Histopathologic correlation with MR and CT
contrast enhancement with stereotactic biopsy. Radiology
166:823–827

Ehlers N, Kae S, Rasmussen K, Rabjer, E (1983) Hereditary
bilateral retinoblastoma, pinealoma and normal chromo-
somes. A case report. Acta Pathol 61:838–843

Enzmann DR, Krikouian J, York C, Hayward R (1978a) Computed tomography of leptomeningeal spread of tumour. J
Comput Assist Tomogr 2:448–455

Enzmann DR, Norman D, Levin V, Wilson C, Newton,
TD (1978b) Computed tomography in the follow-up of
medulloblastomas and ependymomas. Radiology 128:57

Enzmann DR, Kirkorian J, Norman D, Kramer R, Pollock J,
Faer M (1979) Computed tomography in primary reticulum
cell sarcoma of the brain. Radiology 130:165–170

Erlich SS, Davis RC (1978) Spinal subarachnoid metastasis
from primary intra cranial glioblastoma multiforme. Cancer
42:2854–2864

Felix R, Schorner W, Laniado M et al. (1985) Brain tumours:
MR imaging with Gadolinium DTPA. Radiology 156:681–
688

Flannigan BD, Bradley WG, Maziotta JC (1985) Magnetic resonance of the brain stem: normal structure and basic functional anatomy. Radiology 154:375–383

Freeman MP, Kessler RM, Allen JH, Price AC (1987) Craniopharyngioma: CT and MR Imaging in 9 cases. J Comput
Assist Tomogr 11:810–814

Fujisawa I, Asato R, Nishimura K et al. (1987a) Anterior and
posterior lobes of the pituitary gland: Assessment by 1.5T
MR imaging. J Comput Assist Tomogr 11:214–220

Fujisawa I, Kikuchi K, Nishimura K et al. (1987b) Transection

of the pituitary stalk : Development of an ectopic posterior
lobe associated with MR imaging. Radiology 165:485–489

Ganti SR, Hilal SK, Stein BM, Silver AJ, Mawad M, Sane P
(1986) C.T. of pineal region tumours. AJNR 7:97–104

Gentry LR, Jacoby CG, Turski PA, Houston LW, Strother CM,
Sackett JF (1987) Cerebellopontine angle – petromastoid mass
lesions: Comparative study with MR and CT imaging.
Radiology 162:513–520

Graif MM, Bydder G, Steiner R, Niendorf P, Thomas DGT,
Young IR (1985) Contrast enhanced MR of malignant brain
tumours. AJNR 6:855–862

Graus F, Rogers LR, Posner JB (1985) Cerebrovascular complications in patients with cancer. Medicine 64:16–35

Hackney DB, Grossman RI, Zimmerman RA et al. (1987) Low
sensitivity of clinical MR Imaging to small changes in the
concentration of non paramagnetic protein. AJNR 8:1003–
1008

Han JS, Huss RG, Benson JE et al. (1984) MR imaging of the
skull base. J Comput Assist Tomogr 8:944–952

Hardy J (1973) Transsphenoidal surgery of hypersecreting pituitary tumours. In: Kohler PO, Ross GT (eds) Diagnosis and
treatment of pituitary tumours. Excerpta Medica, Amsterdam, p 179

Haughton VM, Rimm AA, Sobocinski KA et al. (1986) A
blinded clinical comparison of MR imaging and CT in neuroradiology. Radiology 160:751–757

Hayes WS, Sherman JL, Stern BJ, Citrin CM, Pulaski PD (1987)
MR and CT evaluation of intracranial sarcoidosis. AJR
149:1043–1049

Healey ME, Hesselink JR, Press GA, Middleton MS (1987)
Increased detection of intracranial metastases with intravenous Gd-DTPA. Radiology 165:619–624

Hefelfinger MJ, Dahlin DC, MacCarthy CS, Beabout JW (1973)
Chordomas and cartilaginous tumours of the skull base.
Cancer 32:410–420

Helle TL, Conley FK (1980) Haemorrhage associated with meningioma: a case report and review of the literature. J Neurol
Neurosurg Psychiatry 43:725–729

Hibi I, Fujiwara K (1987) Precocious puberty of cerebral origin:
A cooperative study in Japan. Prog Exp Tumour Res 30:224–
238

Ho K, Hoschner JA, Wolfe DE (1981) Primary leptomeningeal
gliomatosis. Symptoms suggestive of meningitis. Arch Neurol
38:662–666

Horton WA, Wong V, Eldridge R (1976) Von Hippel Lindau
disease. Arch Intern Med 136: 769–772

Hughs PG (1984) Cerebellar medulloblastoma in adults. J
Neurosurg 60:994–997

Jaeckle KA, Krol G, Posner JB (1985) Evolution of computed
tomographic abnormalities in leptomeningeal metastases.
Ann Neurol 17:85–89

Johnson MA, Pennock JM, Bydder GM et al. (1983) Clinical
NMR imaging of the brain in children: normal and neurological disease. AJR 141:1005–1018

Kao SCS, Yuh WTC, Sato Y, Barloon TJ (1987) Intracranial
granulocytic sarcoma (chloroma): MR findings. J Comput
Assist Tomogr 11:938–941

Kart BH, Reddy SC, Rao GR, Porveda H (1986) Choroid plexus
metastasis: CT appearance. J Comput Assist Tomogr 10:537–
540

Kazner E, Wende S, Grumme T, Lanksch W, Stochdorph (1982)
Computed tomography in intracranial tumours. Springer,
Berlin, Heidelberg, New York

Kelly JK, Laxo A, Metes J, Wilner HI, Watts FB (1985) Intracranial haemorrhagic dissemination of acute myelocytic leukaemia. AJNR 6:113–114

Kendall BE, Tatler GLV (1978) Radiological findings in neurosarcoidosis. Br J Radiol 51:81–92

Kendall BE, Jakoubowski J, Pullicino P, Symon L (1979)

Difficulties in the diagnosis of supratentorial glioma by CAT scan. J Neurol Neurosurg Psychiatry 42:485–492

Kilgore DP, Starshak RJ, Strother CM, Haughton VM (1986) Pineal germinoma: MR imaging. Radiology 158:435–438

Kjos BO, Brant-Zawadzki M, Kucharczyck W, Kelly W, Norman D, Newton TH (1985) Cystic intracranial lesions: magnetic resonance imaging. Radiology 155:363–369

Kortman KE, Van-Dalsen WJ, Bradley WG (1985) MR Imaging of epidermoid tumours. Radiology 157:17

Kucharczyck W, Davis DO, Kelly WM (1986) Thin section, high resolution imaging of pituitary adenomas at 1.5 Tesla. Radiology 161:761–765

Kucharczyk W, Peck WW, Kelly WM, Norman D, Newton TH (1987) Rathke cleft cysts: CT, MR imaging and Pathologic features. Radiology 165:491–496

Kulkarni MV, Lee KF, McArdle CB, Yeakley JW, Haar FL (1988) 1.5T MR Imaging of pituitary microadenomas: technical considerations and CT correlation. AJNR 9:5–11

Lanzieri CF, Som PM, Sacher M, Solodnik P, Moore F (1986) Post craniectomy site: C.T. appearance. Radiology 159:165–170

Latack JT, Kartack JM, Kemork JL, Graham MD, Knake JE (1985) Epidermoidomas of the cerebellopontine angle and temporal bone: CT and MR aspects. Radiology 157:361–366

Latchaw RE, Gold LHA, Moore JS, Payne J (1977) The non-specificity of absorption coefficients in the differentiation of solid and cystic tumours. Radiology 125:141–145

Lee BCP, Kneeland JB, Cahill PT, Cahill MDF (1985) MR Recognition of supratentorial tumours AJNR 6:871–878

Lee DH, Norman D, Newton TH (1987) MR Imaging of pineal cysts. J Comput Assist Tomogr 11:586–590

Lee YY, Lin SR, Horner F (1979) Third ventricle meningioma mimicking a colloid cyst in a child. AJR 132:669–671

Lee YY, Posner JB, Chernik NL, Glass JP, Geoffray A, Wallace S (1984) Cranial Computed tomographic abnormalities in leptomeningeal metastases. AJR 143:1035–1039

Lee Y–Y, Castillo M, Nauert C, Moser RP (1985) Computed tomography of gliosarcoma. AJNR 6:527–530

Levin VA, Hoffman WF, Heilbron DL, Norman D (1980) Prognosis of pretreatment CT scan on time to progression. J Neurosurg 52:642–647

Mackay IM, Bydder GM, Young IR (1985) MR Imaging of central nervous system tumours that do not display increase in T1 or T2. J Comput Assist Tomogr 9:1055–1061

Mamourian AC, Towfight J (1986) Pineal cysts: MR imaging. AJNR 7:1081–1086

Masdeu JC (1983) Infarct vs neoplasm on CT: Four helpful signs. AJNR 4:522–523

Max MB, Deck MDF, Rottenburg DA (1981) Pituitary metastases in cancer patients and clinical differentiation from pituitary adenoma. Neurology 31:998–1002

Mikhael MA (1979) Radiation necrosis of the brain: correlation between patterns on computed tomography and dose of radiation. J Comput Assist Tomogr 3:241–249

Miller MH, Tucker WS, Bilbao JM (1986) Supratentorial haemangioblastoma associated with Von Hippel Lindau disease: Case report and review of the literature. J Can Assoc Radiol 37:33–37

Morrison G, Sobel DF, Kelley WM, Norman D (1984) Intraventricular mass lesions. Radiology 53:435–442

Nakamura T, Schorner W, Bittner R Ch, Felix R (1988) The value of paramagnetic contrast agent gadolinium DTPA in the diagnosis of pituitary adenomas. Neuroradiology 30:481–486

Nass R, Whelan M (1981) Gangliogliomas. Neuroradiology 22:67–71

Nemoto Y, Inoue Y, Fukuda T et al. (1988) MR appearances of Rathkes cleft cysts. Neuroradiology 30:155–159

New PFJ, Hesselink RJ, O-Carrol CP, Kleinmann GM (1982) Malignant meningiomas: CT and histological criterion including a new CT sign. AJNR 3:267–276

Numaguchi Y, Conolly ES, Kumra AK, Vargas EF, Gum GK, Mizushima A (1987) Computed tomography and MR imaging of thalamic neuroepithelial cysts. J Comput Assist Tomogr 11:583–585

Okamata S, Handa H, Yamashitu J (1985) Computed tomography in intra- and suprasella epithelial cysts (symptomatic Rathke cleft cysts). AJNR 6:515–519

Paganii JJ, Libshitz HI, Wallace S, Hayman LA (1981) Central nervous system leukaemia and lymphoma involvement: Computed tomographic manifestations. AJR 137:1195–1201

Palma L, Guidetti B (1986) Cystic pilocystic astrocytomas of the cerebral hemispheres: surgical experience with 51 cases and long term results. J Neurosurg 62:811–815

Patronas NJ, Di Chiro G, Brooks SA (1982) Work in progress: [^{18}F] fluorodeoxyglucose and positron emission tomography in the evaluation of radiation necrosis of the brain. Radiology 144:885–889

Pearl BC (1984) Xanthogranuloma of the choroid plexus. AJR 143:401–402

Pechora-Peterova V, Kalvach P (1986) C.T. findings in cerebral metastases. Neuroradiology 28:254–258

Peyster RG, Ginsberg F, Hoover ED (1986) Computed Tomography of familial pineoblastoma. J Comput Assist Tomogr 10:32–33

Pojunas KW, Daniels DL, Williams AL, Haughton VM (1986) MR imaging of prolactin-secreting microadenomas. AJNR 7:209–213

Powers WJ, Miller EM (1981) Sarcoidosis mimicking glioma: Case report and review of intracranial sarcoid mass lesions. Neurology 31:907–910

Priest JR, Ramsey NK, Latchaw RW et al. (1980) Thrombotic and haemorrhagic strokes complicating early therapy for childhood acute lymphoblastic leukaemia. Cancer 46:1548–1554

Pusey E, Kortman KE, Flannigan EB, Tfurunda J, Bradley WG (1987) MR imaging of craniopharyngiomas. AJNR 8:439–444

Quencer RM (1980) Lymphocytic adenohypophysitis: Autoimmune disorder of the pituitary gland. AJNR 1:343–345

Reith KG, Di-Chiro G, Cromwell LD et al. (1981) Primary demyelinating disease simulating glioma of the corpus callosum. J Neurosurg 55:620–624

Romero FJ, Ortega A, Ibaura B, Pomes J, Rovira M (1987) Craniocervical neuroepithelial cyst (colloid cyst). AJNR 8:1000–1002

Rumack CM, Guggenheim MA, Fasules JW, Burdick D (1980) Transient post postictal computed tomographic scan. J Pediatr 97:263–264

Russell EJ, George AE, Kricheff II, Budzilovich GN (1980) Atypical computed tomographic features of intracranial meningioma: radiological–pathological correlation in a series of 130 cases. Radiology 135:673–682

Russell EJ, Geremia GK, Johnson CE et al. (1987) Multiple cerebral metastases: Detectability with Gd-DTPA-enhanced MR imaging. Radiology 165:609–617

Sartor K, Karnaze MG, Winthrop JD, Gado M, Hodges FJ (1987) MR Imaging of infra-, para- and retrosellar mass lesions. Neuroradiology 29:19–29

Sato Y, Waziri M, Smith W et al. (1988) Hippel–Lindau disease: MR imaging. Radiology 166:241–246

Scheithaeur BW (1978) Symptomatic subependymoma. Report of 21 cases with review of the literature. J Neurosurg 49:689–696

Shadir J, Coblenz C, Malanson D, Eyhier R, Robitaille Y (1985) New CT findings in aggressive meningioma. AJNR 6:101–102

Sherwin RP, Grassi JE, Sommers SC (1962) Hamartomatous malformation of the postero-lateral hypothalamus. J Lab Invest 11:89–97

Shoenberg BS, Christine BW, Wishant JP (1975) Nervous system neoplasms and primary malignancies at other sites. The unique association between meningiomas and breast cancer. Neurology 25:705–712

Shungshotti S, Kasantikul V, Suwanwela N, Suwanwela C (1984) Solitary primary intracranial extracerebral glioma. Case report. J Neurosurg 61:772–781

Sigbee B, Deck DF, Posner JB (1979) Nonmetastatic superior sagittal sinus thrombosis complicating systemic cancer. Neurology 29:139–146

Silverman C, Marks JE (1981) Prognostic significance of contrast enhancement in low grade astrocytomas of the adult cerebrum. Radiology 139:211–213

Smith AS, Weinstein MA, Modic MT et al. (1985) Magnetic resonance with marked T2 weighted images: improved demonstration of brain lesions, tumour and edema. AJR 145:949–955

Spangoli M, Goldberg HI, Grossman RI (1986) High field MR imaging of intracranial meningiomas. Radiology 161:369–375

Stevens JM, Ruiz JS, Kendall BE (1983) Observations on peritumoural oedema in meningioma Part II: Mechanisms of oedema production. Neuroradiology 25:125–131

Stevens JM, Kendall BE, Love S (1984) Radiological features of subependymoma with emphasis on computed tomography. Neuroradiology 26:223–228

Swartz JD, Russel KB, Basile BA, O'Donnell PC, Popky GL (1983) High-resolution CT appearance of the intrasellar contents in women of child-bearing age. Radiology 147:115–117

Sze G, Shin J, Krol G, Johnson C, Liu D, Deck MDF (1988) Intraparenchymal brain metastases: MR imaging versus contrast enhanced CT. Radiology 168:187–194

Tapp E, Huxley M (1972) The histologic appearance of the human pineal gland from puberty to old age. J Pathol 108:137–144

Teasdale E, Teasdale G, Mohshen F, Macpherson P (1986) High resolution computed tomography in pituitary microadenomas: Is seeing believing? Clin Radiol 37:227–232

Tsuruda JS, Kortman KE, Bradley WG, Wheeler DC, Van-Dalsen W, Bradley TP (1987) Radiation effects on cerebral white matter: MR evaluation. AJNR 8:431–437

Vaquero J, Cabezudo JM, Nombela L (1983) C.T. scan in subependymoma. Br J Radiol 56:425–426

Vaquero J, Martinez R, Rossi E, Lopez R (1984) Primary cerebral lymphoma: the "ghost tumour". Case report. J Neurosurg 60:174–176

Vassilouthis J, Ambrose J (1979) Computerised tomographic appearances of intracranial meningiomas. J Neurosurg 50:320–327

Vonofakos D, Marcu H, Hacker H (1979) Oligodendroglioma: CT Patterns with emphasis on features indicating malignancy. J Comput Assist Tomogr 3:783–786

Waal MJ, Peyster SD, Finklestein SD, Pistone WR, Hoover ED (1985) Unique case of neurosarcoidosis with pineal and suprasellar involvement: CT and pathological demonstration. J Comput Assist Tomogr 9:381–383

Wasserstrom WR, Glass JP, Posner JB (1982) Diagnosis and treatment of leptomeningeal metastases from solid tumours: Experience with 90 patients. Cancer 49:759–772

Weiner SN, Pearlstein AE, Eiber A (1987) MR Imaging of arachnoid cysts. J Comput Assist Tomogr 11:236–241

Weinstein MA, Pavlicek MS, Scott AR, Duchesnau MD (1986) Differentiation of tumour and oedema with magnetic resonance. In: Runge VM, Claussen C, Felix R, James AE (eds) Contrast agents in magnetic resonance imaging. Excerpta Medica, Amsterdam, pp 111–113

Weisberg LA (1985) Solitary cerebellar metastases. Arch Neurol 42:336–341

Wong BY, Steinberg GK, Rosen L (1989) Pre-operative diagnosis of Lhermitte–Duclos disease by magnetic resonance imaging. Case report. J Neurosurg 70:135–137

Yanashita J, Handor H, Yumitoris K, Abe M (1980) Reversible delayed radiation effect on the brain after radiotherapy of malignant astrocytoma. Surg Neurol 13:413–417

Yuh WTC, Barloon TJ, Jacoby CG (1987) Case report: Trigeminal lipoma, MR findings. J Comput Assist Tomogr 11:518–521

Yuh WTC, Wright DC, Barloon TJ, Schultz DH, Sato Y, Cervantes CA (1988) MR Imaging of primary tumours of trigeminal nerve and Meckels cave. AJNR 9:665–670

Zimmerman RD, Fleming CA, Saint-Louis LA, Lee BCP, Manning JJ, Deck MDF (1985) Magnetic resonance imaging of meningiomas. AJNR 6:149–150

Chapter 3

Hydrocephalus and Degenerative Cerebral Disease

W. St Clair Forbes

Hydrocephalus

Introduction

Hydrocephalus is a pathological condition in which there is dilatation of part or all of the ventricular system due to an increase in the volume of cerebrospinal fluid (CSF) resulting from a disturbance of its secretion, flow or absorption. The condition is accurately diagnosed by means of computed tomography (CT) which may frequently identify its cause.

The condition may be either "active" or "arrested". In active hydrocephalus there is a progressive increase in intraventricular pressure. Arrested hydrocephalus implies that the intraventricular pressure has returned to normal and is no longer a stimulus for further ventricular enlargement (Faerber 1986).

There are two main causes of ventricular enlargement: hydrocephalus and cerebral atrophy. The accumulation of CSF in hydrocephalus implies an increase in intraventricular pressure causing compression and displacement of the adjacent brain parenchyma. Ventricular shunting is required to prevent irreversible changes in the parenchyma. In cerebral atrophy the enlargement of the ventricles is secondary to loss of brain substance and is accompanied by enlargement of the extracerebral CSF spaces of the basal cisterns, fissures and cortical sulci. The CT differentiation of atrophy from obstructive hydrocephalus is straightforward.

There are two types of hydrocephalus: the obstructive form and the much less common non-obstructive form (Haughton 1985). In obstructive hydrocephalus there is interruption of the flow of

CSF whereas non-obstructive hydrocephalus is the result of excessive CSF production, usually due to a choroid plexus papilloma.

Cerebrospinal Fluid Circulation: Anatomical and Physiological Considerations

The total CSF volume is between 50 and 150 ml and is produced at a rate of about 0.35 ml/min. This is equivalent to approximately 500 ml/24 hours, and represents a turnover every 6 hours. This rate is not significantly reduced by the elevated hydrostatic pressure of hydrocephalus (Lorenzo et al. 1970). As a result, therefore, even hydrocephalic patients turn over their complete CSF volume several times each day.

The major portion of CSF production is from the choroid plexi of the lateral ventricles, with a small contribution by the choroid plexi of the third and fourth ventricles. The choroid plexus includes the choroidal epithelium, blood vessels and interstitial connective tissues. There are no anatomical differences between the choroid plexus of the lateral, third or fourth ventricles. Furthermore, a significant proportion of CSF is produced into the extracellular spaces of the brain from the cerebral vasculature (Milhorat 1975), thence flowing towards the ependyma and diffusing into the ventricle.

Ventricular CSF flows sequentially from lateral to third and fourth ventricles and exits into the basal subarachnoid cisterns through the foramina of Luschka and Magendie. The CSF then passes into the basal cisterns and then anteriorly through the chiasmatic cisterns, Sylvian fissures and pericallosal cisterns, laterally over the cerebral hemispheres, posteriorly around the cerebellum via the quadrigeminal plate cistern and posterior callosal cistern. It then passes over the cerebral hemispheres. Additional CSF passes inferiorly to the spinal subarachnoid space, where it may be absorbed directly or may re-ascend to the parasagittal arachnoid villi. Absorption of CSF occurs primarily at the arachnoid villi and granulations (Pacchionian bodies). The villi represent herniations of the arachnoid membrane which penetrate into the dura and protrude into the lumen of the superior sagittal sinus and other venous structures. The exact mechanism of absorption is unknown.

This directional flow of CSF is maintained by the continuous elaboration of newly formed CSF into the ventricles, by the action of the ependymal cilia sweeping the CSF outward, vascular pulsations, transmitted variations in these pulsations and a nearly constant downhill pressure gradient between the subarachnoid spaces and the dural venous sinuses. Ultimately much of the CSF enters the superior sagittal sinus by passive pressure-dependent resorption through the arachnoid villi. Obstruction to the flow of CSF at any point within the system causes dilatation of the CSF spaces proximal to that blockage.

The CT criterion for the site of obstruction is the point of transition from dilated to non-dilated CSF spaces (Naidich et al. 1976). Table 3.1 correlates the site of the obstruction with the CT scan appearances.

Table 3.1. Sites of obstruction and CT appearances

CT appearances	Site of obstruction
Single temporal horn ("Trapped temporal horn")	Ipsilateral atrium
Single lateral ventricle	Ipsilateral Foramen of Monro
Both lateral ventricles	Bilateral obstruction at the Foramen of Monro
Lateral and third ventricles	At or near the aqueduct
All the ventricles but not the basal cisterns	Exit foramen of the fourth ventricle
All the ventricles and basal cisterns	Incisural block
All the ventricles, basal cisterns, Sylvian fissures and low-convexity sulci	Mid-convexity subarachnoid spaces
All the ventricles and basal cisterns including the high convexity parasagittal cisterns	At or near the arachnoid villi

Ventriculography using positive contrast water-soluble media may be required in some cases to demonstrate the patency of the ventricular system and to differentiate a mass with an attentuation value similar to CSF from simple ventricular dilatation. Magnetic resonance imaging (MRI) may

enable this differentiation to be achieved non-invasively. Furthermore, MRI may have a useful role in demonstrating the dynamics of the CSF pathways in vivo.

CT Evaluation of the CSF Spaces

The volume of the normal adult lateral ventricle measures 15–17 ml, the third ventricle, aqueduct and fourth ventricle combined measure 1–1.5 ml. CT estimates of ventricular size correlate well with those obtained following air encephalography. Both quantitative measurements and subjective assessment are valuable.

Quantitative Measurements (Meese et al. 1980)

1. Absolute measurements of the ventricular system, corrected for computer minification and patient age (Fig. 3.1)
2. Ratios
   a) Frontal horn index
   b) Evan's index
   c) Ventricular size index
   d) Cella media index
   e) Huckman number

The Huckman number (HN) is a useful parameter of anterior horn width. The relation of this

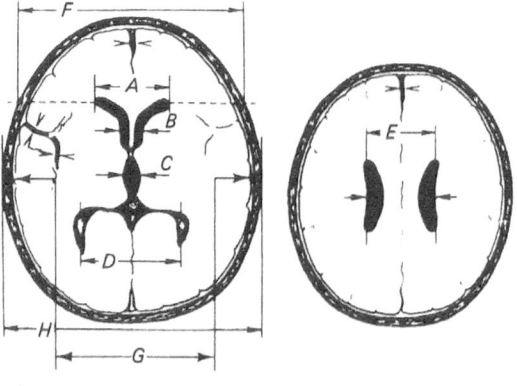

Fig. 3.1. Quantitative measurements of the ventricular system. A: Maximum distance between frontal horns. B: Distance between caudate nuclei. C: Width of third ventricle. D: Distance between choroid plexi. E: Maximum distance between the lateral ventricles at the level of the cella media. F: Maximum external diameter of the frontal bone (at the level of the frontal horns). G: Maximum internal diameter between the temporal bones. H: Maximum external diameter between the temporal bones. F/A: Frontal horn index. A/G: Evans index. B/A: Ventricular index. H/E: Cella media index. A + B: Huckman number. (After Meese et al. 1980.)

section of the ventricle to the width of the skull justifies an additional parameter – the Evans' index – which has the same diagnostic value as the frontal horn index (FHI) but which is more easily determined. The cella media index (CMI) is particularly well suited for evaluation of the lateral ventricles in the area of the ventricular bodies.

The ventricular index (VI) provides supplementary information. It is related to the ventricular system alone and is especially helpful in cases of cranial asymmetry and atypical skull morphology. The third and fourth ventricles can be measured directly.

Of the aforementioned, the cella media index of Schiersmann, mean value 4.0, and Evans' index (Evans 1942; Pedersen et al. 1979), mean value 3.0, are the most useful indices of ventricular size.

Normal CSF Spaces in Adults and Children (Gyldenstedt 1977)

The left lateral ventricle is larger than the right lateral ventricle in both sexes. Both lateral ventricles are larger in the male. There is a statistically significant increase of all ventricular parameters with increasing age and there is a small decrease in the cella media index with advancing years. The linear measurements of the lateral ventricles demonstrate positive correlation to cranial size, whereas the widths of the third ventricle and sulci are independent of the size of the skull.

A statistically highly significant increase in sulcal size was shown with increasing age, but no sex difference was found in the above study.

Generalisations are evident when all values are considered.

1. Values in the first two decades of life are significantly different from those for all other ages, and a separate set of normal values for the younger age group is justified. The relative sizes of the frontal horns, bodies of the lateral ventricles and third ventricle decrease with brain growth (Pedersen et al. 1979). The subarachnoid cisterns are relatively larger in children and decrease to adult size by the mid-teens.

2. The normal values in adults up to the age of 60 years are relatively constant, and a single set of values for this age span is adequate.

3. Normal values after the age of 60 would appear to fall into a third natural group. The significant increase in ventricular size could be regarded as an expression of normal ageing and therefore need not imply an underlying pathological process.

The following subjective observations relating to an increase in ventricular size can be made (Naidich et al. 1982):

1. Conditions producing an increase in ventricular size result in a greater proportion of the intracranial volume occupied by the lateral, third and fourth ventricles.

2. There is a progressive increase in the size and degree of dilatation of the temporal horns of the lateral ventricles. Disproportionately large temporal horns usually indicate hydrocephalus but may be a feature of atrophy (Svendson and Duro 1981).

3. A progressive rounding and bulging of the superolateral angles of the frontal horns is noted.

4. Progressive compression and inferior displacement of the thalami is shown on the appropriate sections.

Types of Hydrocephalus

Non-obstructive Hydrocephalus

This is the result of excessive CSF production for which a papilloma of the choroid plexus is the main cause. The ventricle near the papilloma enlarges and CT readily demonstrates the ventricular enlargement and the intraventricular tumour mass.

In newborn infants an intraventricular haematoma might produce similar features with ventricular enlargement. This type of hydrocephalus may also be seen in cases of grossly elevated CSF protein content which may accompany some spinal tumours where patients will present with papilloedema and hydrocephalus on CT.

Obstructive Hydrocephalus

Obstruction to CSF flow is the commonest form of hydrocephalus. Hydrocephalus is initially associated with increased intraventricular pressure but may later reach a state of equilibrium resulting in the condition of arrested hydrocephalus.

The terms communicating and obstructive have been in use since the early days of neuroradiological diagnosis (Dandy and Blackfan 1913). However, these terms are misleading and have been superseded by the subdivision of hydrocephalus into (a) intraventricular obstructive hydrocephalus, and (b) extraventricular obstructive hydrocephalus.

CT Findings in Hydrocephalus (George and deLeon 1988)

1. Early dilatation and rounding of the temporal

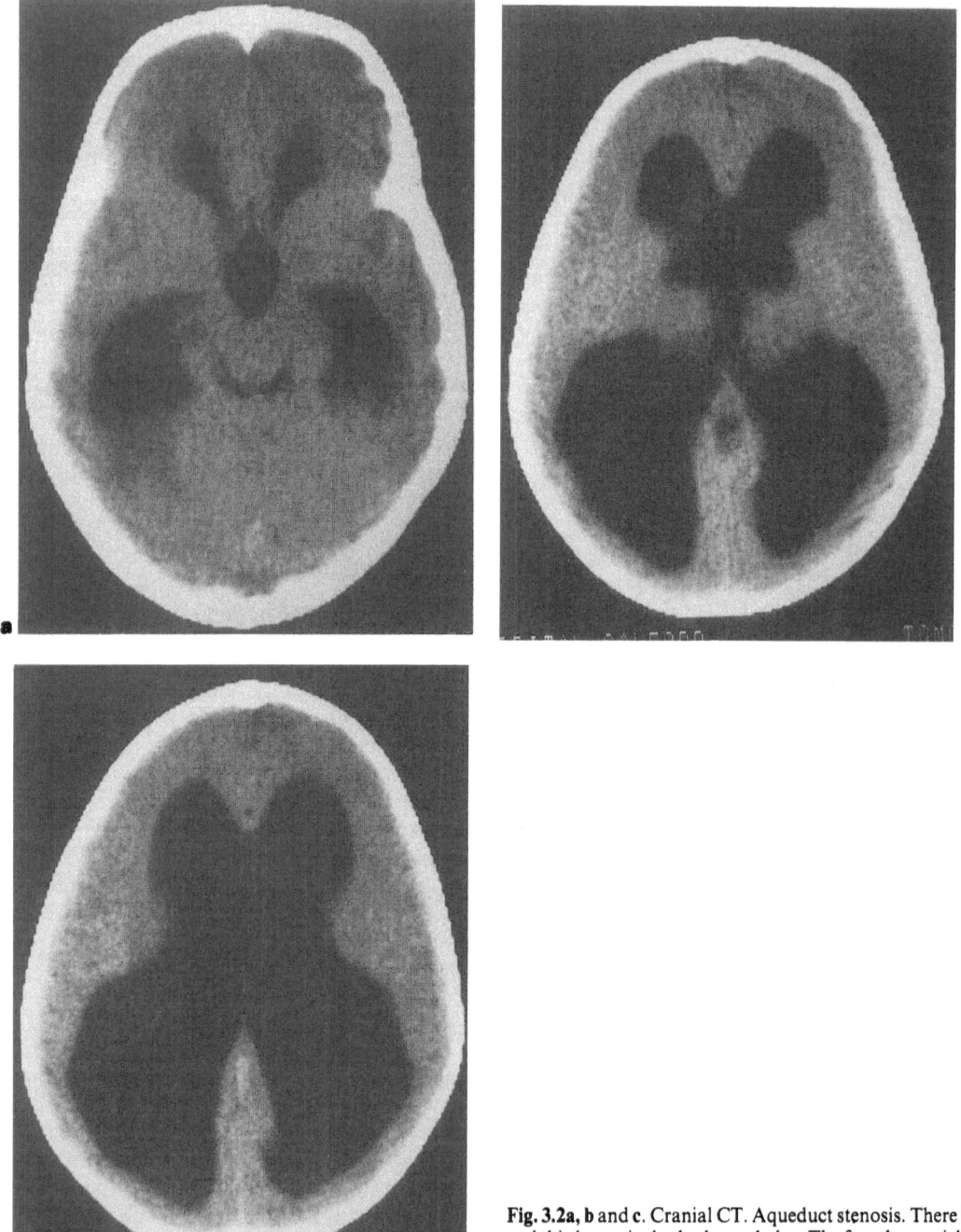

Fig. 3.2a, b and **c**. Cranial CT. Aqueduct stenosis. There is lateral and third ventricular hydrocephalus. The fourth ventricle cannot be identified. Note the acute septal angle (see text).

horns is the earliest sign and may be seen before obvious enlargement of the bodies of the lateral ventricles (Fig. 3.2). The early dilatation of the temporal horns in hydrocephalus is readily differentiated from temporal horn dilatation occurring as a manifestation of temporal lobe

atrophy in which condition it is invariably associated with enlargement of the Sylvian fissures and other signs of temporal lobe atrophy (see later).

2. Rounding and enlargement of the frontal horns with an acute angle formed by the medial walls

of the dilated frontal horns, the septal angle. In atrophy the frontal horns are enlarged but not ballooned and the angle is typically obtuse.

3. Enlargement and ballooning of the third ventricle.

4. Dilatation of the bodies of the lateral ventricles tends to be greater than that occurring secondary to atrophy.

5. Enlargement of the fourth ventricle suggests extraventricular obstructive hydrocephalus.

6. Preservation or accentuation of grey/white matter differentiation.

7. Sulcal effacement, when present, is a diagnostic sign of hydrocephalus, particularly in the elderly age-groups because cortical atrophy is almost invariably present as part of the ageing process. It should be remembered, however, that the sulci may dilate when the obstruction is at the level of the Pacchionian granulations.

8. Periventricular oedema occurs mainly in the periventricular matter of the frontal horns in the acute and subacute phases of hydrocephalus (Fig. 3.3) (see p. 71).

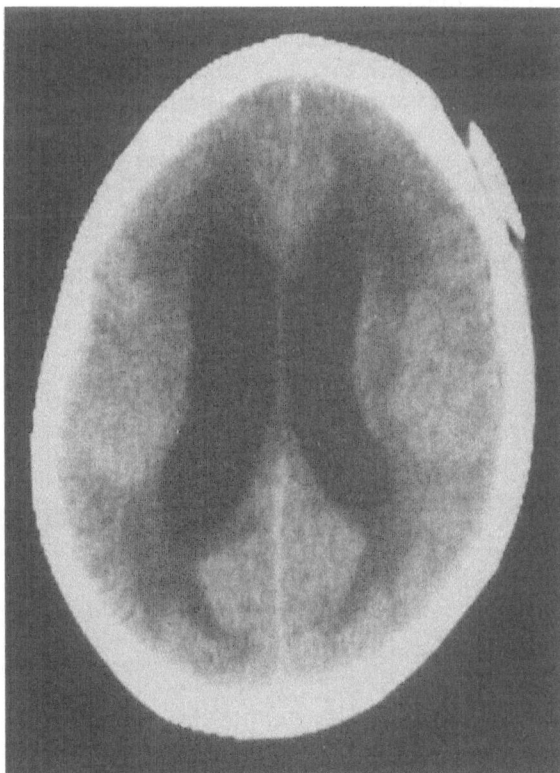

Fig. 3.3. Cranial CT. Hydrocephalus following subarachnoid haemorrhage. Note the periventricular lucencies.

Intraventricular Obstructive Hydrocephalus (IVOH)

Accurate classification of IVOH is possible, because the ventricles dilate proximal to but not distal to the obstruction. Periventricular oedema is a frequent finding and can usually be differentiated from other causes of periventricular low density such as multiple sclerosis or ischaemic lesions which are less symmetrical, better defined and usually multifocal.

Obstruction can occur at a number of sites.

Lateral Ventricles

Congenital coarctation is a rare form of obstruction, occurring usually at the trigone or within the temporal horn. The narrowing may be a congenital maldevelopment or a consequence of intra-uterine ventriculitis with adhesion formation (Harwood-Nash and Fitz 1976). Obstruction of the atrium by an intraventricular tumour produces enlargement of the temporal horn.

Foramen of Monro

Obstruction of the foramen of Monro is rare. Obstruction of CSF flow between the lateral and third ventricles causes lateral ventricular enlargement and usually third and fourth ventricular contraction on CT. The most common cause of an obstructed intraventricular foramen is a third ventricular colloid cyst (see Chap. 2). Less commonly the foramen of Monro may be obstructed by an ependymoma, teratoma, adjacent glioma, a tuber, papilloma or meningioma. The foramen of Monro may be partially obstructed by extra-axial suprasellar masses and arachnoid cysts of the suprasellar cistern. Other causes are intraventricular haemorrhage and infection. Obstruction of one intraventricular foramen where one ventricle enlarges to displace the midline structures to the opposite side may be seen in some cases of tumour (Fig. 3.4).

Third Ventricle

The commonest obstructive lesions are extrinsic to the third ventricle (Harwood-Nash and Fitz 1976). These include craniopharyngioma and paraventricular glioma (thalamus, optic chiasm, hypothalamus) and mass lesions related to the posterior third ventricle (gliomas of the posterior hypothalamus and thalamus), tumours of the pineal region, arteriovenous malformations, aneurysms of the basilar artery and of the vein of Galen.

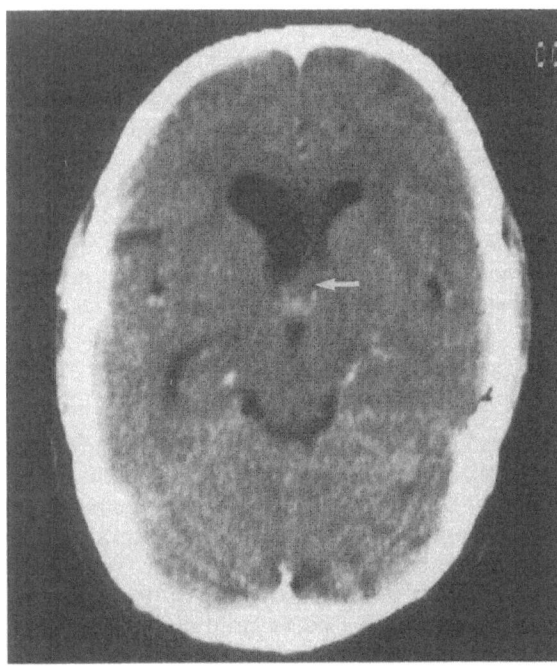

Fig. 3.4. Cranial CT after IV contrast. Glioma within the third ventricle (*arrow*). unilateral obstruction of the foramen of Monro.

Aqueduct

When CSF flow is obstructed at the aqueduct, the third and lateral ventricles enlarge, whereas the fourth usually shrinks. Aqueduct stenosis (Fig. 3.2) is the commonest cause of IVOH. The causes of obstruction are a congenital web or atresia often in association with an Arnold–Chiari malformation or a tumour of the mesencephalon or pineal gland.

Congenital aqueduct stenosis more commonly occurs with the Chiari II malformation. Four main types of anomaly have been described by Russell (1949):

1. Stenosis
2. Forking – two main channels of greatly reduced dimension found side by side
3. Septum formation
4. Gliosis

If the Arnold–Chiari type II malformation is present the CT appearances of the malformation will be seen on the lower sections (vide infra).

Once aqueductal stenosis is detected, benign congenital obstruction must be distinguished from that due to tumour. In these patients, magnetic resonance imaging, positive CT cisternography or possibly ventriculography combined with CT may be necessary to demonstrate the obstructing lesion.

MRI is also of value in assessing aqueductal patency since it is able to identify flowing CSF (Atlas et al. 1988).

Fourth Ventricle

Obstruction at the fourth ventricular level may be congenital (e.g. Dandy–Walker cyst) or acquired. The Dandy–Walker syndrome has a characteristic CT appearance. The main features are cystic enlargement of the fourth ventricle, hypoplasia of the cerebellum, and enlargement of the third and lateral ventricles. Inflammation and scarring in the ependyma from haemorrhage or infection can cause acquired obstruction of the fourth ventricular outlets. CT then shows the enlarged fourth, third and lateral ventricles but without hypoplasia of the cerebellum. This condition may be difficult to differentiate on CT from extraventricular obstructive hydrocephalus since the pattern of ventricular enlargement is the same in the two conditions. Many mass lesions can cause fourth ventricular obstruction, including extraventricular intra-axial neoplasms (astrocytoma, medulloblastoma, brain-stem glioma), abscess, cerebellar oedema, and extra-axial masses such as arachnoid cysts, chordoma and subdural haematoma (Harwood-Nash and Fitz 1976).

If both the aqueduct and fourth ventricular outlets are obstructed, as a complication of ventriculitis or intraventricular haemorrhage, the

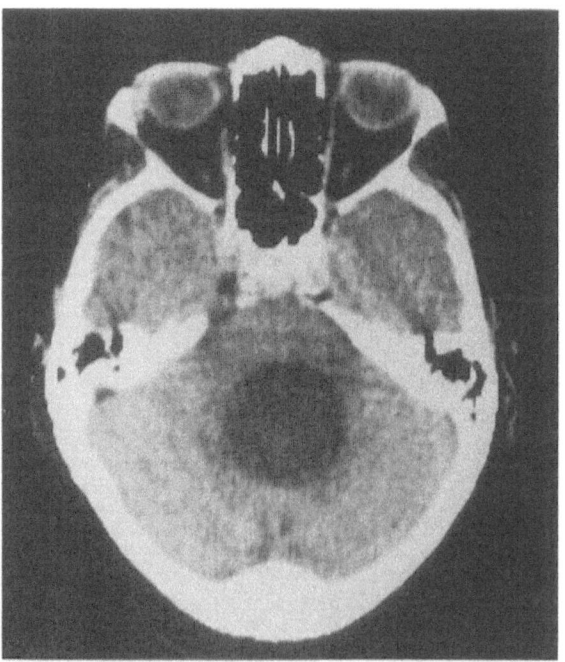

Fig. 3.5. Cranial CT. 'Trapped' fourth ventricle.

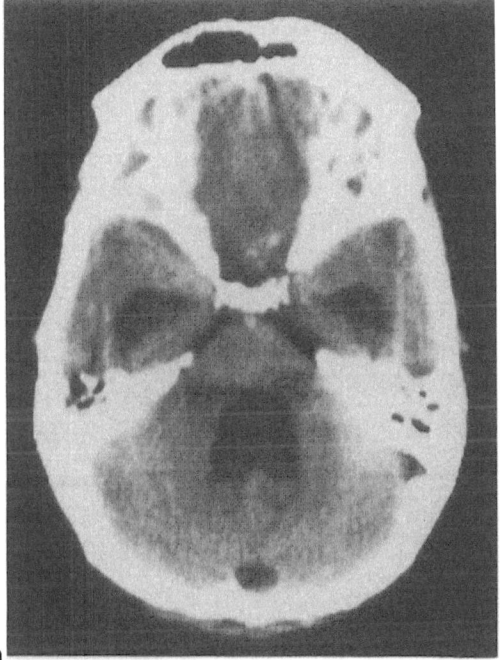
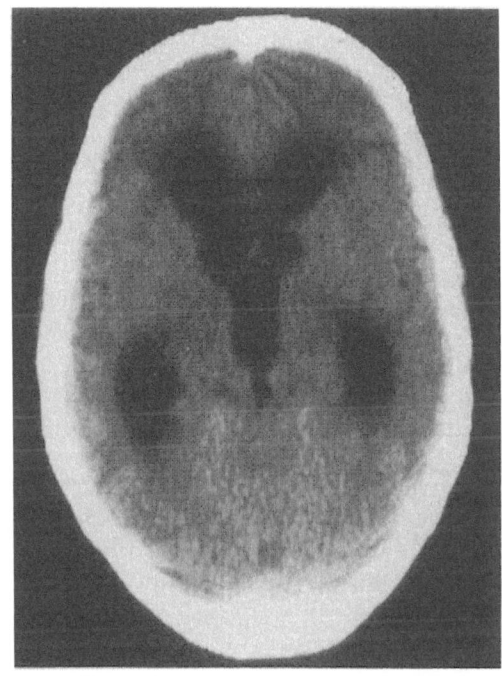

Fig. 3.6a and **b.** Cranial CT. Extraventricular obstructive hydrocephalus. There is enlargement of lateral, third and fourth ventricles.

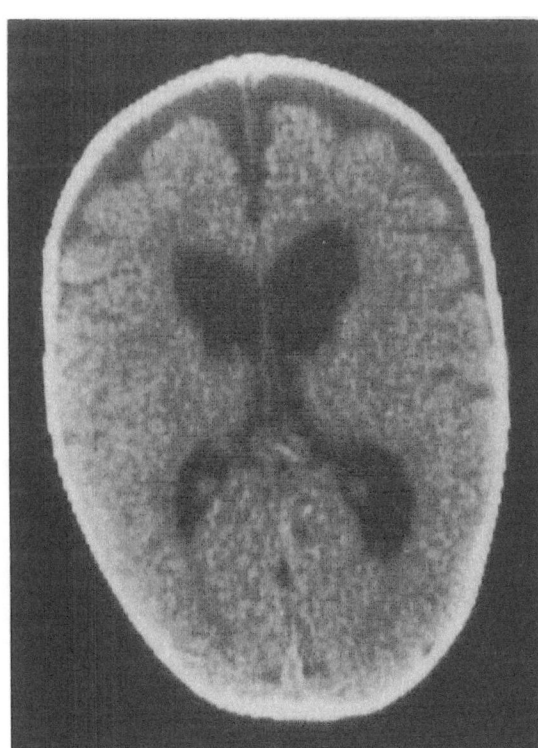

Fig. 3.7. Cranial CT. Bilateral subdural fluid collections.

fourth ventricle may enlarge even after the lateral ventricles are successfully shunted. This is referred to as an isolated or "trapped" fourth ventricle (Fig. 3.5).

Extraventricular Obstructive Hydrocephalus (EVOH)

In extraventricular obstructive hydrocephalus the block to CSF flow is distal to the ventricular system and occurs either at the skull base or at the Pacchionian granulations. Formerly the hydrocephalus was described as communicating hydrocephalus, that is, the ventricular system communicates with the extraventricular subarachnoid spaces. EVOH is a more accurate term. The aetiology is usually obliteration of the subarachnoid space or alteration of the arachnoid villi. In most cases the CT diagnosis of EVOH is not difficult. CT shows symmetrical enlargement of the lateral, third and often fourth ventricles and effacement of the cortical sulci (Fig. 3.6). There is, however, one area of potential diagnostic difficulty in children with bilateral subdural fluid collections who show enlarged cortical subarachnoid spaces and ventricles (Fig. 3.7). With this exception, the demonstration of enlarged sulci and ventricles usually excludes the diagnosis of hydrocephalus. The differentiation of cerebral atrophy from hydrocephalus and bilateral hygromas in children requires clinical information. A small head and a low tension fontanelle support the diagnosis of atrophy whilst an enlarging head and bulging fontanelle will suggest the diagnosis of a subdural haematoma.

Causes of EVOH (See Table 3.2)

The CT scan may show evidence of meningeal enhancement in meningitis (Fig. 3.8) or carcinomatosis, subarachnoid haemorrhage, evidence of trauma, or the classical defect in the enhanced straight or sagittal sinus in cases of sagittal sinus thrombosis (see Chap. 1). The deformed cranial vault in craniosynostosis, Hurler's syndrome (Fig. 3.9) or achondroplasia is readily detected. However, in the majority of patients with hydrocephalus CT provides no specific clues to the diagnosis.

Table 3.2. Causes of extraventricular obstructive hydrocephalus

Prior or current meningitis
Post-haemorrhagic
Trauma
Subarachnoid haemorrhage
Surgery
Subdural haemorrhage
Congenital lesions
Arnold–Chiari malformation
Lissencephaly
Basilar impression
Achondroplasia
Craniosynostosis
Hurler's syndrome
Meningeal carcinomatosis
Venous obstruction
Sagittal sinus or cortical vein thrombosis

"Normal Pressure" Hydrocephalus

This form of extra-ventricular obstructive hydrocephalus is a distinct clinical entity described originally by Adams et al. (1965). In their series a clinical triad of gait impairment, dementia and urinary incontinence was accompanied by evidence of hydrocephalus as shown on air encephalography.

The patients are usually between 50 and 70 years of age and are characterised on CT by ventricular enlargement without commensurate enlargement of the sulci. Unlike other types of obstructive hydrocephalus, the intraventricular pressure as observed at lumbar puncture is not usually elevated. However, intraventricular pressure monitoring shows intermittently raised pressure with a charac-

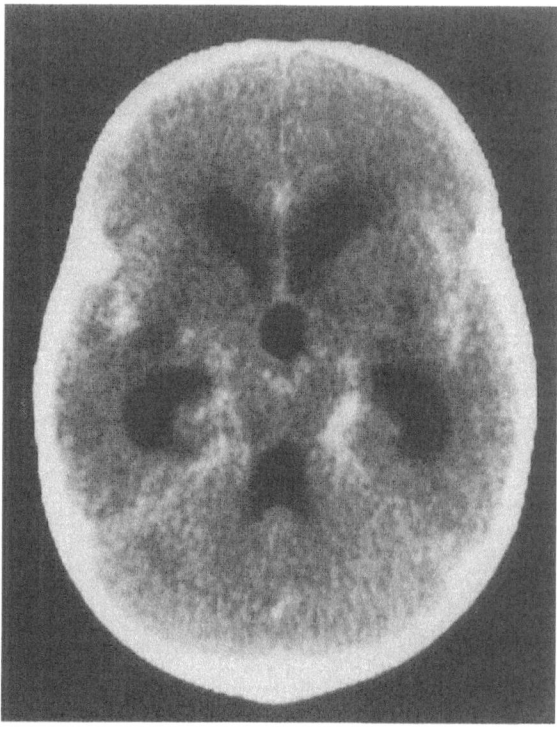

Fig. 3.8. Cranial CT after IV contrast. Tuberculous meningitis. Note the meningeal enhancement.

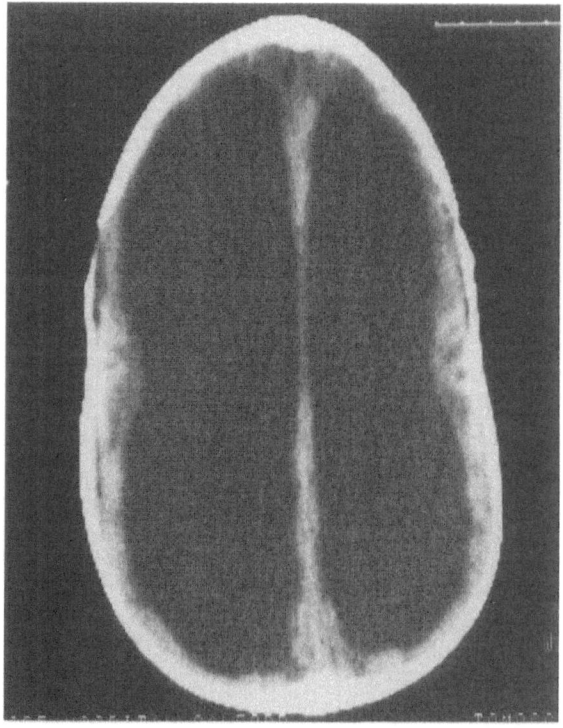

Fig. 3.9. Cranial CT. Hurler's syndrome.

teristic waveform. The CT diagnosis is made by evaluating the disproportion between ventricular and sulcal enlargement. Relatively prominent temporal horns are another typical feature but periventricular oedema is seen less commonly in normal pressure hydrocephalus than in other types of obstructive hydrocephalus. Additional studies using radioactive isotope cisternography and perhaps CT cisternography (Fig. 3.10) are occasionally required, in addition to continuous intraventricular pressure monitoring.

The symptoms may be relieved by ventricular shunting, with the most dramatic improvement usually seen in the gait impairment. Nevertheless, some patients do not respond to shunting and in these cases, the CT appearances are probably confused with those of cerebral atrophy. Therefore, cases lacking definitive CT and clinical findings are better classified as atrophy rather than hydrocephalus, since the best response to shunting is obtained in the unequivocal cases.

Untreated Hydrocephalus

The white matter is affected more than grey matter by the extent of hydrocephalus, as the latter is to some extent protected by its glial structure. The periventricular white matter becomes infiltrated with extracellular oedema fluid which is most marked in the immediate periventricular region (Fitz and Harwood-Nash 1978) (Fig. 3.3).

This extracellular periventricular oedema represents transependymal flow of CSF or ventricular CSF extravasation. The white matter resists damage for an uncertain period but then suffers disruption with axonal swelling and fragmentation, loss of axons and secondary loss of myelin. Ultimately there is severe white matter loss and gliosis.

Periventricular oedema is recognised on CT as blurring or loss of the normally sharp ventricular margins where the ventricles lie against the white matter (Pasquini et al. 1977). The blurring is usually most severe near the superolateral angles of the frontal horns, but may also be seen along the other portions of the ventricles that are adjacent to the white matter. The ventricular margins adjacent to the grey matter of the caudate nucleus are relatively spared until very late. Clinically, periventricular oedema is associated with acute and subacute hydrocephalus with high intraventricular pressures and impaired levels of consciousness, rather than with normal pressure hydrocephalus or chronic, relatively compensated hydrocephalus, e.g. aqueduct stenosis.

The ventricular dilatation is determined, in part, by the distensibility of the brain, dura, and cal-

varium that surround and support the ventricle. Greater distensibility of the ventricular walls (low "yield pressure") is associated with more rapid ventricular enlargement, earlier cessation of ventricular enlargement and larger final ventricular size, more rapid decline of intraventricular pressure and lower final pressure after compensation. Greater rigidity of the ventricular walls (high "yield pressure") is associated with slower ventricular enlargement, smaller final ventricular size, later decline of intraventricular pressure and higher final pressure after compensation.

The atria and occipital horns are often disproportionately dilated when compared to the frontal horns (Fig. 3.11). This has been attributed to the varying effects of hydrocephalus on grey and white matter and the variable distensibility of the vertex and skull base. The relative rigidity of the skull base restrains expansion of the frontal horns, whereas the vertex is distensible and thus permits dilatation of the atria and occipital horns. The grey matter surrounding the frontal horns is only slightly affected by the axonal fragmentation, myelin destruction and gliosis which occur with severe hydrocephalus. The atria and occipital horns are surrounded by white matter which is more susceptible to the effects of hydrocephalus. Progressive thinning of the cerebral mantle occurs with increasing ventricular dilatation. This change is attributed to stretching of axon fibres and sheaths passing around the dilated ventricles.

Attentuation of the ependyma and cerebral mantle by hydrocephalus may lead to focal dehiscence of the ventricular wall with formation of unilateral or bilateral pulsion diverticula of the ventricular wall (Fig. 3.12).

Treated Hydrocephalus

Successful intraventricular shunt therapy leads to a number of changes on the brain parenchyma which can be recognised on CT (Naidich et al. 1982).

1. Periventricular oedema regresses significantly or even disappears in the first few weeks after shunting. In cases of acute onset hydrocephalus this occurs more rapidly than in chronic hydrocephalus. The resolution of periventricular oedema, however, lags behind the clinical recovery.

2. The decrease in ventricular size after shunting is often asymmetrical, the shunt-containing ventricle being smaller (Fig. 3.13). Ventricles that are asymmetrically small secondary to shunting may return to an equal or larger size when the shunt system is removed or malfunctions. Shunt-

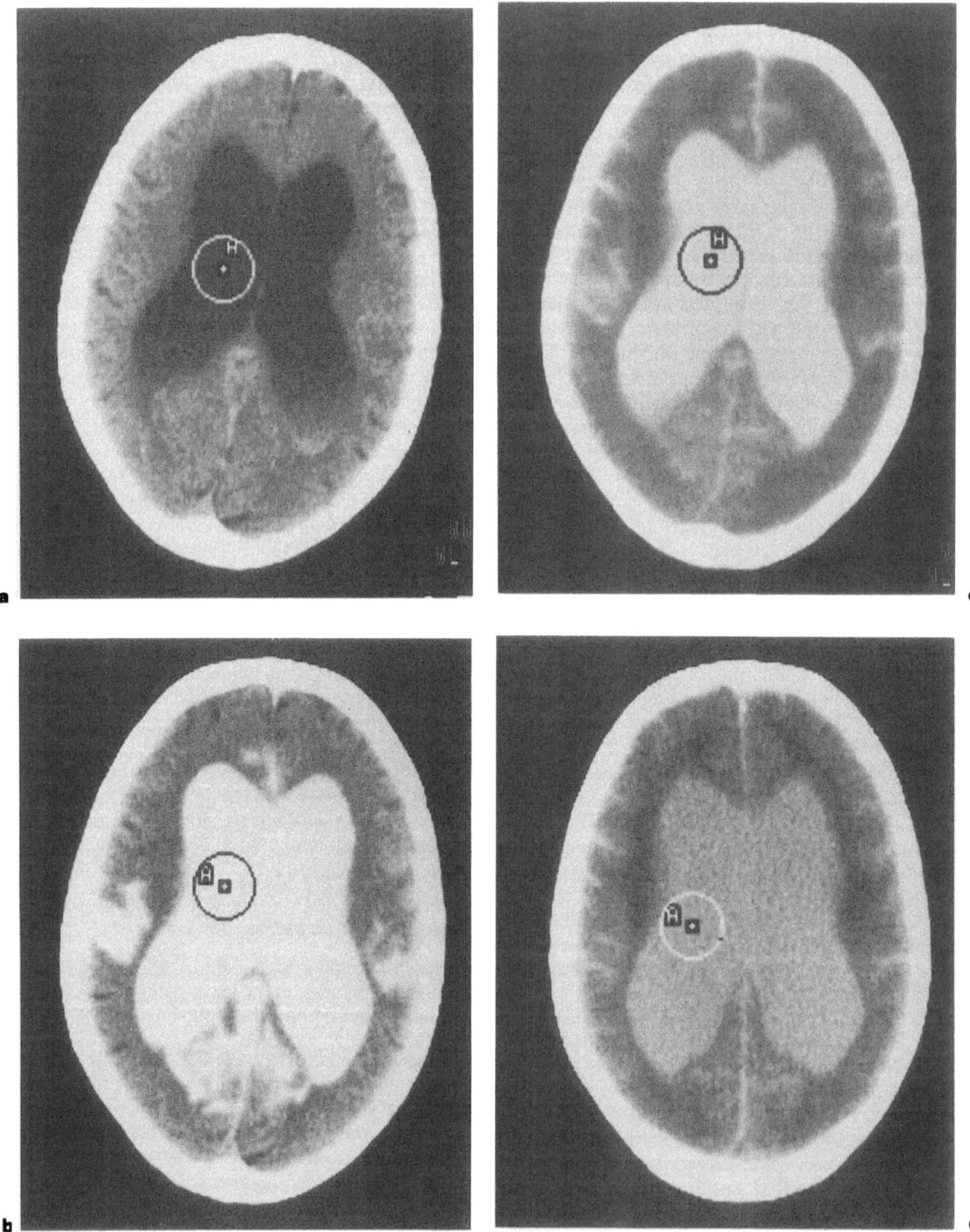

Fig. 3.10. CT cisternography. Normal pressure hydrocephalus: **a** 12 minutes, **b** 4 hours, **c** 24 hours and **d** 48 hours after an intrathecal injection of water-soluble iodinated contrast medium. There is abnormal retention of contrast within the ventricles at 24 and 48 hours.

induced haemorrhage with fibrosis may contribute to the inequality in ventricular size and may not permit symmetrical ventricular enlargement with shunt malfunction.

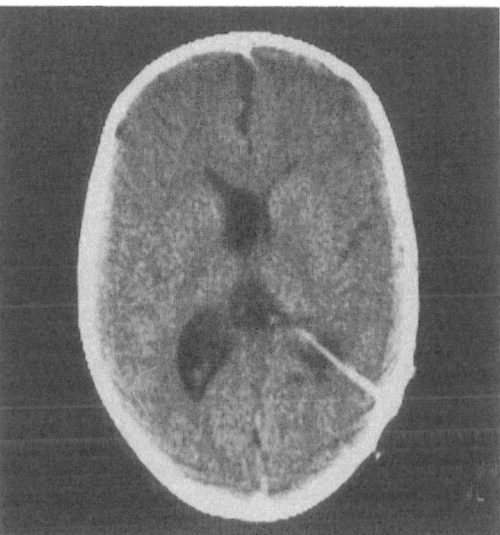

Fig. 3.13. Cranial CT. Hydrocephalus treated by shunting. The shunt-containing ventricle is smaller.

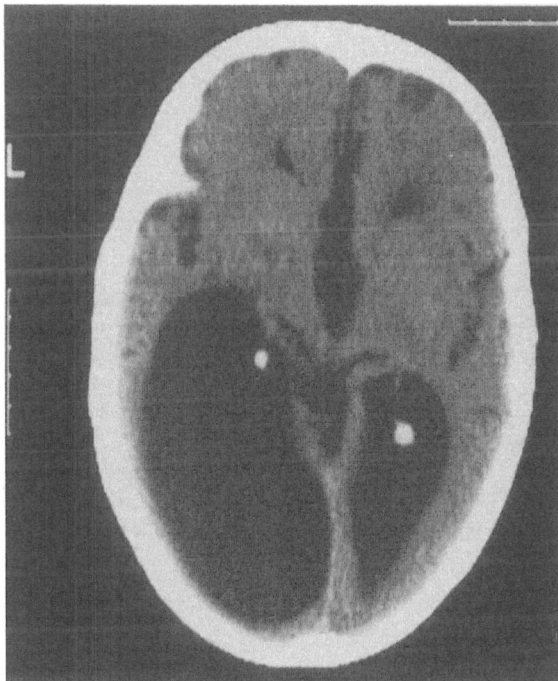

Fig. 3.11. Cranial CT. Untreated hydrocephalus. The occipital horns are grossly dilated, the frontal horns are minimally enlarged.

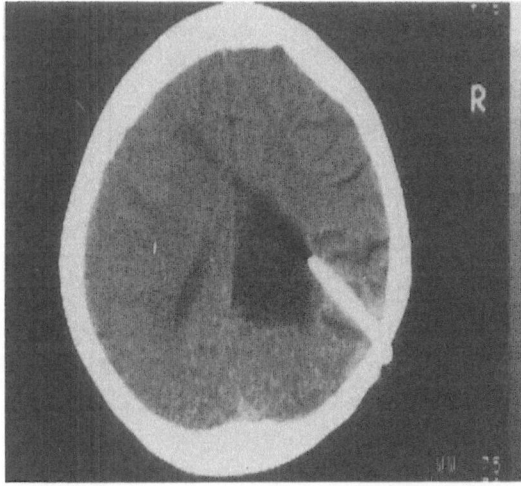

Fig. 3.12. Cranial CT. Treated hydrocephalus. The ventricular end of the shunt is within a pulsion diverticulum. The extracerebral CSF spaces of the shunt-containing hemisphere are larger.

3. The reduction in size of the frontal horns is often greater than that of the atria and occipital horns, as the grey matter rapidly returns to normal compared with the more severely damaged white matter. Shunting therefore often increases the disparity in size between the frontal horns and atria.

4. The cerebral mantle may increase in thickness after shunting in early hydrocephalus (Fig. 3.14). However, if treatment is delayed, irreversible changes occur which prevent the increase in mantle size despite effective reduction in intraventricular pressure.

5. The thalami move superomedially. The corpus callosum folds downwards. These changes result in small ventricles with sharpened lateral angles and an acute callosal angle, which is the angle subtended by lines drawn along the roofs of the lateral ventricle in the coronal plane.

6. The lateral ventricles may become nearly invisible. In such instances, there is absence of cortical sulci and formation of a diamond-shaped CSF space at the apex of the incisura, composed of the dilated confluent superior vermian and velum interpositum cisterns (Fig. 3.15). Patients with meningomyelocele and Chiari II malformation frequently exhibit upward transincisural growth of the so-called cerebellar pseudotumour (Fig. 3.15).

7. Fissures and sulci may appear to be widened, with focal or diffuse invagination of the cortical surfaces. The interhemispheric fissure widens

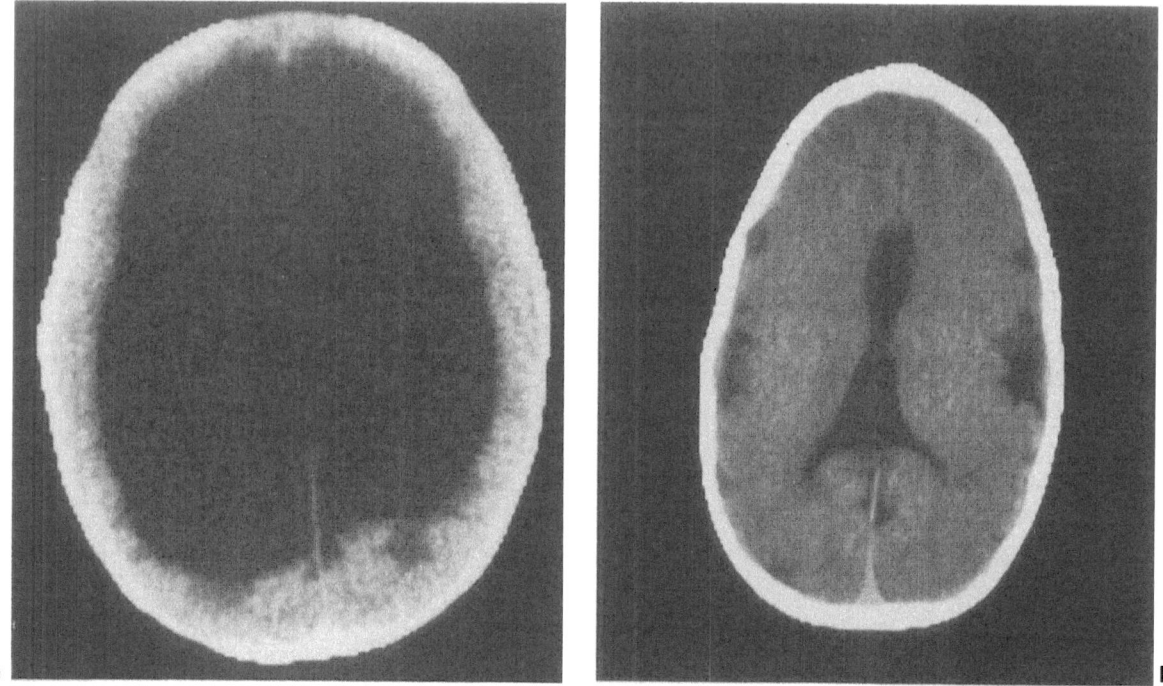

Fig. 3.14. Cranial CT. Lobar holoprosencephaly: **a** before and **b** 14 months after shunt insertion. The cerebral mantle has increased in size.

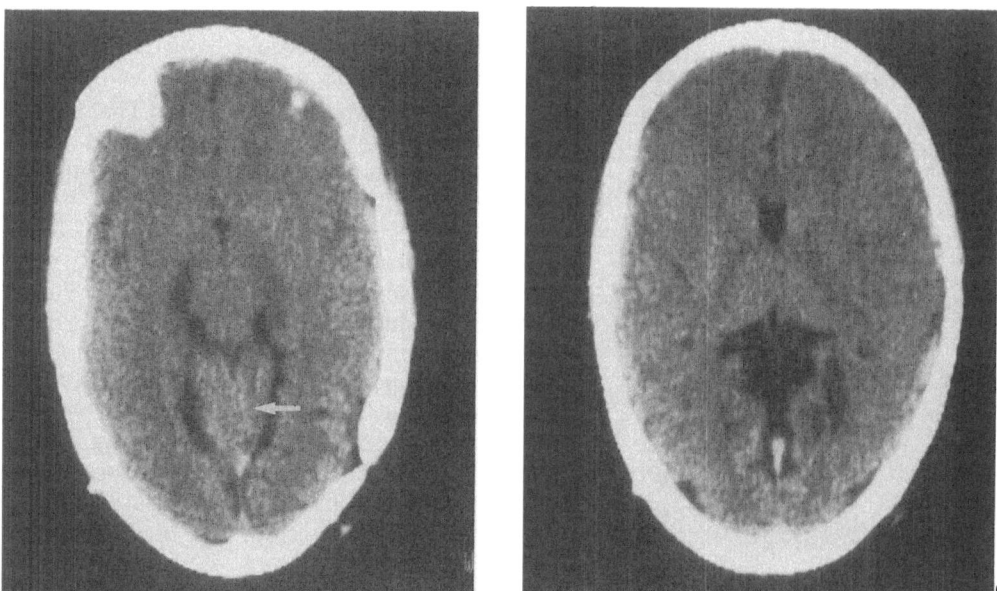

Fig. 3.15a and **b.** Cranial CT. Chiari II malformation. Note the cerebellar "pseudotumour" (*arrow*) due to upward herniation of the cerebellum and the diamond shaped CSF space formed by the superior vermian cistern and the cistern of the velum interposition.

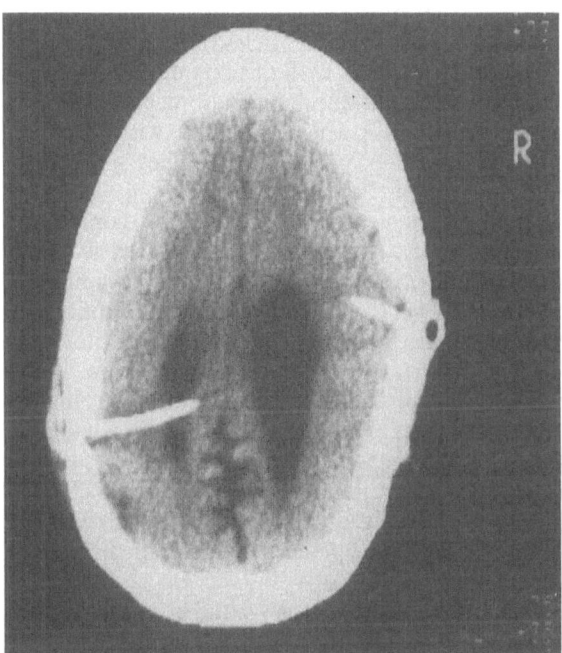

Fig. 3.16. Cranial CT. Treated hydrocephalus. The dilated posterior interhemispheric fissure is shown.

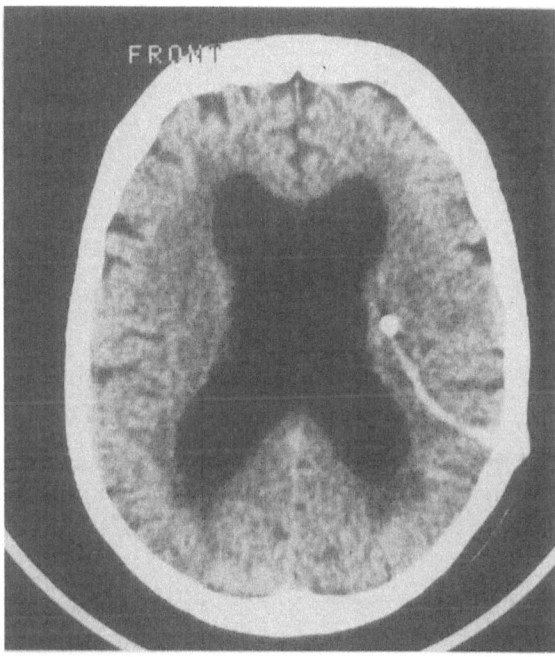

Fig. 3.17. Cranial CT. Extraventricular shunt.

just above the corpus callosum (Fig. 3.16). Large pools of CSF over the convexities usually signify that the brain cannot fill the intracranial volume created by previous calvarial expansion.

Intracranial Complications of Shunts

The shunt system consists of a proximal ventricular catheter that extends from the lateral ventricle through a burr-hole and a distal portion that continues into the superior vena cava, pleural or peritoneal cavities. The proximal portion is usually placed in the ventricle through the frontal or posterior parieto-occipital lobes to avoid inducing significant neurological deficit. Because hydrocephalic patients frequently have a fenestrated or absent septum pellucidum, it is not unusual to see the shunt catheter across the midline into the opposite lateral ventricle. Multiple intraventricular shunts may lead to ventricular loculation.

Shunt malfunction is not infrequent and is recognised by:

1. Renewed separation and bulging of sutures and fontanelles in children
2. Renewed periventricular oedema
3. Fullness of ventricular contours
4. Increasing size of the ventricular system

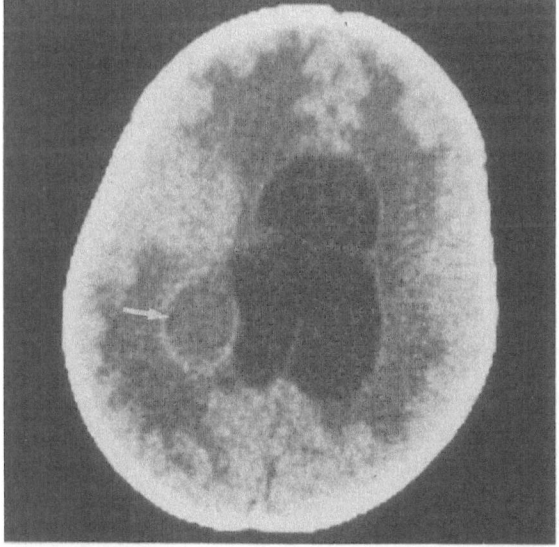

Fig. 3.18. Cranial CT. Shunt infection. The ventricular system is loculated and there is a periventricular abscess (*arrow*).

The causes of shunt malfunction include perforation of brain, haemorrhage, inspissated CSF and debris or adhesions following ventriculitis. The shunt may come to lie in the cerebral parenchyma (Fig. 3.17).

Shunt infection occurs in 2%–15% of patients which may lead to extensive intracranial sepsis (see Chap. 5) (Fig. 3.18).

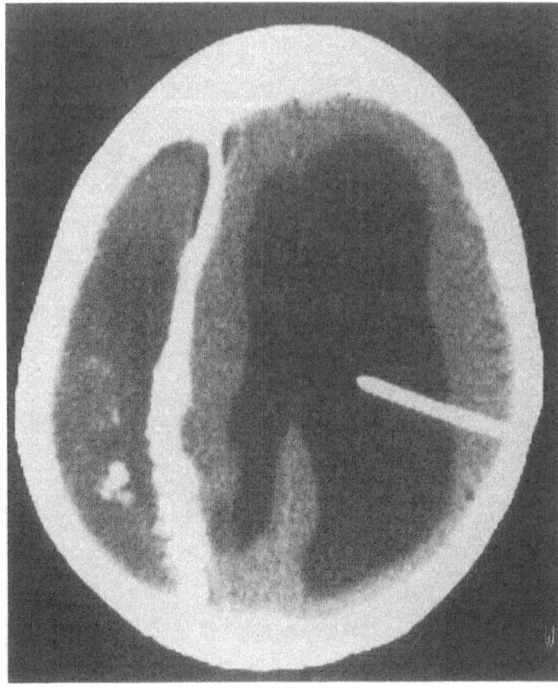

Fig. 3.19. Cranial CT. Calcified subdural haematoma.

the dependent posterior horns in 10% of patients. Rapid collapse of the ventricles may cause rupture of the bridging veins with ensuing development of small or large subdural haematomas. These are usually self-limiting but may enlarge with time and subsequently calcify (Fig. 3.19). They may also become infected (Fig. 3.20).

Subnormal ventricular size is commonly observed in asymptomatic patients after shunt insertion and does not necessarily signify shunt malfunction. However, patients who exhibit subnormal ventricular size at the time of a symptomatic increase in intraventricular pressure from shunt malfunction constitute a special group with higher ventricular yield pressures, and often subependymal fibrosis ("slit ventricle syndrome"). Since there is little ventricular dilatation in these patients, serial CT scans show little change from pre-revision to post-revision. These patients are predisposed to frequent shunt revisions.

Premature closure of sutures may follow decreased intracranial pressure and ventricular size. The calvarial plates abut or may override at the sutures (before the sutures fuse). Thickening of the calvarium occurs with premature fusion of the sutures if shunting is performed near the end of the

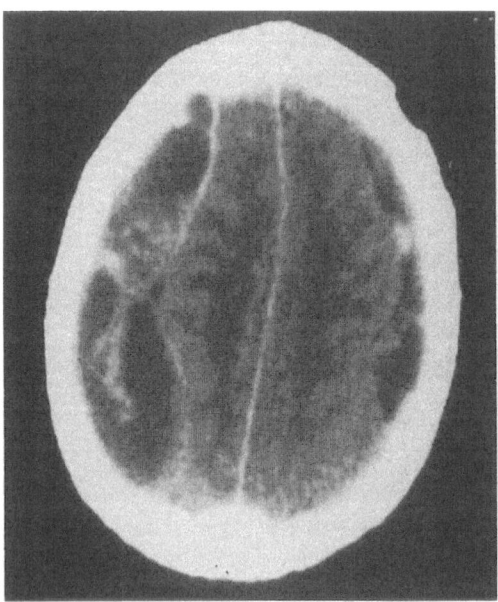

Fig. 3.20. Cranial CT after IV contrast. Infected bilateral subdural haematomas.

Adhesions may lead to trapping of the fourth ventricle or temporal horns.

Haemorrhage may occur at any point along the shunt track. Small pools of blood are found in

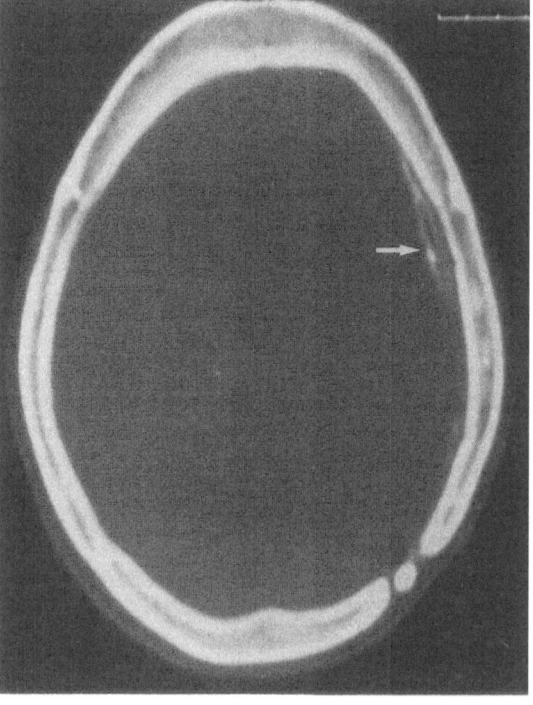

Fig. 3.21. Cranial CT. Calvarial thickening following prolonged shunting. There is also a calcified right subdural haematoma (*arrow*).

period of rapid brain growth or because of prior damage to the brain (Fig. 3.21). The bony changes are frequently accompanied by enlargement of the paranasal sinuses and other air-containing cavities.

Cerebral Atrophy

Diffuse

Cerebral atrophy is an irreversible loss of brain substance that results in enlarged ventricles and sulci (Hughes and Gado 1981). The physiological loss of brain substance with age is distinguished from the pathological processes resulting in cerebral atrophy by comparing the size of the ventricles and sulci with controls matched for age and sex.

The CT features of atrophy are non-specific and may be seen in a variety of conditions (Table 3.3). Sequential examinations may show rapid shrinkage in Alzheimer's disease and following severe closed-head injuries (see Chap. 4). Generalised enlargement of sulci and fissures with associated generalised ventricular enlargement produces the typical "cracked walnut" appearance of the brain (Fig. 3.22). In young and middle-aged patients, this appearance is assumed to represent degenerative disease. However, over the age of 65 years there is no relationship between dementia and measurements of ventricular or sulcal size as demonstrated on CT. Despite studies of ventricular volumes, diameters and indices, no CT criteria have been accepted for diagnosing dementia. The main benefit for performing CT in dementia is to distinguish cases of "normal pressure" hydrocephalus that may be treated by shunting, from atrophy or rare cases of an intracerebral mass lesion, e.g. a frontal tumour presenting with dementia. In most cases, hydrocephalus and atrophy are easily distinguished. The cases with enlarged ventricles and minimally enlarged sulci are probably better classified as atrophy if the false-positive diagnosis of hydro-

Table 3.3. Causes of cerebral atrophy

Normal
Alzheimer's disease
Creutzfeldt–Jacob disease
White matter degeneration
Cerebrovascular disease
Alcoholism
Trauma
Inflammation
Radiation
Chemotherapy
Hypoxia
Certain drugs e.g. phenytoin

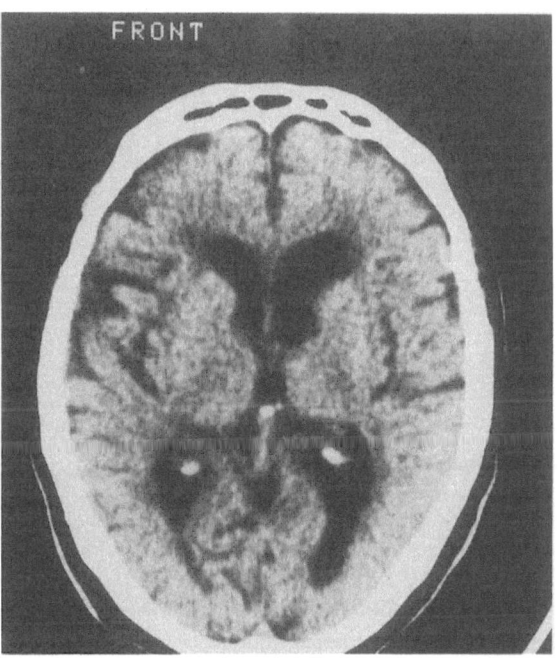

Fig. 3.22. Cranial CT. Cerebral atrophy.

cephalus is to be avoided. Atrophy appears to be the end stage of a wide variety, if not all, of white matter diseases.

Alzheimer's Disease

The commonest CT abnormality in this condition is the non-specific appearance of generalised ventricular and sulcal dilatation. The atrophic changes accentuate those of normal ageing. Recent studies have shown that ventricular changes are more sensitive to the degenerative effects of Alzheimer's disease than cortical changes, and that specific changes in the temporal lobes can be detected on CT and MRI (Le May 1986). Temporal lobe changes are highly sensitive markers of Alzheimer's disease, with a sensitivity as high as 97% and an overall accuracy as high as 80%. These changes include dilatation of the temporal horns, the presence of medial, lateral cortical atrophy and the presence of an area of decreased attenuation in the parahippocampal gyrus (Fig. 3.23). Pathologically this correlates with the memory disorder characteristic of Alzheimer's disease. Poor grey/white matter differentiation is another feature seen in Alzheimer's disease (George et al. 1981). However, the attenuation values of the brain parenchyma are not changed significantly in Alzheimer's disease.

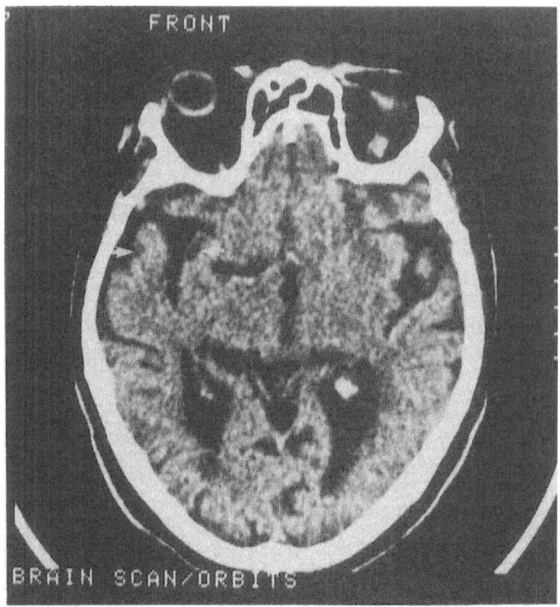

Fig. 3.23. Cranial CT. Alzheimer's disease. Note the symmetrical temporal lobe atrophy with areas of low density (*arrows*).

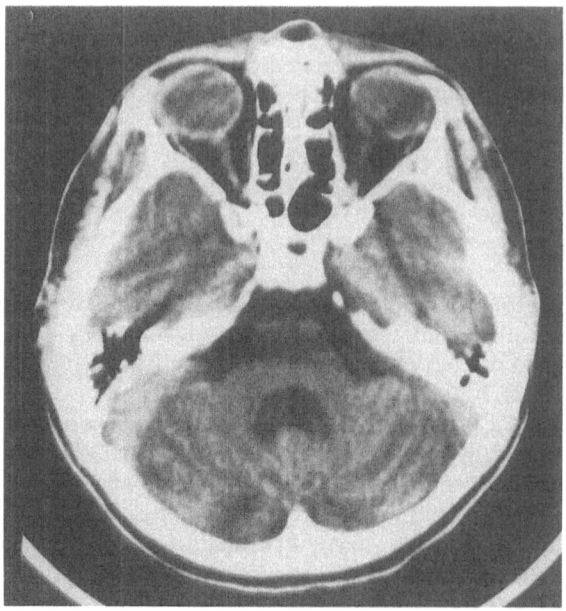

Fig. 3.24. Cranial CT. Cerebellar atrophy.

Reversible Changes Simulating Atrophy

In younger people, some cases of enlarged ventricles and sulci may be reversible and therefore, by definition, not attributable to atrophy. These conditions include anorexia nervosa, alcoholism, catabolic steroid treatment and some paediatric malignancies. These processes probably interfere with cerebral metabolism to produce a reversible loss of substance or water from the brain. There is a good correlation between the dosage of prolonged corticosteroid therapy and the degree of atrophy in young people (Bentson et al. 1978). Similarly ACTH and dexamethasone therapy in children result in changes of severe "cerebral atrophy" which is reversible on cessation of the therapy.

The "atrophy" seen in anorexia nervosa may be reversible if normal nutrition is restored.

Cerebellar Atrophy

Atrophy of the cerebellum and brainstem may occur independently of atrophy of the cerebral cortex and may not be clinically significant. The CT signs include enlargement of the superior cerebellar and cerebellopontine angle cisterns and lateral posterior fossa spaces, enlargement of the fourth ventricle and prominence of sulci over the cerebellar hemispheres. Atrophy of the brainstem and quadrigeminal plate is manifested by enlargement of the perimesencephalic and quadrigeminal cisterns respectively (Fig. 3.24). Cerebellar atrophy may be seen in the congenital cerebellar syndromes. The CT demonstration of cerebellar atrophy is particularly useful in patients with suspected masses of the posterior fossa.

Olivopontocerebellar atrophy produces atrophy of the inferior olives, pons and central cerebellar white matter. There may be associated lesions of the basal ganglia, dentate nuclei and spinal cord. Cerebellar parenchymal atrophy may result from the prolonged use of phenytoin and alcohol abuse.

Atrophy of the midbrain, brainstem and cerebellum may be seen in many degenerative conditions such as Pick's disease, Alzheimer's disease, Tay-Sach's disease, Wilson's disease and multiple sclerosis, etc.

Cerebellar atrophy may precede the diagnosis of Hodgkin's disease and may also be seen in other malignancies, particularly carcinoma of the bronchus.

Focal Atrophy

Focal changes may result from vascular, chemical, metabolic or traumatic injury to the brain. Without the history it may be difficult to determine the cause. The term focal atrophy implies contraction of a hemisphere or lobe with compensatory enlargement of the adjacent ventricle and sulci.

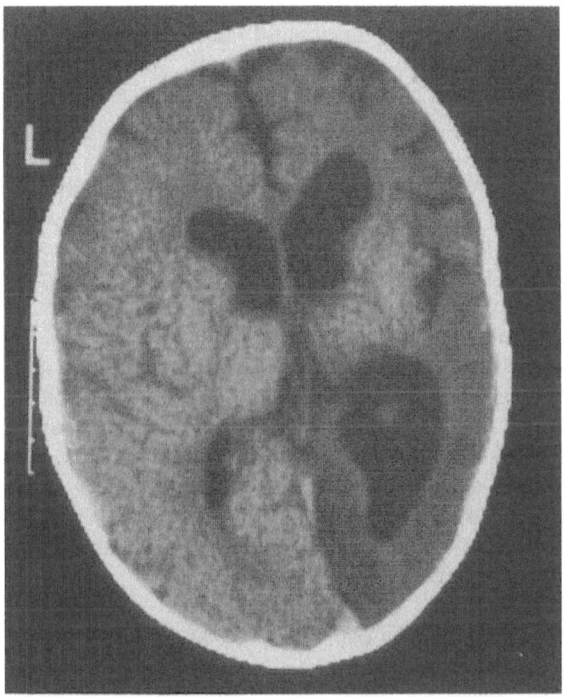

Fig. 3.25. Cranial CT. Right cerebral hemiatrophy. Male aged 8 years. Presumed perinatal vascular occlusion.

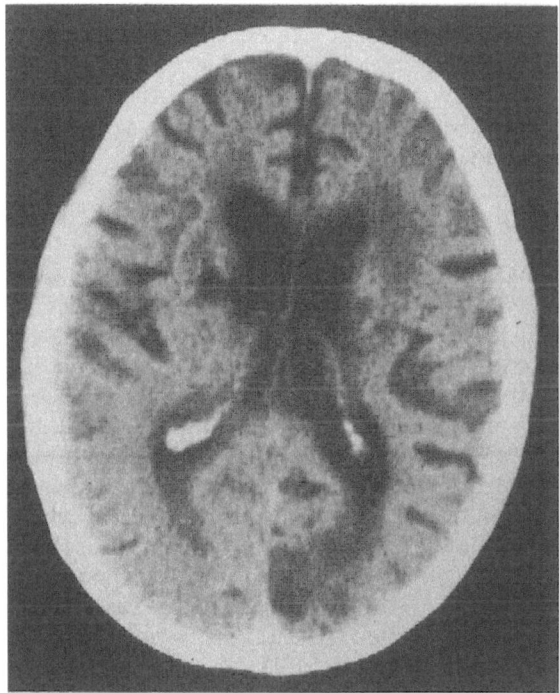

Fig. 3.26. Cranial CT. Multi-infarct atrophy.

The *Dyke–Davidoff syndrome* (atrophy of one hemisphere), may be the result of a subdural haematoma or other cerebral injury in early life. CT shows loss of brain parenchyma in the affected hemisphere. The ventricle and adjacent sulci are commensurately enlarged (Fig. 3.25).

Infarctions that occur in the distributions of the major intracerebral arteries usually cause atrophy limited to those territories.

Hemi-atrophy in later life also results from acute trauma, infection or vascular occlusion. CT shows a dilated lateral ventricle in the hypoplastic hemisphere and there may be dilatation of the third ventricle. The lateral ventricle, falx and pineal are shifted to the atrophic side. If the atrophy has been present for a long time, there may be calvarial thickening and enlargement of the paranasal sinuses. A large CSF-filled porencephalic cyst in continuity with the ventricle may be seen.

In *multi-infarct atrophy* there are multiple small areas of infarction in the white and grey matter with associated multifocal sulcal enlargement and generalised ventricular enlargement (Fig. 3.26). Multi-infarct dementia is usually associated with hypertension and dementia progresses in a stepwise or episodic fashion as opposed to the slow steady progression of Alzheimer's disease.

Pick's disease, which is a hereditary condition, presents as focal cerebral atrophy (McGeachie et al. 1979) with symmetrical areas of atrophy in the frontotemporal region sparing the posterior third of the superior temporal gyrus. The parietal cortex is seldom involved and the occipital cortex is always spared. The ventricular dilatation corresponds to the zones of cortical atrophy. This characteristic distribution of the focal atrophic changes should suggest the possibility of Pick's disease in the appropriate clinical setting.

Degenerative Brain Disease

The degenerative disorders of the central nervous system encompass a wide spectrum of diseases, in many of which a specific aetiology or biochemical basis has yet to be established. These diseases result in the loss or alteration of one or more components of the brain. They may be progressive or characterised by exacerbations and remissions.

The role of CT is twofold (Huckman 1982):

1. In some disorders the appearance may be diagnostic, precluding the necessity for brain-biopsy.
2. Specific disease processes, e.g. infarction or

tumour, which may initially produce similar clinical symptoms, can be excluded. CT may distinguish diseased grey and white matter from normal brain tissue. Almost all degenerative diseases will eventually demonstrate ventricular enlargement.

White Matter Degeneration

Demyelinating disorders result in increased water content of the white matter because myelin (rich in solids) is lost, leaving behind more hydrated material. The magnitude of change depends on the severity of the disease. The abnormally increased water content causes reduced attenuation values that can be detected as low density changes in the white matter on CT. In the late stages of demyelination, extreme shrinkage of the affected white matter may result, accompanied by gross cerebral atrophy. This may preclude the CT diagnosis of white matter disease in many advanced cases, since the final, common pathway is severe atrophy (Barnes and Enzmann 1981).

The high lipid content of normal adult white matter is responsible for its lower CT attenuation values (29–33 Hounsfield Units (HU)) compared to grey matter (35–40 HU). The white matter is less vascular than grey matter and contrast infusion increases the difference in attenuation values only slightly. White matter in the infant is significantly different from in the adult. Immature myelin has a much greater water content and demonstrates a typical low density on CT. Extensive myelination occurs in the first few months after birth and is virtually complete by the end of the second year, with identical attenuation values to those of adults. Magnetic resonance imaging has also contributed to the understanding of normal myelination in neonates and infants (Barcovich et al. 1988). After middle-age the total amount of certain myelin lipids decreases, and the cerebral hemispheres show increased water content. These changes appear as decreased attenuation of the cerebral white matter in CT scans of elderly patients.

Patterns of White Matter Degeneration

Degenerative disease of white matter may be detected on CT by changes in the frontal lobes, occipital lobes, the centrum semi-ovale and the internal capsule. Three patterns of CT abnormality in diseases of the white matter have been described (Heinz et al. 1979): demyelination, dysmyelination and a combination of these two.

In demyelinating disease (e.g. multiple sclerosis, anoxia, under-nutrition, progressive multifocal leu-

koencephalopathy) there is formation of normal myelin, which is subsequently destroyed.

In dysmyelinating diseases (e.g. metachromatic leukodystrophy and Alexander's disease) there is abnormal formation and maintenance of myelin as a result of enzymatic disturbance. Adrenoleukodystrophy has features of both types of disease.

The CT appearances of demyelinating disease is that of diminished white matter density, mass effect, and enhancement following high dose intravenous contrast, presumably due to inflammation at sites of active demyelination. Dysmyelinating diseases are less likely to demonstrate mass effect or abnormal contrast enhancement. Adrenoleukodystrophy shows large areas of low attenuation with peripheral advancing zones of gliosis that may show enhancement. The patterns of white matter degeneration which may be recognised on CT are listed in Table 3.4.

Table 3.4. Patterns of white matter degeneration

Focal symmetrical degeneration of white matter
e.g. adrenoleukodystrophy (see Chap. 6)
        disseminated necrotising leukoencephalopathy (see Chap. 6)
Focal asymmetrical degeneration of white matter
e.g. progressive multifocal leukoencephalopathy (see Chap. 5)
Periventricular degeneration of white matter
e.g. multiple sclerosis
Centrum semi-ovale pattern of white matter degeneration
e.g. chronic subcortical ischaemic encephalopathy
        hypertensive encephalopathy
Generalised white matter degeneration
e.g. Alexander's disease (see Chap. 5)
        anoxic encephalopathy
Basal ganglial degeneration
e.g. Wilson's disease
        Huntington's disease
        Parkinson's disease
        Leigh's disease
Central pontine myelinolysis

Multiple Sclerosis

This is the most common demyelinating disease. Three forms of the disease process are recognised: acute, chronic or relapsing. Clinically the condition presents initially with optic neuritis with subsequent paralysis, numbness, ataxia and tremor. The disease is characterised by frequent remissions and exacerbations.

CT abnormalities have been demonstrated in 33%–85% of published series. Three groups of CT abnormalities are recognised.

First, focal areas of reduced attenuation in the periventricular white matter (Fig. 3.27) which are

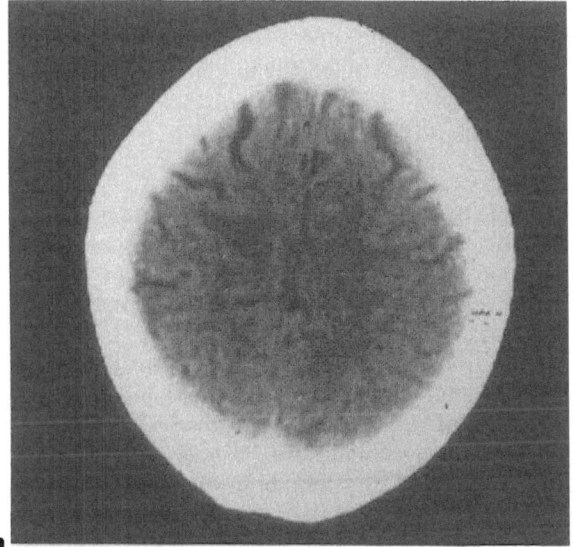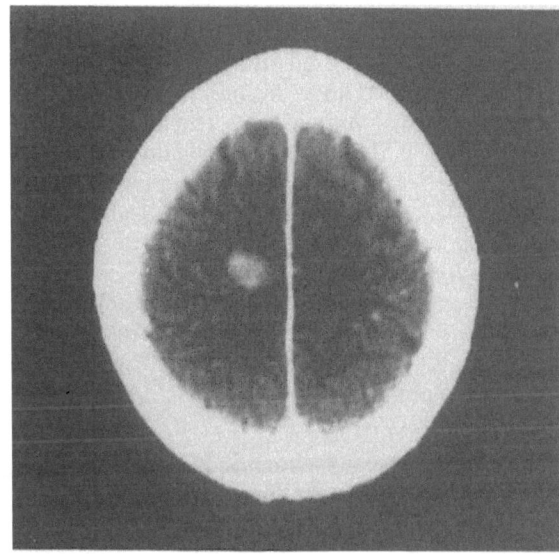

a   b

Fig. 3.27. Cranial CT. Multiple sclerosis: **a** before and **b** after IV contrast.

due to the plaques of demyelination. The attenuation value may be as low as CSF. The plaques are usually multiple and measure 5–70 mm. Multiple small confluent plaques may produce the larger lesions. In the acute phase a significant mass effect may occur. Many of the smaller periventricular lesions may be missed because of the partial volume effect (Haughton et al. 1979). Some plaques are permanent sclerotic lesions, unvarying over time, whereas others may resolve completely on subsequent CT scans.

Second, focal areas of contrast enhancement, which almost always correspond to the acute phase. This blood–brain barrier breakdown resolves spontaneously within days or weeks and is markedly ameliorated or abolished by administration of steroids. Usually small, round or ovoid and homogeneous but thick-walled ring-like lesions with associated mass effect have been seen (Van der Velden et al. 1979). These enhancing foci are located in the same general areas as the hypodense plaques and are most often of low attenuation precontrast (Fig. 3.27). Some may be isodense and are only shown by contrast infusion. Plaques that were only detectable on delayed or high-dose contrast enhancement have been reported (Morariu et al. 1980).

Silent asymptomatic lesions may be shown on CT. Conversely, severe neurological deficits may not have a demonstrable anatomical correlation because of the limited resolution of CT in certain sites, e.g. optic nerve, brainstem and cord.

Magnetic resonance imaging has a much more specific role in demonstrating the plaques of demyelination and is preferred to CT (Young et al. 1981). T2 weighted images are especially sensitive to the detection of plaques (Fig. 3.28) but such high signal

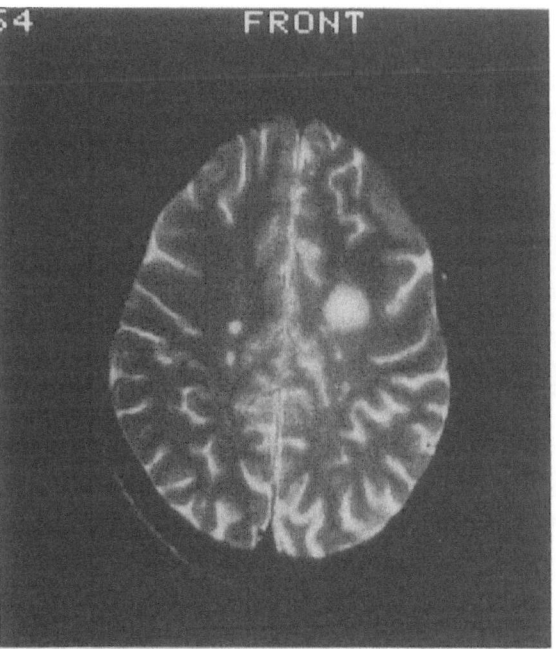

Fig. 3.28. Cranial MRI. Multiple sclerosis. Multiple periventricular high signal lesions consistent with plaques are seen on this T2 weighted image. (P.B.)

lesions are by no means specific for multiple sclerosis. Vascular or infective lesions can appear similar (see Chap. 1) and "unidentified bright objects" ("UBOs") are sometimes found coincidentally in ostensibly normal individuals. The diagnosis of demyelination is therefore an amalgam of clinical and investigative features. Enhancement with gadolinium DTPA may enable active lesions to be identified which are responsible for abnormal clinical findings (Grossman et al. 1986).

Third, cerebral atrophy – generalised ventricular dilatation – which is caused in part by diffuse, white matter shrinkage. Generalised sulcal dilatation is another common feature.

Chronic Subcortical Ischaemic Encephalopathy (Binswanger's Disease) (Binswanger 1894)

Binswanger's disease is a diffuse or multifocal destructive process in the central white matter, resulting from generalised ischaemic or vascular conditions and is associated with hypertension and dementia, and seizures. Pathologically the symmetrical and diffuse white matter lesions are associated with severe arteriosclerosis of the small penetrating arteries. CT demonstrates a diffuse, severe, incompletely symmetrical hypodensity of the white matter (Fig. 3.29), especially in the centrum semi-ovale and frontal lobes (Zeumer et al. 1980). There is no mass effect or contrast

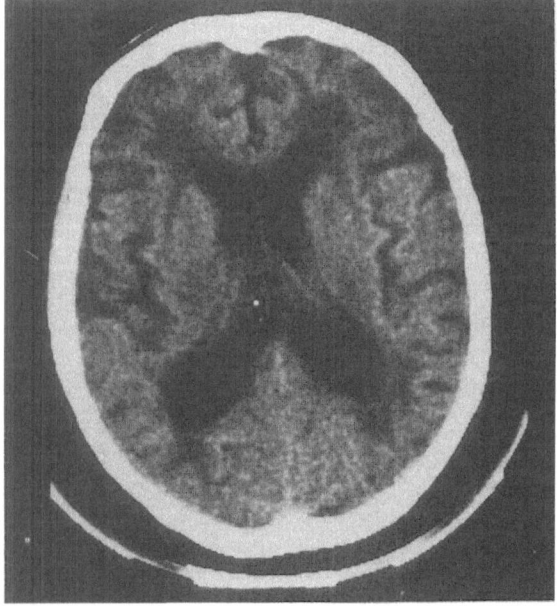

Fig. 3.29. Cranial CT. Chronic subcortical ischaemic encephalopathy (Binswanger's disease).

enhancement. Moderate generalised cerebral atrophy is invariably present, and lacunar infarcts in the basal ganglia and thalami are common.

Hypertensive Encephalopathy

CT shows extensive, symmetrical, well-defined hypodensity in the centrum semi-ovale, internal and external capsules and periventricular white matter. The ventricles are smaller than normal and may be effaced. These appearances are caused by the diffuse cerebral oedema.

In addition to these, decreased density in the centrum semi-ovale may be seen in most demyelinating or dysmyelinating diseases, storage diseases, viral encephalitides, progressive multifocal leukoencephalopathy metabolic disorders, intoxications, cerebral oedema, the ageing brain and hydrocephalus with periventricular translucencies.

Degeneration of the Basal Ganglia

Degenerative basal ganglionic diseases primarily involve the caudate nucleus, putamen and globus pallidus. These nuclei are readily visualised on CT.

Wilson's Disease (Hepatolenticular Degeneration)

CT findings are more frequent in patients with neurological signs. Dilatation of the frontal horns is seen in most cases. Areas of low attenuation are seen in the basal ganglia in 50%. This association is most characteristic of Wilson's disease (Nelson et al. 1979).

Huntington's Disease

This is a familial condition and affects primarily the caudate nucleus and putamen. The frontal and parietal cortex may also be involved but to a lesser degree. The most severe change is first neuronal loss and then atrophy of the caudate nuclei that gives the ventricles a characteristic appearance. CT scanning shows flattening of the lateral margins of the lateral ventricles, because the normal caudate nucleus impression on the ventricle is absent. When the cerebral hemispheres are not atrophic, the flattened caudate nuclei are easily recognised.

Parkinson's Disease

Although parkinsonism produces degeneration in the basal ganglia, CT shows no specific findings in the basal ganglia. Cerebral atrophy is often seen and is associated with a poor prognosis.

Leigh's Disease

This is a rare hereditary, progressive disease of infancy and childhood. Pathologically there is a spongy degeneration of the brain. CT findings of bilateral, symmetrical slit-like or irregular low attenuation regions in the basal ganglia or centrum semi-ovale without contrast enhancement are characteristic.

Central Pontine Myelinolysis (CPM)

This is a special category of white matter degeneration involving acute, pontine, demyelination (Messert et al. 1979). Patients have a history of alcoholism associated with hyponatraemia. CPM is also caused by overhydration and the administration of diuretic medications. The patients present with a rapidly progressive, pontine-level, neurological deficit (quadriparesis and pseudobulbar symptoms).

The characteristic CT appearance is of a central pontine low attenuation abnormality (Telfer and Miller 1979) (Fig. 3.30). High resolution CT is often required for its demonstration. The CT abnormality correlates with the pathological appearances of oedematous demyelination of the central ventral pons, with characteristic sparing of the tegmentum. The demyelination may extend cephalocaudally from the superior cerebellar peduncle to the inferior olive.

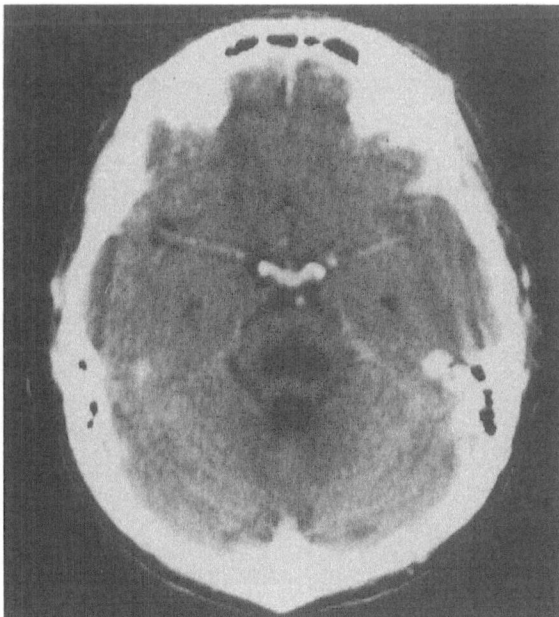

Fig. 3.30. Cranial CT after IV contrast. Central pontine myelinolysis.

MRI discloses similar pontine abnormalities which may be mimicked by infarction, tumour, demyelination or post-irradiation change (Miller et al. 1988).

References

Adams RD, Fisher CM, Hakim S (1965) Symptomatic occult hydrocephalus with "normal" cerebrospinal fluid pressure: a treatable syndrome. N Engl J Med 273:117–126

Atlas SW, Mark AS, Fram EK (1988) Aqueductal stenosis: Evaluation with gradient-echo rapid MR imaging. Radiology 169:449–453

Barcovich AJ, Kjos BO, Jackson DE, Norman D (1988) Normal maturation of the neonatal and infant brain: MR imaging at 1.5T. Radiology 166:173–180

Barnes DM, Enzmann DR (1981) The evolution of white matter disease as seen on computed tomography. Radiology 138:379

Bentson JR, Reza M, Winter J, Wilson G (1978) Steroids and apparent cerebral atrophy on computed tomography scans. J Comput Assist Tomogr 2:16–23

Binswanger O (1894) Die abrengzung der allgemeinen progressiven paralyse. Berl Klin Wochenschr 31:1103–1105, 1137–1139, 1180–1186

Dandy WE, Blackfan KD (1913) An experimental and clinical study of internal hydrocephalus. JAMA 61:2216

Evans WA Jr (1942) An encephalographic ratio for estimating ventricular enlargement and cerebral atrophy. Arch Neurol Psychiatry 47:931–937

Faerber EN (1986) In: Cranial computed tomography in infants and children. Spastics International Medical Publications, pp 82–98 (Clinics in developmental medicine no. 93)

Fitz CR, Harwood-Nash DC (1978) Computed tomography in hydrocephalus. Comput Tomogr 2:91–108

George AE, DeLeon MJ (1988) In: Haaga JR, Alfidi RJ (eds) Computed tomography of the whole body, 2nd edn, vol. 1. CV Mosby, St Louis, pp 313–333

George AE, DeLeon MJ, Ferris SH, Kricheff II (1981) Parenchymal CT correlates of senile dementia loss of gray/white matter discriminability. AJNR 2:205–213

Grossman RI, Gonzalez-Scarano F, Atlas SW, Galetta S, Silberberg DH (1988) Multiple sclerosis: gadolinium enhancement in MR imaging. Radiology 161:721–725

Gyldenstedt C (1977) Measurements of the normal ventricular system and hemispheric sulci of 100 adults with CT. Neuroradiology 14:183–192

Harwood-Nash DC, Fitz CR (1976) Hydrocephalus. In: Neuroradiology in infants and children. CV Mosby, St Louis, pp 609–667

Haughton VM (1985) Hydrocephalus and atrophy. In: William AC, Haughton VM (eds) Clinical computed tomography. CV Mosby, St Louis, pp 240–256

Haughton VM, Ho KC, Williams AL, Eldevik OP (1979) CT detection of demyelination plaques in multiple sclerosis. AJR 132:213–215

Heinz ER, Drayer BP, Haenggeli CA, Painter MT, Crumrine P (1979) Computed tomography in white matter disease. Radiology 130:371–378

Huckman MS (1982) Computed tomography in the diagnosis of degenerative brain disease. Radiol Clin North Am 20:169–183

Hughes CP, Gado M (1981) Computed tomography and ageing of the brain. Radiology 139:391–396

LeMay M (1986) CT changes in dementing diseases: a review. AJNR 7:841–853

LeMay, M, Stafford JL, Sandor T, Albert M, Haykal H, Zamani

A (1986) Statistical assessment of perceptual CT scan ratings in patients with Alzheimer type dementia. J Comput Assist Tomogr 10:802–809

Lorenzo AV, Page LK, Walters GV (1970) Relationship between cerebrospinal fluid formation, absorption and pressure in human hydrocephalus. Brain 93:679–692

McGeachie RF, Fleming JO, Sharer LR, Hyman RA (1979) Diagnosis of Pick's disease by computed tomography. J Comput Assist Tomogr 3:113–116

Meese W, Kluge W, Grumme T, Hopfenmuller W (1980) CT evaluation of the CSF spaces of healthy persons. Neuroradiology 19:131–136

Messert B, Orrison WW, Hawkins MJ, Quagliere E (1979) Central pontine myelinolysis: Considerations on aetiology, diagnosis and treatment. Neurology 9:147–160

Milhorat, TH (1975) The third circulation revisited. J Neurosurg 42: 628–645

Miller GM, Baker HL, Okazaki H, Whisnant JP (1988) Central pontine myelinolysis and its imitators: MR findings. Radiology 168:795–802

Morariu MA, Wilkins DE, Patel S (1980) Multiple sclerosis and serial computed tomography: Delayed contrast enhancement of acute and early lesions. Arch Neurol 37:189–190

Naidich TP, Epstein F, Lin JP, Kricheff II, Hochwald G (1976) Evaluation of paediatric hydrocephalus by computed tomography. Radiology 119:337–345

Naidich TP, Schott LH, Baron RL (1982) Computed tomography in evaluation of hydrocephalus. Radiol Clin North Am 20:143–167

Nelson RF, Guzman DA, Grahovac Z, House DCN (1979) Computerised cranial tomography in Wilson's disease. Neurology 29:866–868

Pasquini U, Bronzini M, Gozzoli E et al. (1977) Periventricular hypodensity in hydrocephalus: A clinico-radiological and mathematical analysis using computed tomography. J Comput Assist Tomogr 1:443–448

Pedersen H, Gyldensted M, Gyldenstedt C (1979) Measurement of the normal ventricular system and supratentorial subarachnoid space in children with computed tomography. Neuroradiology 17:231–237

Russell DS (1949) Observations on the pathology of hydrocephalus. MRC special report series no. 265. HMSO London, p 138

Svendson P, Duro O (1981) Visibility of the temporal horns on computed tomography. Neuroradiology 21:139–144

Telfer RB, Miller EM (1979) Central pontine myelinolysis following hyponatraemia demonstrated by computerised tomography. Ann Neurol 6:455

Van Der Velden M, Bots GTAM, Endtz LJ (1979) Cranial CT in multiple sclerosis showing a mass effect. Surg Neurol 12:307–310

Young IR, Hall AS, Pallis CA, Legg NJ, Bydder GM, Steiner RE (1981) Nuclear magnetic resonance imaging of the brain in multiple sclerosis. Lancet ii:1063–1066

Zeumer H, Schonsky B, Sturm KW (1980) Predominant white matter involvement in subcortical arteriosclerotic encephalopathy (Binswanger disease). J Comput Assist Tomogr 4:14–19

Chapter 4

Radiological Aspects of Head and Spinal Trauma

Evelyn Teasdale

Head Injury

Head injury is very common; most injuries are mild but severe head injury is a leading cause of death and disability in young men between the ages of 15 and 25. As many as 50% of severely head-injured patients die and many of the survivors have permanent neurological sequelae. It is estimated that one in a thousand of the population is disabled, to some extent, as a result of head injury. Accident and emergency departments, neurosurgeons, orthopaedic and general surgeons are primarily involved in the acute care of these patients but many will seek neurological advice at a later date due to persistent or new symptoms.

The criteria for both neurosurgical referral and computed tomographic (CT) scanning of head-injured patients are given in Table 4.1.

Skull Fractures: Significance

In an analysis by Teasdale et al. (1990) of 180 000 patients the presence or absence of a fracture and the patient's clinical state at the time of assessment in the primary hospital were related to whether or not the patient developed an intracranial haematoma. The results show that for all levels of consciousness, from fully conscious to deep coma, the presence of a fracture significantly increases the risk of the chance of a treatable intracranial haematoma (Table 4.2). In the group who are fully conscious with no history of post-traumatic altered consciousness and who do not have a fracture, the risk of haematoma is less than one in 30 000. If a fracture is present, the chance of a haematoma is increased to one in 81. Clinically these groups are identical and would fall into the "low-risk" group identified by Thornbury et al. (1987), but clearly the "real"

Table 4.1. Criteria for neurosurgical referral and CT

1. Fractured skull accompanied by any neurological sign or symptom
2. Coma continuing *after* resuscitation (even in the absence of a fracture)
3. Neurological deterioration
4. Confusion or other neurological disturbances persisting for more than 6–8 hours whether or not there is a skull fracture
5. Compound depressed fracture of the skull vault
6. Suspected skull base fracture or penetrating injury

Patients in categories 1–3 should be referred urgently

Note: In all cases the diagnosis and initial treatment of serious extracranial injuries takes priority over transfer to the neurosurgical unit.

Table 4.2. Risk rates for the development of an intracranial haematoma with the presence or absence of a fracture and the clinical state in adults and children

| | GCS 15 | | GCS 9–14 | GCS 3–8 |
	PTAC−	PTAC+		(coma)
No fracture	1:31 000	1:7000 (1:13 000)	1:180 (1:580)	1:27 (1:65)
Fracture	1:81	1:29 (1:160)	1:5 (1:25)	1:4 (1:12)

GCS, Glasgow Coma Scale: 8 or less = coma, 15 = fully conscious (Teasdale and Jennett 1974).
( ), Value of risk for children aged 2–15 years.
PTAC, History of post-traumatic altered consciousness.

risk of patients in this group varies widely; only those without a fracture can properly be described as "low risk". In patients who attend casualty with altered consciousness, but who are not in coma, the risk of an intracranial haematoma increases from one in 180 for those without fracture, to one in five for those with a fracture.

It seems clear that information about the presence or absence of fracture can significantly change the management of conscious patients or those with mild neurological impairment. Skull radiography is perhaps of least use in determining the management of patients in coma who should probably be referred for urgent CT whether or not the skull films show a fracture.

Various groups have attempted to identify the patients in whom skull radiography is indicated, in terms of cost and contribution to management (Royal College of Radiologists 1980; Thornbury et al. 1987). The guidelines, given in Table 4.3, were issued after discussion by a multidisciplinary group which agreed in principle with the findings of the Royal College of Radiologists (Fenton Lewis 1983). These guidelines do not specifically identify a group of patients in whom skull radiography is *not* advised, that is a "low risk" group, but give positive advice on who should be radiographed. The absence of such a "low risk" group is sometimes taken as a limitation of the guidelines. However, it is most important that for any individual patient there should be a careful assessment of the degree of force applied to the head. By so doing it is possible to identify a group of patients whose injury has been so trivial that significant head injury could not have resulted and the patient may be discharged, without skull radiography, into the care of a responsible adult, with the advice that they should return to hospital if any deterioration occurs. The advice concerning the value of skull radiography in the UK is very different from that in the USA (Cooper 1987) because of the vast difference in the availability of CT scanning. In the UK it is necessary to select high risk groups who are likely to benefit from neurosurgical care and skull films provide a much cheaper way of doing this than would scanning all head injuries.

Table 4.3. Criteria for skull radiography after recent head injury

Clinical status	Recommendation
Asymptomatic	No skull radiography – discharge with advice to responsible second person
No loss of consciousness (i.e. "low risk")	
Loss of consciousness or amnesia at any time	Skull radiography or immediate CT if appropriate
Neurological symptoms or signs	
CSF or blood from nose or ear	
Suspected penetrating injury	
Scalp bruising or swelling	
Difficulty in assessing the patient (e.g. alcohol, intoxication, epilepsy, children)	

A detailed discussion of the radiology of skull fractures is given in standard textbooks of radiology (e.g. Du Boulay 1980) and it is also noteworthy that CT scanning cannot be relied upon for the diagnosis particularly of linear vault fractures, although basal skull fractures are better demonstrated than on plain films (Macpherson and Teasdale 1989).

Complications of Skull Fractures

Cranial Nerve Palsies

Cranial nerve palsies are common after head injury.

Anosmia is present in about 7% of head-injured patients; it is temporary in about half the cases and can occur with or without a fracture of the anterior fossa. It may go unnoticed for many months and radiology is not indicated unless there is a co-existing leak of cerebrospinal fluid (CSF).

Blindness is less common. If there is marked proptosis then a haematoma within the orbit may be responsible and CT is indicated. A fracture at the level of the optic foramen is difficult to detect, even with CT, and disruption of the optic nerve itself is rare. Occipital injury can give rise to cortical blindness which may be detected only once the acute phase has passed and the patient can be properly assessed.

Skull base fracture may result in *ophthalmoplegia* due to nerves damaged by a fracture involving the superior orbital fissure. Third or sixth nerve palsies, if present, must be assumed to represent the secondary compressive effects of a mass lesion in the acute phase and urgent scanning is indicated. Facial palsy and deafness may be complications of petrous fracture and are dealt with in Chapter 9. An acute Horner's syndrome can be caused by a skull base fracture or trauma to the internal carotid artery with disruption of the sympathetic chain.

An *arteriovenous fistula or pseudoaneurysm* can develop in relation to tears of the meningeal vessels. These are usually of no significance but rarely can result in delayed or recurrent intracranial haematomas. The intracavernous segment of the carotid artery, damaged by a skull base fracture, can form a fistula between the carotid artery and the cavernous sinus (see Chap. 1) or more rarely a pseudoaneurysm. These may develop either in the acute phase of injury or some weeks later.

Meningitis is a common complication of compound fractures and fractures involving the skull base or paranasal sinuses. Radiology is rarely of value except to confirm the presence of a fracture, either by CT or plain film. *Cerebral abscess* can be a complication of penetrating injury particularly when this was not suspected initially, and so the patient may present some days or weeks later with signs and symptoms of an intracranial mass. The thin bone of the orbital roof is particularly vulnerable to unsuspected penetration in association with eye injuries. *Bony infection* is an uncommon primary complication although it may affect the edges of a craniotomy. A wound discharge will often be the first indication. Plain films show abnormalities only after there is established infection and isotope scanning may be the most useful test if the fracture or craniotomy is more than a year old.

A fistulous connection may develop between the subarachnoid space and either the paranasal sinuses, the Eustachian tubes, the external auditory meatus or the mastoid air cells. CSF *rhinorrhoea* may be present from the time of injury and in some instances will heal spontaneously. In others it develops sometime after the injury, or an *aerocele* may be produced after a bout of coughing or sneezing. Here air is forced through the fracture either into the subarachnoid space, parts of the brain weakened by contusions or haematoma, or into the ventricular system. In some cases repeated attacks of meningitis indicate the presence of an underlying fistula. Surgical repair is required if the CSF leak persists, if there is an aerocele or if there is repeated infection. Plain films and complex motion tomography may show a fracture but they cannot identify the site of the CSF leak. Isotope cisternography may be used especially when a leak is intermittent (see Chap. 11) but the simplest and most accurate method of determining the site of a CSF leak is by CT cisternography following the introduction of intrathecal contrast (Marel et al. 1982).

Bone Lesions

Most linear fractures undergo spontaneous healing and in children the skull remodelling is such that even depressed fractures may completely disappear. Sometimes bone fragments or the edges of a fracture are resorbed causing an area of lucency. Occasionally areas of skull lucency develop after head injury due either to an intradiploic haematoma or to fibrosing osteitis, an idiopathic and benign condition. Cephalohaematomas are a particular complication peculiar to the neonate. Blood clot forms under the periosteum, the raised edges of which may calcify. A history of birth or other trauma gives the diagnosis and radiology is not indicated.

Rarely a fracture will increase in size and a soft fluctuant swelling bulges through the defect. Such a "growing fracture" has a typical radiographic appearance with widening and smoothing of the previous fracture line although the edges may be

slightly sclerotic. The lesion is thought to result from tearing of the underlying dura and either a local arachnoid cyst develops or the pulsation of the CSF on the unprotected bone causes widening of the fracture. The CT scan may show areas of cerebromalacia with local porencephalic dilatation of the ventricle or arachnoid cyst; in other cases there is evidence of hydrocephalus. Clinical and radiological follow-up are required in such cases and surgical intervention may be necessary.

Primary Cerebral Injuries

Patterns of cerebral injury are indicated in Fig. 4.1.

Contusions. Contusions are cerebral bruises, usually found on the inferior frontal and inferior temporal lobes, and caused by contact of the brain against the skull base. They are the most common abnormality seen on CT in head-injured patients. They can occur on the same side as the impact, on the opposite side (contre coup), or locally under a fracture. They have a very varied radiological and pathological appearance which changes with time. Minor lesions may not be identified on the CT performed on admission but a few days later areas of reduced attenuation with slight local swelling can be seen in the typical sites. If the contusions have been more severe, areas of haemorrhage develop, involving the cortex, and if more severe still, the haematoma will extend more deeply into the white matter (Zimmerman et al. 1977). On CT these are seen as areas

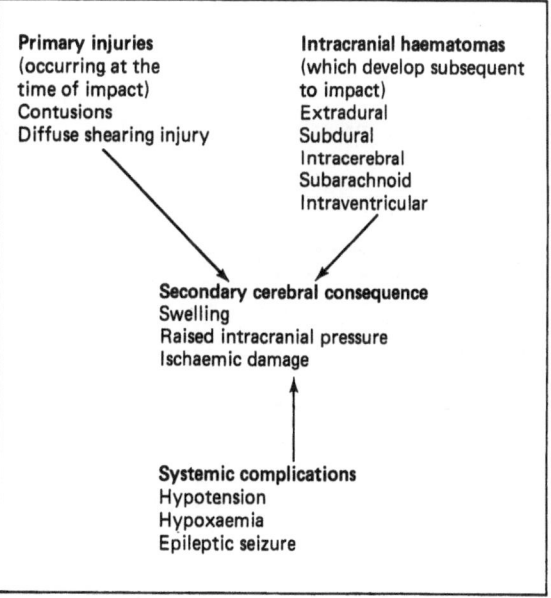

Primary injuries
(occurring at the
time of impact)
Contusions
Diffuse shearing injury

Intracranial haematomas
(which develop subsequent
to impact)
Extradural
Subdural
Intracerebral
Subarachnoid
Intraventricular

Secondary cerebral consequence
Swelling
Raised intracranial pressure
Ischaemic damage

Systemic complications
Hypotension
Hypoxaemia
Epileptic seizure

Fig. 4.1. Patterns of cerebral injury

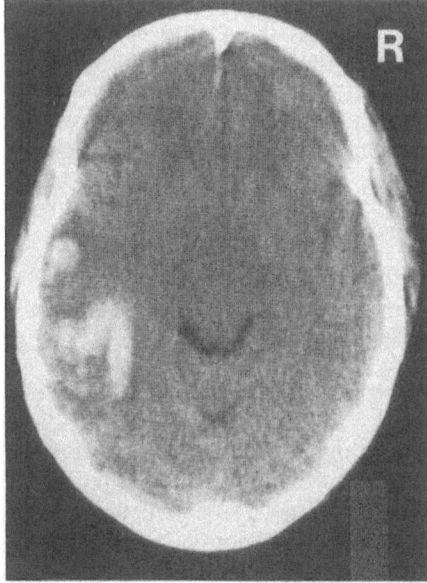

Fig. 4.2. Cranial CT. Haemorrhagic contusion.

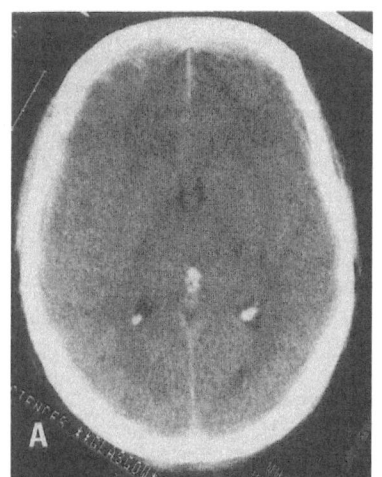

Fig. 4.4. Cranial CT. Right frontotemporal haemorrhagic contusion with adjacent extracerebral collections typical of the "burst lobe". The basal cisterns are compressed (*arrowheads*) and there is temporal horn entrapment (*arrow*) consistent with tentorial herniation.

of mixed high and low attenuation (Fig. 4.2). All contusions undergo increasing swelling which is maximal by 7–10 days, and this swelling may cause deterioration (Fig. 4.3). An extracerebral haematoma often accompanies severe contusion. This is usually a subdural or a large subarachnoid collection, and the lesion is called a "burst lobe" (Fig. 4.4). Surgical intervention is often urgently required.

Diffuse Shearing Injury. White matter axonal shearing injury was first identified by Strich (1961), and in severe fatal cases lesions can be seen histologically throughout the white matter of the hemispheres and brainstem. Small macroscopic haematomas may be found in the corpus callosum, the rostral brainstem and the cerebellar peduncle (Adams et al. 1977). Haematomas in the basal ganglia region, and small haematomas in the subcortical areas of the hemi-

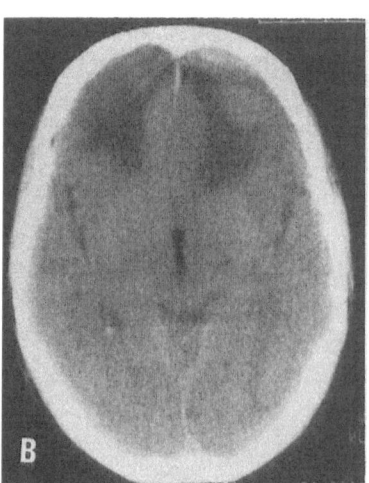

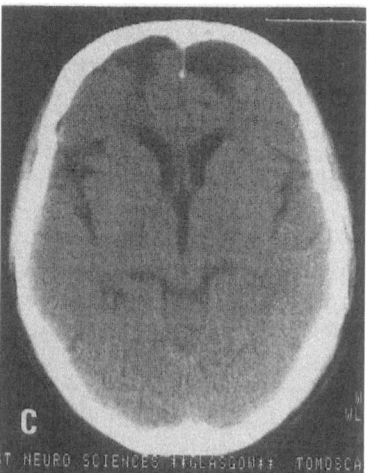

Fig. 4.3. Cranial CT. **a** Admission scan; **b** at 5 days; **c** at 6 months, showing bifrontal contusion which becomes more hypodense with the ultimate development of focal cerebromalacia and generalised cerebral atrophy.

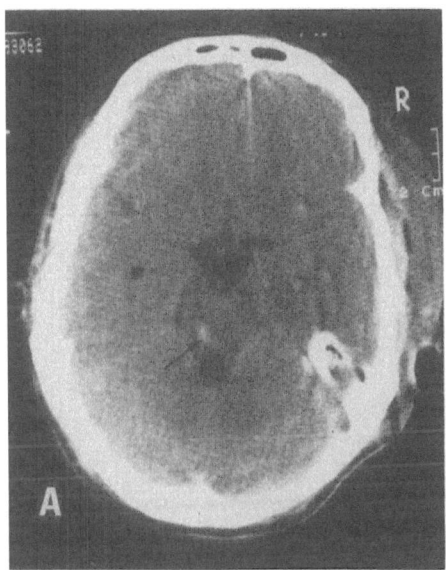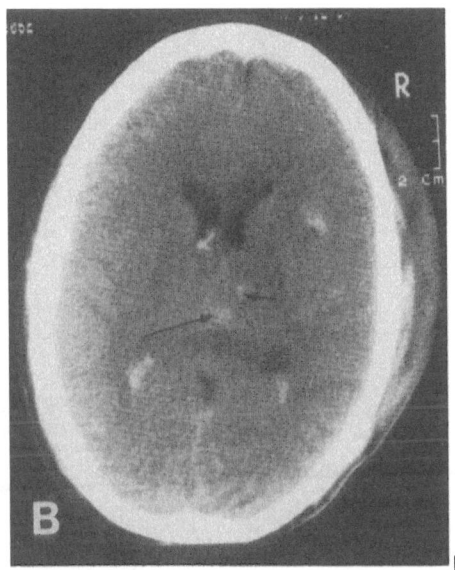

Fig. 4.5a and **b.** Cranial CT. Diffuse shearing injury. Small haematomas are *arrowed.*

spheres at the junction of the grey and white matter, ("gliding contusions") are frequently found in association with diffuse shearing injury (Zimmerman et al. 1978; Macpherson et al. 1986).

Severe shearing damage to the brain results from high-velocity injury, usually from road traffic accidents or falls from a height causing immediate coma or altered consciousness. The axonal disruption itself cannot be visualised on CT but the small haematomas may be. The pattern of lesions allows a presumptive diagnosis of diffuse shearing injury (Fig. 4.5). The haematomas in relation to the basal ganglia may be small or large but only rarely is evacuation undertaken because the patient's condition is due to the underlying diffuse primary damage.

Intracranial Haematomas

Extradural Haematomas

Extradural haematomas are the result of bleeding between the bone and the dura mater as a result of tearing of the meningeal arteries or veins or the dural venous sinuses. The haematoma is contained and defined by the displaced dural margin and almost 90% are associated with an ipsilateral fracture. Extradural haematomas are uncommon and account for only 5% of all traumatic intracranial clots. A patient suffering from an extradural haematoma was classically thought to show initial concussion then a lucid interval followed by deterioration. This is now known to be an excep-

tional pattern. Radiologically these haematomas show as biconvex uniformly hyperdense lesions based against the skull vault usually in the midtemporal and temporoparietal regions. They may occur in the floor of the temporal or anterior fossa and here, because of the axial plane of section of CT, may be confused with an intracerebral clot (Fig. 4.6). Occasionally low density is seen within the haematoma; this indicates that fresh bleeding is occurring (Fig. 4.7) (Paterson and Esperson 1984). Data from magnetic resonance imaging (MRI) indicates that tiny extradural collections are present with many vault fractures. Small clots demonstrated on CT may not require immediate evacuation but can be managed by observation and repeat scanning.

Subdural Haematomas

Subdural haematomas account for 50% of all intracranial clots, and almost half have an associated intracerebral clot. A fracture occurs in 70% but is ipsilateral in only half the cases. The haematoma occurs because of tearing of the veins bridging from the surface of the brain to the dura. The acute blood clot forms a crescent around the cerebral hemisphere lying within the potential space between the dura and the arachnoid. The pattern of ventricular compression produced is typical and diagnostic of a subdural collection even if the clot itself cannot be identified (Fig. 4.8). The anterior horn of the ipsilateral ventricle is displaced posteriorly, the

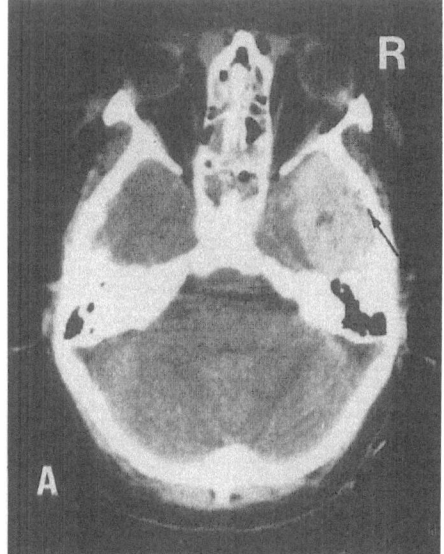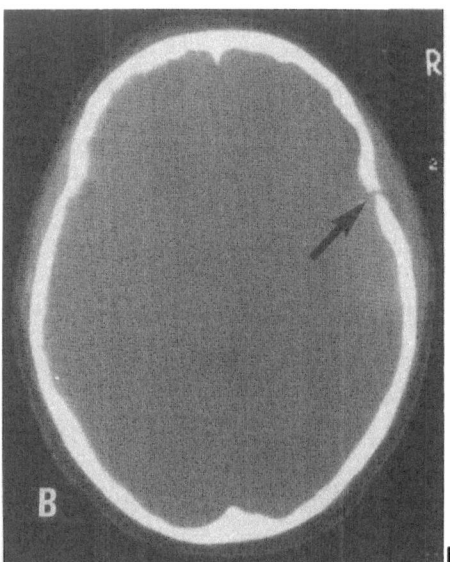

Fig. 4.6. Cranial CT. **a** Right subtemporal haematoma with small collection of gas (*arrow*) with **b** an associated fracture (*arrow*). The soft tissue in the ethmoid and sphenoid sinuses is blood and indicates a skull base fracture.

occipital horn or trigone is displaced anteriorly, and the whole ventricle is displaced towards the contralateral side. In the acute phase the haematoma is hyperdense on CT, but if removal is not required, or if the patient presents later, then the haematoma becomes isodense with normal brain at approximately two weeks; as the clot ages further, it becomes hypodense (Fig. 4.9). Rarely if the patient is anaemic or has suffered multiple injuries with much blood loss, the acute subdural haematoma can be isodense or hypodense. In a young patient a very thin subdural haematoma can be present with disproportionate midline shift. This is due to swelling of the ipsilateral hemisphere which can appear slightly hypodense and probably reflects ischaemic change. Removal of the subdural haematoma can also be associated with uncontrollable hemisphere swelling.

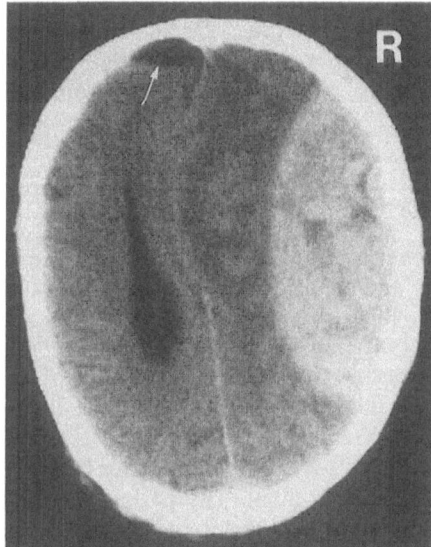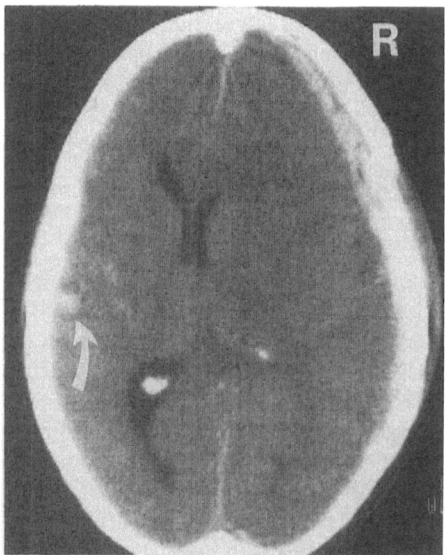

Fig. 4.7. Cranial CT. Extradural haematoma with low density indicative of active bleeding. Intracranial air is present (*arrow*).

Fig. 4.8. Cranial CT. Acute subdural haematoma in association with contralateral temporoparietal contusions (*arrow*).

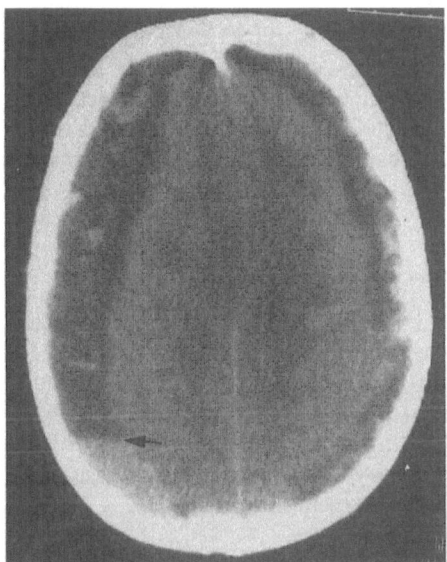

Fig. 4.9. Cranial CT. Bilateral subdural haematomas. Hyperdense clot is seen within the collections. A fluid level is *arrowed*.

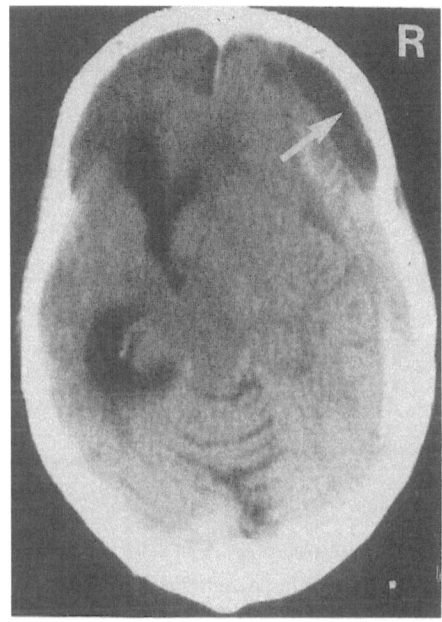

Fig. 4.10. Cranial CT. Acute on chronic subdural haematoma. The chronic hypodense collection is superficially placed (*arrow*).

Chronic Subdural Collections

The classical presentation of a fluctuating conscious level and increasing headache is rarely seen. Most patients present with progressive intellectual deterioration, progressive hemipharesis or with symptoms of raised intracranial pressure. In only half the cases is there a history of trauma and they are six times more common in men than women. They are associated with atrophy, epilepsy, alcohol abuse, or an intraventricular shunt and may be found in a patient with a congenital arachnoid cyst. At the time of presentation, CT usually demonstrates the chronic clot as a hypodense collection, but some show evidence of fresh bleeding, probably from the friable new vessels that form in the capsule of the haematoma (Fig. 4.10). Some of the collections are isodense with brain at the time of presentation and are identified primarily because of the pattern of ventricular displacement. As many as 17% may be bilateral and care must be taken not to misinterpret the scan as normal because the midline is central. The diagnostic signs are the absence of cerebral sulci, the absence, or compression, of the third ventricle, the posterior displacement of the anterior horns, and the medial displacement of the bodies of the lateral ventricles to give what are said to look like "rabbits' ears". All these CSF spaces would be expected to be large in the elderly atrophic brain prone to these lesions. Screening can be successfully undertaken with isotope scanning which is readily available in most hospitals and is accurate in detecting more than 90% of chronic collections. As with CT, unilateral clots are more obvious on the scan than bilateral collections.

Intracerebral Haematomas

Intracerebral haematomas have three main origins. They may develop within an area of contusion either acutely or over a period of 25–48 hours but, rarely, later. In severe acute contusions the haematoma may become the major feature (Fig. 4.11). The haematomas associated with diffuse shearing injury have already described above (p 88). The third type of haematoma is due to rupture of blood vessels within the cerebral substance. These haematomas are not related to surface contusions or collections and in many cases, on purely radiological grounds, are indistinguishable from spontaneous clots. A history of trauma, the presence of a skull fracture, and occasionally angiography, may point to the true nature of the collection. Clots developing after an initially "normal" scan are termed "delayed haematomas". This definition may depend on how soon after the injury the patient is scanned although this does not seem to be a practical problem. The great majority of all intracranial haematomas are present within hours of the injury and only very rarely does a delayed haematoma develop in a site which was completely normal on the initial scan (Gentleman et al. 1989). In any event

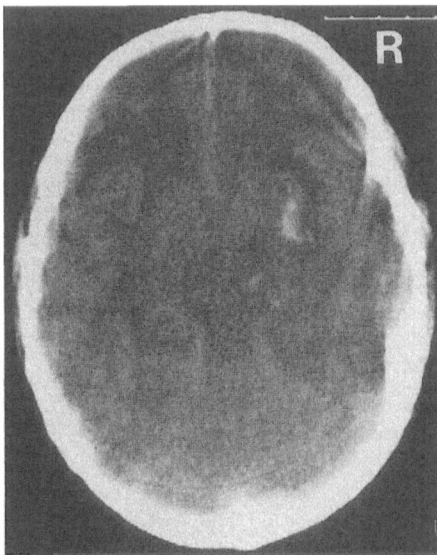

Fig. 4.11. Cranial CT. Haemorrhagic contusion and effacement of ventricles and basal cisterns due to cerebral swelling.

the development of a haematoma is associated with clinical deterioration; follow-up scanning is not indicated as a routine but only if there is deterioration or failure to improve as expected (Kobayashi et al. 1983; Statham et al. 1989).

Haematomas within the posterior fossa are uncommon (2%–3%) and the majority are associated with occipital fracture. Each type of haematoma can occur although most commonly there is a combination of cerebellar contusion/ haematoma with a surface collection. Small haematomas of the cerebellar peduncle are seen uncommonly even with high resolution scanning because of the artefact caused by the petrous bone. Cerebellar contusion can lead to subtle CT appearances (Fig. 4.12).

Subarachnoid Haemorrhage

Subarachnoid haemorrhage is a common consequence of head injury. The exact aetiology is unknown but is probably related to surface contusions or rupture of surface veins. Subarachnoid haemorrhage is a relatively common finding in the old and in the very young and it may be the only radiological sign of head injury.

Intraventricular Haemorrhage

Intraventricular haemorrhage is a common finding in severe head injury. It may result from contusions or intracerebral haematomas adjacent to the ventricle, from rupture of the choroid plexus or its attachments, or from tearing of the fornix or septum (Fig. 4.5). Hydrocephalus and raised intracranial pressure are common complications.

Secondary Consequences of Head Injury

Cerebral Swelling

Focal cerebral swelling is commonly associated with contusions and intracerebral haematomas. It is thought to be due to ischaemia secondary to local pressure. Unilateral hemisphere swelling is an uncommon occurrence but can be seen with extracerebral collections in young patients and is also thought to represent ischaemic change (Fig. 4.13). Focal or unilateral swelling is seen on imaging as an area of reduced attenuation with a secondary compressive effect. Diffuse swelling affecting both hemispheres is also uncommon and may be caused by either intra- or extracranial causes. Seizures, episodes of hypoxia or hypotension may all cause general swelling. The condition is commoner in children than in adults and it is not clear if it is due to an increase in blood volume (Bruce et al. 1981) or an increase in intracellular water; it probably results from a combination of these factors. Diffuse swelling is very difficult to diagnose by assessment of changes in the attenuation of the brain and is best determined by the mass effect produced.

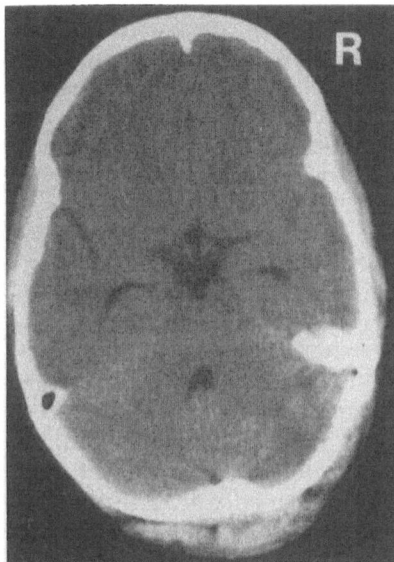

Fig. 4.12. Cranial CT. Right cerebellar contusion with compression and displacement of the fourth ventricle.

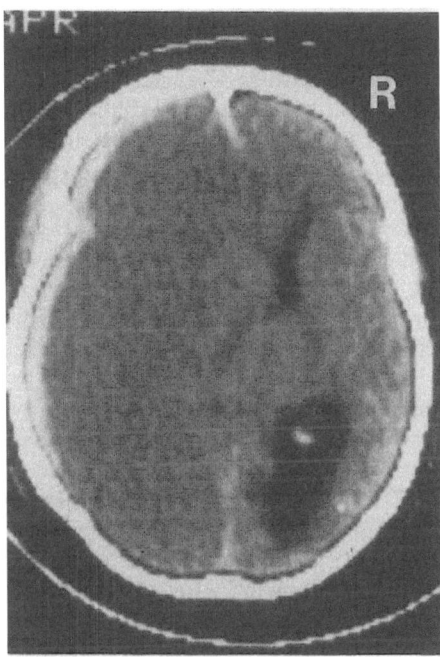

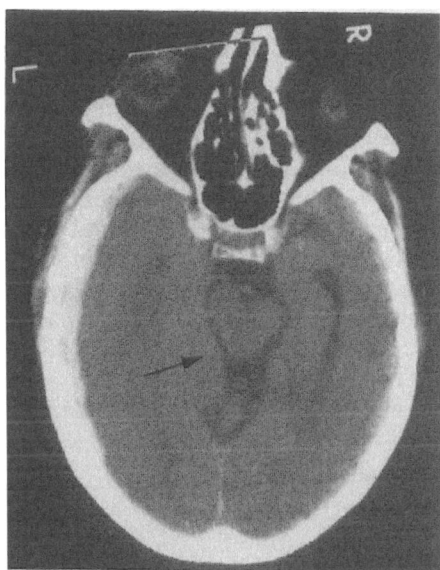

Fig. 4.14. Cranial CT. Left subdural haematoma with uncal herniation (*arrow*).

Fig. 4.13. Cranial CT. Diffuse left hemisphere hypodensity due to oedema and ischaemic change. There is a thin overlying crescent of subdural blood.

Raised Intracranial Pressure

Raised intracranial pressure (ICP) is a frequent consequence of head injury. It may be secondary to mass lesions or cerebral swelling or to the development of hydrocephalus. CT can detect shift of the cerebral contents, both laterally or in a craniocaudal direction and less commonly in the caudocranial direction.

Unilateral mass lesions cause lateral and downward displacement of the cerebral contents. As the midline is pushed over the brainstem rotates and is compressed against the tentorial notch on the contralateral side: the ipsilateral third nerve and brainstem are compressed by the uncus (Fig. 4.14). Transcallosal herniation is frequently found in association with increases in the mass effect. There is obstruction to the drainage of the CSF at the level of the foramen of Monro and the body of the contralateral ventricle dilates.

These changes accurately reflect the clinical signs of brainstem compression (Stovring 1977). The most sensitive first sign of such dilatation is enlargement of the normally small and crescent-shaped temporal horn. When there is generalised brain swelling or diffuse bilateral lesions there is craniocaudal shift but no side-to-side shift. The earliest sign of this is obliteration of the third ventricle, followed by obliteration of the basal cisterns. These appearances correlate with an ICP equal to or greater than 20 mmHg determined by intraventricular monitoring (Teasdale et al. 1984). Posterior fossa mass lesions or intraventricular haemorrhage commonly cause hydrocephalus with consquent increase in the intracranial pressure.

Ischaemic Brain Damage

Adams et al. (1977) found ischaemic brain damage in 90% of patients dying after severe head injury. Probably, with the exception of diffuse shearing injuries, all the other complications of head injury can result directly in some form of ischaemic damage but this can also occur in the absence of any other intracranial lesion. The ischaemic effect of local mass lesions and raised pressure are aggravated by systemic hypotension or hypoxaemia. CT is very poor at detecting the kind of diffuse ischaemic change usually seen at autopsy but focal arterial territory ischaemia is relatively common. This is usually in the distribution of the posterior cerebral artery if it has been compressed by an ipsilateral mass lesion. Much less commonly pericallosal artery ischaemia results from subfalcine herniation. The risk of developing such ischaemic change is increased in the presence of pre-existing arterial disease with prolonged tentorial compression, and by reduced cerebral perfusion from any cause. Arterial damage to the vertebral or carotid arteries in the neck or in the skull base can also cause focal arterial territory ischaemia. This is usually reflected by reduced attenuation in the distribution of the middle cerebral artery territory if the carotid artery is damaged. Angiography is not indicated unless there is evidence of continuing swelling in the neck (North et al. 1986). When there is severe reduction in the cerebral perfusion or oxygenation, areas of ischaemia develop along the boundary zones between the anterior and middle, and the middle and posterior cerebral arteries. These areas of ischaemia, in the frontotemporal, temporo-occipital and high parafalcine areas are rarely seen in the acute phase although haemorrhage into them may occur after resuscitation. They are most commonly seen in the late follow-up scans of head-injured patients as well-defined, low density areas of established ischaemic change. The pattern of ischaemia most commonly found at autopsy consists of small areas of cortical damage scattered throughout the hemispheres. Such ischaemic change is found in patients who have survived some time after cardiorespiratory arrest, severe hypoxia or severe elevations of ICP. CT can almost never identify these changes in head-injured patients which have also been reported in abused infants and in cases of near drowning (Cohen et al. 1985).

Imaging and Prognosis

The availability of CT has improved overall outcome in head injury, and so improved prognosis. Turazzi et al. (1987) reported on a large series of patients which showed that since the advent of CT there had been a reduction from 30% to 16% in the proportion of patients who had deteriorated from being conscious to being in coma at the time of operation.

A number of CT appearances have been shown to give information about the likely outcome and prognosis for the patient. Only the review by Van Dongen et al. (1983) gives information about the accuracy of these predictions. Both these authors and Lipper et al. (1985) considered that the combination of radiological appearances and clinical information gave a more accurate prediction of outcome than radiological features alone.

Focal abnormalities have some predictive value: unilateral lesions have a better outlook than bilateral lesions as do lesions without radiological signs of pressure. Lobato et al. (1983) have shown that features associated with a favourable outcome are (a) an isolated extracerebral haematoma, (b) a single contusion, (c) general brain swelling and (d) a normal CT scan. Poor outcome was associated with (e) cerebral hemisphere swelling after removal of an extracerebral haematoma, (f) multiple contusions, unilateral or bilateral and (g) evidence of

diffuse shearing injuries. Of patients in coma with a normal CT scan, only about one-third make a good recovery and a normal CT scan can occur with severe diffuse brain damage. The difference in outcome in these cases is not predicted by the CT scan but by the length of time for which the patient is in coma.

The state of the basal cisterns is a powerful predictor of outcome, with or without a mass lesion. This is presumably because it reflects the intracranial pressure which can itself be a good predictor of outcome. In one series (Toutant et al. 1984) 77% of patients with effacement of the cisterns died as did 39% of those with compressed cisterns but only 22% of those with normal cisterns. This study was performed on a single scan taken on admission. Van Dongen et al. (1983) looked at sequential CT scans taken over the period of the acute admission and also found the condition of the basal cisterns was an important prognostic factor. Another CT appearance which has been shown to be a predictor of poor outcome is the presence of intraventricular blood (Cordobes et al. 1983).

These studies suggest the most significant CT scan predictor of outcome is the detection of raised ICP. The "best" prediction will probably be obtained from a combination of the clinical and radiological appearances, observed serially over the first few days following injury.

Long-term Sequelae

Epilepsy is much commoner in patients who have had a depressed fracture or an operation, or who have had fits during the acute phase of their head injury. Radiological follow-up in these patients is usually unhelpful although the history of their acute episode may be very relevant.

Post-concussional syndrome comprises symptoms of headache, dizziness, failure of concentration and memory. These are increasingly recognised as reflecting minor diffuse injury but this cannot be determined from CT. Follow-up scans may show abnormalities in both these patients and in head-injured patients who have no complaints. There is thus no clear relationship between late CT abnormalities and the patient's complaints following head injury.

Cerebromalacia is the name given to areas of focal atrophy which occur at the sites of previous contusions or haematoma. It affects the cortex and the underlying white matter and lesions are found in the low frontal regions and at the temporal poles (Fig. 4.3). They may occur deep within the brain at the site of an intracerebral clot and can be seen related to fractures particularly if they were depressed.

Atrophy is one of the most common findings following diffuse head injury. Generalised cerebral atrophy involves not just focally traumatised areas but the entire cerebrum and often the cerebellum. There is sulcal enlargement and generalised ventriculomegaly without evidence of obstructive hydrocephalus. This is secondary to diffuse ischaemic or shearing injury (Fig. 4.3). Atrophy can also be seen in areas of the arterial watershed and arterial territory infarction may develop (p. 93).

Hydrocephalus is an uncommon late complication of head injury and is more likely if there was evidence of subarachnoid or ventricular haemorrhage in the acute stages. The condition is diagnosed on CT when there is disproportionate enlargement of the lateral and third ventricles compared to the size of the cerebral sulci. The temporal horns should also be involved in this dilatation, but this can be a local complication of temporal contusions and so may be a misleading finding. Reduced attenuation in the periventricular white matter is another radiological sign which may indicate the presence of obstruction to CSF flow.

Head Injury in Infants: Accidental and Non-Accidental

If severe head injury occurs in the first few years of life then the arrest or alteration of brain growth later causes secondary maldevelopment of the skull and plagiocephaly. Altered skull vault growth can also be associated with a subdural hygroma which is thought to result from tearing of the arachnoid membrane which allows CSF to accumulate in the subdural space. The fluid is unable to re-enter the subarachnoid space because of a valve-like mechanism. Hygromas occur mainly in the temporal regions in young children and result in local expansion of the temporal fossa with marked thinning of the bone. Although they may also occur in adults after head injury they almost never give rise to complications.

It is unfortunate but true that the major cause of head injury in children under the age of two is abuse by adults or other children. Unless there is clear objective evidence of accidental injury to a child who is not yet walking, non-accidental injury must be suspected. Physically abused children frequently suffer repeated episodes of injury and the majority of those who die do so as a result of the head injury. There appear to be poorly understood differences between the way that an infant brain responds to injury when compared to the older child or adult. Once the infant brain is damaged, growth in that area is severely retarded although function may be transferred elsewhere. The mechanisms of head injury in physical abuse also differ from those of accidental trauma. Severe shaking results in a 'whiplash' cerebral injury because the head is disproportionately large for the weak neck, and this alone can produce severe damage (Caffey 1974). Repeated insults and neglect of an abused child in coma make it more prone to the additional complications of hypoxia and hypotension from associated injuries.

There are CT appearances which may be accepted as virtually pathognomic of shaking injuries. Before high-resolution CT scanning, collections of blood seen along the falx were thought to be subdural in location (Zimmerman et al. 1979). With improved resolution it can be seen that many of these collections are in fact in the subarachnoid space, and diffuse subarachnoid haemorrhage is one of the commonest findings in such children. The parafalcine collections are almost certainly the result of shaking. Cerebral swelling, either focal or diffuse, can be found in over 60% of patients (Cohen et al. 1985). Occasionally the effects of very severe hypoxic injury can be seen when CT shows a diffuse reduction in attenuation of the cortical grey matter but with preservation of the grey matter in the basal ganglia region, cerebellum and brainstem. If these patients survive, marked gross central atrophy and ventricular dilatation develop rapidly which reflect irreversible brain damage. Cerebral lacerations associated with intra- and extracerebral haematomas result from impact and are equally common with or without a fracture. The cerebral contusion, so common in accidental head injuries in older patients, is much less frequent in abused children. Acute or chronic subdural haematomas should also suggest abuse, particularly in a child whose head diameter is above the 90th centile and whose developmental milestones are delayed (Figs 4.15 and 4.16).

Many of the surviving children go on to develop mental retardation, blindness, hydrocephalus and focal neurological deficits. The CT scan indicates much more severe and diffuse general atrophy than would be expected to have developed in an older child or adult after a similar insult and children over the age of five have a better prognosis than younger children or infants.

Other Radiological Investigations in Head Injury

Angiography may be required very occasionally to confirm the presence of bilateral subdural collections or to exclude aneurysmal rupture as a cause

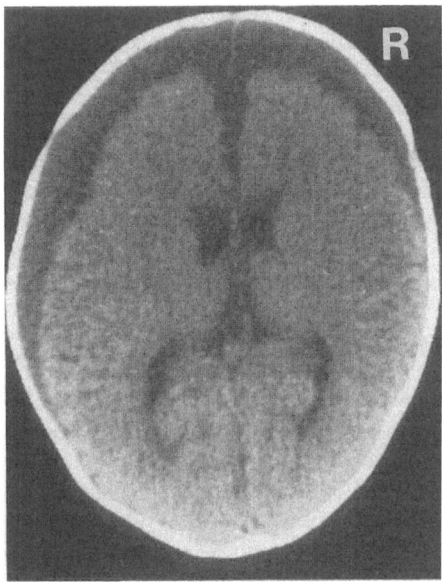

Fig. 4.15. Cranial CT. Child of 14 months. Bilateral large chronic subdural collections suspicious of non-accidental injury.

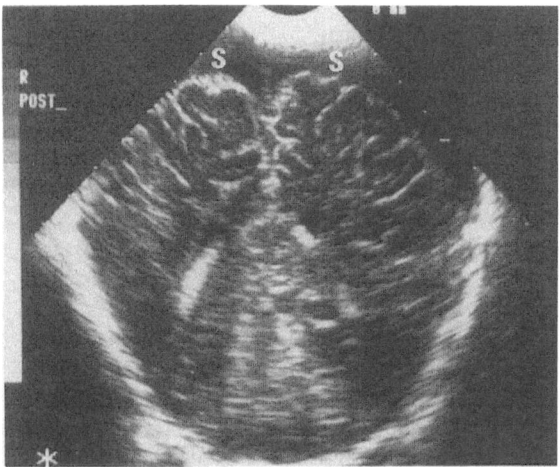

Fig. 4.16. Cranial ultrasound (same patient as Fig. 4.15). The bilateral subdural collections (s) are seen as hypoechoic regions.

of intracerebral or subarachnoid haemorrhage. It will also be necessary if a pseudoaneurysm or caroticocavernous fistula is suspected. In cervical injuries angiography is indicated in presence of a locally expanding mass (North et al. 1986) or if arterial dissection is suspected.

Radioisotope studies are of limited value in acute head injury because bruising of the scalp results in areas of increased uptake. They remain useful in screening for chronic subdural haematomas in the predominantly elderly population in whom this diagnosis is suspected.

Transcranial Doppler ultrasound of the middle cerebral artery may become more widely used as a method to monitor intracranial pressure in head-injured patients since changes in the waveform of the middle cerebral artery occur in raised intracranial pressure (Kirkham et al. 1987).

In the neonatal period ultrasound can be used through the patent fontanelle (Fig. 4.16). It is, however, much less informative than CT and many haematomas may be missed (Cohen et al. 1985).

Magnetic Resonance Imaging in Head Injury

If CT is available it is inappropriate to suggest MRI as the "first choice" examination in acute head injury. However, the few studies of MRI in acute head injury that are available (Zimmerman et al. 1986; Hadley et al. 1988; Hesselink et al. 1988) confirm that it can detect all the soft tissue lesions shown by CT. Indeed, because cortical bone has a low free water content and a stable lattice structure, it gives a negligible MRI signal so that contusions at all sites close to the bone are more clearly seen by MRI than by CT. Areas of acute haemorrhage were previously thought to be difficult to identify but can now be seen within a contusion by using carefully selected pulse sequences. Oedema in and around contusions is shown as areas of hypointensity on T1 and hyperintensity on T2 weighted images. The acute haematoma is identified as a hypointense area within the contused region of the T2 weighted images but by 7 days, in the subacute stage, clot is hyperintense on both T2 and T1 weighted images (Fig. 4.17).

In diffuse shearing injuries T2 weighted images often show many more areas of hyperintensity than are suggested by CT (Fig. 4.18). These are seen in the white matter of the hemispheres especially at their interfaces with grey matter, and corpus callosum and the long white matter tracts. Areas which appear normal on CT may show abnormalities on MRI. With high field high resolution systems some, but not all, of these tiny lesions have been shown to contain not only oedema but petechial haemorrhages. In some patients who have only briefly been unconscious after head injury, subcortical areas of hyperintensity are seen on the T2 weighted images. These observations support the view that diffuse hemisphere damage is responsible for transient unconsciousness after head injury (Jenkins et al. 1986; Levin et al. 1988).

The display of extradural and subdural haematomas by MRI is superior to that of CT (Fig. 4.19). This is because the clot never becomes isointense on all sequences and imaging can be carried out in direct coronal and sagittal planes

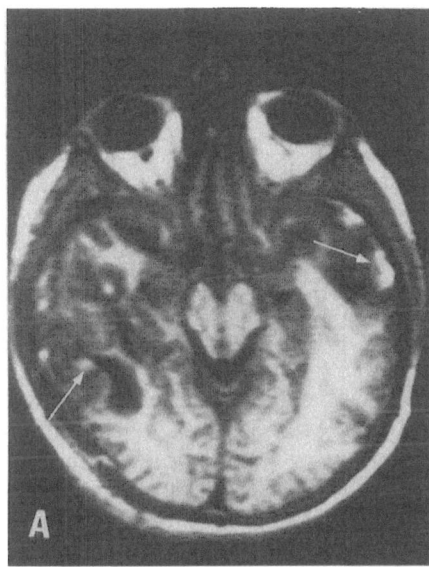 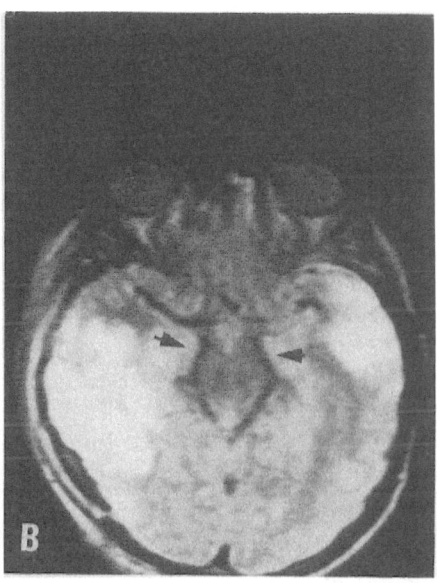

Fig. 4.17. Cranial MRI. Head injury. **a** T1 weighted scan showing hypointense oedema with hyperintense haematomas (*arrows*). **b** T2 weighted scan showing the oedematous contusion as hyperintense with bilateral uncal oedema (*arrows*).

without repositioning the patient. Subfalcine and uncal herniation can be easily seen in the coronal view.

MRI has also shown that small extradural haematomas are very commonly present in relation to fractures and that many more thin subdural collections are present than were found by CT. This is

because the difference in density of the peripheral high density clot adjacent to the high density bone may not be appreciated on CT, whereas on MRI the signal differences are such that the clot is readily discriminated against the very low signal from cortical bone. Despite the increased sensitivity of detection of MRI, surgically significant lesions are not missed by CT. If MRI is so sensitive for the diagnosis of subdural collections it may be argued that

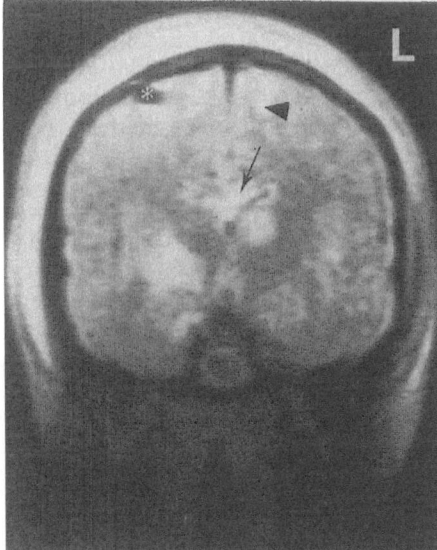

Fig. 4.18. Cranial MRI. Head injury. The T2 weighted coronal scan shows a hyperintense corpus callosum shearing lesion (*arrow*) with bilateral basal ganglial lesions. A left parafalcine gliding contusion is also seen (*arrowhead*). The *asterisk* indicates a subdural pressure monitor.

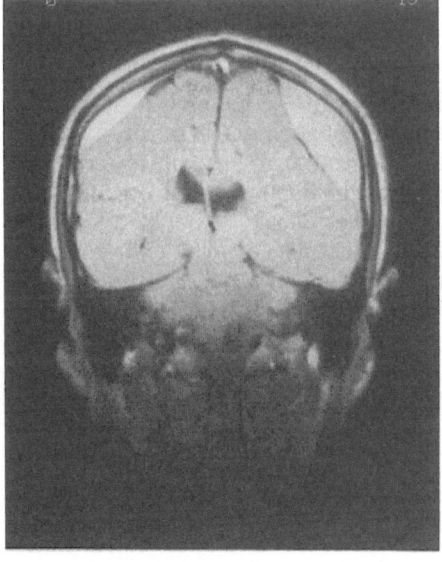

Fig. 4.19. Cranial MRI. This slightly T2 weighted coronal image shows bilateral subdural collections of different ages.

it should be the examination of choice when they are suspected, particularly as the subacute lesions may be isointense and difficult to diagnose on CT. It is unlikely that MRI will become so universally available as to become the examination of choice when screening for these lesions at least in the near future. The role of MRI in the diagnosis of intra-cerebral haemorrhage is discussed in Chapter 1.

It has proved difficult to demonstrate basal cistern obliteration with MRI. Because flowing CSF and venous blood cause a signal void, MRI only rarely shows no hypointensity on the T2 weighted image of the basal cisterns or third ventricle. Because of this MRI may be less good than CT at determining early elevation in ICP in patients who have generalised swelling but no midline shift.

The increased sensitivity of MRI to small areas of cerebral damage, contusions and cerebromalacia may mean that MRI will correlate more accurately with the neurological findings after severe head injury than CT, which shows only non-specific atrophy. Further, in the acute phase MRI may again detect many more abnormalities and show the presence of diffuse injury not seen on CT. It therefore may suggest a poorer prognosis for outcome. MRI is less sensitive to the detection of small rises in ICP; CT is superior in the assessment of this prognostic factor.

What are the indications for MRI on a head-injured patient? In the acute stages MRI may be used as an alternative to CT if this is not available (e.g. due to breakdown or service). This has been done successfully at the Institute of Neurological Sciences, Glasgow, when, on rare occasions, no CT was available. Special care must be taken to ensure that no loose ferrous metal objects are brought within the 5 gauss limit of the magnet and specially modified ventilators, anaesthetic monitoring and resuscitation equipment are required if MRI is to be used in acutely ill patients. If a diffuse injury is suspected clinically and the CT scan is normal then MRI may confirm the diagnosis, but it is not able to exclude the diagnosis since diffuse axonal injury can be identified pathologically in patients in whom both CT and MRI are completely normal. If uni-lateral or bilateral isodense subdural haematomas are suspected but not satisfactorily shown by CT, when MRI is available, it is preferable to angi-ography. MRI may also be a better predictor of eventual outcome because of its greater sensitivity in detecting the full spectrum and total number of acute lesions (Kelly et al. 1988; Gentry et al. 1988).

Spinal Injury

Spinal cord injury, like other forms of trauma, is a disease of the young and the majority are the result of road traffic accidents. It is unfortunate that the outcome of the cord damage is little influenced by therapy. Between 10% and 40% of quadriplegics die within a year of the injury but the true mortality rate is masked by the large number who die at the scene of the accident.

The pattern of injury to the bony spine is import-ant because the radiological appearances imply the direction and size of the force applied to the spine. They also indicate if the fracture is stable and there-fore not liable to cause further neurological deterio-ration, or unstable, when neurological damage may be exacerbated by movement. The purpose of radio-logical investigations is to show and to determine if there is compression of the cord or cauda equina. This can be inferred from plain film findings but a more complete demonstration requires myel-ography with or without CT or MRI.

Spinal cord injury may be present from the time of the accident or develop later if there is an unstable fracture. Intrinsic cord damage includes oedema, contusion and haematoma (Mirvis et al. 1988). Extrinsic compression may result from subdural and extradural haematomas and bony fragments. Complete cord transection can occur with severe injuries. The treatment of structural instability entails immobilisation of unstable fractures and dis-locations, which might otherwise cause progressive deformity, pain or neurological deterioration. The management of neurological deficit may involve laminectomy and decompression in addition to a stabilising procedure. CT has little impact on improving the neurological outcome of these patients and while the results of MRI are promising, its value remains to be proven. The approach to the radiological assessment of a patient with acute spinal injury depends upon the philosophy of the local management team and the neurological con-dition of the patient.

Neurological deterioration may develop weeks after injury if an unstable fracture is unrecognised. Moreover, some patients with complete and long-standing paraplegia can develop additional pro-gressive signs and symptoms. Radiology is frequently of value in assessing such post-traumatic progressive meylopathy.

Mechanisms of Spinal Injury

The mechanisms of spinal injury have implications for stability and treatment. A fracture is stable if only the anterior or posterior elements of the spinal canal are disrupted, and unstable if both are involved. Spinal injury can be caused by flexion, flexion with rotation, extension, vertical compression or by shearing forces. Flexion fractures are the most complex and vary according to the relationship between the longitudinal spinal axis and the fulcrum around which the force acts. If this is centred on the vertebral body then a crush fracture of the body results and the posterior elements are not damaged. This fracture is common and stable and is infrequently associated with cord damage. If the fulcrum for flexion is anterior to the vertebral body, then the posterior ligaments may be disrupted or there may be fracture of the neural arch in addition to vertebral body fractures. Combined flexion and rotation can result in unilateral or bilateral fracture/subluxations of the apophyseal joints, fractures of the laminae, and anterior and posterior ligamentous damage.

Fractures of the Cervical Spine

Fractures of the spine occur in the most mobile regions, i.e. the cervical and dorsolumbar areas. In the cervical spine the apophyseal joints may be almost horizontal and so more susceptible to subluxation and pure ligamentous damage associated with flexion/rotation. Of all cervical fractures 70% occur below the level of C3 in the older child and adult, whereas the upper cervical spine is most commonly injured in infants. In children the fracture often occurs through the epiphyseal end plate and plain films may show no bony injury in the presence of severe cord damage (Hill et al. 1984). Imaging of the soft tissues and the performance of flexion/extension views may be required to assess these injuries accurately. With extension injuries of the cervical spine, where there is disruption through the disc and anterior longitudinal ligament, the abnormally widened anterior disc space may only be evident on the extension view.

Fracture dislocations of the craniocervical junction and C1 on C2 are frequent but rarely seen clinically because in most cases death occurs at the scene of the accident. Fractures of the odontoid peg and burst fractures of the second cervical vertebra (Hangman's fracture) are rarely associated with neurological deficit because they do not result in spinal compression, but they are unstable.

Facet subluxation may be unilateral or bilateral and oblique views may be required to confirm this (Fig. 4.20). The injuries are most frequent at the level of the sixth and seventh vertebrae.

Fractures of the Thoracolumbar Spine

The lumbar and thoracic spines are relatively immobile and have a steep angle at the apophyseal joints. This portion of the spine is therefore intrinsically more stable and resistant to injury than is the cervical region. Pure flexion injuries produce anterior wedging of the vertebra, which is rarely associated

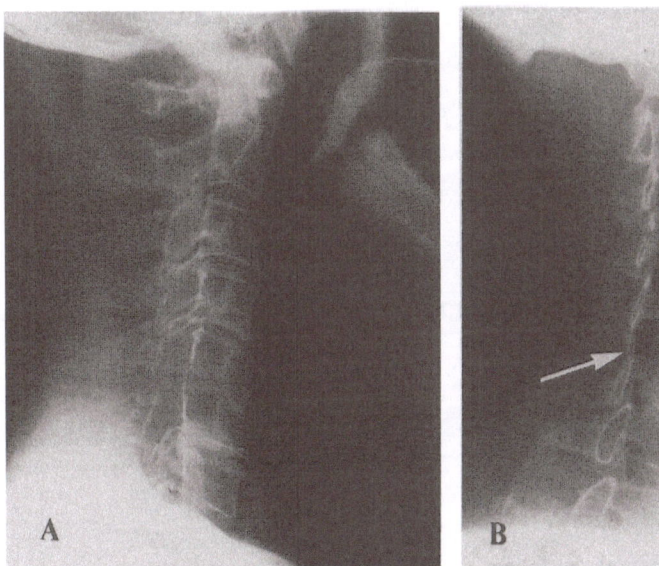

Fig. 4.20. Cervical spine. The lateral view (**a**) shows a loss of height of C5/6 disc and distraction of the spinous processes. The oblique view (**b**) confirms facet subluxation in which one articular facet is positioned directly on top of the other (*arrow*) rather than being interleaved. This is an unstable injury which may become fixed.

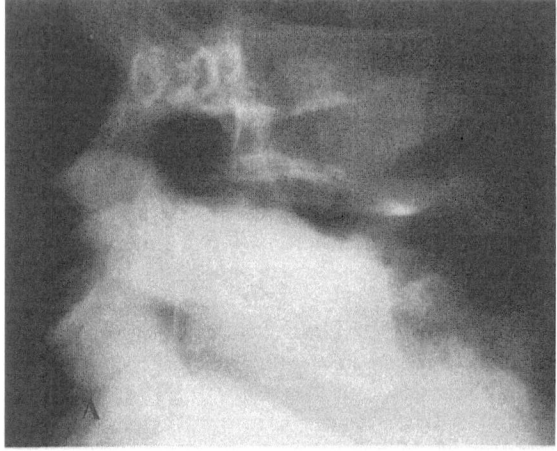
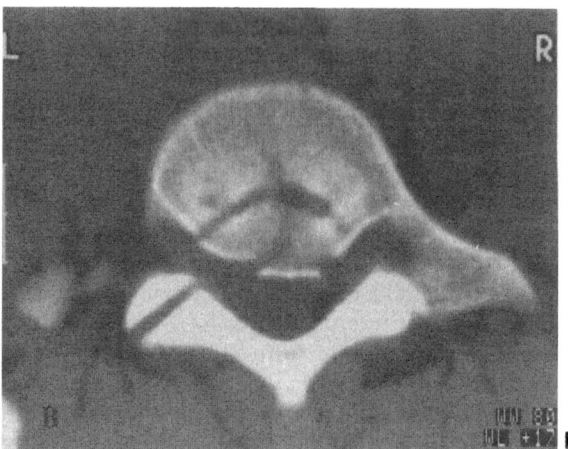

Fig. 4.21. Lumbar spine. Burst fracture L5. The lateral film (**a**) shows fragments driven posteriorly into the spinal canal. Axial CT (**b**) demonstrates the multiple fractures more clearly.

with neurological deficit. Conversely, complete fracture/dislocation is not uncommon in the thoracic region and is associated with cord transection. Forced flexion/rotation caused by lap-only seat belts gave rise to facet subluxation injuries similar to those already described for the cervical spine. Burst fractures from vertical compression frequently result in neurological deficits because bony fragments are forced into the spinal canal (Fig. 4.21). These fractures can also be associated with fractures of the posterior elements and may be unstable.

Radiological Investigations

Plain Films

Plain films of the spine are indicated in all patients with possible spinal trauma. Anteroposterior and lateral films should include the entire region of interest. Cervical spine views should include the skull base and the cervicodorsal junction and similarly the lumbar region should include the thoracolumbar and lumbosacral spine. Plain films will show the vast majority of spinal fractures and detect bony fragments which may encroach upon the canal.

Apophyseal subluxation both in the anterior and lateral direction, and anterior or posterior body subluxation can all be identified. Oblique views of the cervical or lumbar spine may be indicated to confirm apophyseal subluxation. Close scrutiny of the soft tissues may show disruption of the normal fat line anterior to the vertebral bodies indicating significant trauma even in the absence of bony injury (Fig. 4.22). Small bony fragments or avulsed

osteophytes can be seen in hyperextension injuries and indicate anterior ligamentous injury. Flexion and extension views are of value in assessing craniocervical trauma or when there is no evidence. of bony injury in the presence of either soft tissue injury or neurological deficit. Tomography is not necessary if plain films are abnormal and most

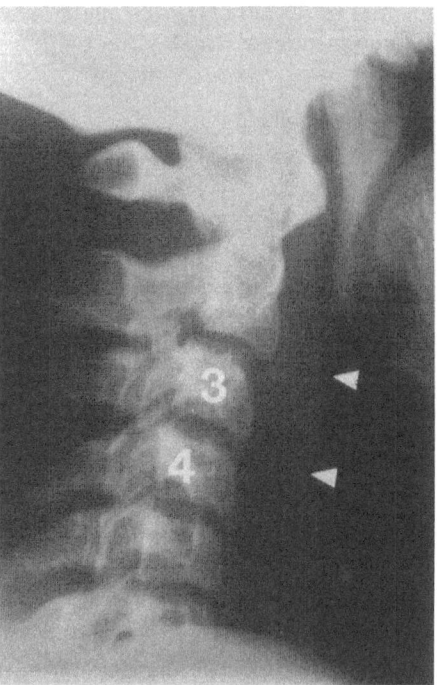

Fig. 4.22. Cervical spine (lateral view). Ligamentous injury. There is swelling of the soft tissue anterior to the vertebral bodies (*arrowheads*) and anterior angulation of C3 on C4 with widening of the interspinous distance but no fracture.

unlikely to show an abnormality if plain films are normal. CT has largely replaced conventional tomography because it provides more information.

Myelography

Myelography is rarely indicated in acute spinal trauma unless there is progressive neurological deficit. It may then be undertaken as an emergency to exclude treatable cord compression and is particularly important in the absence of bony injury, or if the neurological deficit is inappropriate for the level of the fracture. If there is clinical evidence of root avulsion then myelography will determine if this is pre- or postganglionic; reparative surgery is often indicated in the latter case (Chap. 10). Myelography in acutely injured patients should be performed by direct lateral cervical puncture with the patient in the supine position to minimise patient movement.

Computed Tomography

CT is superior to both plain films and standard tomography in the identification of fracture and therefore may be used if there is doubt about the extent of a fracture, particularly of the neural arch, or if a small bony spicule is thought to compress the cord (Fig. 4.23) (Brant-Zawadzki et al. 1981).

An accurate assessment of extraspinal soft tissue swelling is achieved but CT myelography is usually required to examine the contents of the spinal canal. Occasionally CT will demonstrate a high attenuation haematomyelia or a crescentic extradural haematoma.

Magnetic Resonance Imaging

MRI is superior to CT because it can identify the thecal sac, the spinal cord, the CSF space, and disc and other soft tissue. It can also identify ligamentous injury in the absence of swelling, and disruption of the normal fat lines in the absence of bony displacement (McArdle et al. 1986) (Fig. 4.24) There is experimental and clinical evidence which indicates that changes within the cord itself can be demonstrated within hours of a cord injury (Chakeres et al. 1987; Kadoya et al. 1987). Cord contusion appears as an area of prolonged T2 which resolves some weeks after injury. These lesions have been confirmed histologically in an experimental study (Chakeres et al. 1987) and clinically (Mirvis et al. 1988). MRI was found to be superior to CT in demonstrating haematomyelia in two of three clinical cases; the acute haematoma showed as an area of hyperintensity on a T1 weighted sequence (McArdle et al. 1986). Extradural haematomas were identified both by CT and MRI. In patients assessed soon after injury CT and MR are probably equally sensitive to acute haemorrhage, but in the more chronic cases MRI should be superior because it permits identification of a blood clot which will have become isodense on the CT. Fractures can be identified by MR but CT is superior in the detection

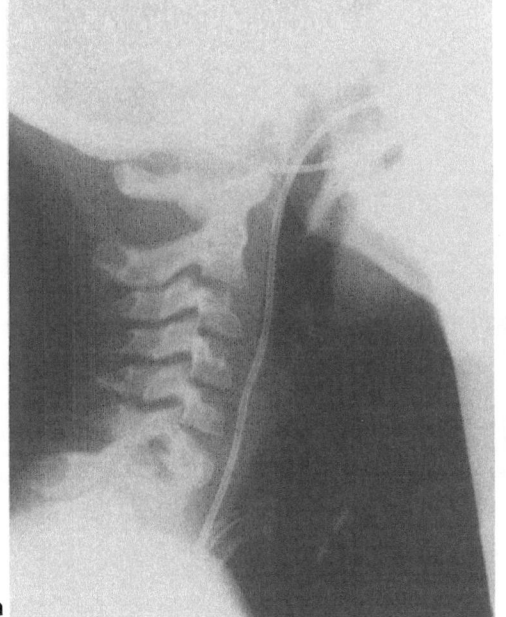
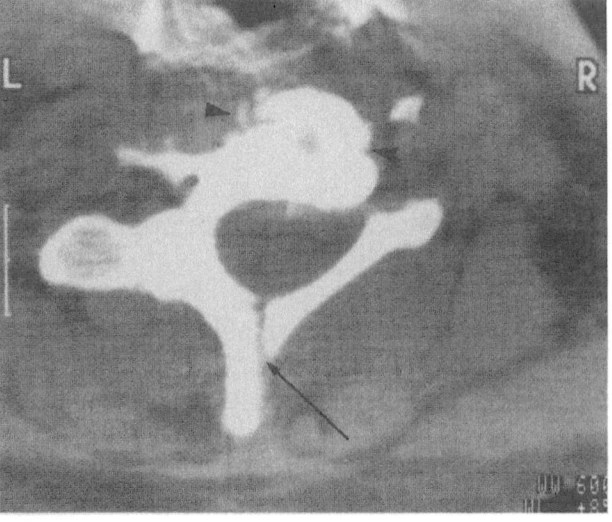

Fig. 4.23. Cervical spine. Fracture/subluxation of C6/7. **a** Lateral view. **b** Axial CT of C6 showing an oblique fracture through the body (*arrowheads*) and one through the neural arch (*arrow*).

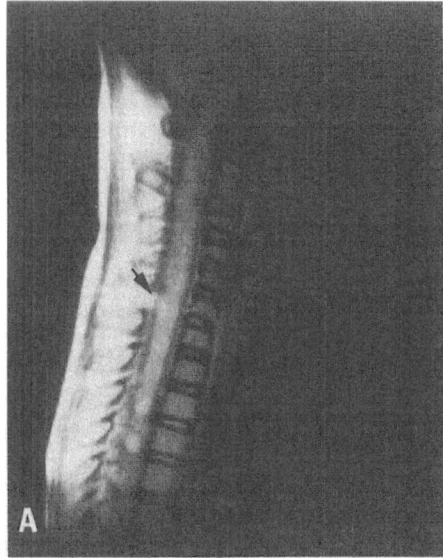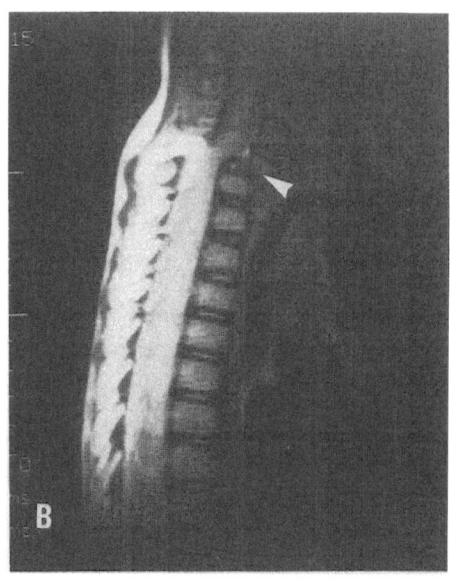

Fig. 4.24. Cervical spine. Sagittal MRI (T2 weighted). Hyperextension injury. **a** A small extramedullary haematoma (*black arrow*) is seen. **b** At 1 week follow-up and with some clinical improvement, complete subluxation of C6 body on its inferior end plate is present (*arrowhead*).

of small neural arch fractures. A further advantage of MRI is that it can be used to examine the entire cord when the exact level of spinal injury is not clear. This is impractical with CT and would otherwise require myelography. Spinal traction is not a contraindication to MRI although modifications to standard equipment are required.

Radiological Protocol for Acute Spinal Trauma

An excellent review of the role of radiology in spinal trauma is given by Djang (1987) which includes a flow chart for investigation. A modified version of this chart is given in Fig. 4.25. As with all flow charts it is intended to be a guide only and each patient must be assessed as an individual.

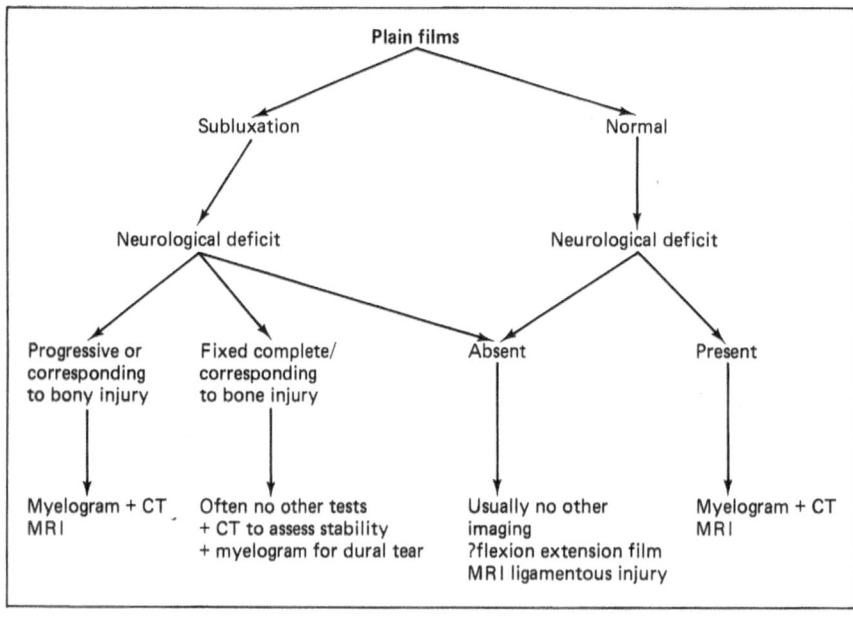

Fig. 4.25. The radiological assessment of spinal trauma.

If plain films are normal but the patient has a neurological deficit then myelography perhaps with CT is indicated. MRI is a suitable alternative to this established investigation and is likely to replace it. If there is a fixed complete or incomplete neurological deficit appropriate to the bony injury and the degree of stability is known then CT is not necessary. If decompression is contemplated, then CT or MR may be indicated pre-operatively to provide additional information. If the neurological deficit is progressive or does not correlate with the bony level of injury, myelography with CT, or preferably MRI, is indicated.

Despite advances in imaging technology and surgical technique, the outlook for many patients with acute spinal cord trauma is depressingly bleak. Such injuries may be best cared for in a specialised spinal trauma unit and it is hoped that MRI will be readily available and so obviate the need for invasive and potentially hazardous examinations.

Late Effects of Spinal Cord Injury and Their Investigation

Bony Effects

Progressive bony changes occur as an unstable fracture or subluxation "settles" into a stable position and fuses. Exuberant osteophyte formation can result due to secondary degenerative change which may result in nerve root compression, often above the level of injury. Wedge fractures may continue to collapse and produce neurological deterioration and new fractures, due to disuse osteoporosis, can also occur. Loss of muscle tone may result in increasing kyphoscoliosis which will exacerbate pre-existing bony compression. These changes are usually obvious on plain films but myelography or MRI may be required to assess the spinal cord.

Neurological Sequelae

Patients with varying degrees of paraplegia may later go on to develop increasing pain or sensory disturbance, and hyperhidrosis. This clinical syndrome of post-traumatic progressive myelography may develop at any time after the injury and has a variety of causes. Arachnoid adhesions are common at the site of injury resulting in narrowing of the subarachnoid space and tethering of the cord, usually posteriorly. In addition, extradural fibrosis and bony compression can result in obstruction to CSF pathways and progressive cord atrophy not confined to the level of previous injury. A cyst or syrinx may form, within the cord, proximal or distal to the area of trauma, but unlike congenital syr-

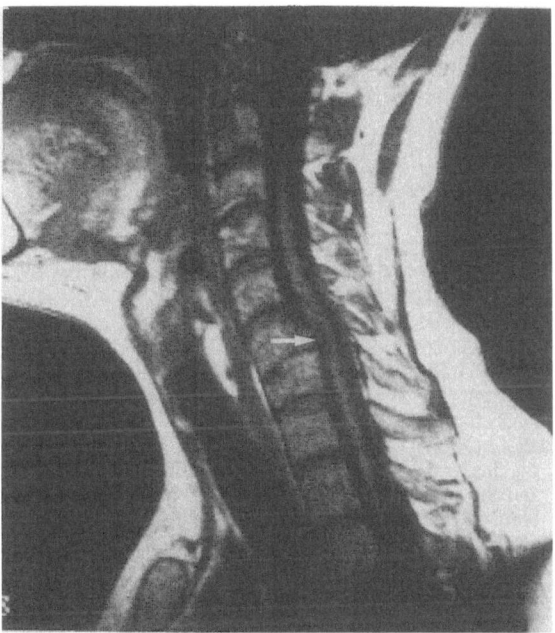

Fig. 4.26. Cervical spine. Sagittal MRI (T1 weighted). Post-traumatic syrinx (*arrow*) in association with a C6/7 wedge compression fracture. (P.B.)

ingomyelia, the dimensions of the cord usually remain normal (Fig. 4.26). Myelomalacia is another late effect of haematomyelia and/or contusion of the cord: the cord becomes atrophic and contains many small areas of cystic degeneration within the length of cord originally damaged. Very occasionally an arachnoid cyst will develop causing displacement and compression of the cord. In a study by Osborne et al. (1982) all these lesions could be identified radiologically and MRI has proved useful (Gebarski et al. 1985) with good correlation between the radiological and the operative findings. CT performed 4–8 hours after myelography will usually confirm the presence of a syrinx within the cord because the contrast medium becomes concentrated within the cyst. Surgery is beneficial in the former case but not in myelomalacia and so it is important to be able to differentiate between these two conditions.

MRI studies in post-traumatic progressive myelopathy (Quencer et al. 1986) indicate that it is less sensitive than myelography in the detection of adhesions, but more sensitive to the diagnosis of a traumatic syrinx and can identify these cysts because they contain fluid with the same signal characteristics as CSF. In patients with myelomalacia the T1 weighted images showed hypointensity within the cord. On a moderately T2 weighted image these areas became isointense or slightly hyperintense compared to the surrounding cord. These changes did not exactly parallel the signal from CSF. MRI may thus differentiate a treatable syrinx from the cysts of myelomalacia.

References

Adams JH, Mitchell DE, Graham DI, Doyle D (1977) Diffuse brain damage of immediate impact type. Brain 100:489–502

Brant-Zawadzki M, Miller E, Federle M (1981) CT in the evaluation of spine trauma. AJR 136:369–375

Bruce DA, Alari A, Bilaniuk L, Dolinskas C, Obrist W, Uzzell B (1981) Diffuse brain swelling following head injuries in children: The syndrome of "malignant brain oedema". J Neurosurg 54:170–178

Caffey J (1974) The whiplash shaken infant syndrome: manual shaking by the extremities with whiplash-induced intracranial and intra-ocular bleedings linked with residual permanent brain damage and mental retardation. Paediatrics 54:396–403

Chakeres D, Flickinger F, Bresnahan J, Beattie M, Weiss K, Stokes B (1987) MR imaging of acute spinal cord trauma. AJNR 8:5–10

Cohen RA, Kaufman RA, Myers PA, Towbin K (1985) Cranial computed tomography in the abused child with head injury. AJNR 6:883–888

Cooper PR (1987) Skull fracture and traumatic cerebrospinal fluid fistulas. In: Cooper PR (ed) Head injury, 2nd edn. Williams and Wilkins, Baltimore, pp 89–107

Cordobes F, De La Fuente M. Lobato R et al. (1983) Intraventricular haemorrhage in severe head injury. J Neurosurg 58:217–222

Djang W (1987) In: Albin M (ed) Radiology of acute spinal trauma in Critical Care Clinics: Acute spinal cord injury. Saunders, Philadelphia, vol 3, pp 495–518

Du Boulay EPGH (1980) Principles of X-ray diagnosis of the skull, 2nd edn. Butterworths, London

Fenton Lewis A (1983) Management of acute head injury. Harrogate seminar report 8. HMSO, London

Gebarski S, Maynard F, Gabrielsen T, Knake J, Latack J, Hoff J (1985) Post traumatic progressive myelopathy. Radiology 157:379–385

Gentleman D, Nath F, Macpherson P (1989) Diagnosis and management of delayed traumatic haematomas. Br J Neurosurg 3:367–372

Gentry LR, Godersky JC, Thompson B (1988) MR Imaging of head trauma: review of the distribution and radiopathologic features of traumatic lesions AJNR 9:101–110

Hadley MDM, Teasdale GM, Jenkins A et al. (1988) Magnetic resonance imaging in acute head injury. Clin Radiol 39:131–139

Hesselink JR, Dowd CF, Healy ME, Hajek P, Baker LL, Luerssen TG (1988) MR imaging of brain contusions: a comparative study with CT. AJNR 9:269–278

Hill S, Miller C, Kosnike F, Hunt W (1984) Paediatric neck injuries. A clinical study. J Neurosurg 60:700–706

Jenkins A, Teasdale G, Hadley MDM, Macpherson P, Rowan JO (1986) Brain lesions detected by magnetic resonance imaging in mild and severe head injuries. Lancet ii:445–446

Kadoya S, Nakamura T, Kobayashi S, Yamamoto I (1987) Magnetic resonance imaging of acute spinal cord injury. Report of three cases. Neuroradiology 29:252–255

Kelly A, Zimmerman R, Snow R, Gandy S, Heier L, Deck M (1988) Head trauma: comparison of MR and CT experience in 100 patients. AJNR 9:699–708

Kirkham FJ, Levin SD, Padayachee TS (1987) Transcranial

pulsed Doppler ultrasound findings in brainstem death. J Neurol Neurosurg Psychiatry 50:1504–1513

Kobayshi S, Makazawa S, Otsuka T (1983) Clinical value of serial computerised tomographic scanning of the prognosis of severe head injury. Surg Neurol 20:25–29

Levin HS, Williams, D, Crofford M et al. (1988) Relationship of depth of brain lesions to consciousness and outcome after closed head injury. J Neurosurg 69:861–866

Lipper M, Kishore P, Enas G, Domingues da Silva A, Choi S, Becker D (1985) Computed tomography in the prediction of outcome in head injury. AJNR 6:7–10

Lobato R, Cordobes F, Rivas J et al. (1983) Outcome from severe head injury related to the type of intracranial lesion. A computerized tomography study. J Neurosurg 50:762–774

Macpherson P, Teasdale E (1989) Can computed tomography be relied upon to detect skull fractures? Clin Radiol 40:22–24

Macpherson P, Teasdale E, Dhaker S, Allerdyce G, Galbraith S (1986) The significance of traumatic haematoma in the region of the basal ganglia. J Neurol Neurosurg Psychiatry 49:29–34

Marel C, Cellerier P, Sobel D, Prevost C, Bonafe A (1982) Cerebrosipinal fluid 'rhinorrhoea: Evaluation with metrizamide cisternography. AJR 138:471–476

McArdle C, Crofford M, Mirfakhrace M, Amparo E, Colhoun J (1986) Surface coil of MR spinal trauma: preliminary experience. AJNR 7:885–886

Mirvis S, Geisler F, Jelinek J, Joslyn J, Gellad F (1988) Acute cervical spine trauma: evaluation with 1.5T MR imaging. Radiology 166:807–816

North CM, Ahmadi J, Segall H, Zee C-S (1986) Penetrating vascular injuries of the face and neck: clinical and angiographic consideration AJNR 7:855–859

Obsorne R, Vavoulis G, Nashold B, Dubois P, Drayer B, Heinz R (1982) Late sequelae of spinal cord trauma. Myelographic and surgical correlation. J Neurosurg 57:18–23

Paterson OF, Esperson JO (1984) How to distinguish between bleeding and coagulated extradural haematomas on the plain CT scanning. Neuroradiology 26:285–292

Quencer R, Sheldon J, Post M et al. (1986) Magnetic resonance imaging in the chronically injured cervical spinal cord. AJNR 7:457–464

Royal College of Radiologists (1980) A study of the utilisation of skull radiography in nine accident and emergency units in the UK. Lancet ii:1234–1236

Statham P, Johnston R, Macpherson P (1989) Delayed deterioration in patients with traumatic frontal contusions. J Neurol Neurosurg Psychiatry 52:351–354

Stovring J (1977) Contralateral temporal horn widening in unilateral supratentorial mass lesions: A diagnostic sign indicating tentorial herniation. J Comput Assist Tomogr 1:319–323

Strich SL (1961) Shearing of nerve fibres as a cause of brain damage due to head injury. Lancet ii:443–448

Teasdale E, Cardosa E, Galbraith S, Teasdale G (1984) CT scan in severe diffuse head injury: physiological and clinical correlations. J Neurol Neurosurg Psychiatry 47:600–603

Teasdale G, Jennett B. (1974) Assessment of coma and impaired consciousness. A practical scale. Lancet ii:81–84

Teasdale G, Galbraith S, Murray L, Ward P, Gentleman D, McKean M (1982) Management of traumatic intracranial haematoma. Br Med J 285:1695–1697

Teasdale G, Murray G, Anderson E, Mendelow, D, Jennett B (1990) The risks of intracranial haematoma after head injury in adults and children. Br Med J in press

Thornbury JR, Masters SJ, Campbell JA (1987) Imaging recommendations for head trauma; a new comprehensive strategy. AJR 149:781–783

Toutant S, Klauber M, Marshall L et al. (1984) Absent or

compressed basal cisterns on first CT scan: ominous predictors of outcome in severe head injury. J Neurosurg 61: 691–694

Turazzi S, Bricola A, Pasut ML, Formenton A (1987) Changes produced by CT scanning in the outlook of severe head injury. Acta Neurochir (Wien) 85:87–95

Van Dongen K, Braakman R, Gelpke G (1983) The prognostic value of computerised tomography in comatosed head-injured patients. J Neurosurg 59:951–957

Zimmerman RA, Bilaniuk LT, Dolinskas C (1978) Computed tomography of acute intracranial haemorrhagic contusion.

Axial Tomogr 1:271–280

Zimmerman RA, Bilaniuk LT, Gennarelli T (1978) Computed tomography of shearing injuries of the cerebral white matter. Radiology 127:393–396

Zimmerman RA, Bilaniuk LT, Bruce D, Schut L, Uzzell B, Goldberg H (1979) Computed tomography of craniocerebral injury in the abused child. Radiology 130:687–690

Zimmerman RA, Bilaniuk LT, Hackney DB, Goldberg HI, Grossman RI (1986) Head injury: early results of comparing CT and high field MR. AJNR 7:757–765

Chapter 5

Infections of the Central Nervous System
John M. Stevens

CRANIAL INFECTIONS

Infections of the Meninges

Acute Bacterial Meningitis

Pathogenesis

1. *Bacteraemia.* Most meningitis is contracted in this way and indeed the probability of developing meningitis is proportional to the magnitude of a preceding bacteraemia (Kroll and Moxon 1987). There is a peak incidence in neonates due to reduced immunity in this period where the agents are commonly *Escherichia coli* or other Gram-negative rods. In infants and young children, the commonest agent is *Haemophilus influenzae* whereas in young adults the agents are most commonly *Neisseria meningitidis* or *Streptococcus pneumoniae* (Harriman 1984).

2. *Parameningeal sepsis.* Infection of the paranasal sinuses and petromastoid, and osteomyelitis of the calvarium, may be associated with intracranial empyema and brain abscess as well as leptomeningitis.

3. *Septic emboli.* Infective endocarditis and right to left cardiac shunts are more usually associated with brain abscess but occasionally meningitis occurs.

4. *Infected ventricular and subarachnoid shunts.* These and other neurosurgical procedures may be complicated by meningitis. *Pseudomonas aeruginosa* and *Staphylococcus aureus* are commonly involved.

5. *Cerebrospinal fluid fistula.* About 70% of these result from craniofacial trauma. About 70% close

spontaneously within a week and most of the rest usually within 6 months. Leakage from spontaneous fistulae on the other hand tends to be both copious and prolonged. The agents are usually Gram-negative rods, including *Pseudomonas*, and the risk of developing severe meningitis is of the order of 2% per year while the fistula remains (Ommaya 1976).

6. *Malformations.* These include malformations of the middle and inner ear as well as dermal sinuses, encephaloceles and meningomyeloceles.

Radiology

The following are situations in which imaging may be desirable:

1. Diagnostic uncertainty at presentation and prior to lumbar puncture, especially when there is suspicion of raised intracranial pressure.
2. The development of focal neurological signs during treatment.
3. Suspicion of hydrocephalus or severe ependymitis.

Imaging modalities which are appropriate are computed tomography (CT) and magnetic resonance imaging (MRI), and ultrasound in infants.

Computed Tomography. Scans are often normal although pronounced contrast enhancement of the meninges may be seen especially in those bordering the basal cisterns. In severe cases the attenuation of cerebrospinal fluid (CSF) may be increased, and in exceptional cases may even resemble subarachnoid haemorrhage (de Slegte et al. 1988).

Low attenuation in brain substance is common; seen in over half the children scanned acutely by Cockrill et al. (1978). Grey and white matter were usually involved, and in over 70% of children with meningitis due to *H. influenzae* it was located near the frontal poles bilaterally. However, it can occur in any location and may not conform to a major artery territory. The outcome in Cockrill's material was resolution (29%), no change (10%) and progression to severe atrophy and/or encephalomalacia (70%). Gyral enhancement may occasionally be shown after intravenous contrast administration and brain abscesses have also developed during treatment (Fig. 5.2), although Cockrill recorded this development in only four of his 47 cases.

Hydrocephalus is seen in about 20% of cases scanned acutely, although it is present in over half the cases requiring scanning during treatment (Cockrill et al. 1978; Marrie et al. 1984). In most it resolves or remains static, only about one-third show definite progression and less than 10% of patients require shunting.

Subdural effusions are especially frequent in children and are usually present on scans made during treatment. Although often sterile the medial membrane usually, but not always, enhances markedly (Cockrill et al. 1978; Zimmerman et al. 1986). Arachnoid and subependymal cysts have also been shown to develop during treatment (Marrie et al. 1984), the latter only in infants.

Ependymitis, when severe, manifests as diffuse enhancement of the ventricular walls. Sometimes there is also diffuse periventricular low attenuation in the cerebral white matter.

Cortical vein and dural sinus thrombosis may complicate meningitis (see Chap. 1).

Magnetic Resonance Imaging (MRI). The abnormalities shown by CT are also shown by MRI. Increased signal in the periventricular white matter which is frequently seen is usually due to ventriculitis but may sometimes result from interstitial oedema of hydrocephalus or occasionally widespread vasculitis. Large areas of signal change are frequent, and sometimes MRI shows evidence of recent haemorrhage (Davidson and Steiner 1985; Zimmerman et al. 1986; Moseley 1987).

Ultrasound. This is only of value in neonates and infants where the fontanelles are wide enough to facilitate an adequate "window" on the brain. It will detect most of the complications occurring in this age group including the various forms of severe parenchymal damage. However, it may not detect all extracerebral effusions or posterior fossa abnormalities. CT or MRI may also be required (London et al. 1980; Enzmann et al. 1982).

Acute Viral Meningitis

In this condition MRI and CT will only be required if the diagnosis is in doubt or if encephalitis is suspected.

Subacute and Chronic Meningitis

Tuberculous Meningitis (TBM)

Meningitis is by far the commonest form of neurotuberculosis. The incidence peaks in children aged between 6 months and 6 years (Dastur and Lalitha 1973; Kocen 1987), and infection has often been noted to follow measles (Kocen 1987).

Pathogenesis. TBM is nearly always a reactivation disease months or years after prior haemotogenous dissemination and seeding in the brain. Meningitis arises when a superficial parenchymal tuberculoma, termed a Rich focus, ruptures into the subarachnoid space (Rich 1951). Therefore well over 80% of intracerebral tuberculomata are associated with tuberculous meningitis, and meningitis is rare in miliary tuberculosis (Kocen 1987).

Hydrocephalus is a common complication including unusual forms such as the encysted fourth ventricle (see Chap. 3) and is due to organised subarachnoidal exudates and ependymitis (Kingsley et al. 1987). About 40% of autopsied cases show cerebral infarcts. A border zone encephalitis and a tuberculous encephalopathy may be found, the latter usually in children (Dastur and Lalitha 1973; Kocen 1987).

Spirochaetal Infections

Infections by the spirochaetes *Treponema, Borrelia* and *Leptospira* commonly result in a non-pyogenic meningitis, after a variable latency, which is characterised by a high frequency of vasculitis and cerebral invasion by organisms.

Parasites

Many parasitic diseases involve the nervous system. The subject is complex and varied and the reader is referred to Brown and Voge (1982) for a detailed account.

Neurocysticercosis. *Taenia solium* infestation is by far the commonest parasitic disease of the nervous system in man (Sotelo 1987; Zee et al. 1980). The brain is involved in 60%–90% of cases and "symptomatic" involvement of muscle occurs in 5%, although many other tissues are infested. Neurocysticercosis is predominantly a disease of the subarachnoid space, only 13%–20% of lesions being truly parenchymal (Carbajal et al. 1977; Sotelo 1987; Lotz et al. 1988). In over 85% of cases, intracranial cysts are multiple and between 1% and 17% of cases have intraventricular cysts. Sulcal sequestration may result in large multiseptate cysts invaginating brain substance. Marked basal granulomatous meningitis resulting in hydrocephalus is an infrequent complication (Lotz et al. 1988).

Fungi

Many of the haematogenously disseminated fungi may cause either meningitis, brain granulomas or abscesses, and patients suffering from these diseases often have significant medical disorders (Wiles and MacKenzie 1987).

Radiology in Chronic Meningitis

Neuroimaging is usually indicated during the course of chronic meningitis. Plain films have no role except perhaps occasionally to increase the clinical suspicion of cysticercosis in a doubtful case, by showing calcified larvae in muscles which may be inconspicuous or invisible on plain skull films (see Chap. 10, Fig. 10.1). Calcification on plain X-ray films occurs in only 13.6% cases of neurocysticercosis and takes about 10 years to develop (Carbajal et al. 1977).

Angiography often shows evidence of arteritis. This is best recognised in the more common forms

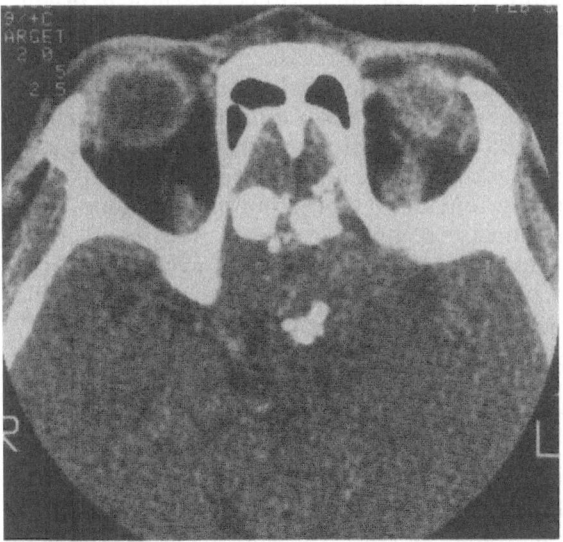

Fig. 5.1. Cranial CT. Tuberculous meningitis. Note the densely calcified basal exudates in this patient with visual failure.

of chronic meningitis. It is usually due to a Heubner's type of arteritis affecting the internal carotid and its branches and appears as areas of narrowing or short segment ectasias (Holland et al. 1986). In tuberculous meningitis vascular narrowing is seen especially in the branches of the middle cerebral artery in the Sylvian cisterns (Casselman et al. 1980). Such changes have been seen in 50%–70% of cases (Dastur and Lalitha 1973; Bhargava et al. 1982), and indicate severe meningeal exudation and a poor eventual outcome.

Local vascular ectasias and beading of the supraclinoid carotid, proximal middle and anterior cerebral arteries and their distal branches were shown in a proven case of meningovascular syphilis (Holland et al. 1986), and correlated with the presence of brain infarction. Similar appearances have been described in leptospirosis (Reik 1987), cysticercosis (Zee et al. 1980), coccidioidomycosis (Wiles and MacKenzie 1987) and other fungal diseases.

Computed Tomography

1. *Tuberculous meningitis* (Fig. 5.1). Only about 5% of scans made in this condition will be normal (Casselman et al. 1980; Bhargava et al. 1982; Kingsley et al. 1987). The most frequent abnormality in children is hydrocephalus, which is usually mild and occurs in 87% of cases. In over 70% the fourth ventricle is enlarged indicating obstruction at the level of the cerebellopontine angle cisterns and vallecula; in the remainder the appearances are those of aqueduct stenosis. Hydrocephalus may appear early in the disease, but is more usual in cases of long duration. It frequently increases during treatment (Casselman et al. 1980; Kingsley et al. 1987; Kocen 1987). On the other hand hydrocephalus is observed in only about 12% of adults with the disease (Bhargava et al. 1982). Loculation within the ventricles is very occasionally found.

The meningeal exudates are frequently shown. The cisterns may be invisible, or outlined by high density material which eventually calcifies in about 75% of cases (Casselman et al. 1980). Enhancement of the exudates after administration of intravenous contrast is present in over 80%, usually in the chiasmatic, ambient and Sylvian cisterns (Bhargava et al. 1982). Enhancement may appear during treatment and only diminish after many months – in many cases persisting indefinitely (Kingsley et al. 1987). Cerebral infarcts have been shown in 28% of cases. Over 80% are in middle cerebral artery territory with frequent involvement of the basal ganglia (Bhargava et al. 1982; Kingsley et al. 1987).

Tuberculomas, shown in 10%–25% of cases (Bhargava et al. 1982; Kingsley et al. 1987), are most frequently seen near the Sylvian cisterns. Far more are found pathologically than are shown even on contrast-enhanced CT (Bhargava et al. 1982; Kocen 1987). New tuberculomas may appear up to seven months after initiation of treatment (Kingsley et al. 1987).

Tuberculous encephalopathy may have been shown in 3% of the cases of Bhargava et al. (1982), as low attenuation in the cerebral white matter. This is far below the incidence of 27% reported by Dastur and Udani (1966) in autopsy material.

2. *Neurocysticercosis.* It is desirable to distinguish active disease from the effects of now quiescent disease. Brain odema and contrast enhancement indicate actively degenerating cysts (Sotelo 1987), whereas viable cysts appear as low density structures in which the protoscolix is usually not visible, and bladders may be difficult to differentiate from sulcal sequestration and complex arachnoid cysts. Six types of abnormality are described (Lotz et al. 1988; Chang et al. 1988):

1. Multiple or single viable cysts 8–20 mm in size. Enhancement and oedema may or may not be present.

2. Enhancing nodules, thin walled abscesses, thick walled granulomas.

3. Complex arachnoid cysts, often multilocular and involving Sylvian cisterns or other cerebral sulci.

4. Mineralised nodules, usually associated with negative seroconversion and representing long dead and inactive larvae (Fig. 5.7).

5. Basal meningitis appearing as loculated, often enlarged cisterns with or without enhancement. Hydrocephalus may be present.

6. Intraventricular larvae, not usually recognisable on plain CT, but computed myelography and ventriculography usually show them well. Contrast medium may penetrate the cuticle and form a layer in the cyst. Mobility of the cysts within the ventricle may be demonstrable (Zee et al. 1980). Ependymal enhancement and periventricular oedema may be found when the cysts degenerate and become adherent to the ependyma (Sotelo 1987).

The fourth ventricle is a frequent site in which to find a solitary cysticercus. Indeed if a patient is found to have hydrocephalus on CT and serology is positive for *Cysticercus cellulosae* the cause is likely to be intracranial cysticercosis, and in the absence of any visible abnormality, intraventricular cysts should be sought (Chang et al. 1988).

Finally, viable cysticerci can be killed by specific chemotherapeutic agents, especially Praziquantel and Albendazole. The most susceptible are those within or invaginating into the brain. Death and degeneration may cause marked reaction with brain oedema and enhancement, and should not be misinterpreted as progression despite treatment. Intraventricular bladders are not susceptible (Sotelo 1987) and usually require surgical removal.

3. *Other subacute and chronic meningitides.* Infarcts, both deep and superficial, may be seen in the other conditions discussed, such as the spirochaetal infections, and many of the parasitoses. Haemorrhages may occur with many of them, especially leptospirosis and some of the parasites. Low density areas in the brain may also represent parenchymal involvement by the organism. Hydrocephalus is the commonest abnormality seen in cryptococcosis.

Magnetic Resonance Imaging. It has become axiomatic to state that MRI shows all that is visible on CT only with greater sensitivity. In diseases characterised by profuse subarachnoid exudates, signal alterations in the cisterns reflecting the raised protein content, increased solid component and especially reduced pulsatile CSF movements would be expected, but although increased signal in the basal cisterns has been documented on spin-echo images (Moseley 1987), MRI has been disappointing in this area (Zimmerman et al. 1986). Infarcts and other parenchymal lesions are shown with great sensitivity however, and sometimes are shown to contain unexpected haemorrhage, appearing as areas of high signal on T1 weighted images. Many of the diseases have been found to be associated with patchy subcortical signal abnormalities which seem identical to multiple sclerosis, and their nature, though presumed to be vasculitic in origin, is usually unproven (Reik et al. 1985).

Cysticercosis is one disease in this group in which MRI may contribute specificity. Viable cysts have a central signal paralleling CSF; in more T1 weighted images the protoscolex may be clearly visible as a high signal mural nodule. Racemose cisternal cysts usually contain no scolex, but mural nodules may be shown in complex arachnoid cysts representing intact bladders within it, or the convoluted walls of a racemose cyst may be recognisable within the thickened meningeal envelope (Zimmerman et al. 1986; Lotz et al. 1988).

Intraventricular cysts are infrequently shown as rounded or multilocular structures; the cuticular wall may be visible as a low signal rim. High signal in the periventricular tissues suggests degeneration of the cyst and ependymal adhesions (Zimmerman et al. 1986). Surgical excision of intraventricular cysts is usually required, and ependymal adhesions can significantly hinder safe excision.

Intracranial Empyemas and Other Infections of the Extradural Spaces

Empyemas are collections of pus in the extradural or subdural space. About 25% of intracranial suppurations are empyemas (Danziger et al. 1980; Zimmerman et al. 1984), of which about half are extradural and half subdural (Moseley and Kendall 1984). The mortality of this condition used to be over 40%, but has fallen to about 12% since the advent of CT. The infective agents are nearly always pyogenic bacteria.

Pathogenesis

Sinusitis and otitis are the commonest overall causes. According to Kaplan (1976) 80% of intracranial empyemas were associated with face and scalp infections.

Meningitis is the commonest cause in children, accounting for all the childhood cases of subdural empyema reported by Weisberg (1986).

Trauma is a relatively frequent cause accounting for between 12% and 33% of cases (Moseley and Kendall 1984; Zimmerman et al. 1984). Empyema may complicate intracranial surgery, especially following the insertion of ventricular shunts which cause subdural collections and may complicate wound infections even in the absence of osteomyelitis (Lanzieri et al. 1988). Delayed development of an empyema months or years after surgical or accidental trauma is well recognised (Harriman 1984; Tokoro et al. 1987); the trauma may be superficial but more often involves a compound fracture of the cranium.

Haematogenous spread from lung abscess, thoracic empyema and intravenous drug abuse has been identified in 2%–4% of cases.

No cause is identified in 4%–8% of cases, compared with 20% in the case of intracerebral abscess.

Pathology

Epidural abscess almost always arises near an infected frontal sinus or mastoid. It tends to be localised by natural adhesions of the dura to the inner table of the skull, but may be extensive when underlying an osteomyelitis. Subdural empyema on the other hand is diffuse, and frequently bilateral. Loculations may develop later in the process to form walled abscesses. Empyemas usually form at the site of their pathogenesis, but loculations are frequently found in remote locations. They occur anywhere in the subdural space but especially posteriorly, presumably due to the patient's supine position (Borovich et al. 1981).

Complications are:

1. Cerebral compression by extracerebral mass
2. "Brain oedema", the origin and nature of which are unclear
3. Parenchymal involvement of a focal nature: cerebritis, abscess and very occasionally venous and arterial infarcts

Radiology

In the early stages of a subdural empyema the thin film of exudate may be impossible to see on CT. Clinical features may be profound even at this stage, and other imaging tests have been advocated such as angiography and radionuclide studies to aid early detection.

Computed Tomography of Empyemas (Fig. 5.2)

In proven cases of empyema the initial CT may not show the collection in up to 18% of cases and may be entirely normal in 10% (Moseley and Kendall 1984; Zimmerman et al. 1984). Subsequent CT studies may not be expected to show the collection within 12 hours but certainly within 4 days (Zimmerman et al. 1984).

Opacity of the frontal sinuses and overlying soft tissue swelling is frequently present. This finding in a patient with severe acute neurological dysfunction should alert one to the diagnosis. Wide window settings may show an early epidural abscess (Carter et al. 1983). It should be noted, however, that the collections appeared on the side contralateral to the sinus disease in 50% of the cases of Moseley and Kendall (1984).

Osteomyelitis of the calvarial bones may arise adjacent to chronic sinusitis or otitis, although occasionally it is unrelated to the sinuses; it results in permeative bone destruction and sclerosis but infrequently sequestra, which when present are usually small.

About 70% of empyemas are found over the cerebral convexities and 28% are parafalcine. Parafalcine collections are usually located posterosuperiorly and in 10% may be the only collections visible (Zimmerman et al. 1984). A small proportion lie adjacent to the tentorium (Moseley and Kendall 1984).

The attenuation of the collection is similar to or slightly greater than the CSF and bubbles of air may be seen within it. The medial membrane is denser than adjacent brain but is clearly visible in only a minority of cases. Somewhere between 40% and 60% of convexity collections are crescentic in

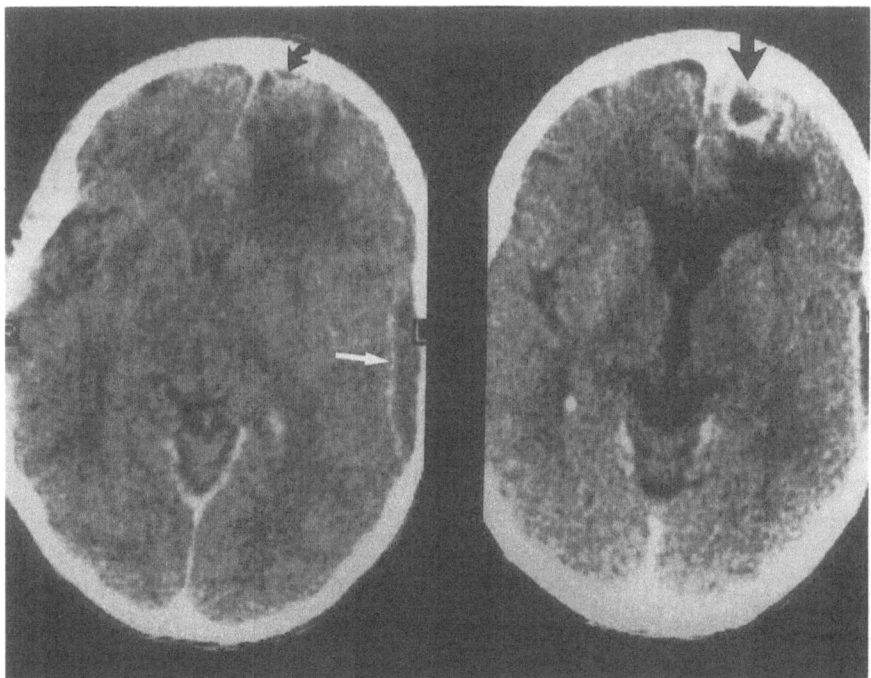

Fig. 5.2. Cranial CT after IV contrast. Complicated frontal sinusitis. A cerebral abscess (*black arrow*), an epidural abscess (*curved black arrow*) and a subdural empyema (*white arrow*) are shown.

shape, but most parafalcine collections are flat. Localised, lentiform subdural collections with rounded medial surfaces constitute the remainder, making it impossible to distinguish extradural or intradural location by the shape of the collection, although anterior midline extradural collections may be seen to displace the superior sagittal sinus away from the vault (de Slegte et al. 1988). About 60% of collections are multilocular and appear lobulated even on the initial scan (Zimmerman et al. 1984).

Considerable emphasis is often placed on enhancement of the medial membrane after intravenous contrast. However in 16% of the cases of Zimmerman and co-workers there was little or no enhancement, and over half of these were not acute. Moseley and Kendall observed that only 36% of convexity collections and 75% of parafalcine collections showed an enhancing membrane. Therefore the belief that the appearance of the medial membrane after intravenous contrast administration indicates whether an extracerebral collection is infected or not is groundless.

Abnormalities may be visible in the brain before extracerebral collection is recognised. Mass effect may be greater than expected from the size of the collection but dislocation of midline structures is present in less than 40% of cases.

An area of low attenuation in the brain adjacent to the extracerebral collection is present in about 25% of cases. In some it resembles vasogenic oedema, and in others grey and white matter are both involved. Enhancement of gyri beneath an empyema is said to be very common, although this has not been the author's experience. In 12% of the cases of Zimmerman and co-workers this was intense enough to suggest infarction. Deep patchy or ring enhancement which develops in 10%–16% of cases is usually interpreted as indicating cerebritis or cerebral abscess. Moseley and Kendall consider all focal parenchymal changes to represent inflammation rather than ischaemia. Superficial venous and dural sinus thrombosis are not a feature of intracranial empyemas in the postantibiotic era but the presence of cerebral lesions considerably increases the likelihood of sequelae or an eventually fatal outcome.

Magnetic Resonance Imaging of Empyemas

Thin extracerebral collections may be easily overlooked on T1 weighted images. However, on T2 weighted images the increased signal from even small collections is usually well shown even when the adjacent brain appears oedematous (Zimmerman et al. 1986). Changes in adjacent cortex and underlying white matter are shown with great sensitivity, as is attendant disease in paranasal sinuses or diploe (Lanzieri et al. 1988; Zimmerman et al. 1986; Moseley 1988; Weingarten et al. 1989).

Less Common Organisms Causing Empyemas

Actinomycosis may produce a suppurative osteomyelitis with epidural empyema and meningitis.

MRI in *aspergillosis* and *rhinocerebral mucormycosis* will show the sinus disease, intracerebral abscesses and the usually haemorrhagic brain infarcts. Signal change in the brain abutting the involved sinuses is frequently present. Signal changes in the cavernous sinuses and internal carotid arteries may indicate thrombosis in these structures.

Echinococcosis typically causes bone destruction. On CT an associated low density non-enhancing but well-circumscribed soft tissue mass is shown. A large low density cyst-like structure in the epidural space was shown by Ba'assiri and Haddad (1984) without any involvement of the calvarium. The cyst contents may yield a homogeneous high signal on MRI but the spectrum of appearances on this modality still awaits adequate description.

Septic Dural Sinus Thrombosis

The cavernous sinuses are usually involved and paranasal sinus disease and orbital cellulitis are the most frequent underlying causes. Orbital cellulitis may be difficult to distinguish from septic cavernous sinus thrombosis itself on clinical grounds (Clifford-Jones et al. 1982). Septic thrombosis rarely occurs in primary intracranial infections, although it may be found as a terminal event and was frequent in the pre-antibiotic era.

Radiology

The signs of cavernous sinus thrombosis on contrast-enhanced CT have been described by various authors (Ford and Sarwar 1981; Clifford-Jones et al. 1982; Ahmadi et al. 1985; de Slegte et al. 1988). These may be listed as follows:

1. Filling defects in the cavernous sinuses (distinguished from normal structures within the sinus by their irregularity and side to side asymmetry)
2. Bulging of the cavernous sinuses to produce a convex lateral margin (usually asymmetrical and visible in only about 20% of established cases)
3. Enlargement of superior and inferior orbital veins (relatively infrequent and indicative of extensive thrombosis)

4. Cerebral infarction, usually involving middle cerebral artery territory and including the striatum
5. Other evidence of intracranial infection such as meningitis, brain abscess and occasionally intracranial empyema

MRI may be expected to show areas of abnormally high signal within the cavernous or sigmoid sinus on spin-echo sequences especially with T2 weighting. However, it should be remembered that patches of high signal may occur in this region due to artefacts, and that on occasion flow-related enhancement may be indistinguishable from the thrombosis (Stevens and Valentine 1987).

Intracerebral Infections

These may be either focal or diffuse. Focal infections with tissue necrosis usually develop into pyogenic abscesses but when the response is mainly cellular and chronic, granulomas result. Widespread tissue responses with mainly perivascular cellular infiltrates or microabscesses are referred to as encephalitis.

Brain Abscesses

Pathogenesis

Brain abscesses arise as a result of parameningeal sepsis or haematogenous dissemination. A source of infection is identifiable in only about 80% of cases (Legg 1983; Chun et al. 1986; Danziger et al. 1980).

Parameningeal Sepsis. About 50% of cases are associated with chronic middle ear disease. Abscesses are found in the white matter of the ipsilateral temporal lobe (60%) or cerebellar hemisphere. The route of spread is probably direct. According to Harriman (1984) there is always adhesion between brain and infected dura over the petrous bone, and in many cases a scar can be found within the adhesion which traverses all cortical layers, representing the site of penetration by organisms. A similar mechanism possibly occurs in brain abscesses associated with subdural empyema and chronic sinusitis which are nearly always in the frontal lobe.

Haematogenous Spread. The most frequent extracranial source of infection is in the thorax, usually either bronchiectasis or pleural empyema. Occasionally osteomyelitis, cutaneous infection or dental sepsis are identified as sources.

Children with cyanotic heart disease are also particularly at risk, constituting about 10% of all cases (Kagawa et al. 1983).

Agents. Organisms are successfully isolated from only about 80% of brain abscesses (Chun et al. 1986). Most infections are mixed, and sometimes only obligate anaerobes (bacteroides, fusobacterium) are present.

Pathology

Recent reviews of case material have indicated that the commonest sites of abscesses are the frontal and parietal lobes, together accounting for about two-thirds of cases. Most parietal lesions result from haematogenous spread. Cerebellar abscesses are rare and temporal lobe abscesses less frequent than they used to be (Danziger et al. 1980; Chun et al. 1986). About 75% of abscesses are solitary, especially those arising from parameningeal sepsis. Most abscesses are unilocular and the wall is thinner on their medial aspects.

Histopathological Development (Staging). The experimental work of Enzmann and Britt carried out mainly on mongrel dogs has developed a system of abscess staging correlated with modern imaging techniques (Enzmann et al. 1982a; Britt and Enzmann 1983). This is important because surgical intervention is best delayed until encapsulation has taken place and because when brain abscesses are detected earlier than this medical therapy may be effective. The two main stages are cerebritis and encapsulation, the first evolving over about 10 days and the second progressing to a coherent collagen-based rim within a further 4 or 5 days. Each of these is subdivided into early and late phases.

Radiology

Since the advent of CT several studies have reported a significant decline in the mortality from brain abscess (Claveria et al. 1976; Rosenblum et al. 1978). In the study by Moseley and Zilkha (1983) the mortality was only 10%. Clinical features are usually suggestive but nearly half the cases are afebrile. Lumbar puncture rarely yields useful information and results in clinical deterioration in 30% of cases (Legg 1983). CT and MRI are the most sensitive imaging modalities and may be expected to detect virtually all intracranial abscesses. However, appearances may be non-specific, and indium-111-labelled leucocyte brain scans may occasionally provide definite information. Ultrasound is capable of accurately staging an abscess but is limited by acoustic access.

Computed Tomography (Figs 5.3 and 5.4). A typical brain abscess is a circumscribed round or oval mass of homogeneous low density surrounded by a slightly hyperdense, enhancing thin and smoothly curved rim. Oedema is present in the surrounding brain. The appearance is non-specific and may be seen in tumours, infarcts and organising haematomas. A firm diagnosis is often not made on the first scan (Moseley and Zilkha 1983). The appearance of an abscess varies according to its stage (Enzmann et al. 1983):

1. Early cerebritis stage: CT shows a poorly circumscribed low density and patchy enhancement occurs after intravenous contrast.

2. Late cerebritis stage: A ring appears after contrast enhancement representing inflammatory reaction in viable tissue surrounding a devascularised and partially necrotic central zone. This ring thickens with time as contrast slowly penetrates the partially necrotic central area.

3. Early capsule stage: Plain CT still shows no definite rim, but ring enhancement occurs after contrast administration. The enhancement is now due in part to neovascularity and tends to diminish in intensity after about 5–10 minutes,

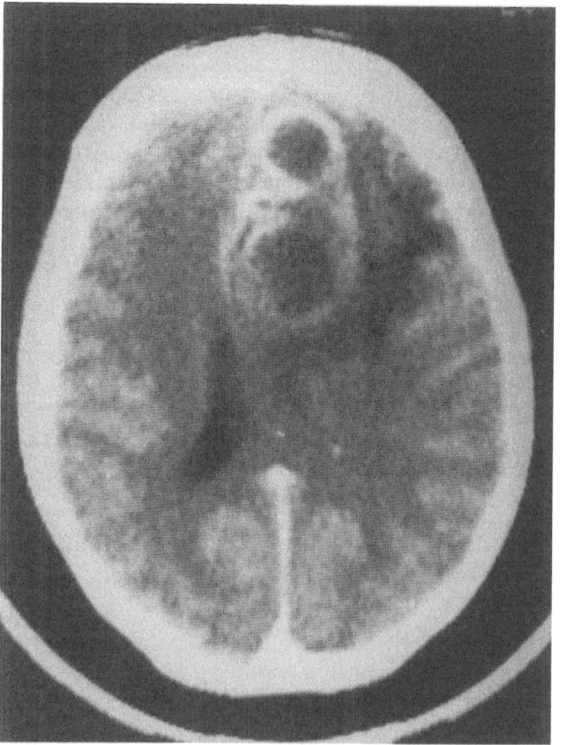

Fig. 5.3. Cranial CT after IV contrast. Cerebral abscess in a patient with cyanotic congenital heart disease. (P.B.)

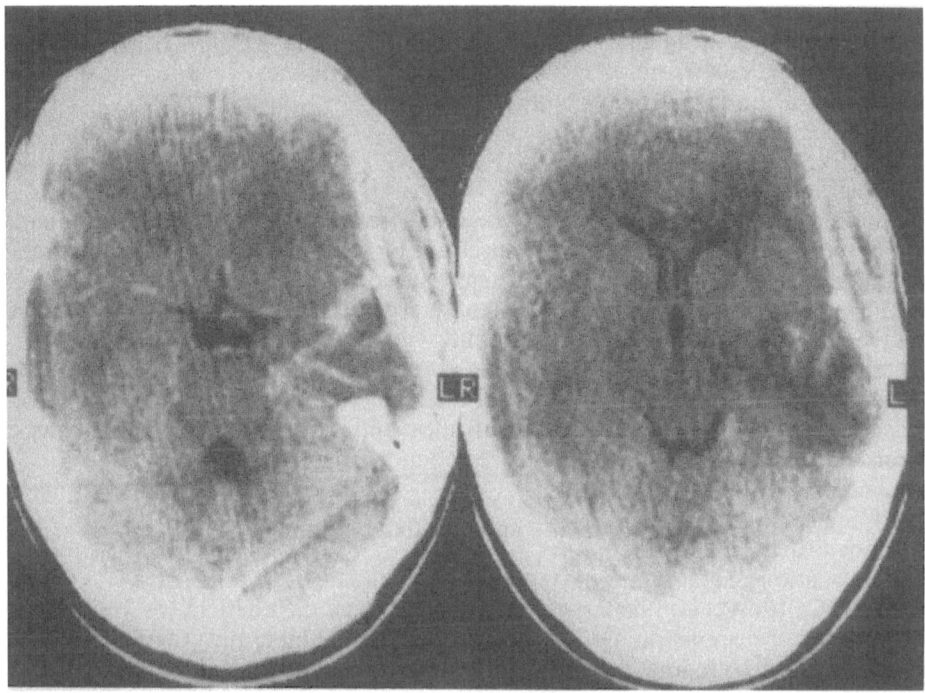

Fig. 5.4. Cranial CT after IV contrast. Infected left craniectomy with an epidural empyema and an irregular temporal lobe abscess.

whereas in the cerebritis stage the intensity of enhancement is sustained for an hour or more. Enhancement does not extend into the central area with time.

4. Late capsule stage: On plain CT a thin isodense rim is clearly visible. This represents the collagenous capsule and is the most reliable indicator of effective encapsulation. After intravenous contrast it enhances, appearing as a somewhat thinner rim than in the previous stage, and the intensity of enhancement declines more rapidly with time.

The time course of these events is variable, being dependent on the type of organism and the ability of the host to respond. Healing is indicated by reduction in size of the central hypodensity. Oedema diminishes and eventually disappears but contrast enhancement around a small hypodense centre may persist indefinitely. Contrast enhancement in the wall is valueless as an indicator of persisting activity; the overriding consideration in making this judgement should be the condition of the patient.

It is customary to scan patients at frequent intervals during treatment although it is doubtful that this is necessary in every case. In a review of over 100 CT examinations for which the indication given was "routine", Moseley and Zilkha (1983) found only 10 which showed any unexpected feature, usually enlargement of the abscess. They also argued that a check CT scan immediately after surgical intervention was unnecessary unless haemorrhage had occurred or drainage was unsatisfactory.

There is an increasing tendency to treat brain abscesses medically using antibiotics and steroids. The effect of steroids alone on the CT appearance has been investigated by Enzmann et al. (1982b) who found that the main effect was to reduce enhancement in the cerebritis and early encapsulation stages but not in the late encapsulation stage. As a caution, Dobkin et al. (1984) have shown that some medically cured "abscesses" were actually misdiagnosed cerebral infarcts. It is therefore desirable to obtain proof of diagnosis by aspiration biopsy. The frequent variability in shape, thickness of the wall, degree of contrast enhancement and surrounding oedema in intracerebral abscesses on CT should be emphasised, and diagnosis may be difficult.

Magnetic Resonance Imaging. The relatively large area of increased signal visible on T2 weighted spin-echo images has been shown accurately to delineate the oedema (Grossman et al. 1985). The necrotic centre of a developing abscess has a prolonged T1 which becomes increasingly prolonged as liquefaction proceeds. In T1 weighted images therefore the pus returns a uniform low signal; on increasingly T2 weighted images it returns a higher signal and may appear as bright as or brighter than the surrounding oedema if the repetition time is long. The capsule usually returns the same signal as normal brain and may not be seen on T2 weighted sequences. On T1 weighted images it is usually visible and sometimes the capsule returns a very high signal on T1 weighted images suggesting that it is haemorrhagic (Zimmerman et al. 1986). The administration of intravenous gadolinium DTPA greatly improves the visibility of the capsule and may reveal loculations or additional abscesses not suspected on the pre-enhanced study (Grossman et al. 1985; Davidson and Steiner 1985; Moseley 1988). If gadolinium is not available then more precise information about loculation and local multiplicity may be obtained from CT (Post et al. 1986), although MRI remains superior at demonstrating the full extent of the abnormality including the detection of remote lesions.

Neurosonography. Because of the difficulty of acoustic access, sonography in adults is only established as an intraoperative tool. In experimental brain abscess Enzmann et al. (1982a) concluded that sonography was more sensitive to some of the histological features of encapsulation than CT, in particular to the early deposition of collagen. The central necrosis is hypoechoic becoming more so as encapsulation proceeds. Collagen appears as multiple relatively low level echoes on the inner margin of the capsule which increase as encapsulation progresses.

Sonographic localisation and guided aspiration of brain abscesses is now an accepted technique, and haemorrhagic complications can be recognised by the appearance of high level echoes. Some workers have found that injecting saline microbubbles as a sonographic contrast agent was helpful in identifying unsuspected loculi and monitoring response to treatment (Scatamachia et al. 1987).

Radiolabelled Leucocyte Brain Scanning. This is a recently developed technique based on labelling white cells from the patient with indium-111. These are reinjected into the patient who is then scanned by a Gamma camera at 4 and 24 hours. In one study in children, which included abscesses in all locations, the overall accuracy was 86%, and sensitivity 85% (Gordon and Vivian 1984). The major cause of false positives in the brain is infarction which sometimes has intense leucocyte infiltration.

Other causes include any of the non-infective inflammations, including primary demyelination. Nevertheless, the technique can be of value in the author's experience.

Other Types of Abscess

Abscesses and granulomas represent different ends of a spectrum of focal response to infection. Some organisms usually produce granulomas but occasionally even with these the response may be to produce a non-granulomatous capsule surrounding a cavity containing purulent necrotic material best referred to as an abscess. Radiologically these appear identical to abscesses caused by more common organisms.

Intracerebral Granulomas

A granuloma consists of a solid mass of mainly mononuclear cells and their derivatives. Epithelioid giant cells often predominate and granulation tissue and fibroblasts are usually present. Granulomas often surround a central zone or zones of necrosis which can consist of either solid, purulent or caseous material. Sometimes the central portion is a solid mass of organisms.

Granulomas Due to Eubacteria

The organisms involved here are the filamentous bacteria of the group actinomycetes, comprising the genera *Mycobacterium*, *Nocardia* and *Actinomyces* (Millan et al. 1985). Some species resemble fungi more than others because of their tendency to filamentous growth but nevertheless are true bacteria. Granulomas may also result from spirochaetes.

Tuberculoma. Up to 80% of patients with intracerebral tuberculosis also have tuberculous meningitis. The remainder have good immunity and the granulomas do not discharge into the subarachnoid space. Only about 10% are associated with miliary tuberculosis. The lesions are between 2 and 10 mm in diameter and in about a third of patients are multiple (Bhargava and Tandon 1980). Large studies have shown no particular site predilection, although most lesions in adults are supratentorial (Dastur and Lalitha 1973). Pathologically the lesions usually consist of a firm caseous central zone surrounded by a thick capsule consisting of fibrous tissue in which are embedded multiple tubercles. Surrounding gliosis and oedema are also usually present.

In the early stages CT shows an area of poorly circumscribed low density suggestive of vasogenic

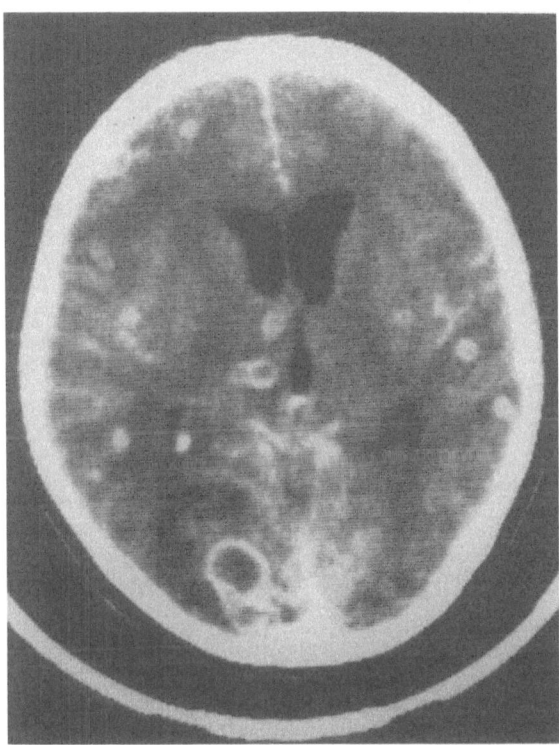

Fig. 5.5. Cranial CT after IV contrast. Multiple tuberculomata. (P.B.)

alarming increase in oedema may occur in the first few weeks (Kocen 1987).

MRI of tuberculomas shows areas of low signal on T1 weighted and high signal on T2 weighted images. The tuberculoma may be distinguishable from surrounding oedema on T1 weighted and mildly T2 weighted sequences and the pattern of enhancement with gadolinium DTPA parallels that seen on CT (Davidson and Steiner 1985; Moseley 1988). Some tuberculomas have appeared as nodules of high signal on T1 weighted images (Zimmerman et al. 1986). They probably represent the cystic type of tuberculoma (or tuberculous pseudoabscess) which Dastur and Lalitha state always involve a blood vessel and represent haemorrhagic ischaemic necrosis of the central part of the tuberculoma.

MRI shows more areas of focal change in the brain than are evident on CT both in the subcortical and periventricular white matter. Most of these probably represent further areas of tuberculous cerebritis and perhaps the occasional tuberculoma which is not shown by CT. However, some presumably represent ischaemic changes and others perhaps the border zone and tuberculous encephalitides which are vasculitic and demyelinating (Dastur and Lalitha 1973).

Granulomas and Abscesses due to Eufungi

1. *Aspergillus* (Fig. 5.6). Cerebral lesions usually arise only in the disseminated form of the disease, although direct vascular invasion reaching the subarachnoid space and cavernous sinuses may occur from the paranasal sinuses. *Aspergillus fumigatus* is another ubiquitous saprophyte and most often becomes pathogenic in an immunosuppressed patient. Granulomas may coalesce to form large masses or large thin-walled abscesses may occur in the brain (Scaravilli 1984; Wiles and MacKenzie 1987). On computed tomography large ring lesions, thick-walled irregular lobulated rings or near solid masses may occur and the usual diagnosis is of a malignant neoplasm (Coccia-Portugal et al. 1987). Angiography often shows vasculitis, with major vessel occlusions and mycotic aneurysms, as well as mass. MRI may show a high signal mass on T2 weighted sequences, but available descriptions are few (Zimmerman et al. 1986).

2. *Cryptococcus.* Intracerebral cryptococcomas may arise by extension of yeasts from the subarachnoid into the Virchow–Robin spaces, or by haematogenous dissemination. They consist of a mass of organisms surrounded by a giant cell granulomatous reaction. In an analysis of 55 cases with intracerebral masses, Fujita et al. (1981) noted that

oedema, in which ring enhancement appears after intravenous contrast (Fig. 5.5). Later the tuberculoma becomes visible as an isodense or hyperdense disc or ring which also enhances, though rarely becoming as dense as calcium. The rings may be small with thick walls and only images of good quality may reveal the central rather punctate hypodensity. Less common forms include larger rings enclosing central material of somewhat higher attenuation than is usually seen in abscesses, and large lobulated solid or inhomogeneous masses resembling a neoplasm. Such masses when located on the surface of the brain can resemble a meningioma (Bhargava and Tandon 1980; Whelan and Stern 1981).

An unusual pattern of gyral enhancement with underlying vasogenic oedema has been described which histologically proved to be due to a conglomeration of tubercles in the grey matter unrelated to meningitis, and termed focal tuberculous cerebritis. Five such lesions followed by serial CT did not resolve even on antituberculous therapy; they either remained unchanged or progressed to focal cortical atrophy (Jinkins 1988). Successful treatment is attended usually by reducing size of the lesion and reducing oedema. This may be delayed (Bhargava and Tandon 1980) and occasionally an

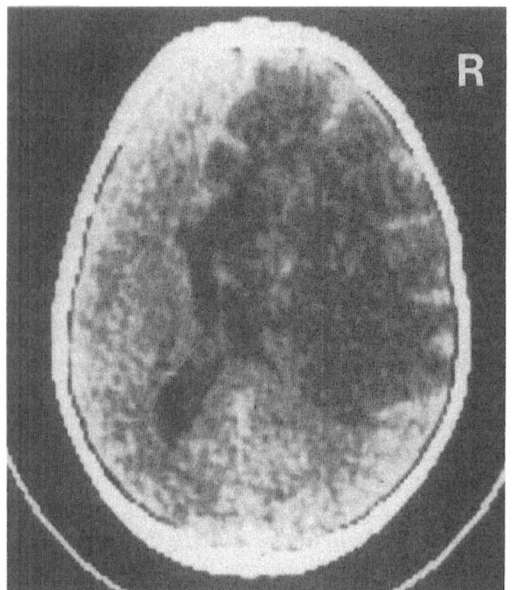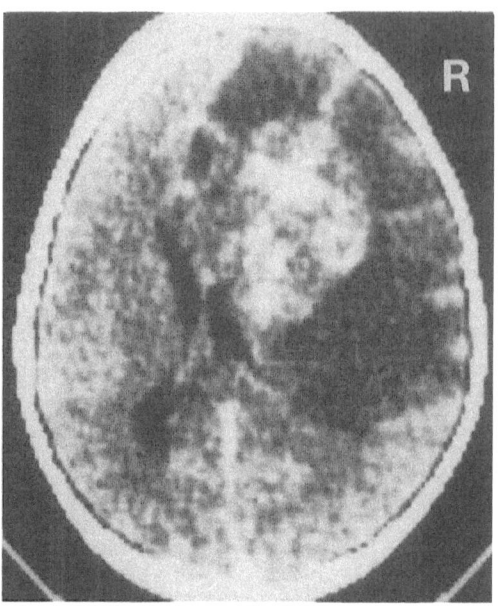

Fig. 5.6. Cranial CT before (**a**) and after (**b**) IV contrast. Aspergilloma.

35% were multiple, and that each mass could represent either an abscess (9%), a gelatinous mass with little host reaction (24%), or a fibro-granulomatous mass (15%). Forty-three per cent were mixed in type and 58% of the cases in their material had no associated meningitis. On computed tomography cryptococcomas usually appear as low-density lesions with or without thin- or thick-walled ring enhancement, or as solid enhancing nodules. Lesions in the basal ganglia are common and some have been shown to protrude into a ventricle and to be associated with extensive ependymal enhancement. Others have involved the optic chiasm (Cornell and Jacoby 1982; Arrington et al. 1984; Garcia et al. 1985).

3. *Mucormycosis.* A primary nasal infection is usually present and vascular invasion results in haematogenous dissemination directly to the brain. Computed tomography demonstrates a large and rapidly growing low-density lesion representing the necrosis caused by the hyphae and a surrounding rim of variable enhancement and oedema although these may be entirely absent. Angiography usually indicates a severe vasculitis, and sometimes a mycotic aneurysm is shown proximal to the intracerebral mass, suggesting this to be a source of embolising hyphae (Gamba et al. 1986; Wiles and MacKenzie 1987).

4. *Candida.* Candida infections of the brain are among the most frequent fungal infections found at autopsy. Patients are ill for other reasons and have disseminated candidiasis as a contributory terminal event. Early vascular involvement is prominent, producing multiple relatively small haemorrhagic infarcts which organise into abscesses or granulomas if survival time permits (Scaravilli 1984; Wiles and MacKenzie 1987).

Granulomas Due to Parasites

1. *Neurocysticercosis* (Fig. 5.7). Most superficially placed cysts lie within cortical sulci although occasionally true intraparenchymal cysts are seen. Only about 14% calcify heavily enough to be seen on plain X-ray films. The viable lesions appear on CT as low-density cysts usually without contrast enhancement. After cyst degeneration, a granuloma may result with nodular contrast enhancement. Sometimes large lobular masses develop which consist of multiple cysts resembling a malignant cerebral neoplasm. Very occasionally fragments of a degenerative cyst becomes incorporated in a region of encapsulated purulent necrosis – a brain abscess.

2. *Echinococcosis.* Cerebral hydatid cysts are usually solitary, spherical and unilocular. The cyst wall is 2–3 mm thick and characteristically there is little or no reaction in the surrounding brain. On CT they appear as circumscribed rounded low-density lesions typically with no contrast enhancement in the wall and no oedema. Calcification occurs only rarely. Daughter cysts and multilocular forms have

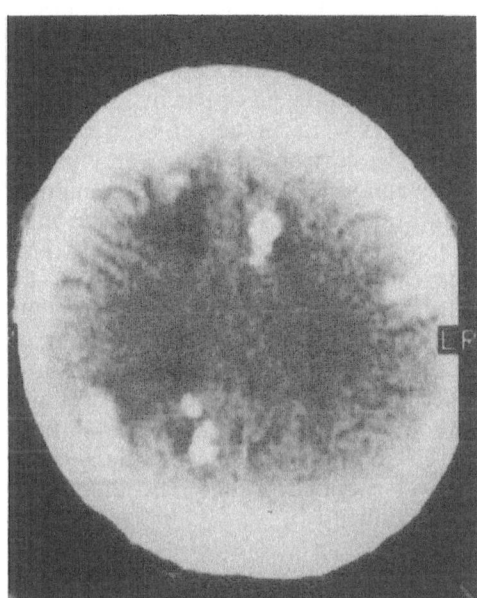

Fig. 5.7. Cranial CT. Neurocysticercosis. Multiple calcified granulomas are shown.

been seen in the brain but are also rare. Sonographic examination of the liver for evidence of other cysts is an important investigation. Surgical excision is usually required.

3. *Paragonimiasis*. This disease is produced by the lung fluke, *Paragonimus westermani*. It is a disease of Asia, Africa and Latin America and is especially prevalent among the Japanese. It is acquired by eating infected fresh water snails. The flukes develop in the intestine whence they invade the peritoneal cavity and migrate to many sites but mainly to the lungs. Flukes may also invade the cranial cavity through the jugular or carotid canals. They penetrate the meningeal barrier, and lodge in the basal regions of the brain, mainly the occipital and temporal lobes. Pairs of flukes develop a cyst, as in the lung, but rarely survive after producing ova. The cyst degenerates, resulting in a host reaction which produces either numerous granulomas or abscesses containing ova in the central necrotic zone. Fresh lesions often appear as haemorrhagic foci. On computed tomography a variety of appearances are found:

1. Multiple rounded structures within heavy peripheral calcification
2. Large low density areas surrounding or linked to calcified zones often with the appearance of porencephalic cysts
3. Diffuse cerebral atrophy (Udaka et al. 1988; Sinycharcen et al. 1988)

Encephalitis

Encephalitis is caused by viral, bacterial and parasitic agents and often distinction between infective and postinfective forms is not clear. Radiological evaluation is imprecise, because CT is either normal or shows very non-specific and poorly localised abnormalities. The appearances may also resemble an infiltrating glioma. MRI reveals an even greater spectrum of non-specific abnormalities but appearances may closely resemble those of multiple sclerosis.

Acute Viral Encephalitis

The commonest agents are the arbo- and roboviruses and some herpes viruses, notably Herpes simplex.

Herpes Simplex Encephalitis (Adult Type). Herpes simplex virus (HSV) type 1 is the commonest cause of sporadic acute encephalitis (acute necrotising encephalitis) and affects previously fit adults. It is very uncommon in patients with recurrent "cold-sores", but because many patients have pre-existing antibodies it probably does represent a reactivation disease. The latent virus may reside in (a) the olfactory bulb, which may explain the distribution of lesions in the limbic system (the olfactory bulb is involved in only 40% of cases) or (b) the trigeminal nerve, from which the brain is invaded via the meningeal distribution of its sensory nerves (Brownell and Tomlinson 1984; Davis 1987).

The pathological findings are highly characteristic with widespread necrosis usually maximal in the temporal lobes. One hemisphere is usually affected more than the other. Mortality is about 70% and nearly half the survivors are severely disabled. Early diagnosis is crucial as treatment is possible with acyclovir and, because necrosis is a progressive phenomenon, early treatment may significantly reduce morbidity. Serological diagnosis takes 10–12 days to establish. A positive diagnosis can be made by brain biopsy in 2–3 hours (Lunsford et al. 1984).

Computed tomography (Fig. 5.8) shows abnormalities which are clear and unequivocal in 95% of cases, but only in 78% in the first 5 days (Zimmerman et al. 1980; Ketonen and Koskiniemi, 1980; O'Neil et al. 1987). The earliest abnormality is subtle low density in one temporal lobe. Later this becomes more definite with additional involvement of the inferior frontal lobe and insula. In 90% the insula has a distinctive sharp medial margin indicating sparing of the striatum. Over 80% of patients eventually show bilateral changes, whereas the earliest scans show bilateral change in only 10%.

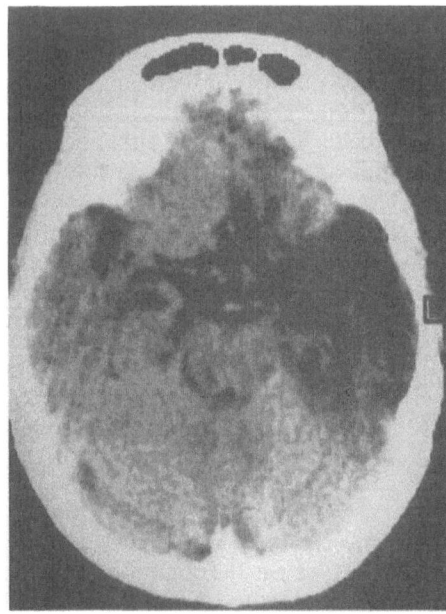

Fig. 5.8. Cranial CT. Herpes simplex encephalitis.

Local mass effect develops with time, but becomes prominent in only 75%. Diffuse mass has also been reported (Zimmerman et al. 1980). Contrast enhancement is present in 70% of cases though is rarely present on early scans and is seldom marked (Ketonen and Koskiniemi 1980).

Haemorrhage is recognisable at some stage in about 15%. It is most common in the medial part of the temporal lobe bordering the crural cistern and can be mistaken for subarachnoid haemorrhage. In about 5% of cases extensive haemorrhage in the temporal lobe is seen. The end result is severe atrophy, indistinguishable from mature infarction.

MRI shows great promise in providing clear evidence of the disease and bilateral involvement at an earlier stage than CT. Extensive signal changes are often present also in the periventricular white matter. T1 weighted images often fail to reveal any abnormality unless haemorrhage or extensive necrosis have occurred (Zimmerman et al. 1986; Moseley 1988) or unless mass effect is marked.

Angiography is not indicated but may be performed because of an erroneous diagnosis. Vascular changes including occlusions are often shown, closely resembling infarction.

Neonatal Herpes Simplex Encephalitis. Herpes simplex virus (HSV) type 2 (genital herpes) may cause a mild self-limiting meningitis in adults. In neonates and infants a severe generalised encephalitis with a high morbidity results. Premature babies are especially at risk. The disease is presumed to be acquired from the birth passages but sometimes also via the placenta. Computed tomography shows the progressive development of patchy low attenuation in the deep white matter of both cerebral hemispheres. The cortex and central grey matter may become abnormally dense, due to multiple small haemorrhages initially and calcification later. Atrophy becomes obvious within about three weeks. The early development of extensive calcification in gyri (especially along the grey–white matter junctions), basal ganglia, and in the germinal matrix around the ventricles is a distinctive feature. Later this becomes visible even on plain X-ray films. Marked ventricular dilation and heavy periventricular calcification is found especially when the disease was acquired in utero (Benaton et al. 1985; Noorbehesht 1987).

Cytomegalovirus (CMV). Cytomegalic inclusion disease is a disseminated disease of neonates, acquired during delivery or at any stage in intrauterine life. Severe congenital anomalies occur when infection occurs early, and a disseminated viral illness when inoculation is late. The brain is not invariably involved but the commonest abnormalities are hydrocephalus and extensive periventricular calcification. Both are the result of extensive subependymal necrosis. It is the second most common infective cause of intracerebral calcification in infants and young children on plain X-ray films after toxoplasmosis. The disease also occurs in patients with AIDS.

Acute Postinfectious Encephalomyelitis. This includes acute disseminated (perivenous) encephalomyelitis and the more severe form, acute haemorrhagic leucoencephalitis (Allen 1984; Johnson and Griffin 1987). The disease is monophasic and develops 2–7 days after a preceding illness, most often an upper respiratory tract infection. However, other sensitising illnesses are, in descending order of importance: measles, vaccinia (in the recent past), varicella, rubella, type A influenza, EB virus (infectious mononucleosis) and *Mycoplasma pneumoniae*.

It is the commonest neurological complication of measles and about 50% of children with uncomplicated measles show electroencephalographic abnormalities. Minor behavioural problems are common for weeks or months after an apparently uncomplicated exanthematous illness. The disease develops when cell-mediated immunity has matured, and is virtually unknown in children under the age of 2 years.

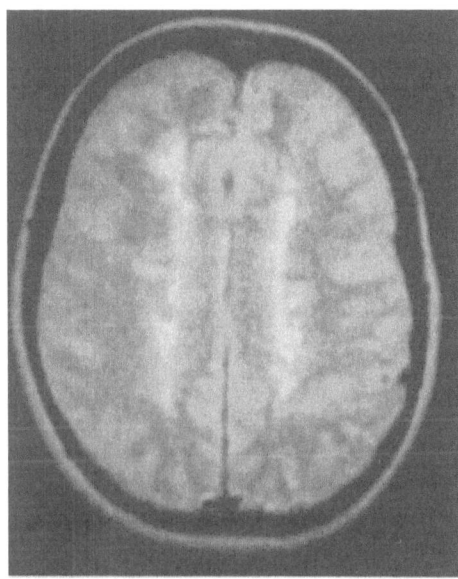

Fig. 5.9. Cranial MRI (T2 weighted image). Postinfectious encephalitis (varicella). The patient was asymptomatic at the time of this scan, 4 months after the onset of the disease.

MRI shows multifocal involvement mainly involving white matter but on occasion only the brain stem is abnormal (Atlas et al. 1986). However, since CT is usually unremarkable the MRI changes may strongly suggest multiple sclerosis (Moseley 1988) (Fig. 5.9). In some cases which have been followed by MRI, many but not all of these white matter lesions have resolved within 3–6 months (Belman and Anand 1985).

Acute haemorrhagic leucoencephalitis is usually shown by CT and certainly by MRI. Mixed density large white matter masses were shown by CT in the examples reported by Valentine et al. (1982) in which patchy contrast enhancement occurred and the lesions were initially diagnosed as malignant gliomas. MRI may show evidence of haemorrhage in various stages of evolution (Atlas et al. 1986), but this has not been evident on CT.

Chronic Encephalopathies Due to Slow Viruses

Spongiform encephalopathy. The term includes Creutzfeldt–Jacob disease, kuru (mainly cerebellar) and scrapie (affecting sheep). There is also a transmissible form of the Gerstmann–Staussler syndrome (spinocerebellar) which is now regarded as a variant of Creutzfeldt–Jacob disease.

The agent is likely to be a novel one, for there is no inflammatory reaction in involved tissue and no antibodies are produced. The evidence has pointed to an agent consisting exclusively of protein, for

which the term prion has been coined and a strong contender has been found recently and designated PrP or Pr27–30 (Prusiner 1982; Matthews 1987).

Computed tomography in Creutzfeldt–Jacob disease is normal in the early stages but later there is a marked generalised cortical atrophy (Matthews 1987). Progression of this process over a few months has been well documented by serial CT and may also show the cerebellum to be affected (Westphal and Schachenmayne 1985). Cases with a long clinical course have also shown white matter changes (Le May 1987); however, care should be exercised in interpreting an individual case because of the high prevalence of cortical atrophy and ischaemic rarefaction of the white matter in the elderly.

Progressive Multifocal Leucoencephalopathy. Papovaviruses are ubiquitous and not pathogenic to man. They exist in latent form in lymphocytes especially in the bone marrow (Houf et al. 1988). When activated by other diseases such as AIDS, lymphoproliferative disorders, sarcoidosis and also by iatrogenic immunosuppression lymphocytes carry the agent to the brain where it develops into a lytic infection of oligodendrocytes. Occasional cases have been reported in fit individuals (Zochodne and Kaufmann 1987).

Computed tomography shows areas of low attenuation in the cerebal white matter, often in the occipitotemporal regions, but lesions can be found anywhere including the brainstem and cerebellum (Fig. 5.10). The grey matter is usually but not

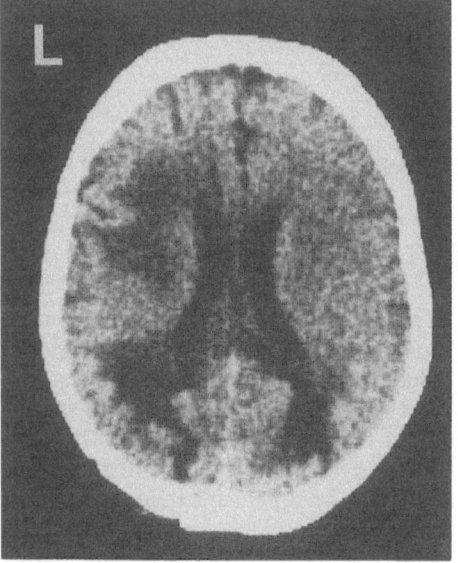

Fig. 5.10. Cranial CT. Progressive multifocal leucoencephalopathy.

always spared, and when there is evolving necrosis the similarity to infarction can be close. Contrast enhancement may be present in the lesions, and there may be an appearance of multifocal enhancement. Sometimes the lesions are solitary and exhibit sufficient mass to simulate a tumour. Not all the patients die, and arrest of the disease may occur when immunosuppressive therapy is discontinued (Krupp et al. 1985; Shafran et al. 1987; Vanneste et al. 1984). MRI shows the lesions well and reveals lesions not detected by CT (Zimmerman et al. 1986; Moseley 1987).

Subacute Sclerosing Panencephalitis. The agent is the measles virus. Over 90% of cases are children 4–16 years old, and 75% are boys. The disease progresses over months and myoclonus is a common feature. The onset is several years after classical measles, and the risk is greatest if the latter occurs in the first year of life. The pathogenesis of reactivation and the reason for the slow course are not understood.

Computed tomography is often normal, but may show evidence of brain swelling. Areas of low attenuation in the white matter and progressive cortical atrophy have also been documented (Krawiecki et al. 1984), and these abnormalities have been shown to progress on CT even when the clinical picture is improving.

A clinically similar disease has been caused by rubella virus, chronic progressive rubella panencephalitis. Pathological differences are present, in that the brain stem and cerebellum are heavily involved, and there is widespread vasculitis with fibrinoid necrosis. CT and MRI can resemble Herpes simplex encephalitis (Davidson and Steiner 1986).

INFECTIONS OF THE SPINE

Bacterial Osteomyelitis

Vertebral osteomyelitis is most commonly a consequence of spinal surgery but may arise "spontaneously" due to a bacteraemia in which the primary focus is often trivial. The organisms usually lodge initially in the spongy bone beneath a vertebral endplate where there is a hyperaemic zone (Wiley et al. 1959). The organisms then invade the endplate itself and eventually destroy the intervertebral disc. Atypical patterns of involvement are seen which are more common in tuberculosis. Infection can arise in the appendages, especially the apo-

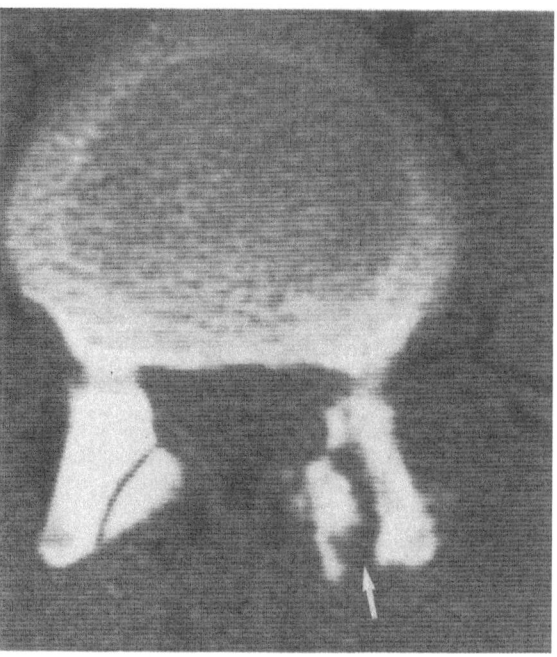

Fig. 5.11. Spinal CT. Tuberculous arthritis of a lumbar apophyseal joint (*arrow*).

physeal joints (Fig. 5.11) or in the anterior part of a vertebral body and spread beneath the anterior longitudinal ligament from vertebra to vertebra without destroying the intervening discs (Chapman et al. 1979). Paravertebral abscess formation is common, especially in tuberculosis.

The usual agents are *Staphylococcus aureus* and *Mycobacterium tuberculosis* but many others have occasionally been isolated, notably *Salmonella typhi* and *Brucella abortus*.

Radiology

Plain films show loss of the vertebral end plate on each side of the intervertebral disc space, which rapidly becomes narrowed. Sclerosis in the subchondral bone as well as an erosive type of bone destruction become conspicuous and substantial vertebral collapse may occur. The thoracic and lumbar spine are most often involved. Osteophytes and exuberant new bone are features during treatment and bony ankylosis often with some degree of gibbus is the frequent result. Sometimes a large calcified psoas abscess is evident which is pathognomonic of tuberculosis.

Infections of the spine can occur anywhere, and cervical spine is not infrequently involved. The radiological features described above may not appear for several weeks, and paraspinal and epidural sepsis may occur early. Thickening of the pre-

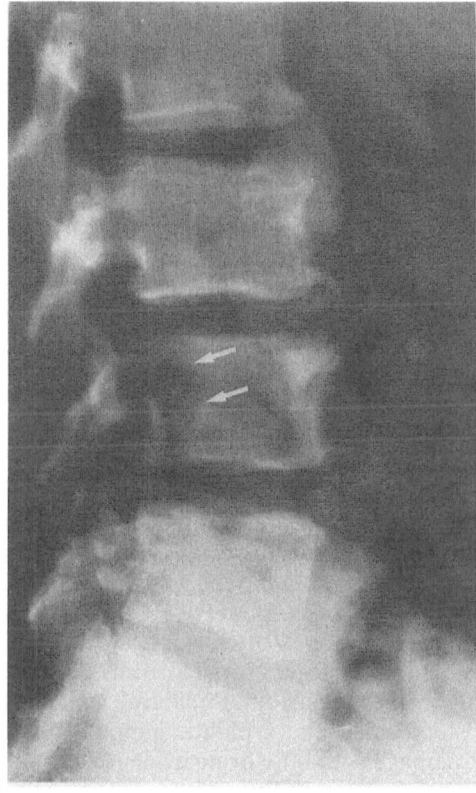

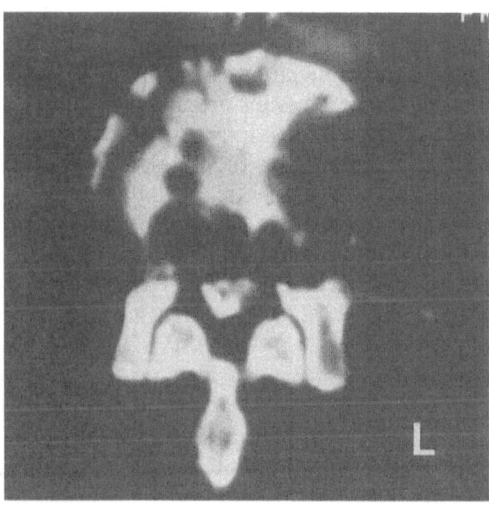

Fig. 5.12. Lumbar spine: **a** lateral radiograph; **b** axial CT. Tuberculous spondylitis. Inconspicuous bone destruction seen on the plain radiograph (*arrows*) is much more evident on CT which shows a moth-eaten bony appearance.

vertebral soft tissues of the neck on a lateral radiograph can be an important early sign.

Computed tomography is far more sensitive at detecting the early changes in spongy bone and the paravertebral swelling. Often marked erosions are shown which are barely visible on plain radiographs although they would be shown by conventional tomography (Fig. 5.12) (Golimbu et al. 1984).

MRI may be abnormal at an even earlier stage than CT (Fig. 5.13). On T1 weighted images there is signal reduction in the intervertebral disc and adjacent vertebral body, with loss of definition of the cortical margin between. On T2 weighted images there is increased signal in all or part of the disc and in the adjacent vertebrae the normal central lamina becomes invisible or disrupted early (Modic et al. 1985; de Roos et al. 1986).

Other techniques can be helpful. Bone scanning using ⁹⁹ᵐTc–disphosphonate or its analogues is positive in virtually all cases of pyogenic osteomyelitis but may be negative in some non-pyogenic cases.

Tissue diagnosis is usually required to identify the causative organism, and needle aspiration biopsy under fluoroscopic or CT control of the disc, vertebral body or preferably the paraspinal abscess (Adapon et al. 1981) is usually adequate.

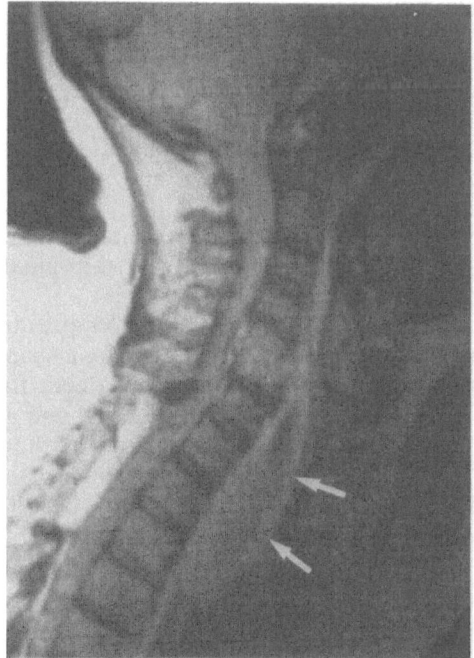

Fig. 5.13. Cervical MRI (T1 weighted image). Pyogenic osteomyelitis of the 5th and 6th cervical vertebrae with a large prevertebral abscess (*arrows*).

Differential Diagnosis. Normal postoperative changes after discectomies and fusions can be difficult to distinguish from infection especially in the early stages when the soft tissues are swollen. This is particularly true of MRI (Zimmerman et al. 1986; Moseley 1987). Occasionally a focal destructive spondyloarthropathy can be identical to infective disco-vertebral spondylitis on plain radiographs and may be seen in rheumatoid arthritis, ankylosing spondylitis, calcium pyrophosphate deposition disease and in patients on long-term haemodialysis (Deramond et al. 1987).

Changes in the intervertebral discs also occur after chemonucleolysis. There is loss of height of the intervertebral disc and on MRI many cases develop increased signal in the adjacent vertebral bodies but the disc itself persistently returns a low signal which should distinguish it from infection (Masaryk et al. 1986). On CT a mottled appearance in the bone adjacent to a disc may represent local reaction to chymopapain, but a moth-eaten appearance usually indicates infection (Deeb et al. 1985).

Non-bacterial Osteomyelitis

Fungal osteomyelitis is similar in appearance to that due to tuberculosis and often involves disc spaces. The fungi most often isolated are *Aspergillus fumigatus*, *Blastomyces dermatitidis*, and *Coccidioides immitis* (Wiles and MacKenzie 1988).

The main parasitic disease affecting the vertebrae is echinococcosis, either *E. granulosis* and *E. multicocularis* (alveolaris). The lesion begins in the vertebral body and the cyst becomes lobulated as it burrows through the spongiosa and into the appendages. Cortical breaches appear and the multilocular cyst extends into the paraspinal tissues. Liver cysts are usually associated with the spinal cysts which are always multilocular.

Plain radiographs show bone destruction spreading to the neural arches, sometimes having a soap bubble appearance. Spread from one vertebra to another or into the costal elements is usual and a soft tissue mass can often be recognised. Pathological fractures and vertebral dislocations can occur. These features are also well shown by CT (Claudon et al. 1987). The soft tissue masses are of low attenuation and show no peripheral enhancement after intravenous contrast (Braithwaite and Lees 1981). On MRI the signal from the cysts is variable (Mikhael et al. 1985).

Epidural Infection

Unlike the situation in the cranium where the majority of empyemas are subdural, most spinal empyemas are epidural. By 1987, only 18 cases of spinal subdural empyema had been reported (Knudsen et al. 1987). Most cases of epidural empyema arise from vertebral osteomyelitis although this may be inconspicuous and remote from the site of maximal epidural sepsis. Occasionally there is no vertebral focus and the infection is acquired from a bacteraemia. Less frequently the epidural space is involved by direct extension from a pleural empyema.

Epidural infections usually spread widely, and in children may involve the entire length of the spinal canal. Haematogenous infection usually loculates posteriorly. Chronic infections due to tuberculosis and fungi characteristically cause marked dural thickening, sometimes sufficient to compress the spinal cord.

The clinical picture is often acute, with pain, toxaemia and paraplegia; surgical drainage is a matter of urgency. Sometimes epidural infections such as tuberculosis and syphilitic gummas cause ligament damage with little or no evidence of bone involvement, and instability results. Severe complications of this have occurred at the craniovertebral junction occasioning sudden death from high spinal cord compression.

Myelography shows an extensive epidural mass, often located dorsal to the theca. An incomplete spinal block is usually shown by water-soluble myelography. The degree of cord compression and precise relationship of the abscess are best shown by computed myelography (Fig. 5.14). MRI can also demonstrate epidural collections (Zimmerman et al. 1986; Moseley 1987).

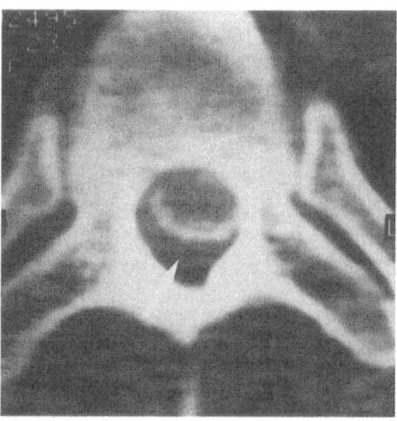

Fig. 5.14. CT myelography. Epidural abscess (*arrow*).

Myelitis and Myelopathy in Infection

Myelopathy is frequently caused by compression which usually originates from the epidural space. This can arise from an epidural abscess and pachymeningitis, or from vertebral or craniovertebral subluxation and dislocation. Pyogenic retropharyngeal abscesses have also been associated with this latter complication, which is usually non-fatal. The cord may be rendered more susceptible to the effects of compression by an associated arteritis which may also cause spinal cord infarcts in the absence of compression.

The myelitis associated with infections is frequently demyelinating in type. Organisms may invade the cord and produce either a myelitis or intramedullary abscess or granuloma. Most sporadic cases of infective myelitis are probably caused by viruses, especially of the enterovirus group.

Some of the previously poorly understood chronic myelopathies are now being found to have an infectious aetiology. One such is tropical spastic paraparesis (West Indian neuromyelitis). The pathology is mainly of a meningitis but perivascular infiltrates also extend into the spinal cord and extensive demyelination occurs. The agent has been identified as the virus HIV I.

Radiology in all these conditions yields nonspecific findings or no abnormality at all. Myelography may show fusiform cord swelling involving several segments, which is usually mild but may cause a partial spinal block. An arachnoiditis may also be present, increasing the degree of spinal block and causing irregularities. Computed myelography shows the cord swelling and delayed imaging frequently shows abnormal uptake and retention of contrast material in central regions of the cord, usually representing necrosis (Fig. 5.15).

MRI is usually more sensitive than CT in detecting these abnormalities, especially T2 weighted images. Areas of high signal which are either focal or extend for multiple segments are shown, but are indistinguishable from acute myelitis in multiple sclerosis.

IMMUNODEFICIENCY STATES AND AIDS

The two conditions which have caused an upsurge in clinical opportunistic infections are organ transplantation and the disease which is outstripping all others in clinical importance, the acquired immu-

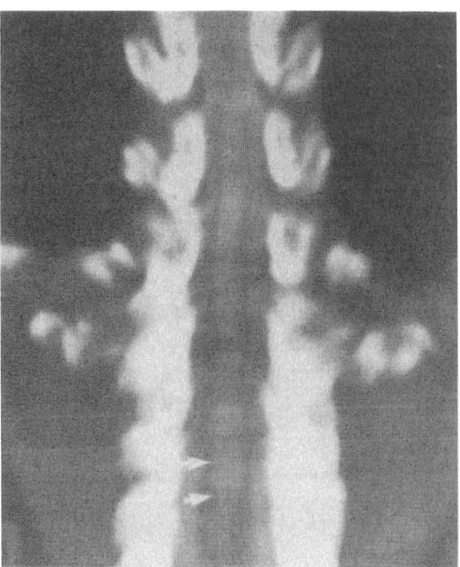

Fig. 5.15. CT myelography. Coronal reformat showing abnormal uptake of contrast medium by the spinal cord (*arrows*).

nodeficiency syndrome (AIDS). A group of three RNA tumour viruses has been identified as having a predilection for infecting T-lymphocytes. These viruses have been designated HIV or human immunodeficiency viruses. HIV III causes suppression of circulating lymphocytes resulting in a slowly and remorselessly progressive suppression of cell mediated and dependent humoral immunity. There develops a marked susceptibility particularly to opportunistic infections.

The hallmarks of immunodeficiency diseases are unusual infections, unusual manifestations of common infections, and depressed host response resulting in unusual pathological and radiological appearances.

The Radiology of HIV III Infection of the Nervous System

Computed Tomography. Cortical atrophy and ventricular enlargement may be seen and sometimes low density is present in the deep white matter. In a recent study of 200 cases with neurological abnormalities, diffuse atrophy only was found in 38% and 40% appeared normal; the rest showed mass lesions of various kinds (Levy et al. 1986). Progression of atrophy is demonstrable, and atrophy has been noted on scans before the appearance of neurological abnormalities. However, other infections have been found in cases showing brain atrophy only, including cytomegalovirus, Herpes viruses, toxoplasmosis and *Cryptococcus*. In children, atrophy, microcephaly and basal ganglia calcification have been documented by CT (Bellman et al. 1985).

Magnetic Resonance Imaging. Ventricular expansion and diffuse or patchy signal changes in the cerebal white matter are shown. Sensitivity is considerably greater than CT, especially for the white matter abnormalities. Abnormalities were shown in 70% of cases of established AIDS, and 50% of cases with AIDS-related complex or just positive seroconversion (Grant et al. 1987). Therefore MRI is very sensitive to early involvement of the central nervous system.

Viral Infections in Immunosuppression

These are Herpes simplex encephalitis, cytomegalovirus (CMV), progressive multifocal leucoencephalopathy (rare in AIDS), Herpes zoster and measles (especially in children with lymphoma). A severe demyelinating or necrotising encephalitis or myelitis may result from any of these (Price and Navia 1987).

CMV is isolated from the brains of about 25% of autopsy cases dying of AIDS. It also causes a dementing disease (Morgello et al. 1987). On computed tomography the usual finding is brain atrophy with enlargement of the cerebral ventricles. About 30% have recognisable focal brain involvement, in the rest it is diffuse. Often CMV infection is not the dominant infection present (Post et al. 1986b). Severe progressive atrophy has been shown due to CMV in a child with AIDS (Post et al. 1986a).

Abscesses and Granulomas in Immunosuppression (Fig. 5.16)

Abscesses and granulomas may be caused by a wide range of parasitic, fungal and bacterial agents, many of which have been considered in other sections. However, in the immunosuppressed patient, lesions are likely to be diffuse or multifocal and difficult to eradicate. Mixed infections are common. Cases with atrophy on an initial scan are more likely eventually to develop mass lesions than those in whom the initial scan was normal (Levy et al. 1986).

About 50% of mass lesions in patients with AIDS are due to *toxoplasmosis* (Levy et al. 1986; Post et al. 1986c). Between 60% and 80% are multiple and 75% of lesions involve the basal ganglia (Handler

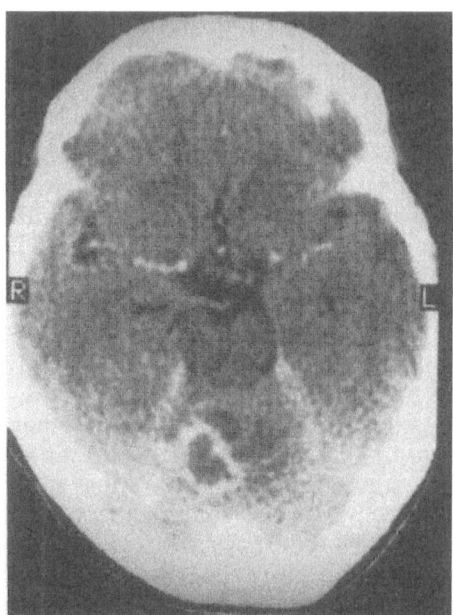

Fig. 5.16. Cranial CT after IV contrast. *Nocardia asteroides* abscess of the cerebellum in a patient with lymphoma.

et al. 1983; Levy et al. 1986). In about 5% of cases the disease is diffuse and CT shows only evidence of atrophy or hydrocephalus. Computed tomography shows several patterns of abnormality (Fig. 5.17):

1. Ring lesions after contrast enhancement (70%)
2. Hypodense areas with no focal enhancement (20%)
3. No oedema, just a small disc or ring of enhancement (10%)
4. Intracerebral haemorrhage (7%)
5. Diffuse periventricular enhancement (one case, Cohen and Koslow 1985)
6. Gyral enhancement with underlying oedema

Response to therapy should be clearly evident on CT within a few days. If there is no response an alternative diagnosis should be considered, and biopsy may be necessary.

Cerebral Neoplasms in AIDS

Lymphoma

About 6% of patients with the neurological complications of AIDS are eventually shown to have cerebral lymphoma. The mass lesions often look atypical on computed tomography, appearing as ring lesions in many cases, often multiple. Diffuse

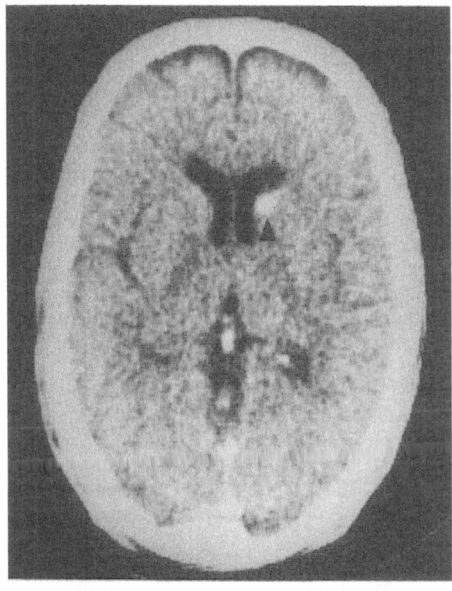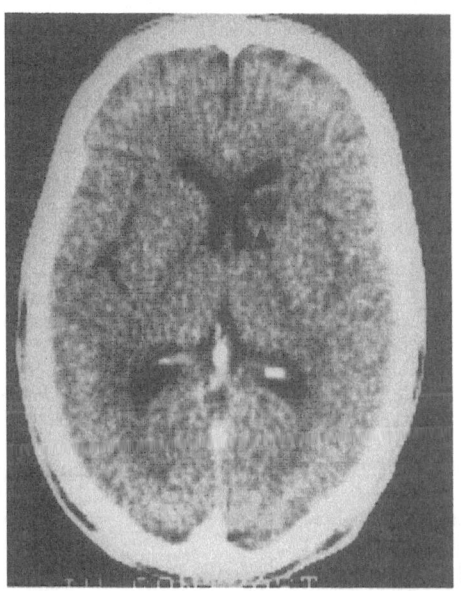

Fig. 5.17 a and **b.** Cranial CT after IV contrast. Cerebral toxoplasmosis in patients with AIDS. Lesions are shown in relation to the head of the caudate nucleus (*arrowheads*).

lymphoma has been found at autopsy which was not evident on CT. Cerebral atrophy is usually associated (Levy et al. 1986; Post et al. 1986c).

Metastatic Kaposi's Sarcoma

This tumour has been seen several times in the brain on computed tomograms. The lesions are usually solitary, in either cerebrum or cerebellum. They have appeared as diffusely enhancing masses (Post et al. 1986c).

References

Adapon BD, Legada B, Eva L et al. (1981) CT guided biopsy of the spine. J Comput Assist Tomogr 5:73–78

Ahmadi J, Keane JR, Segall HD, Zee CH (1985) CT observations pertaining to septic cavernous sinus thrombosis. AJNR 6:755–758

Allen IV (1984) Demyelinating diseases. In: Hume Adams J, Corsellis JAN, Duchen LW (eds) Greenfield's neuropathology. Edward Arnold, London, pp 338–384

Arrington JA, Murthagh FR, Martinez CR, Schnitzlein HN (1984) CT of multiple intracranial cryptococcomas. AJNR 5:472–473

Atlas SW, Grossman RI, Goldberg HI et al. (1986) MR diagnosis of acute disseminated encephalomyelitis. J Comput Assist Tomogr 10:798–801

Ba'assiri A, Haddad FS (1984) Primary extradural intracranial hydatid disease: CT appearance. AJNR 5:474–475

Bellman AL, Anand AK (1985) Magnetic resonance imaging in post-infectious and post-vaccinal encephalomyelitis. Ann Neurol 18:391

Bellman AL, Ultmann MH, Horoupian D et al. (1985) Neuro-

logical complications in infants and children with AIDS. Ann Neurol 18:560–566

Benaton RM, Magill HL, Gerald B (1985) Herpes Simplex Encephalitis: CT findings in the neonate and young infant. AJNR 6:539–543

Bhargava S, Tandon MS (1980) Intracranial tuberculomas: a CT study. Br J Radiol 53:935–945

Bhargava S, Gupta AK, Tandon PN (1982) Tuberculous meningitis – a CT study. Br J Radiol 55:189–196

Borovich B, Braun J, Honigman S et al. (1981) Supratentorial and parafalcine subdural empyema diagnosis by CT. J Neurosurg 54:105–107

Braithwaite PA, Lees RF (1981) Vertebral hydatid disease: radiological assessment. Radiology 140:763–777

Britt RH, Enzmann DR (1983) Clinical stages of human brain abscesses on serial CT scans after contrast infusion. Computed tomography, neuropathological and clinical correlations. J Neurosurg 59:972–989

Brown WJ, Voge M (1982) Neuropathology of parasitic infections. Oxford University Press, Oxford

Brownell B, Tomlinson AH (1984) Virus diseases of the central nervous system. In: Hume Adams J, Corsellis JAN, Duchen LW (eds) Greenfield's neuropathology, 4th edn. Edward Arnold, London

Carbajal JR, Palacois E, Azar-Kia B, Churchill R (1977) Radiology of cysticercosis of the central nervous system, including computed tomography. Radiology 125:127–131

Carter BL, Bankoff MS, Fisk JD (1983) Computed tomographic detection of sinusitis responsible for intracranial and extracranial infections. Radiology 147:739–742

Casselman ES, Hasso AN, Ashwal S, Schneider S (1980) Computed tomography of tuberculous meningitis in infants and children. J Comput Assist Tomogr 4:211–216

Chang KH, Kim WS, Cho SY et al. (1988) Comparative evaluation of brain CT and ELISA in the diagnosis of neurocysticercosis. AJNR 9:125–130

Chapman M, Murray R, Stoker D (1979) Tuberculosis of the bones and joints. Semin Roentgenol 14:266–282

Chun CH, Johnson JD, Hofsetter et al. (1986) Brain abscess: a study of 45 consecutive cases. Medicine 65:415–431

Claudon, Bracard SB, Plenat F et al. (1987) Spinal involvement in alveolar echinococcosis: assessment of 2 cases. Radiology 162:571–572

Claveria LE, du Boulay GH, Moseley IF (1976) Intracranial infections: investigation by computed axial tomography. Neuroradiology 12:59–71

Clifford-Jones RE, Ellis CJK, Stevens JM, Turner A (1982) Cavernous sinus thrombosis. J Neurol Neurosurg Psychiatry 45:1092–1097

Coccia-Portugal MA, Sieling WL, Terblanche APJ et al. (1987) Aspergillous brain abscess. S Afr Med J 71:116–118

Cockrill HH, Dreisbach J, Lowe B, Yamauchi R (1978) Computed tomography in leptomeningeal infections. AJR 130:511–515

Cohen W, Koslow M (1985) An unusual CT presentation of cerebral toxoplasmosis. J Comput Assist Tomogr 9:384–326

Cornell SH, Jacoby CG (1982) The varied computed tomographic appearance of intracranial cryptococcosis. Radiology 143:703–707

Danziger A, Price H, Schechter MM (1980) An analysis of 113 intracranial infections. Neuroradiology 19:31–34

Dastur DK, Lalitha VS (1973) The many facets of neuro-tuberculosis: an epitome of neuropathology. In: Zimmerman HM (ed) Progress in neuropathology, vol 2. Grune and Stratton, New York, pp 351–408

Dastur DK, Udani PM (1966) Pathology and pathogenesis of tuberculous encephalopathy. Acta Neuropathol (Berl) 6:311–326

Davidson HD, Steiner RE (1985) Magnetic resonance imaging in infections of the central nervous system. AJNR 6:499–505

Davis LE (1987) Acute viral meningitis and encephalitis. In: Kennedy PGE, Johnson RT (eds) Infections of the nervous system. Butterworths, London, pp 156–176

Deeb ZL, Schimel S, Daffner RH et al. (1985) Intervertebral disc space infection after chymopapain injection. AJNR 6:55–58

Deramond H, Sebert JL, Rosat P et al. (1987) Destructive spondyloarthropathy in chronic haemodialysis patients. J Neuroradiol 14:27–38

de Roos A, van Persijn van Meerten El et al. (1986) MRI of tuberculous spondylitis. AJR 146:79–82

de Slegte RGM, Kaiser MC, van der Baun S, Smit L (1988) Computed tomography of septic sinus thromboses and their complications. Neuroradiology 30:160–165

Diebler C, Dussen A, Dulac O (1985) Congenital toxoplasmosis. Clinical and neuroradiological evaluation of the cerebral lesions. Neuroradiology 27:125–130

Dobkin JF, Healton EB, Dickson T, Brust JCM (1984) Non-specificity of ring enhancement in medically cured brain abscess. Neurology 34:139–144

Enzmann DR, Britt RH, Lyons B et al. (1982a) High resolution ultrasound evaluation of experimental brain abscess evolution: comparison with computed tomography and neuropathology. Radiology 142:95–102

Enzmann DR, Britt RH, Placone RC (1982b) Effect of short term corticosteroid treatment in the CT appearance of experimental brain abscesses. Radiology 146:79–84

Enzmann DR, Britt RH, Placone RC (1983) Staging of human brain abscess by computed tomography. Radiology 146:703–708

Ford K, Sarwar M (1981) Computed tomography of dural sinus thrombosis. AJNR 2:539–543

Fujita NK, Reynard M, Sapico FL et al. (1981) Cryptococcal intracranial mass lesions. The role of computed tomography and non-surgical management. Ann Intern Med 94:382–388

Gamba J, Woodruff WW, Djang WT, Yeates AE (1986) Craniofacial mucormycosis: assessment with CT. Radiology 160:207–212

Garcia CA, Weisberg LA, Lecorde WSJ (1985). Cryptococcal intracerebral mass lesions: CT and pathological considerations. Neurology 35:731–734

Golimbu C, Firooznia H, Rafii M (1984) CT of osteomyelitis of the spine. AJR: 159–163

Gordon I, Vivian G (1984) Radio-labelled leukocytes: a new diagnostic tool in occult infection/inflammation. Arch Dis Child 59:62–66

Grant I, Atkinson JH, Hesselink JR et al. (1987) Evidence for early central nervous system involvement in AIDS and other HIV infections. Studies with neuropsychologic testing and magnetic resonance imaging. Ann Intern Med 107:828–836

Grossman RI, Joseph PM, Wolf G et al. (1985) Experimental intracranial septic infarction: magnetic resonance enhancement. Radiology 155:649–653

Handler M, Ho V, Whelan M, Budzolovich G (1983) Intracerebral toxoplasmosis in a patient with acquired immunodeficiency syndrome. J Neurosurg 59:994–1001

Harriman DGF (1984) Bacterial infections of the central nervous system. In: Hume Adams J, Corsellis JAN, Duchen LW (eds). Greenfield's neuropathology, 4th edn. Edward Arnold, London, pp 237–259

Holland BA, Perrett LV, Mills CM (1986) Meningovascular syphilis: CT and MR findings. Radiology 158:439–442

Horten B, Price RW, Jimenez D (1981) Multifocal varicella-zoster virus leukoencephalitis temporarily remote from Herpes Zoster. Ann Neurol 9:251–266

Houf SA, Major EO, Katz DA et al. (1988) Involvement of JC virus-infected mononuclear cells from the bone marrow and spleen in the pathogenesis of progressive multifocal leukoencephalopathy. N Engl J Med 318:301–305

Jinkins JR (1988) Focal tuberculous cerebritis. AJNR 9:121–124

Johnson RT, Griffin DE (1987) Post-infectious encephalomyelitis. In: Johnson RT, Kennedy PGE (eds) Infections of the nervous system. Butterworths, London, pp 209–226

Kagawa M, Takeshita M, Yato S, Kitamura K (1983) Brain abscess in congenital cyanotic heart disease. J Neurosurg 58:913–917

Kaplan RJ (1976) Neurological complications of infections of the head and neck. Otolaryngol Clin North Am 9:729–749

Ketonen L, Koskiniemi M (1980) Computed tomographic appearances in Herpes Simplex virus encephalitis. Clin Radiol 31:161–165

Kingsley DPE, Hendrickse WA, Kendall BE (1987) Tuberculous meningitis: role of computed tomography in management and progress. J Neurol Neurosurg Psychiatry 50:30–36

Knudsen LL, Voldby B, Stagaard M (1987) Computed tomographic myelography in spinal subdural empyema. Neuroradiology 29:99

Kocen RS (1987) Tuberculosis of the nervous system. In: Kennedy PGE, Johnson RT (eds) Infections of the nervous system. Butterworths, London, pp 23–42

Krawiecki NS, Dyken PR, el Gamel T et al. (1984) Computed tomography of the brain in subacute sclerosing panencephalitis. Ann Neurol 15:459–493

Kroll JS, Moxon ER (1987) Acute bacterial meningitis. In: Kennedy PGE, Johnson RT (eds) Infections of the nervous system. Butterworths, London, pp 3–22

Krupp LB, Lipton RB, Swerdlow RB, Leeds NE, Llena J (1985) Progressive multifocal leuco-encephalopathy: clinical and radiological features. Ann Neurol 17:344–349

Lane T, Goings S, Fraser DW et al. (1979) Disseminated actinomycosis with spinal cord compression: report of two cases. Neurology 29:890–893

Lanzieri CF, Larkins M, Mancall A et al. (1988) Cranial postoperative site: MR imaging appearance. AJNR 9:27–34

Legg NJ (1983) Intracerebral abscess. In: Harrison M (ed) Contemporary neurology. Butterworths, London

Le May M (1987) CT changes in dementing disease: a review. AJNR 7:841–853

Levy RM, Rosenbloom S, Perrett LV (1986) Neuroradiologic findings in AIDS: a review of 200 cases. AJNR 7:833–839

London DA, Carrol BA, Enzmann DR (1980) Sonography of ventricular size and germinal matrix haemorrhage in premature infants. AJNR 1:295–300

Lotz J, Hewlett R, Alheit B, Bowen R (1988) Neurocysticercosis: correlative pathomorphology and MR imaging. Neuroradiology 30:35–41

Lunsford JD, Martinez AJ, Latchaw R et al. (1984) Rapid and accurate diagnosis of Herpes Simplex encephalitis with computed tomographic stereotactic biopsy. Surg Neurol 21:249–257

Marrie TJ, Riding M, Grand B (1984) Computed tomography in Listeria monocytogenes meningitis. Clin Invest Med 7:355–359

Massaryk TJ, Boumphrey F, Modic MT et al. (1986) Effects of chemonucleolysis demonstrated by MR imaging. J Comput Assist Tomogr 10:917–923

Matthews WB (1987) Slow infections. In: Johnson RT, Kennedy PGE (eds) Infections of the nervous system. Butterworths, London, pp 227–247

Mikhael MA, Ciric IS, Tarkington JA (1985) MR imaging in spinal echinococcosis. J Comput Assist Tomogr 9:398–400

Millan JM, Escudero L, Roger RL (1985) Actinomycotic brain abscess: CT findings. J Comput Assist Tomogr 9:976–978

Modic MT, Feuglin DH, Piriano DW et al. (1985) Vertebral osteomyelitis: assessment using MR imaging. Radiology 157:157–166

Morgello S, Cho ES, Nielsen S et al. (1987) Cytomegalovirus encephalitis in patients with AIDS. Hum Pathol 1987:289–297

Moseley I (1988) Magnetic resonance imaging in diseases of the nervous system. Blackwells, London

Moseley IF, Kendall BE (1984) Radiology of intracranial empyemas, with special reference to computed tomography. Neuroradiology 26:333–345

Moseley IF, Zilkha E (1983) Considerations of radiation dose in the management of intracranial abscesses by computed tomography. Br J Radiol 57:303–307

Noorbehesht B, Enzmann DR, Sullender W et al. (1987) Neonatal Herpes Simplex encephalitis. Correlation of clinical and CT findings. Radiology 162:813–819

Ommaya AK (1976) Spinal fluid fistulae. Clin Neurosurg 23:363–392

O'Neil RA, Albertun LE, Perrett LV, Sage MR (1987) Computed tomography of adult Herpes Simplex encephalitis. Australas Radiol 31:357–360

Post MJD, Curtess RG, Gregorios JB (1986a) Reactivation of congenital cytomegalic inclusion disease in an infant with HTLV–III associated immunodeficiency: a CT-pathologic correlation. J Comput Assist Tomogr 10:533–536

Post MJD, Hensley GT, Moskowitz LB, Fischl M (1986b) Cytomegalic inclusion virus encephalitis in patients with AIDS: CT, clinical and pathological correlation. AJR 146:1229–1234

Post MJD, Sheldon JJ, Hensley GT et al. (1986c) Central nervous system disease in acquired immunodeficiency syndrome: prospective correlation using CT, MRI and pathology studies. Radiology 158:141–148

Price RW, Navia BA (1987) Infections in AIDS and other immunosuppressed patients. In: Johnson RJ, Kennedy PGE (eds) Infections of the nervous system. Butterworths, London, pp 248–274

Prusiner SB (1982) Novel proteinaceous infectious particles cause scrapie. Science 216: 136–144

Reik L (1987) Spirochaetal infections of the nervous system. In: Kennedy PGE, Johnson RT (eds) Infections of the nervous

system. Butterworths, London, pp 43–75

Reik L, Smith L, Khan A, Nelson W (1985) Demyelinating encephalopathy in Lyme disease. Neurology 32:1302–1305

Rich AR (1951) The pathogenesis of tuberculosis, 2nd edn. Blackwell Scientific, Oxford

Rosenblum ML, Hoff JT, Norman D et al. (1978) Decreased mortality from brain abscess since the advent of computed tomography. J Neurosurg 49:658–668

Sandhyarani S, Bhatia R, Mohapatra LN et al. (1981) Cerebral cladosporosis. Surg Neurol 15:431–434

Savoiardo M, Cimino C, Passerini A, La Rantia L (1986) Mobile myelographic filling defects: spinal cycticersosis. Neuroradiology 28:116–169

Scaravilli F (1984) Parasitic and fungal infections of the nervous system. In: Hume Adams J, Corsellis JAN, Duchen LW (eds) Greenfield's neuropathology. Edward Arnold, London, pp 304–387

Scatamachia SA, Raptopoulos V, Davidson RI (1987) Saline microbubbles monitoring sonography assisted abscess drainage. Invest Radiol 22:868–870

Shafran B, Roke ME, Barr RM, Cairncross JG (1987) Contrast enhancing lesions in progressive multifocal leukoencephalopathy: a clinicopathological correlation. Can J Neurol Sci 14:600–602

Sinycharcen T, Rawd-Aree P, Baddeley H (1988) Computed tomography, findings in disseminated paragonimiasis. Br J Radiol 61:83–86

Sotelo J (1987) Neurocysticercosis. In: Johnson RT, Kennedy PGE (eds) Infections of the nervous system. Butterworths, London, pp 23–42

Stevens JM, Valentine AR (1987) Magnetic resonance imaging in neurosurgery: Review article. Br J Neurosurg 1:405–426

Tokoro K, Yamataki A, Nakajima F (1987) Subdural empyema occurring 20 years after trauma: case report. Neurosurgery 21:724–726

Tomlinson BE, Corsellis JAN (1984) Ageing and dementias. In: Hume Adams J, Corsellis JAN, Duchen LW (eds) Greenfields neuropathology, 4th edn. Edward Arnold, London, pp 951–1025

Udaka F, Okuda M et al. (1988) CT findings of cerebral paragonimiasis in the chronic state. Neuroradiology 30:31–34

Valentine AR, Kendall BE, Harding BN (1982) Computed tomography of acute haemorrhagic leukoencephalitis. Neuroradiology 22:225–234

Vanneste JAL, Bellot SM, Stam FC (1984) Progressive multifocal leukoencephalopathy presenting as a single mass lesion. Eur Venerol 23:113–118

Wadia NH, Dastur DK (1969) Spinal meningitis with radiculomyelopathy. Parts 1 and 2. J Neurol Sci 8:239–299

Weingarten K, Zimmerman RD, Becker RD, Heier LA, Haimes AB, Deck MDF (1989) Subdural and epidural empyemas: MR imaging. AJNR 10:81–87

Weisberg L (1986) Subdural empyema: clinical and computed tomographic correlations. Arch Neurol 43:497–500

Westphal KP, Schachenmayne W (1985) Computed tomography during Creutzfeldt–Jacob disease. Neuroradiology 27:362–364

Whelan MA, Stern J (1981) Intracranial tuberculosis. Radiology 138:75–81

Wiles CM, MacKenzie DWR (1987) Cerebral malaria. In: Johnson RT, Kennedy PGE (eds) Infections of the nervous system. Butterworths, London, pp 119–144

Zee C, Segall HD, Miller C et al. (1980) Unusual neuroradiological features of intracranial cysticercosis. Radiology 137:397–407

Zimmerman RA, Bilanikuk LT, Sze G (1986) Intracranial infections. In: Brant-Zawadzki M, Norman D (eds) Magnetic resonance imaging of the central nervous system. Raven Press, New York, pp 235–258

Zimmerman RD, Russell EJ, Leeds NE, Kaufman D (1980) CT in the early diagnosis of Herpes Simplex Encephalitis. AJR 134:61–66

Zimmerman RD, Leeds NE, Danziger A (1984) Subdural empyema: CT findings. Radiology 150:417–422

Zochodne DW, Kaufmann CE (1987) Progressive multifocal leukoencephalopathy without immunosuppression. Can J Neurol Sci 14:603–607

Chapter 6

Paediatric Neuro-imaging

Ian W. Turnbull

Paediatric Brain Tumours

Introduction

Paediatric brain tumours constitute between 15% and 20% of all primary brain tumours and represent almost 15% of all paediatric tumours, being the second most common malignancy of childhood (Farwell et al. 1977; Naidich and Zimmerman 1984; Tomita and McLone 1985). Posterior fossa tumours are more frequent than supratentorial neoplasms when all paediatric ages are grouped together, but the reverse is true in the first two years of life when approximately 60% of brain tumours are supratentorial. Posterior fossa lesions predominate from 4 to 11 years of age and both locations are equally frequent throughout the rest of the paediatric period (Table 6.1).

During the first 12 to 24 months of life, the histology and origin of cerebral neoplasms is different from those encountered in later childhood. The origin of 90% of tumours is neuroectodermal (astrocytoma, medulloblastoma, ependymoma, choroid plexus papilloma and others). These tumours tend to be located along the neural axis with 70% of the lesions occurring in the ventricle or elsewhere along the midline (Jooma et al. 1984).

Table 6.1. Site of tumour

	In first year of life	In second year of life	In children 0 – 16 years
Posterior fossa	33%	44%	55%
Supratentorial	67%	56%	45%

Modified from Jooma et al. (1984), Naidich and Zimmerman (1984) and Tomita and McLone (1985).

Cerebral metastatic tumours account for between 2% and 8% of all intracranial lesions in children and the adrenal gland is the most common primary site. Metastasis may also occur from hepatoblastoma or retinoblastoma.

Macrocrania is the most important physical sign and is present in around 80% of cases being due to hydrocephalus, tumour volume or a combination of both factors. Despite this, in only half of these cases do the parents notice the increased head size. Papilloedema is generally thought to be rare in infants but has been noted in up to 35% of cases (Jooma et al. 1984). Skull sutures in children spread easily and quickly in response to raised intracranial pressure, an abnormality which has been recorded in more of 90% of skull radiographs reviewed.

Computed tomography (CT) is currently the single, most useful method of neuroradiological assessment and all children with a suspected brain tumour should have both non-contrast and contrast-enhanced CT in the transaxial plane with supplementary post-contrast direct coronal and sagittal images depending on the location of the tumour and the ability of the child to cooperate with the examination.

Transcranial ultrasound scanning employs the anterior fontanelles as a "window" for imaging the brain and, as such, is only applicable to the very small baby (Fig. 6.1). It is, of course, possible to use burr holes or craniectomy defects as a means of postsurgical monitoring.

Since many tumours are located in the posterior fossa magnetic resonance imaging (MRI) will be particularly valuable both in tumour detection in this site and also in determining whether such tumours are intra- or extra-axial (Levene et al. 1982; Johnson et al. 1983; Lee et al. 1985; Radkowski et al. 1988). Peterman et al. (1984) studied 25 children

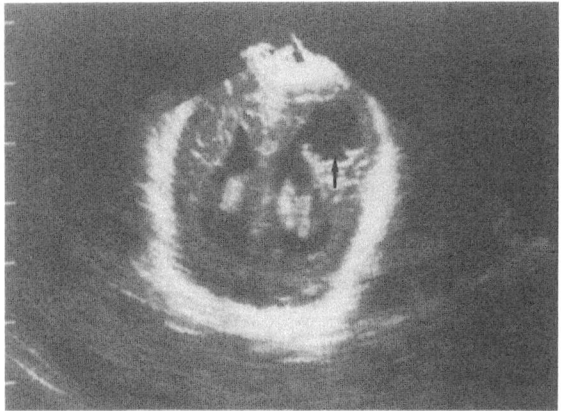

Fig. 6.1. Transcranial ultrasound of neonate demonstrating hydrocephalus with a right frontal porencephalic cyst (*arrow*).

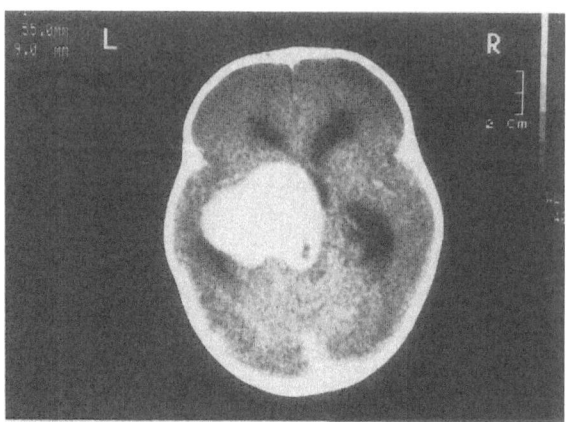

Fig. 6.2. Cranial CT after IV contrast. Astrocytoma. The densely enhancing tumour causes midline shift and hydrocephalus.

and adolescents with a suspected or proven diagnosis of intracranial tumour and compared their findings with CT. MR scans showed more extensive abnormality than did third generation CT scans in eight out of ten cases and mass effects were better demonstrated with MRI in 14 of the 16 cases in whom they were seen. Furthermore, MRI showed cysts or necrosis in the tumours of four patients of which two had no internal structure demonstrated on CT. However, difficulties were encountered. For example, CT demonstrated calcification far better than MRI and the tumour–oedema interface was better shown on CT particularly when there was marked pathological contrast enhancement within the tumour. The use of gadolinium enhancement with MRI should go some way to redress this latter drawback. Thus, although MRI shows more extensive abnormality than does CT, the results of an MR scan are somewhat non-specific and a differential diagnosis of a tumour is primarily dependent on the site of the lesion and the age and gender of the patient. Further disadvantages of MRI include its cost and relatively slow scanning time. Thus, computed tomography remains the most widely used and generally available technique for imaging brain tumours in children and the CT characteristics of the major tumour groups will now be discussed.

Supratentorial Tumours

Hemisphere Astrocytoma

On CT these tumours present as large masses, the majority (55%) having a large cyst with a medially situated mural nodule. A solid tumour is found in

45% of cases. The most frequent sites, in decreasing order of frequency, are:

1. The temporal lobe where cystic tumours are twice as common as solid masses
2. The frontal lobe where cystic and solid lesions are found with equal frequency
3. The parietal lobe where solid tumours are twice as common

CT appearances are enormously variable and may sometimes resemble the adult glioma or glioblastoma (Fig. 6.2).

Primitive Neuroectodermal Tumour (PNET)

This tumour constitutes the major differential diagnosis of a large hemisphere mass and usually occupies the deep white matter where it presents a varied CT appearance. Characteristically, it is sharply marginated and on the non-contrasted scan, the tumour is hypodense in 55%, isodense in 22% and of mixed isodensity/hyperdensity in 22%. It is virtually never purely hyperdense. Calcification, often gross, is a major feature, being seen in 50% to 70% of cases (cf. astrocytoma where this is exceedingly rare) and cyst-like necrotic areas are found within the tumour in 30% to 60% of cases (Altman et al. 1985). Intratumoural haemorrhage is relatively common (10%) and may be a presenting feature (Zimmerman and Bilaniuk 1980). Extensive peritumoural oedema is the rule (90%), a feature which is also usually lacking in astrocytomas. Contrast enhancement may be homogeneous, patchy or ring-like, the pattern having no clinical significance (Fig. 6.3).

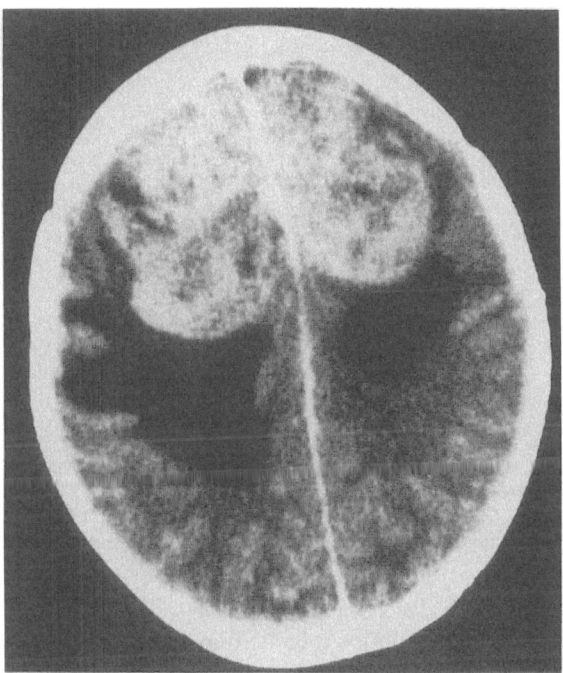

Fig. 6.3. Cranial CT after IV contrast. Primitive neurectodermal tumour. The large bifrontal mass shows heterogeneous enhancement. The plain scan demonstrated foci of calcification.

Seeding into the cerebrospinal fluid (CSF) pathways has been reported in up to 50% of cases.

Ependymoma

Supratentorial ependymomas are rare tumours, occurring most commonly in boys and are typically malignant (86%). Computed tomography generally discloses a single, large tumour of the cerebral white matter, most frequently in the frontal lobe and sometimes within the parietal lobe. Very occasionally, they may be intraventricular. Calcification is seen in 50% of cases and the tumours are cystic in around 70% of cases. Intratumoural haemorrhage has also been recorded. The CT features are not diagnostic and considerable difficulty may arise in distinguishing this tumour from a PNET which also shows calcification in approximately half the cases and has a similar propensity for intratumoural haemorrhage. The only distinguishing feature appears to be the presence of peritumoural oedema which is observed in 90% of cases of PNET and is a rare finding with ependymoma. Both ependymoma and PNET are uncommon tumours, however, and a cerebral hemisphere mass is much more likely to be an astrocytoma.

Optic and Hypothalamic Glioma

Up to one-third of optic gliomas will be associated with symptoms first appearing in children under 2 years of age and 80% of these tumours will occur in the first decade of life. They represent benign hamartomatous tumours of childhood (juvenile pilocytic astrocytoma) which may involve any part of the visual pathways and are associated with neurofibromatosis in 25% to 50% of cases (Stern et al. 1980). They are characterised by slow growth and present with an insidious visual loss in one eye or both eyes with or without proptosis. Over half of these tumours are mainly or entirely intracranial with little or no involvement of the intraorbitial optic nerves. Tumour extension into the hypothalamic and 3rd ventricular area is common and is the typical finding at the time of neuroradiological assessment when distinction from a hypothalamic glioma is one of the diagnostic problems encountered. Such extensive lesions may be associated with a survival of many years, although patients with tumour confined to the chiasm and optic nerves (which many workers regard as hamartomas rather than gliomas) generally have a better prognosis (Fletcher et al. 1986). This contrasts with optic and chiasmatic gliomas encountered in adults which are almost invariably malignant tumours which readily spread to the adjacent neuraxis and are associated with a poor prognosis.

A glioma of hypothalamic origin is more likely to present with diabetes insipidus, a short stature, delayed puberty, the diencephalic syndrome or hydrocephalus. Such tumours may spread to involve the chiasm and visual pathways and, when large, may become indistinguishable from large posterior optic gliomas.

Although CT is the examination of choice, plain radiographs will assist in determining whether one or both optic canals are expanded or eroded which they will do better than CT in many cases. This is an important observation to make, as the majority of optic gliomas will expand the canal, whereas this is an uncommon event even with huge hypothalamic tumours.

With optic chiasm glioma, contrast-enhanced CT typically shows an enhancing mass lesion enlarging the chiasm and extending into the optic nerves on one or both sides. Patronas et al. (1987) evaluated the contributions of CT and MRI in imaging these tumours and concluded that all tumours were identified with both techniques, but in the majority of cases, the posterior extension of the tumour and its relationship to adjacent brain were better shown by MRI.

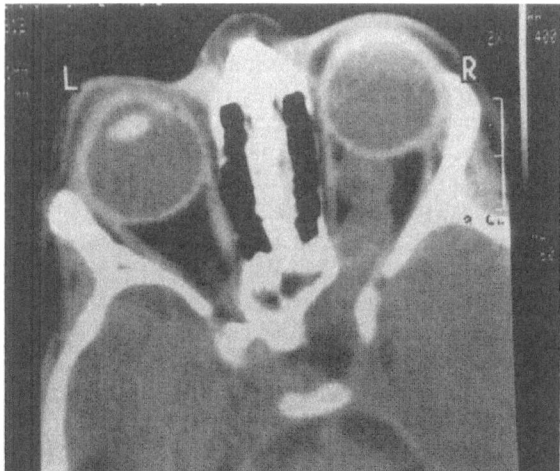

Fig. 6.4. Cranial CT. Right optic nerve glioma.

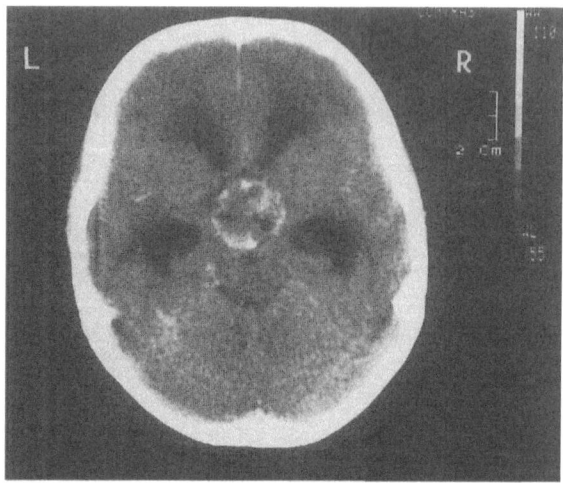

Fig. 6.5. Cranial CT after IV contrast. Craniopharyngioma. A calcified rim encloses a tumour with patchy enhancement.

Hypothalamic gliomas are associated with more subtle contrast enhancement, which is detected in up to two-thirds of tumours, and obliteration of the third ventricle with resultant hydrocephalus is the rule rather than the exception.

Calcification is rare in either tumour except after radiotherapy (Savoiardo et al. 1981), a feature which distinguishes these lesions from craniopharyngiomas, especially in older children. When the intraorbital optic nerves are involved, CT will show a fusiform enlargement of a part of the optic nerve which is generally homogeneous in density and which usually enhances following intravenous contrast (Fig. 6.4).

Craniopharyngioma

This is an epithelial tumour believed to originate from nests of squamous epithelial cells in the pars tuberalis or Rathke's pouch. CT reveals a lobulated mass within the suprasellar cistern associated with prominent tumoural calcification in 80% of cases (cf. 30% in adults), being ring-like in two-thirds and nodular in the remainder (Fig. 6.5). The presence of calcification is not related to the size of the tumour nor to whether it is solid or cystic (Cabezudo et al. 1981). At least 60% of craniopharyngiomas presenting in childhood contain cystic areas (cf. 15% in adults), but the incidence rises to almost 100% with giant tumours (Al-Mefty et al. 1985) and with recurrent disease (Cabezudo et al. 1981). Pathological contrast enhancement occurs in 50% to 75% of lesions and may be seen within the tumour wall or consist of an ill-defined blush throughout the whole tumour mass. Recurrent tumours, however, virtually always display some enhancement.

When CT discloses a suprasellar mass which is (a) cystic, (b) contains calcification and (c) displays contrast enhancement, a correct diagnosis of craniopharyngioma can be assumed in virtually 100% of cases. When any two of three criteria are present, the accuracy falls to 85% and on the rare occasions when only one of them is evident, accuracy falls to 50% with difficulty in distinguishing craniopharyngioma from other lesions such as hypothalamic or chiasmal gliomas, dermoids or intraventricular meningiomas. A further diagnostic difficulty arises in respect of the 20% of craniopharyngiomas which have an intrasellar origin. Fortunately, the majority of these tumours occur in adults where, unless the tumour is calcified, it may be indistinguishable from a pituitary adenoma.

Infratentorial Tumours

Medulloblastoma

Medulloblastoma is a malignant tumour composed of primitive embryonal cells capable of differentiating into glial or neuronal elements (Camins et al. 1980). The tumour originates from primitive glial cells most frequently found in the germinative zone of the posterior medullary velum. As these cells migrate from the roof of the fourth ventricle to form the external granular layer of the cerebellar hemisphere, medulloblastomas may develop anywhere along the path of migration. Together with cerebellar astrocytomas, they are the commonest posterior fossa tumours in children, affecting boys twice as often as girls.

Medulloblastomas are found within the cerebellar vermis in 93% of cases, being confined to the vermis in 30%, extending from the vermis into the cerebellar hemisphere in 31% and invading the brainstem by direct extension across the 4th ventricle in 32%. In 7% of cases, the tumour is confined to the cerebellar hemispheres (Naidich and Zimmerman 1984). Spontaneous intratumoural haemorrhage may be seen in around 5% of cases at presentation and can also occur spontaneously after radiotherapy or following pre-operative ventricular drainage (Park et al. 1983). Tumour dissemination is frequent and often widespread, with subarachnoid seeding and direct arachnoid invasion being commonly observed pre-operatively or at post-mortem (McComb et al. 1981; Tomita and McLone 1983). Spinal cord and an equina metastases are reported in between 10% and 45% of patients. The majority are intradural/extramedullary lesions but true intramedullary metastases have been described. Systemic metastases are found in about 10% to 15% of patients and may occur prior to surgical intervention, although the incidence rises to almost 20% when pre-operative ventricular shunts are performed without a millipore filter (Park et al. 1983). The most frequent site of distal metastasis is the skeleton (86%), followed by the peritoneum (via shunt) (43%), lymph nodes (30%), lung (7%) and liver.

On non-contrast CT, medulloblastomas tend to appear uniformly hyperdense (70%) and less often isodense (20%) or of mixed density (10%). They are very rarely hypodense. Typically they are large, round to oval, discretely marginated, non-calcified, midline masses situated in the inferior vermis behind the fourth ventricle. Contrast enhancement occurs in 95% and is typically homogeneous (Fig. 6.6). The mass may, of course, arise within a cerebellar hemisphere or extend from the midline into it and lateral growth into an adjacent cerebellopontine angle cistern may be observed. Brainstem compression or frank invasion can be discerned in just under a third of cases. Differential diagnosis is mainly from ependymoma, especially in the very young infant. The principal features characterising an ependymoma are the presence of dense calcification in 50%, a greater frequency of mixed or low-density tumours before contrast and the relative smallness of the tumour compared with medulloblastomas which are nearly always very large at presentation.

CT is ideal for demonstrating early intracranial subarachnoid seeding which is usually manifest as intense leptomeningeal enhancement around the base of the brain and into the sylvian fissures. Occasionally, nodular masses may be seen within the cisterns or ventricles (North et al. 1985).

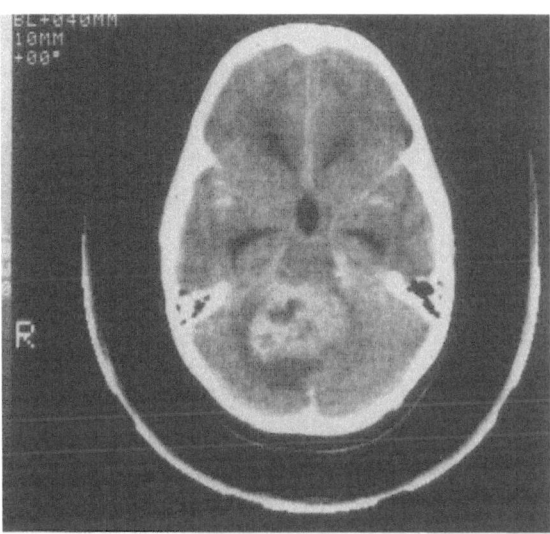

Fig. 6.6. Cranial CT after IV contrast. Medulloblastoma. (P.B.)

MRI has clear advantages over CT in the posterior fossa and is especially valuable in demonstrating midline and deep-seated lesions. It shows more extensive abnormality than CT and provides greater detail about potential cystic or necrotic areas (Peterman et al. 1984). MRI may display a greater accuracy in determining the extent of infiltration, although a possible disadvantage lies in the relative inability of MRI to identify the tumour–oedema interface (Johnson et al. 1983). When a medulloblastoma encroaches upon the brainstem or appears to invade it on computed tomography, distinguishing it from a brainstem glioma can be difficult but in this circumstance, MRI is undoubtedly superior to CT in disclosing the true origin of the tumour (Heafner et al. 1985).

Cerebellar Astrocytoma

As the name suggests, this tumour is composed of astrocytes which display varying degrees of maturity usually subcategorized into ascending grades of malignancy from 1 to 4. Fortunately, most are grade 1. They may be further classified as juvenile type which form the great majority of those seen in children (25 year survival rate, 94%), or diffuse/adult type which may occasionally be seen in this age group and have a much poorer prognosis (25 year survival rate, 38%) (Gjerris and Klinken 1978). They may arise in any part of the cerebellum but, classically, the juvenile type will occur in the midline, possibly extending into one or both hemispheres (80%). The tumours may be solid or cystic, the incidence being approximately equal for midline

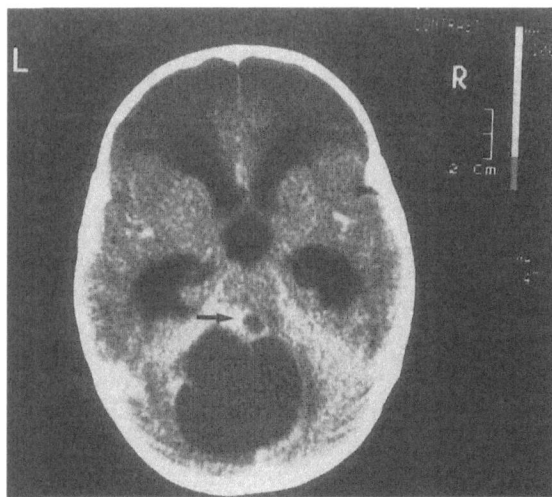

Fig. 6.7. Cranial CT after IV contrast. Juvenile cerebellar astrocytoma. A mural nodule is seen anteriorly (*arrow*).

Brainstem Glioma

The term is used to encompass a group of glial tumours intrinsic to the medulla, pons or midbrain. A few represent a subgroup of a typical benign glioma (Hoffman et al. 1980). Girls and boys are equally affected, with a peak incidence between 4 and 13 years. Although specific subgroups may achieve a 5-year survival of 55%, the great majority of patients show a steady deterioration to death with a median survival of 4 to 15 months (Epstein 1985; Stroink et al. 1986, Albright et al. 1986, Epstein and McCleary 1986; Jenkin et al. 1987). Thus, despite being a relatively common tumour, management remains controversial because of the differing biological behaviour of these tumours and this has prompted several workers to seek a CT classification of these lesions based on:

1. Their location
2. Whether they are focal or diffuse
3. Whether they are solid or cystic
4. Whether they have any specific contrast enhancing features

Epstein (1985) and Epstein and McCleary (1986) initially proposed a staging system based mainly on tumour location describing these as:

1. Intrinsic
2. Exophytic
3. Disseminated

He showed that all diffuse neoplasms were malignant and had an extremely poor prognosis. The great majority of anterolateral and posterolateral exophytic tumours were also malignant and shared a similarly poor outcome. The best results appear to be related to tumours found at the cervical–medullary junction. Substantially similar results were reported by Albright et al. (1986) and these workers were also unable to show any relationship between the pattern or extent of tumour enhancement and prognosis.

Possibly the best CT classification of brainstem tumours as it relates to prognosis has been set out by Stroink et al. (1986) where the following groups were recognised based on CT criteria:

Group 1. Tumours which were isodense or slightly hypodense and extended posteriorly from the brain stem into the fourth ventricle which they filled. All tumours in this group enhanced brightly. This group had the best outcome.

Group 2(A). Diffuse tumours intrinsic to the brainstem which are hypodense and do not enhance. All these tumours are of high-grade malig-

lesions, whereas lateral tumours are cystic in over 80% of cases. The cyst wall may consist of non-neoplastic compressed glial cerebellar tissue, in which case the tumour itself lies along the cyst wall as a mural nodule; in other cases, necrosis within solid tumour creates a true neoplastic cavity lined entirely by tumour. This distinction can be recognised on CT by the presence or absence of contrast enhancement within the wall. The author's experience would suggest that contrast enhancement of the wall only occurs when it is composed of tumour elements.

On CT, cerebellar astrocytomas are usually large and their solid or cystic characteristics readily determined (Fig. 6.7). Because of the high protein content of the fluid within these cysts, the attenuation of the cyst contents is generally well above that of cerebrospinal fluid (CSF). On non-contrast CT the mural nodule is virtually always solitary, tends to be isodense with cerebellum and shows a well-defined, intense homogeneous enhancement with contrast. Solid astrocytomas are usually round, lobulated and well-defined. They are of variable density relative to brain and show variable patterns of pathological enhancement including ring-like, dense, homogeneous or hardly any at all. Calcification is not a feature of either solid or cystic astrocytomas. In the typical cystic tumour with an intratumoral nodule, the CT diagnosis poses very little diagnostic problem in the majority of cases; but with solid tumours, the differentiation from medulloblastoma and ependymoma can be difficult.

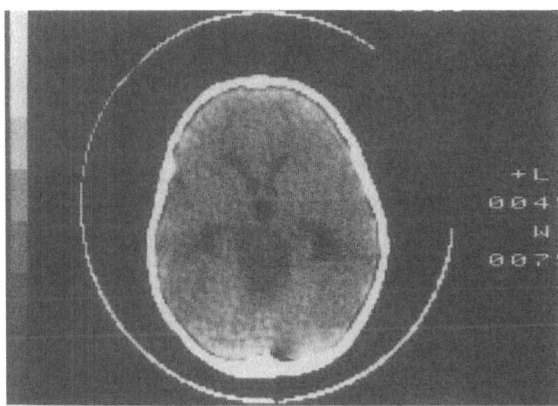

Fig. 6.8. Cranial CT. Brainstem glioma (Group 2A). The hypodense tumour failed to enhance with contrast.

nancy and the prognosis is correspondingly poor (Fig. 6.8).

Group 2(B). Diffuse tumour intrinsic to the brainstem with hyperdense, exophytic, contrast-enhancing components extending into the cerebellopontine angle. This group is similarly associated with an exceedingly poor outcome.

Group 3. Tumours intrinsic to the brainstem, focal and cystic with a contrast-enhancing capsule. Despite cyst aspiration and radiotherapy, virtually all the patients in this group are dead within 12 months.

Group 4. Solid, focal isodense tumour intrinsic to the brainstem which showed marked contrast enhancement with margins that were usually well defined. This group had the second best outcome.

CT can, therefore, be most helpful in classifying brainstem tumours into those in which a reasonable outcome might be predicted and who probably warrant surgical intervention, and those in whom the prognosis is so poor that surgery is rarely indicated. Up to 25% of brainstem tumours disseminate throughout the spinal axis at some time between diagnosis and death. This not only has implications for treatment, but may provide a basis for routine myelography in this small group of patients.

If radiotherapy is offered to a patient with a brainstem tumour, most workers agree that the entire tumour volume should be included within the radiation field. The boundaries of these fields should, ideally, be based on MRI, since the extent of paediatric brainstem gliomas on MRI exceeds that visible on CT scan in up to 50% of cases (Packer et al. 1985).

Congenital Structural Abnormalities

Malformations of the Corpus Callosum

Malformations of the corpus callosum include (a) total or partial agenesis, (b) lipoma and (c) midline cysts in the region of the corpus callosum.

The corpus callosum begins to form at about week 12 of gestation and is fully developed by 18 – 20 weeks. Dysgenesis of the corpus callosum, which includes a spectrum of malformations ranging from complete agenesis to minor degrees of deficiency usually involving the splenium, may be an isolated malformation or may be associated with other abnormalities. These include:

1. Other cerebral malformations such as
   a) agyria
   b) heterotopias
   c) porencephalic cysts
   d) cerebellar hypoplasia including the Dandy–Walker syndrome
2. Cranial malformations such as
   a) hypertelorism
   b) encephaloceles (particularly parietal and spheno-ethmoidal encephaloceles – less frequently with nasofrontal encephaloceles)
   c) craniosynostosis
3. Skeletal, cardiac or genital malformations

When the corpus callosum is agenetic, CT shows that the frontal horns and frequently the bodies of the lateral ventricles are widely separated. The dilated third ventricle is interposed between the bodies of the lateral ventricles (Fig. 6.9). Typically, the medial walls of the lateral ventricular bodies are concave because of invagination by the lateral callosal bundles and the occipital horns are dilated. Irregularity of the lateral ventricular margins is probably a result of heterotopia (collections of cells in abnormal locations as a result of arrested radial migration). If an interhemispheric cyst is present, CT demonstrates a sharply marginated, low-density midline structure superior to the lateral ventricles. On axial scans, a midline CSF-containing structure may be difficult to identify as a third ventricle or interhemispheric cyst – however, on coronal images, the cyst may be recognised as being above the third ventricle.

Lipoma of the Corpus Callosum

This is combined with agenesis of the corpus callosum in nearly half the cases. On plain skull films, the lipoma presents as a mass of low density surrounded by curvilinear calcification projected into the area of the corpus callosum (Fig. 6.10).

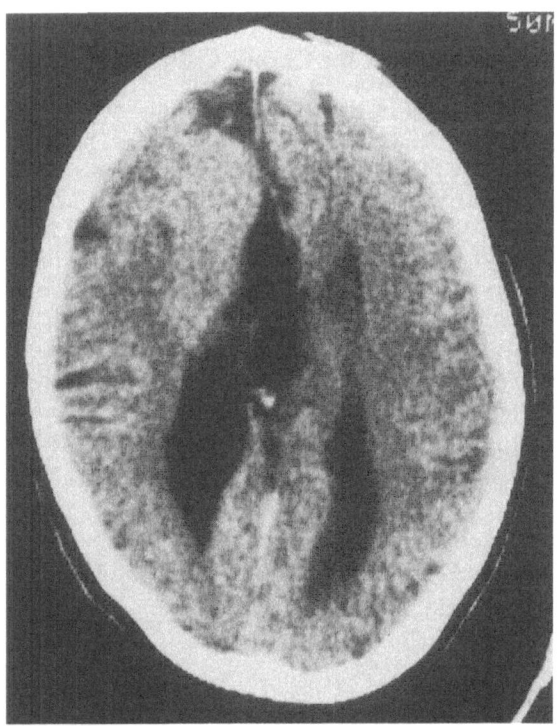

Fig. 6.9. Cranial CT. Agenesis of the corpus callosum. Interposition of a superiorly placed third ventricle between the bodies of the lateral ventricles is shown. (P.B.)

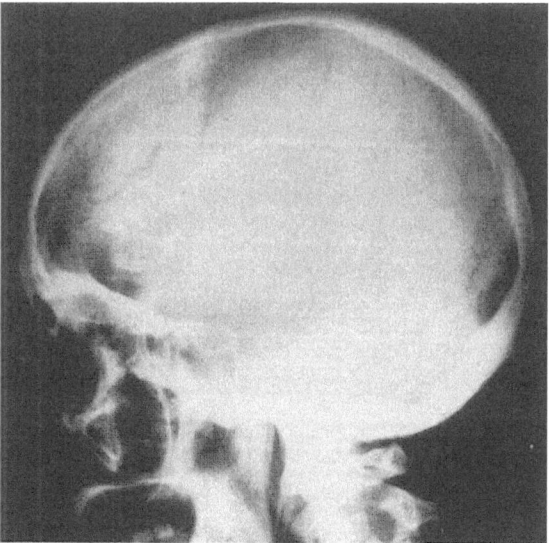

Fig. 6.10. Skull radiograph (lateral projection). Lipoma of the corpus callosum. The pericallosal calcification is well shown.

On CT, the lipoma has the typical low density of fat tissue (Fig. 6.11). It is located in the area of the corpus callosum, but frequently extends into the choroid plexus, the lateral ventricles and the interhemispheric fissure. The calcifications generally surround the anterior part of the lipoma. Large calcifications in the adjacent part of the falx are frequent. The CT scan underestimates the high vascularity of the lipoma which often surrounds abnormal anterior cerebral vessels. On CT, lipomas do not enhance. Corpus callosal lipomas are not infrequently associated with frontal bone defects, usually in the midline and these are easily appreciated on CT.

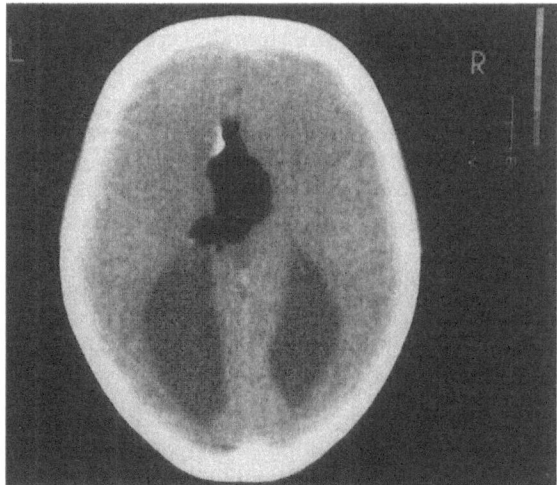

Fig. 6.11. Cranial CT. Lipoma of the corpus callosum. Patchy calcification surrounds the typical low density of a lipoma.

Interhemispheric Cysts

Interhemispheric cysts are most often associated with agenesis of the corpus callosum and may have two possible origins. They may correspond to an abnormal 3rd ventricle with a large dorsal cyst or may represent a median arachnoid cyst which, through its mass effect, tends to progressive thinning and then agenesis of the corpus callosum.

On CT scans, the presentation of agenesis of the corpus callosum with a large dorsal cyst and interhemispheric arachnoid cyst is usually identical and it is not always possible on plain CT to determine whether the cyst is communicating or non-communicating.

The Prosencephalies

Complete or partial lack of separation of the prosencephalon into cerebral hemispheres results in a group of malformations ranging from severe alobar prosencephaly to isolated aplasia of the olfactory bulbs and tracts. A lack of olfactory structures seems to be one of the more constant features of this malformation group (designated arhinencephaly for this reason), but since parts of the rhinencephalon may be found in most cases, the terms holoprosencephaly or prosencephaly are to be preferred.

Depending on the severity of the forebrain anomalies, holoprosencephaly is classified as (a) alobar, (b) semilobar or (c) lobar. A more complete classification of the prosencephalies, detailing and identifying the many subtypes, is available to the interested reader by referring to the monograph of Probst (1979).

Alobar Holoprosencephaly

Alobar holoprosencephaly represents the extreme form of the condition in which the prosencephalon does not divide into the cerebral hemispheres. Virtually all infants with this anomaly die within the first year of life and which is associated with multiple craniofacial anomalies.

The most striking CT feature of alobar holoprosencephaly is the single large 'monoventricle' in place of the lateral and third ventricles. There are no occipital or temporal horns and in the frontal and occipital regions a peripheral rim of cerebral tissue may be identified. Midline palatomaxillary clefts associated with hypertelorism are common accompaniments.

The differential diagnosis of alobar holoprosencephaly includes massive hydrocephalus or hydranencephaly. Unlike hydrocephalus the septum pellucidum, falx cerebri and interhemispheric fissures are absent in alobar holoprosencephaly. In contrast to hydranencephaly in which the thalami are normal, in alobar holoprosencephaly, the thalami are fused.

Semilobar Holoprosencephaly

Semilobar holoprosencephaly is an intermediate form of the disorder that is characterised by incomplete cleavage of the prosencephalon. Facial anomalies, such as midline clefts in lip and palate and hypotelorism, are less severe. Infants with this anomaly frequently survive but are mentally retarded.

CT in semilobar holoprosencephaly demonstrates a single ventricular chamber with partially formed occipital horns but no temporal horns and no Sylvian fissures (Fig. 6.12). The peripheral rim of cerebral tissue is several centimetres thick. The thalami are anteriorly situated, abnormally rotated and fused. The septum pellucidum and corpus callosum are absent. The falx is absent or rudimentary.

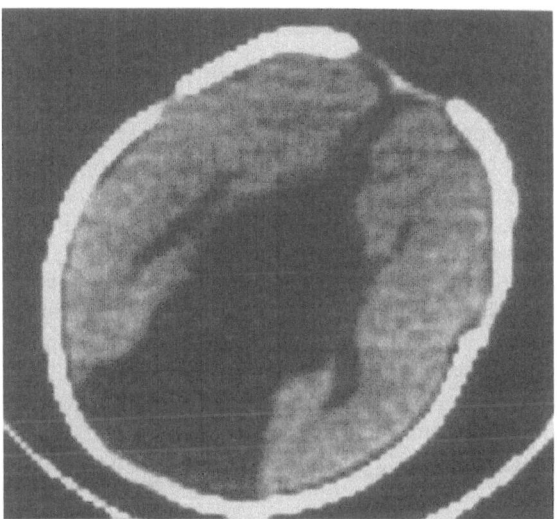

Fig. 6.12. Cranial CT. Semilobar holoprosencephaly. A single midline ventricle is shown.

Lobar Holoprosencephaly

In lobar holoprosencephaly, the mildest form of this disorder, the prosencephalon is divided into two cerebral hemispheres with distinct lateral ventricles. The condition is not usually associated with facial anomalies, although mild forms of cleft lip and palate may be present. Children usually survive into adulthood, but are mentally retarded.

On CT, lobar holoprosencephaly is characterised by reasonably well-formed lateral ventricles and cerebral hemispheres, the lateral ventricles usually having both occipital and frontal horns. Mild dilation of the lateral ventricles is frequently noted, probably secondary to deficient white and grey matter. The falx and corpus callosum are better formed than in the more severe forms of the condition, but still remain rudimentary whilst the septum pellucidum is absent. The main CT differential diagnosis is hydrocephalus. The frontal horns in lobar holoprosencephaly have an angular, flat configuration that is unlike the smooth curvilinear margins observed with hydrocephalus, and with hydrocephalus, the third ventricle is in its normal position. Finally, the septum pellucidum and Sylvian fissures are usually absent in lobar holoprosencephaly.

The CT appearance of septo-optic dysplasia (de Morsier's syndrome) can easily be confused with lobar holoprosencephaly because there is absence of the septum pellucidum and flattening of the roof of the frontal horns. A primitive ventricle further increases the similarity. This condition will be discussed further under the heading of septum pellucidum abnormalities.

Anomalies of the Septum Pellucidum

The septum pellucidum is a thin triangular membrane consisting of two glial layers covered laterally with ependyma, which separates the frontal horns of the lateral ventricles. In the fetus, the two layers of the septum pellucidum are separated by a thin cavity of varying size called the cavum septi pellucidi or "fifth ventricle". The portion of the cavity lying posterior to an arbitrary vertical plane through the columns of the fornix is termed a cavum vergae or "sixth ventricle" (Williams 1985). These cava are not considered part of the true ventricular system, since they are not lined with ependyma and rarely communicate with the lateral or third ventricles, but the anterior and posterior portions of the cavum do communicate freely. The cavum vergae begins to contract posteriorly after about 6 months of gestational age and is absent at term in 70% of infants. A cavum septi pellucidi, although beginning to involute just before term, is seen in about 80% of infants at term and persists in approximately 15% of adults (Williams 1985; Diebler and Dulac, 1987). A cavum septi pellucidi and a cavum vergae are considered developmental anomalies that are seldom of clinical significance.

On CT, a cavum septi pellucidi appears as a midline CSF-containing space separated from the frontal horns by thin septa that are parallel or nearly so and extend posteriorly to the foramina of Monro (Fig. 6.13). Rarely, a cavum septi pellucidi may dilate secondary to fluid production within the cavum, and if sufficiently large, can cause ventricular obstruction at the foramen of Monro.

On CT, a dilated cavum is differentiated from a colloid cyst by the fact that the cavum lies more anterior and superior, is of lower attenuation and does not enhance.

A cavum veli interpositi represents an extension of the quadrigeminal plate cistern which projects anteriorly into the velum interpositum above the third ventricle towards the foramina of Monro. Laterally, it is bounded by the columns of the fornix and the thalamus. This condition may be seen in infants and children, but seldom in adults. There is no association between it and other congenital conditions.

CT shows a cavum veli interpositi as a midline, triangular, CSF-containing structure, located anterior to the quadrigeminal plate cistern above the third ventricle, the anatomy being best appreciated on direct coronal slices. Another cause of a midline cystic structure is an arachnoid cyst in the region of the quadrigeminal plate. However, an arachnoid cyst can usually be distinguished from a cavum by its curvilinear margins and more posterior location.

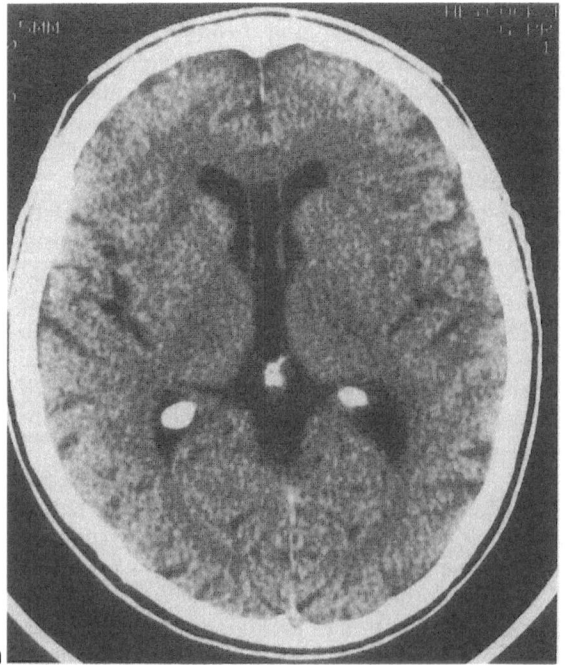
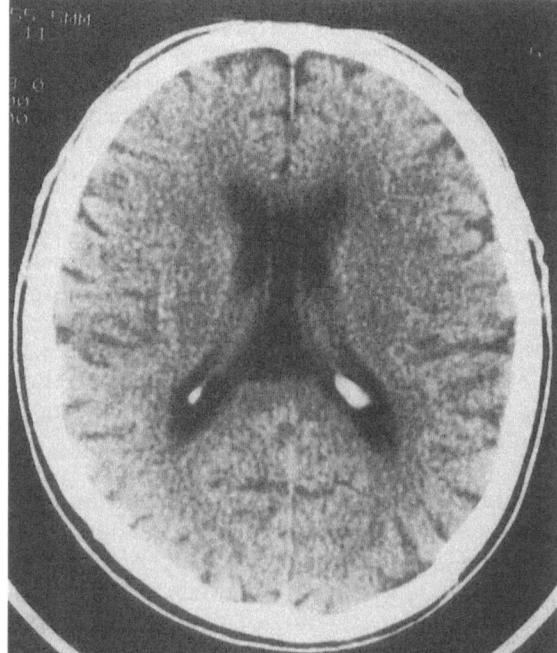

Fig. 6.13. Cranial CT. Cavum septi pellucidi (**a**) and vergae (**b**). (P.B.)

Rupture of the septum pellucidum may be observed in severe hydrocephalus. In the prosencephalies, it is absent by definition. In agenesis of the corpus callosum, the septum may be absent or divided into two sheets.

Absence of the septum pellucidum may be an isolated structural abnormality, possibly associated with mental retardation or epilepsy, but can also occur without any clinical stigmata. More often, absence of the septum pellucidum is linked to other abnormalities, such as porencephalic cysts with heterotopias and abnormalities of gyration, optic nerve hypoplasia or hypothalamic anomalies.

Septo-optic dysplasia combines agenesis of the septum pellucidum with a prominent optic recess of the third ventricle and hypoplasia of the optic nerves, optic chiasm and infundibulum. Distinction from lobar holoprosencephaly can sometimes be difficult on CT, but plain films will reveal small optic canals bilaterally (Diebler and Dulac 1987).

Dandy–Walker Syndrome

The Dandy–Walker syndrome comprises cystic dilatation of the fourth ventricle, aplasia of the cerebellar vermis, and elevation of the lateral sinuses and the tentorum, resulting in a marked enlargement of the posterior fossa which is almost entirely occupied by the dilated fourth ventricle. Dilatation of the third and lateral ventricles and imperforation of the foramina of Luschka and Magendie are frequent, but not constant. The cystic fourth ventricle is lined by a membrane formed by ependymal and pial tissue.

The association of Dandy–Walker syndrome with other cerebral, visceral and skeletal malformations has been described in numerous observations in the literature. The link between agenesis of the corpus callosum and Dandy–Walker syndrome is classic, being as high as 17% in some series (Sanwaya and McLaurin 1981). Occipital encephaloceles may be seen in conjunction with Dandy–Walker syndrome and it seems that the pressure of the cystic fourth ventricle leads to progressive thinning of the occipital vault and then to herniation of the dilated fourth ventricle through the osseous defect.

Plain skull films may suggest a diagnosis by showing the enlarged posterior fossa delimited by the thin, bulging occipital vault, the irregular ridges of the lateral sinuses and the torcula. CT in the Dandy–Walker syndrome reveals the cystic fourth ventricle occupying nearly all of the posterior fossa – its thin membranes cannot in general be differentiated from the occipital vault which constitutes its posterior limits (Fig. 6.14). The anterior

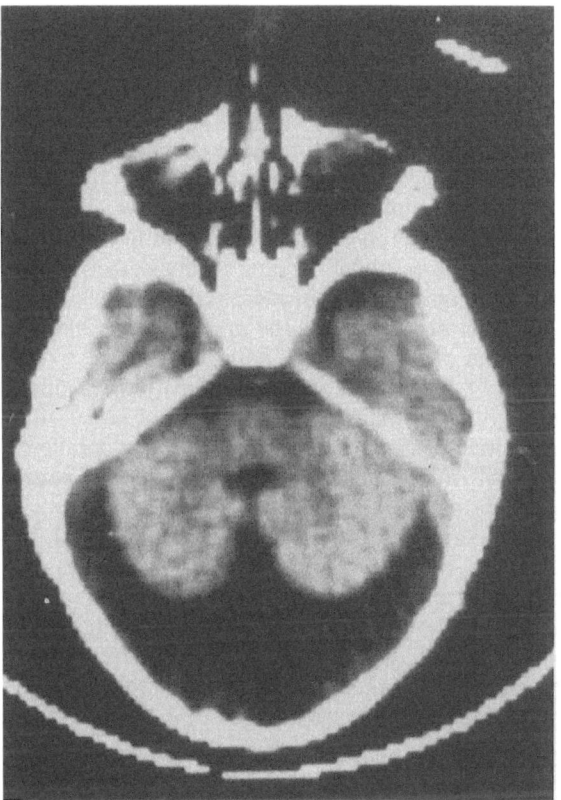

Fig. 6.14. Cranial CT. Dandy–Walker syndrome.

limits are formed by the brainstem, and the floor of the fourth ventricle corresponds to a more-or-less marked ridge between the cerebellar hemispheres, which are displaced laterally and anteriorly. The cerebellar vermis is characteristically hypoplastic or, in about 25% of cases, completely absent. The pons is displaced anteriorly, compressed and deformed. The cerebellopontine angle cisterns are usually effaced. The tentorium, torcula, straight sinus and the vein of Galen are all displaced upwards.

Only in very rare cases will angiography be required nowadays but this will show that the posterior inferior cerebellar arteries (PICAs) are often small or absent in Dandy–Walker syndrome, whereas they are usually normal with a giant cisterna magna and with an arachnoid cyst they are displaced toward the clivus. In a trapped fourth ventricle, the PICAs may be displaced posteriorly and inferiorly (see Chap. 3).

In the Joubert syndrome, which is a rare autosomal recessive condition, there is agenesis of the vermis with normally developed cerebellar hemispheres. In Dandy–Walker syndrome, which is not inherited, these are hypoplastic.

Encephaloceles

Although the word encephalocele is time-honoured, the correct terminology is cephalocele, which represents a herniation of one or more intracranial structures (membranes, brain or ventricles) through a defect in the skull. Encephaloceles may be congenital or acquired. The latter are usually secondary to a traumatic vault defect or most commonly iatrogenic, as the result of a craniectomy defect, often with subsequent raised intracranial pressure.

When it occurs during the first 10 weeks of gestation, an encephalocele is considered to be a disorder of neural tube closure caused by a defective neural tube, a primary osseous defect, or both. This defect may be isolated or form part of a generalised dysplasia or mesodermal abnormality such as neurofibromatosis.

Encephaloceles are midline anomalies that in Europe involve the occipital region in 75% of cases; the frontal and basal regions in 15%; and the vertex in 10%. In South East Asia, nasofrontal encephaloceles are most common. They are frequently associated with other congenital anomalies such as corpus callosum dysgenesis or the Chiari malformation.

In both meningocele and meningoencephalocele, CT shows a well defined defect in the cranium or skull base associated with a soft tissue mass (Byrd et al. 1978) (Fig. 6.15). Density measurements may be used to differentiate brain and CSF within the herniated sac. Basal meningoencephaloceles involving the nasopharynx, sinuses or orbits are rare and frequently overlooked or misdiagnosed on axial CT scans because of the many foramina and canals that are normally present. In these patients, coronal CT sections are usually required to demonstrate the defect in the skull base and the inferior or anterior protrusion of meninges and brain (see Chap. 8).

Hydranencephaly

Hydranencephaly corresponds to a nearly complete destruction of the cerebral hemispheres which are replaced by fluid-filled bubbles. The membrane forming the wall of the bubbles is smooth, translucent and contains attenuated blood vessels, but no convolutions. Islands of glial tissue may be observed along the inner surface, but there is no ependymal layer corresponding to the ventricular walls. Relative preservation of the basal ganglia and the inferior part of the temporal and occipital lobes is frequent. Aetiology most often remains unknown and only in rare cases can a link be established with abdominal trauma, attempted abortion or carbon monoxide intoxication. Many investigators believe,

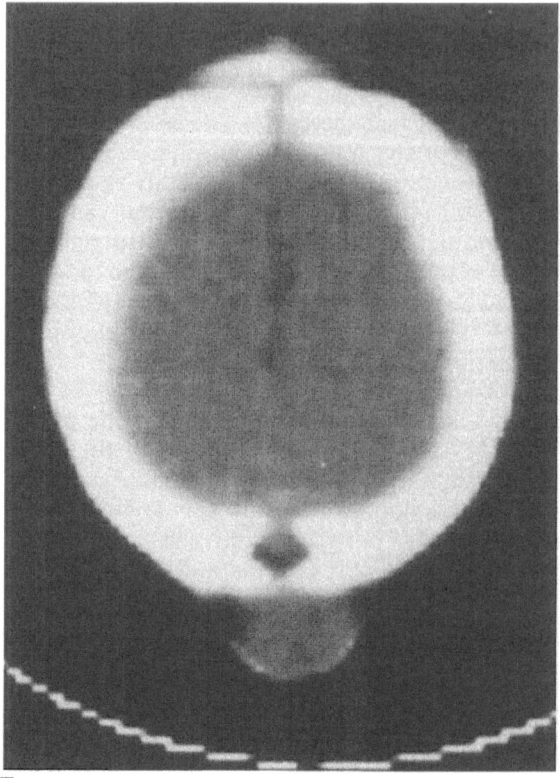

Fig. 6.15. Cranial CT. Occipital encephalocele.

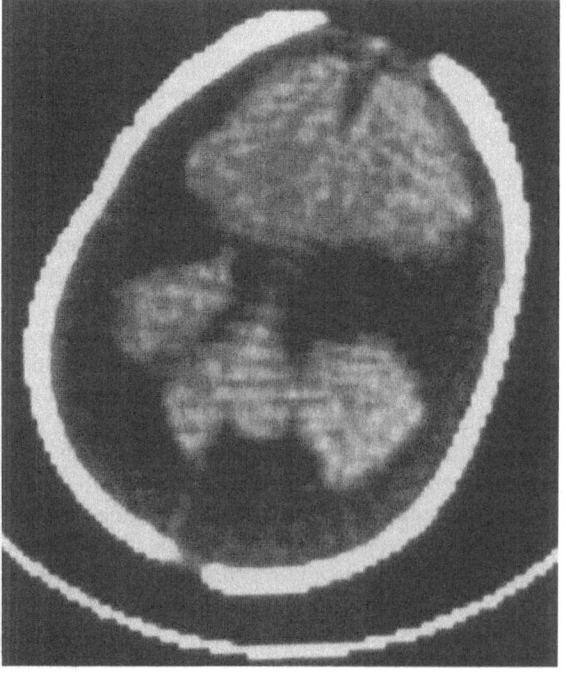

Fig. 6.16. Cranial CT. Hydranencephaly.

however, that it results from intrauterine hemispheric infarction secondary to supraclinoid occlusion of the internal carotid arteries because, typically, there is absence of the portions of the cerebrum supplied by the internal carotid arteries and sparing of the brain supplied by the vertebral basilar system. Lesions similar to hydranencephaly have been observed in toxoplamosis and cytomegalovirus disease. Clinically, the infant is usually normocephalic or microcephalic, but cranial enlargement may be found due to concurrent aqueduct stenosis or to modifications of the convexity preventing the resorption of CSF.

CT shows (Fig. 6.16):

1. A normal posterior fossa, brainstem, thalamus and hypothalamus
2. Persisting basal ganglia
3. Large bubbles of CSF density corresponding to the cerebral hemispheres separated by
4. An intact falx and tentorium

Although hydranencephaly is diagnosed by CT in most cases, angiography is occasionally useful to distinguish between hydranencephaly and severe hydrocephalus. Angiographically, hydranencephaly is characterised by absent or hypoplastic anterior and middle cerebral arteries but with normal external carotid and posterior fossa arteries.

The Neurocutaneous Syndromes

Neurofibromatosis

Neurofibromatosis is a relatively common disease and is inherited as a dominant, autosomal trait, its manifestations resulting from dysplasia of neuroectodermal and mesodermal tissues. It is likely that each patient with neurofibromatosis has or will develop abnormalities of the central nervous system. The brain is often moderately enlarged which accounts for the large head size so frequently seen in these patients. Central nervous system (CNS) neoplasms associated with neurofibromatosis include:

Optic nerve glioma
Cranial nerve tumours
Meningioma
Astrocytoma
Ependymoma
Hamartoma
Glioblastoma

Multiple intracranial tumours are not uncommon and this is particularly true for 8th nerve tumours and for meningiomas. Meningiomas are commonly intraventricular and arise from the choroid of the lateral ventricles where they may be appreciated radiographically as psammomatous calcifications that are usually bilateral and frequently in the temporal horn region. MRI has revealed intraparenchymal lesions in children where no CT abnormality was demonstrated (Hurst et al. 1988). Their nature was uncertain but they may represent either hamartomatous or gliomatous change.

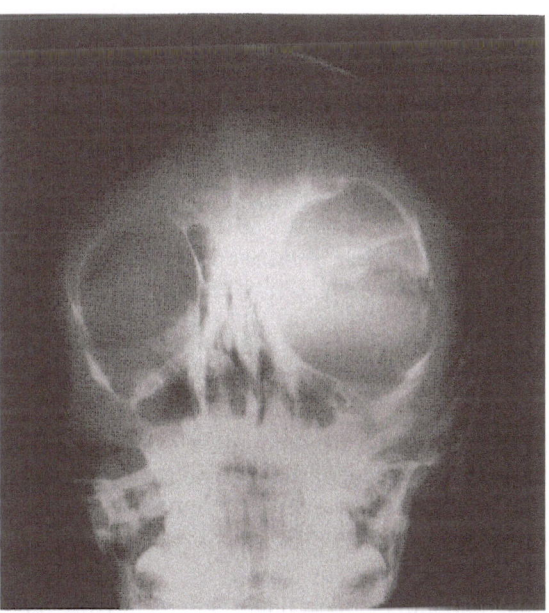

Fig. 6.17. Skull radiograph (frontal projection). Neurofibromatosis. The "bare" left orbit is associated with maxillary and ethmoidal sinus hypoplasia.

Radiology

Skull. A defect in the posterior superior wall of the orbit is one of the characteristic skeletal features of neurofibromatosis (Fig. 6.17). As a result, the subarachnoid space and/or temporal lobe can herniate into the posterior orbit where the constant pulsation of the brain and CSF may enlarge the orbit and even produce pulsating exophthalmos. Radiographic findings related to the orbital defect include:

Hypoplasia of the greater wing of the sphenoid
Elevation of the lesser wing of the sphenoid
Downward tilting of the floor of the sella
Enlargement of the middle cranial fossa
Enlargement of the orbit

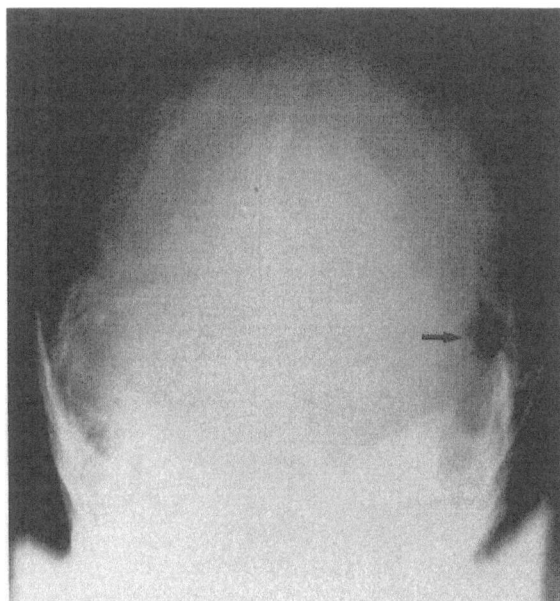

Fig. 6.18. Skull radiograph (semi-axial projection). Neurofibromatosis. A diamond-shaped defect within the lambdoid suture is *arrowed*.

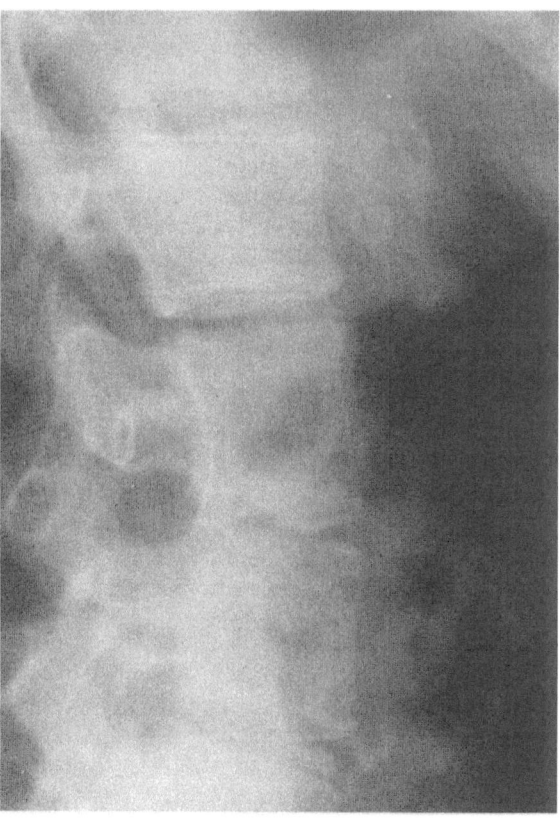

Fig. 6.19. Lumbar spine (lateral projection). Neurofibromatosis. Posterior scalloping of the vertebral bodies is seen.

Hypoplasia of the ethmoid and maxillary sinuses, medial displacement of the cavernous portion of the internal carotid artery and forward displacement of the anterior temporal branches of the middle cerebral artery

An uncommon, but highly characteristic skull defect may be observed in the lambdoid suture, most commonly on the left side (Fig. 6.18). This abnormality probably represents a mesodermal defect of the periosteum and is associated with underdevelopment of the mastoid bone and air cells on the same side.

Spine and Contents. Dural ectasia with enlargement of the spinal canal is a common finding in neurofibromatosis. This may be localised to one or two segments, but more commonly multiple segments are involved, the thoracic and lumbar regions being the most usual sites. The primary underlying abnormality is congenital weakness of the dura. Over a period of years, the constant pulsation of CSF causes progressive enlargement of the dural sac with resultant bony erosion and this, in turn, causes posterior scalloping of the vertebral bodies and erosion of the pedicles (Fig. 6.19). The differential diagnosis of these changes include other connective tissue disorders such as Marfan syndrome and Ehlers–Danlos syndrome. Posterior scalloping

is also observed with slow-growing intraspinal masses such as ependymoma, lipoma and dermoid, but these, and indeed most intraspinal masses that cause scalloping, lie below the level of the spinal cord. (Meningiomas, although commonly found in the thoracic region, rarely cause bony changes.)

A neurofibroma may extend through an intervertebral foramen with erosion of the pedicle and enlargement of that foramen.

Kyphoscoliosis is a common skeletal abnormality in neurofibromatosis, occurring in approximately 10% of patients. It is classically short-segment and angular with a predominance of the kyphotic portion. It may be rapidly progressive. Aetiology is not certain as neurofibromatous tissue is generally not found at the site of the vertebral abnormality. Kyphoscoliosis is virtually always associated with dural ectasia and, thus, enlargement of the canal, posterior scalloping and erosion of the pedicles and laminae (Klatte et al. 1976).

Syringomyelia is also associated with neurofibromatosis.

Tuberous Sclerosis

Tuberous sclerosis is a rare, hereditary disease with the classical clinical triad of (a) adenoma sebaceum, (b) seizures and (c) mental retardation. The disease is characterised by a potential for hamartomatous growth in various organ systems including the brain which is involved in most cases. Hamartomas develop in the cerebral cortex and paraventricular regions.

CNS involvement

Characteristically, the cerebrum is involved, although the cerebellum, medulla and spinal cord may also be affected. The lesions are hamartomatous foci and vary in size and number. The vast majority are found in relation to the CSF pathways and are of two types – cortical foci or tubers and subependymal nodules around the ventricular system. Cortical tubers may involve any portion of the cerebral cortex and are composed of glial and neural elements in disarray. Large astrocytes are frequently present. Subependymal nodules are of a different microscopic appearance and tend to be more discrete and more often contain deposits of calcium.

The giant cell astrocytoma is the commonest neoplasm seen in tuberous sclerosis, but is by no means the only one found, a variety of gliomas and ganglial gliomas having also been reported. Whilst the majority of brain tumours are slow-growing and pursue a benign course, varying degrees of malignancy have been reported in up to 10%–15% of them. The great majority of tumours arise in relation to subependymal hamartomas, particularly those located near the foramina of Monro where they may cause ventricular obstruction and hydrocephalus.

Radiology

Skull films may show characteristic intracerebral calcification and/or cranial vault sclerosis, the latter probably being related to long-term anticonvulsant therapy rather than being a specific feature of the condition. The reported incidence of parenchymal calcification varies from 50% to 80%. Several studies have confirmed that there is no relationship between the existence or extent of cerebral calcification and the presence of seizures.

On CT, the subependymal nodules are the most constant abnormality and are easily recognised (Fig. 6.20). They can be seen from as early as two and a half months, and are located around the lateral ventricles and the third ventricle; only rarely

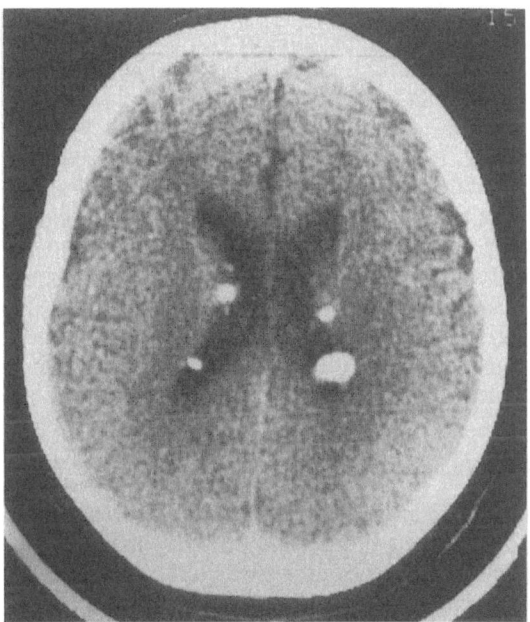

Fig. 6.20. Cranial CT. Tuberous sclerosis. Calcified subependymal nodules are shown.

in the cerebellum or the brainstem. They are most often multiple and round and usually fail to enhance. Their size and degree of calcification progresses with increasing age.

The differential CT diagnosis of tuberous sclerosis includes (a) Intrauterine infection, (b) Sturge–Weber syndrome, (c) Vascular malformation and (d) cerebral heterotopia. Intrauterine infections such as toxoplasmosis or cytomegalovirus disease frequently result in periventricular calcification. However, these postinfectious calcifications are usually smaller than the subependymal nodules of tuberous sclerosis and are associated with significant diffuse cerebral atrophy and microcephaly. Unlike Sturge–Weber syndrome or some vascular malformations, the associated atrophic changes in tuberous sclerosis are not focal. Cerebral heterotopia (islands of normal cortical tissue in a periventricular location), which produces irregularity of the ventricular margins, may resemble subependymal hamartomas; however, heterotopic foci are located along the medial ventricular wall and are isodense with brain, whereas subependymal nodules of tuberous sclerosis are hyperdense and are located along the lateral ventricular wall.

Sturge–Weber Syndrome

The Sturge–Weber syndrome is a non-familial neurocutaneous syndrome that includes (a) trigeminal angioma (90%), (b) pial angioma (100%), (c) epilepsy (88%), (d) focal neurological deficit (50%), (e) mental retardation (55%) and (f) glaucoma (39%) (Diebler and Dulac 1987). The skin angioma is congenital, flat and of port-wine colour. Microscopically, it consists of dilated capillaries with a single endothelial cell layer. The intracranial angioma is usually limited to the pia mater, extending only rarely to involve the dura and the bone. It most often occupies the occipital or parieto-occipital areas and is nearly always unilateral, very exceptionally bilateral. The angioma consists of small tortuous vessels resembling veins that rarely enter the cortex.

Radiology

Plain skull films are generally normal before the age of 1–2 years. In older children, they may reveal curvilinear calcifications which conform precisely to the cerebral convolutions of the occipital or parietal lobe on one side (Fig. 6.21). These parallel lines of calcification were once thought to lie in the walls of vessels, but actually lie in the superficial

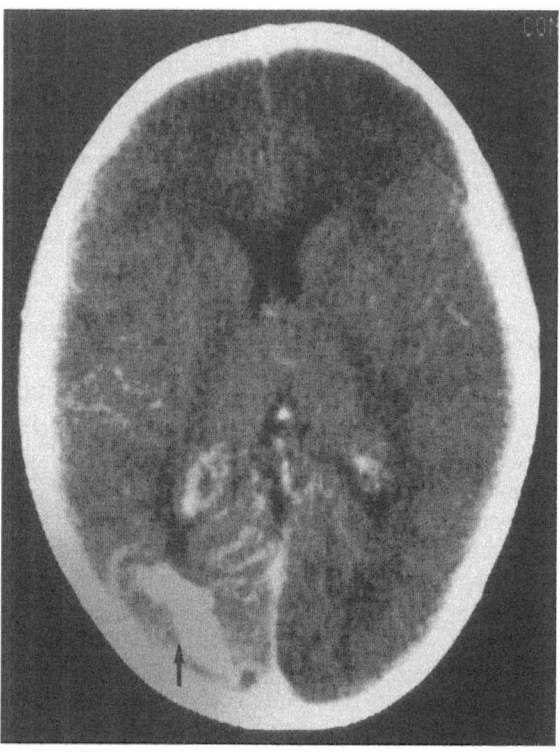

Fig. 6.22. Cranial CT after IV contrast. Sturge–Weber syndrome. The angioma (*arrow*) and adjacent cerebral cortex are enhanced.

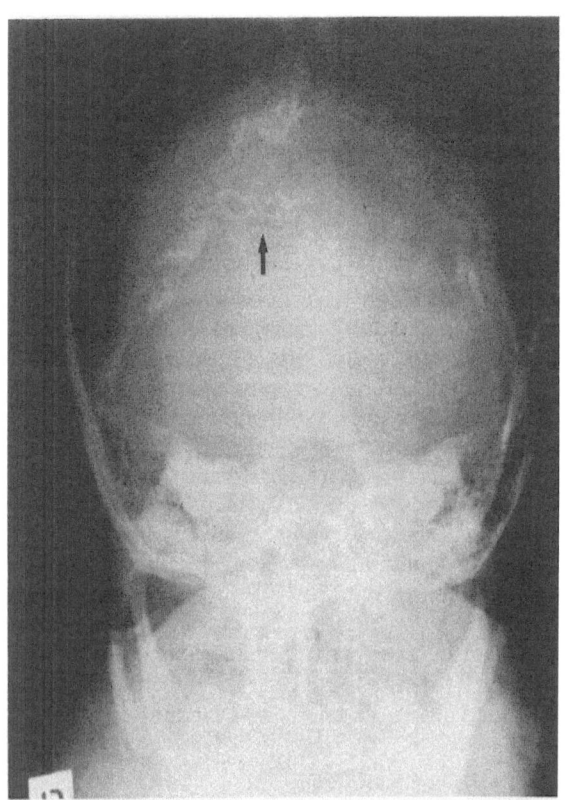

Fig. 6.21. Skull radiograph (semi-axial projection). Sturge–Weber syndrome. Typical curvilinear calcification is arrowed.

layer of cerebral cortex and probably result from repeated anoxic episodes. CT shows the calcification effectively and at an earlier age than radiographs and also demonstrates the underlying cortical atrophy that is commonly associated.

The CT appearance of the intracranial angioma is variable but three typical patterns are encountered. The first two are most often seen in children during the first 24 months of life.

1. CT without enhancement shows a clear asymmetry between the two cerebral hemispheres. On the side of the angioma, the hemisphere is hyperdense and the lateral ventricle and the arachnoid spaces are small. After contrast enhancement, there is opacification of the angioma and the adjacent cerebral tissue (Fig. 6.22). The ipsilateral choroid plexus is dense and sometimes enlarged. There is usually no calcification present.

2. On a post-contrast CT, the angioma appears as an area slightly denser than the surrounding brain. Contrast enhancement outlines the convolutions of the parietal and occipital lobes, possibly extending to involve the entire hemisphere. The adjacent subarachnoid spaces and the ipsilateral

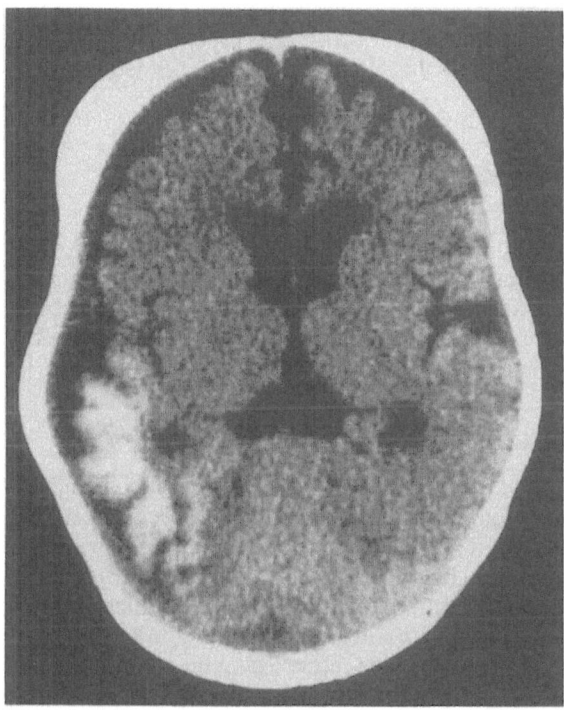

Fig. 6.23. Cranial CT after IV contrast. Sturge–Weber syndrome cortical enhancement and enlargement of the adjacent subarachnoid spaces are shown.

Congenital Infections

Cytomegalovirus (CMV) Infection

Congenital CMV infection affects around 1% of live births. Symptoms typically appear in the neonatal period and include petechiae, jaundice and hepatosplenomegaly; but children who are asymptomatic at birth can present later with neurological disturbance or sudden death.

Central nervous system damage occurs in about 10% of cases and consists of (a) microcephaly (70%), (b) mental retardation (60%), (c) hearing loss (30%), (d) neuromuscular disorders (35%), (e) choreoretinitis or optic atrophy (20%), (f) various seizure disorders including infantile spasms. On neuropathological examination, any or all of the following features may be seen: (a) cerebellar hypoplasia, (b) porencephaly, (c) micropolygyria, (d) periventricular intracerebral calcifications, (e) hydranencephaly.

Radiology

Plain skull films may show characteristic fine curvilinear periventricular calcification (Fig. 6.24).

ventricle are clearly enlarged. (Fig. 6.23). Unilateral or bilateral enlargement of the choroid plexus is a frequent finding. Calcification may be seen within, or at the border of, the angioma.

3. In older children, the angioma may be excluded from the circulation and CT will show large areas of calcification within the adjacent cerebral tissue. The extent and density of the calcification tend to mask any pathological contrast enhancement which might be present within the angiomatous tissue. Focal or general cerebral atrophy is nearly always present.

Less common CT patterns which may occasionally be seen include:

1. An angioma which may have a multifocal appearance interspersed with foci of hyperdensity, the angioma tending to mould itself to the convolutions of the underlying brain.
2. Communicating hydrocephalus which may occur as a result of repeated haemorrhages.
3. The co-existence of hydrocephalus and focal atrophy which may result in the development of a porencephalic cyst, which is an area of cavitation within the brain consequent upon injury due to a variety of causes.

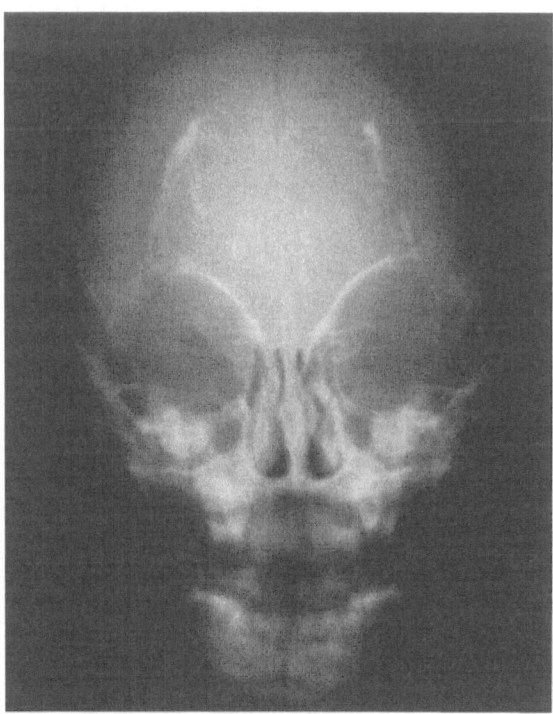

Fig. 6.24. Skull radiograph (frontal projection). Cytomegalovirus infection. The calcification is curvilinear and periventricular in location.

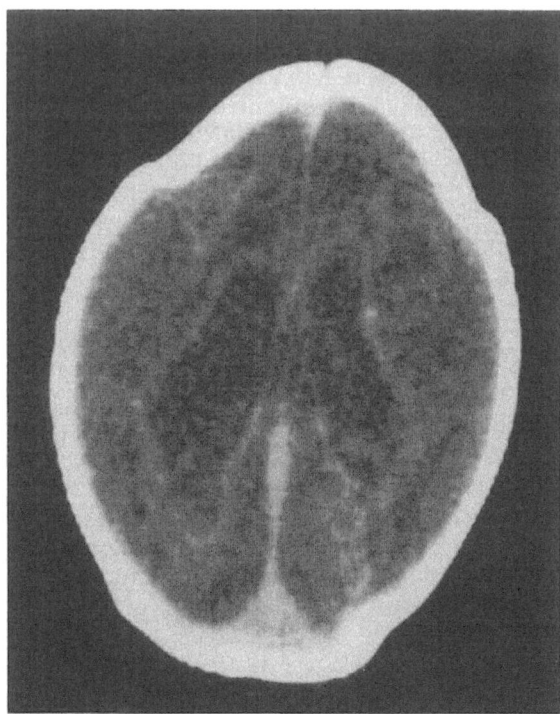

Fig. 6.25. Cranial CT. Cytomegalovirus infection. Fine calcification surrounds enlarged lateral ventricles.

On CT, the lateral ventricles and cortical sulci are enlarged and the ventricles are surrounded by multiple small calcifications (Fig. 6.25). Multiple porencephalic cysts may lead to hydranencephaly. In minor forms, CT may be normal or show areas of low density that will later form porencephalic cysts. Subsequent CT may show progressive cerebral atrophy.

Thus, the hallmarks of CMV infection on CT are (a) periventricular calcification, (b) ventricular dilation due to atrophy and (c) porencephaly. Although brain necrosis is severe, calcifications in the cortex and basal ganglia are not visualised as a general rule and serve to distinguish this disease from toxoplasmosis.

Congenital Rubella Infection

Congenital rubella results from fetal infection prior to week 20 of gestation, most often before week four. The incidental risk is about 10% and the main clinical manifestations are (a) cardiac malformation (52%) including patent ductus arteriosus, pulmonary artery stenosis and atrioseptal or ventriculoseptal defects, (b) hearing loss (50%), (c) cataract, microphthalmos, buphthalmos, or retinopathy (40%), (d) psychomotor retardation often

associated with microcephaly (25%). Hepatosplenomegaly, thrombocytopenia, meningoencephalitis and hepatitis imply persisting viral infection.

Radiology

Plain skull films show microcrania and very occasionally, intracranial calcification. On CT, the brain generally appears small but of normal appearance. Very exceptionally, intracerebral calcifications and areas of low density may be observed.

Congenital Toxoplasmosis

Toxoplasma gondii is a unicellular parasite reproducing in the intestinal mucosa of a specific host, the cat. The cysts are excreted and may infest various occasional hosts, including man. Infection is usually latent or accompanied by minimal clinical symptoms, but severe infection may develop in the fetus or in the immunosuppressed child or adult, and indeed congenital toxoplasmosis is the most frequent infectious disease of the fetus.

Radiology

On plain skull films, calcifications occur which are generally multiple, small and have a grossly periventricular distribution (Fig. 6.26) although many calcifications remain undetected.

Although the CT findings in toxoplasmosis are not pathognomonic, multiple calcifications can usually be observed in (a) the cerebral hemispheres,

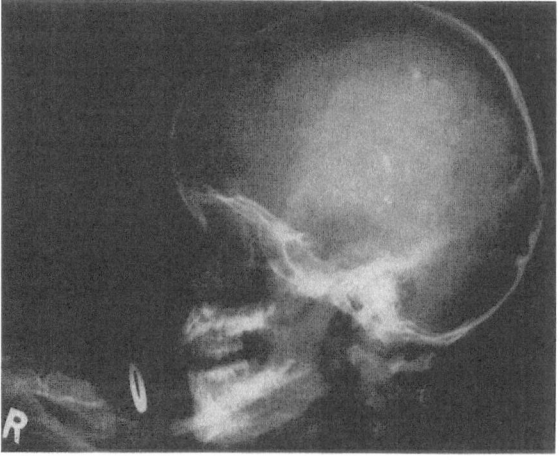

Fig. 6.26. Skull radiograph (lateral projection). Toxoplasmosis. Cerebral parenchymal and basal ganglial calcificaton are evident.

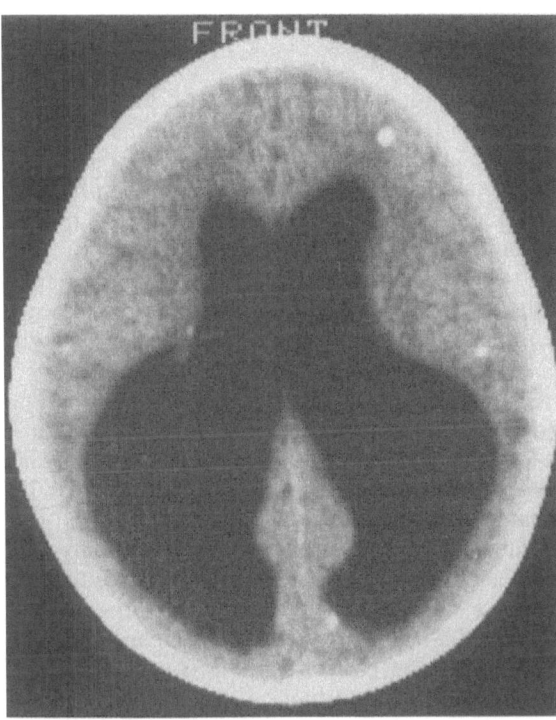

Fig. 6.27. Cranial CT. Toxoplasmosis. (P.B.)

(b) the basal ganglia, (c) the periventricular areas and (d) the choroid plexus. The CT appearance of the disease can be correlated with the time of fetal infection.

With fetal infection occurring during the first 5–6 months of pregnancy, enlargement of the lateral and third ventricles is a more-or-less constant feature (Fig. 6.27). Dilatation of the lateral ventricles nearly always predominates in their posterior half where the cerebral mantle may become very thin. Gross symmetrical, multiple porencephalic cysts (representing cystic encephalomalacia and/or hydranencephaly) may be seen in particularly severe forms. Calcifications are generally multiple and symmetrical and may partly or completely occupy the basal ganglia. There is also a predilection for the periventricular regions, but calcification may also occur within the cerebral tissues. Microphthalmia and ocular calcifications are easily observed on CT.

In cases of fetal infection in the last trimester of pregnancy, CT frequently remains normal. Small periventricular and intracerebral calcifications are occasionally seen but are rarely numerous and the ventricles are usually of normal size.

Together with CMV, toxoplasmosis is the most common cause of intracranial calcifications in children under one year of age. The differential diag-

nosis includes congenital rubella and herpes simplex encephalitis. The cortical and basal ganglia calcifications help to distinguish toxoplasmosis from congenital CMV infection.

Toxic and Metabolic Degenerative Conditions

Diseases included under this heading are generally divided into two major categories: (a) those associated with basal ganglia lesions (Parkinson's disease, Wilson's disease, Huntington's chorea, Hallervorden–Spatz disease and anoxic conditions including carbon monoxide poisoning) and (b) diseases principally affecting the white matter.

The basal ganglia pathologies are most often encountered in adult practice and, thus, our attention is principally drawn to the white matter diseases (leukodystrophies) most of which are recognised in children, often in the very young. Heinz et al. (1979) described three general CT patterns of white matter disease, namely, (a) demyelination, (b) dysmyelination and (c) a combination of these two.

In demyelinating diseases, e.g. multiple sclerosis, anoxia, malnutrition, progressive multifocal leukoencephalopathy (PML), there is formation of normal myelin which is subsequently destroyed. In dysmyelinating diseases, e.g. metachromatic leukodystrophy and Alexander's disease, there is abnormal formation and maintenance of myelin as a result of an enzyme disturbance. Adrenoleucodystrophy has features of both types of disease.

The CT picture of a demyelinating disease is that of diminished white matter density, variable mass effect, and contrast enhancement which is presumably due to inflammation at the site of active demyelination. Dysmyelinating diseases are less likely to demonstrate mass effect or pathological enhancement whereas adrenoleukodystrophy generally exhibits large areas of diminished density with peripheral advancing zones of gliosis that may show some enhancement.

Heinz et al. (1979) have attempted to classify or distinguish patterns of white matter degeneration on CT by documenting the distribution of these changes into the following categories: (a) focal symmetrical, (b) periventricular, (c) focal asymmetrical, (d) centrum ovale and (e) generalised.

Although this approach to the problem has its attractions, the difficulty lies in the fact that there is considerable variation in the CT appearances of individual diseases so that any one condition may have features common to two or more of these groups. With such overlap between the groups, the CT appearance is rarely diagnostic in itself and one has to rely heavily on family history, clinical presentation, and the biochemical and pathological findings in order to arrive at the correct diagnosis.

Table 6.2 sets out a classification of pathological white matter diseases, categorising them according to whether they are demyelinating, diffuse, dysmyelinating or of developmental origin. Only those conditions which are reasonably common and likely to be found in children, will be discussed. CT is the principal method of investigation, but MRI is becoming more widely available and has been used to study these diseases (Nowell et al. 1988).

Table 6.2. Classification of pathological white matter diseases

1. *Primary demyelinating disease*
   Multiple sclerosis
   Acute disseminated encephalomyelitis

2. *Secondary demyelinating disease*
   Progressive multifocal leukoencephalopathy (PML)
   Demyelination secondary to tumour
   Anoxic injury
   Inflammatory disease (see Chap. 5)
      Subacute sclerosing panencephalitis
      Herpes simplex encephalitis
      Cerebritis
   Trauma – localised encephalomalacia
   Radiation and chemotherapy-induced white matter
   changes – disseminated necrotising leukoencephalopathy
   (mineralising microangiopathy)
   Cerebral toxins
      Arsenic
      Bismuth
      Lead
      Alcohol
   Reye's syndrome

3. *Diffuse sclerosis*
   Adrenoleukodystrophy
   Schilder's disease

4. *Dysmyelinating disease*
   Metachromatic leukodystrophy
   Globoid-cell leukodystrophy (Krabbe's disease)
   Spongy degeneration (Canavan's disease)
   Alexander's disease
   Pelizaeus–Merzbacher disease
   Cockayne's syndrome

5. *Developmental disorders unrelated to myelin*
   Mitochondrial cytopathy (Kearns–Sayre syndrome,
   ophthalmoplegia plus)
   Mucopolysaccharidosis (MPS)

Modified from Heinz et al. (1979) and Turnbull (1986).

MRI is more sensitive than CT in demonstrating the extent of disease present and is of proven worth in cases of developmental delay where it is distinctly more useful that CT in demonstrating abnormalities of myelination (Nowell et al. 1988). Thus, MRI may serve to redefine and broaden the spectrum of reported imaging abnormalities in children.

Disseminated Necrotising Leukoencephalopathy

Cerebral irradiation combined with methotrexate therapy for leukaemia produces abnormal CT findings. The original designation of these findings was disseminated necrotising leukoencephalopathy, but subsequent investigations revealed such abnormalities in up to half of all patients receiving this treatment, even when they were asymptomatic. Thus, the term mineralising microangiopathy has been suggested as more appropriate and descriptive of the pathological changes.

CT shows a symmetrical, low-attenuation process in the white matter, especially near the corticomedullary junction, with relative sparing of the deeper white matter (Fig. 6.28). Thin reticular or serrated linear calcification is often present near the corticomedullary junction, especially in the frontal and posterior parietal lobes and in the basal ganglia. Contrast enhancement is usually not present; but several authors have reported low density frontal lesions near the rostrum of the corpus callosum which do show ring enhancement indistinguishable from a brain abscess. Reversal of these changes can occur with steroid treatment.

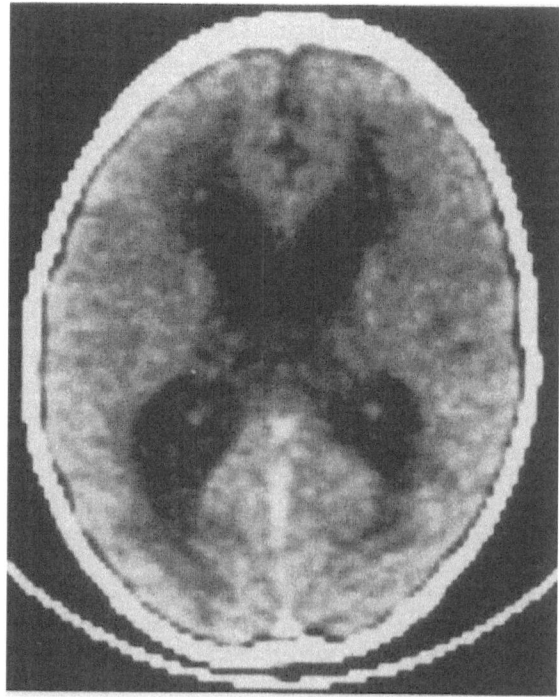

Fig. 6.28. Cranial CT. Disseminated necrotising leuko-encephalopathy. Symmetrical low density is seen within the white matter around both frontal and occipital horns of the lateral ventricles.

Reye's Syndrome

Reye's syndrome, a disease of unknown aetiology most often affecting children and adolescents, is characterised by encephalopathy and fatty degeneration of the viscera following viral infections, notably influenza B and chicken pox. A history of relatively large doses of aspirin ingested during the infection is often elicited. Clinically, Reye's syndrome may mimic acute encephalitis. Mortality is high (75% – 85%) and results from complications of cerebral oedema caused by a direct cytotoxic injury to the brain.

The CT findings are non-specific. Plain scans show diffuse cerebral oedema with hypodense white matter, small compressed ventricles and effaced sulci. Contrast enhancement is rare. In survivors with significant neurological impairment, follow-up scans disclose diminished density of the white matter and diffuse atrophy with dilated ventricles and prominent cisterns, sulci and fissures. The CT features of Reye's syndrome are similar to other leukoencephalopathies such as progressive multifocal leukoencephalopathy, anoxic encephalopathy and possibly even multiple sclerosis or adrenoleukodystrophy. The diagnosis is usually confirmed by liver biopsy.

Adrenoleukodystrophy

Adrenoleukodystrophy is a hereditary, sex-linked disease of young males combining degenerative lesions of the CNS with adrenal insufficiency. The onset is usually between 5 and 10 years of age with a fairly typical clinical presentation including behaviour problems, intellectual impairment, loss of hearing and visual acuity, cerebellar ataxia, pyramidal signs and primary adrenal insufficiency. Recent investigations suggest that the metabolic defect may involve an enzyme system responsible for the oxidation of the very long-chain fatty acids and this abnormality is detectable in the plasma and within fibroblasts, so that antenatal diagnosis is possible. The pathological features in brain include widespread demyelination of the white matter with inflammatory reaction at its periphery.

The CT lesions of adrenoleukodystrophy appear in the month following the apparent onset of the disease and are relatively specific, consisting of grossly symmetrical areas of low density which surround the ventricular trigones and merge with the splenium of the corpus callosum. Demyelination, therefore, characteristically begins in the occipital poles and moves anteriorly (Fig. 6.29). Less typical CT appearances may also be observed, especially at the outset or in the late stages of the disease.

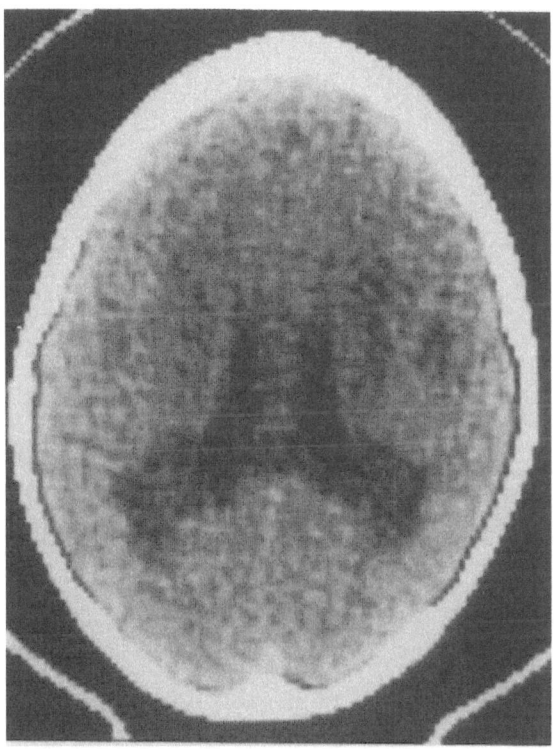

Fig. 6.29. Cranial CT. Adrenoleukodystrophy. Symmetrical occipital lobe white matter hypodensity is present.

Usually, contrast enhancement is absent but the lesions can occasionally demonstrate striking enhancement of the white matter within the internal capsule, corpus callosum, corona radiata, forceps major and cerebral peduncle.

Schilder's Disease (Diffuse Sclerosis)

Diffuse sclerosis occurs sporadically in young adults without a hereditary pattern. The clinical findings include dementia and often deafness.

The CT findings are similar, but not identical, to adrenoleukodystrophy (Fig. 6.30) with low density regions seen in both hemispheres. The lesions are asymmetrical until the late stages and do not normally enhance (Huckman et al. 1977). Differentiation from adrenoleukodystrophy is based on the slightly different CT pattern and, more importantly, the fulminant clinical course and the absence of a family history.

Metachromatic Leukodystrophy

The term metachromatic leukodystrophy designates several disorders due to deficient activity of the enzyme arylsulphatase A. The principal forms

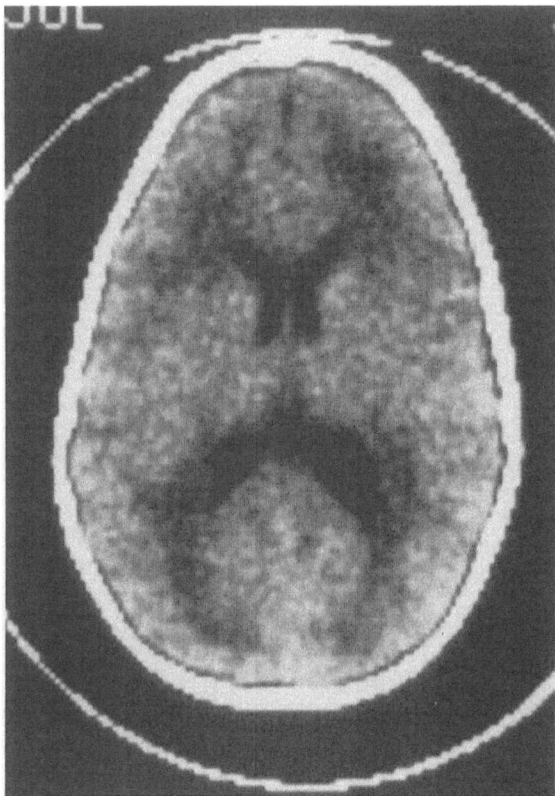

Fig. 6.30. Cranial CT. Schilders disease. Symmetrical low density is present in the white matter of both hemispheres.

of metachromatic leukodystrophy – late infantile, and juvenile – have autosomal recessive transmission. Onset of the late infantile form, usually in the second or third year, is marked by locomotor problems with frequent falls resulting from ataxia and weakness of the legs. Urine sulphatide excretion and leukocyte arylsulphatase A deficiency are the most reliable diagnostic clues. In the juvenile forms, the type with early, (about 4 to 6 years) onset, with gait disturbance and behaviour problems can be distinguished from that with later onset, typified by extrapyramidal signs and behaviour disturbances.

Neuropathological examination shows severe demyelination of the white matter leading to focal areas of cavitation where destruction of the myelin sheaths is accompanied by accumulation of meta-chromatic granules of lipid material rich in sulphatides.

CT is normal in the early stages of the disease. Thereafter, areas of low attenuation appear, initially in the frontal white matter, and show posterior progression. In the late stages of the disease, cerebral atrophy may be marked. There is no pathological contrast enhancement.

Krabbe's Disease (Globoid Leukodystrophy)

Globoid cell leukodystrophy results from B-galactocerebrosidase deficiency and has an autosomal recessive transmission. Pre-natal diagnosis and detection of healthy carriers is possible. Onset is early, between three and six months, or even within the neonatal period. The child begins to cry without any apparent cause and becomes hypersensitive to auditory and tactile stimuli. Feeding difficulties, psychomotor regression and convulsions add to the child's problems and rapid, progressive motor deterioration results in a thrown-back head with extended hypertonic legs, flexed arms, dystonic attitudes and blindness. Children rarely survive longer than two years.

On neuropathological examination, the brain size is grossly reduced with shrunken gyri and widened sulci. The white matter is extemely deficient and of firm consistency, especially in the posterior part of the hemispheres. The white matter lesions comprise marked demyelination in the posterior part of the centrum semi-ovale and the cerebellar white matter with dense fibrous astrocytic proliferation and the presence of a large number of perivascular multi-nucleated cells, called globoid cells.

CT may remain normal in the first months of the disease, with mainly symmetrical areas of low density detected initially in the posterior centrum semi-ovale. Anterior extension of the disease progresses rapidly and, at a late stage of the illness, there may be global involvement of the white matter (Fig. 6.31). There is usually no pathological contrast enhancement. The CT findings are very similar to those seen in metachromatic leukodystrophy as well as some other white matter pathologies, but the pathological and biochemical findings are specific and the genetic history and clinical findings, helpful in diagnosing Krabbe's disease.

Spongiform Degeneration of the White Matter (Canavan's Disease)

This is a rare autosomal recessive disease of unknown cause. Mental handicap, optic atrophy, abnormal eye movements, neck hypotonia and pyramidal signs, appear between two and four months of life. Head enlargement usually becomes evident by six months. The CSF is normal and a definitive diagnosis requires brain biopsy which shows replacement of the white matter by a fine network of fluid-containing cysts giving the characteristic spongy appearance. Spongy degeneration is most marked in the subcortical regions with relative sparing of the internal capsule.

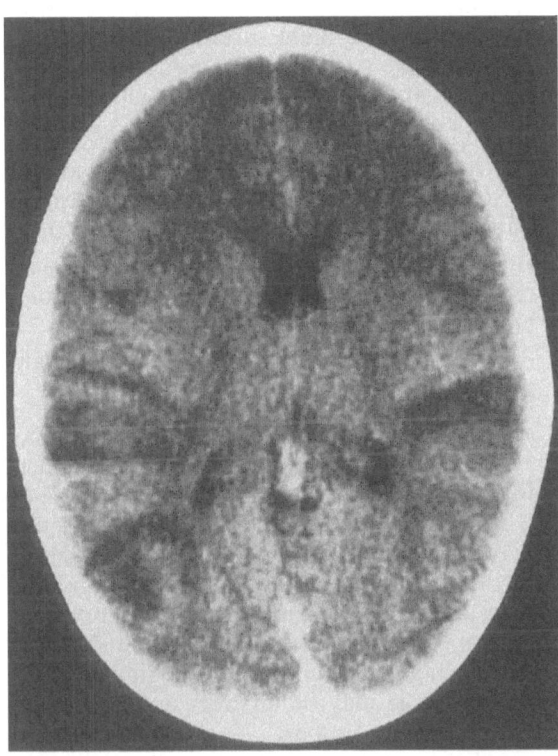

Fig. 6.31. Cranial CT after IV contrast. Krabbe's disease. Extensive white matter involvement closely resembles findings in metachromatic leukodystrophy.

CT appearances vary with the stage of the disease. In the first few weeks following the onset of the illness, the white matter takes on an oedematous, swollen appearance and the lateral ventricles are small and appear compressed. Later, the lateral ventricles become progressively enlarged and the decrease in density of the white matter continues with the appearance of small cavities of CSF density.

Spongy degeneration of the cerebral white matter has been observed in several diseases with a specific metabolic disorder and it seems probable that this condition is a non-specific response of the brain to various metabolic abnormalities. The principal diagnostic feature which distinguishes Canavan's disease from the other leukoencephalopathies is the progressive enlargement of the head. Alexander's disease is also associated with macrocephaly but the distribution, progression and general appearance of the white matter changes are different.

Alexander's Disease

This is a rare neurological disorder which can be classified into infantile, juvenile and adult forms.

Although rare familial causes have been reported, its exact genetic nature remains uncertain. The main clinical manifestations in the infantile and juvenile forms are, slowing of mental development, progressive macrocephaly, hypotonia, corticospinal tract disturbances and seizures from six months of age onwards. The CSF is normal and definitive diagnosis requires cerebral biopsy which will show extensive demyelination and eosinophilic material deposited in the cortex and especially in the white matter.

CT shows diminished density of the white matter with preferential involvement of the frontal lobes where the lesions are extensive and may be associated with compression of the frontal horns of the lateral ventricles. Contrast enhancement is variable, being absent in some children, whilst in others there is a striking symmetrical enhancement within the caudate nuclei and anterior periventricular brain substance.

Kearns–Sayre Syndrome (Oculocraniosomatic Disease)

Kearns–Sayre syndrome is a clinically distinct multisystem disease. Its main clinical manifestations appear during the second decade of life and comprise external ophthalmoplegia, pigmentary retinal degeneration and heart block. Ataxia, deafness, mild mental impairment and hypoparathyroidism may also be observed. The CSF protein level is elevated in the majority of cases. On neuropathological examination, there is a mitochondrial abnormality in various cells with spongy degeneration of cerebral, cerebellar and brainstem white matter.

CT may disclose areas of low density in the white matter and the basal ganglia with scattered hemispheric calcifications resulting from hypoparathyroidism or pseudohypoparathyroidism.

Storage disorders – Mucopolysaccharidoses (MPS)

Genetic transmission is autosomal recessive in all varieties of MPS except Hunter's disease where it is sex-linked recessive. Skeletal and visceral lesions of varying appearance and importance in the different diseases include, dysostosis multiplex with short stature and short limbs, kyphosis, coarse features, depression and widening of the nasal bridge, hypertrichosis, thickened skin, corneal clouding, deafness, hepatosplenomegaly, and umbilical herniation. The most frequent neurological problems observed are mental retardation, hydrocephalus and spinal cord compression.

Neuropathological examination in those diseases with CNS involvement shows storage bodies in the cortical neurones, the astrocytes and the capillary pericytes. In the white matter, the periadventitial spaces are greatly dilated and filled with viscous fluid, gargoyle cells and mesenchymal cells. Pachymeningitis from abnormal deposition of collagen, may cause arachnoid cysts, particularly in the sellar region, and communicating hydrocephalus. Spinal cord compression may be secondary to atlanto-axial subluxation, thoracic gibbus formation, and dural thickening.

CT in MPS with CNS involvement discloses symmetrical areas of low density in the white matter, particularly in the parietal region, that may correlate with cavitation and with dilatation of the perivascular spaces. Follow-up scans may detect progressive hydrocephalus which is a relatively common complication in MPS I, II, III and VII.

Vein of Galen Aneurysm

Aneurysms of the vein of Galen are not true aneurysms but are really deep-seated arteriovenous malformations which drain into a Galenic venous varix. Gomez et al. (1963) and O'Brien and Schechter (1970) maintain that the pathogenesis of this midline vascular malformation is based on a single embryological defect which is possibly related to close contact of the primitive Galenic system with the primitive choroidal arteries. These malformations have been classified into three groups by Litvak et al. (1960);

1. Typical aneurysm of the vein of Galen directly fed by enlarged branches of the carotid and/or vertebro-basilar system, and contiguous with a dilated straight sinus and torcula (Fig. 6.32).
2. Aneurysmal dilatation due to angiomatous malformations of the posterior thalamus and midbrain draining into the Galenic system.
3. Arteriovenous malformations that are transitional between the other two groups.

Several of these categories of malformation may co-exist and this is important to recall when undertaking angiographic evaluation of these lesions, as they have completely different arterial feeders, e.g. a thalamic arteriovenous malforation may take its blood supply from posterior branches of the middle cerebral artery, whereas an associated aneurysm of the vein of Galen may derive its entire blood supply from the posterior cerebral arteries. Similarly, the venous drainage may be different and this might have therapeutic import if a direct surgical approach was contemplated. Clinically, the symptoms are age-dependent. In the first month of life, severe cardiac failure and obstructive hydrocephalus are the main presentations, whereas in infants aged one to fifteen months, clinical symp-

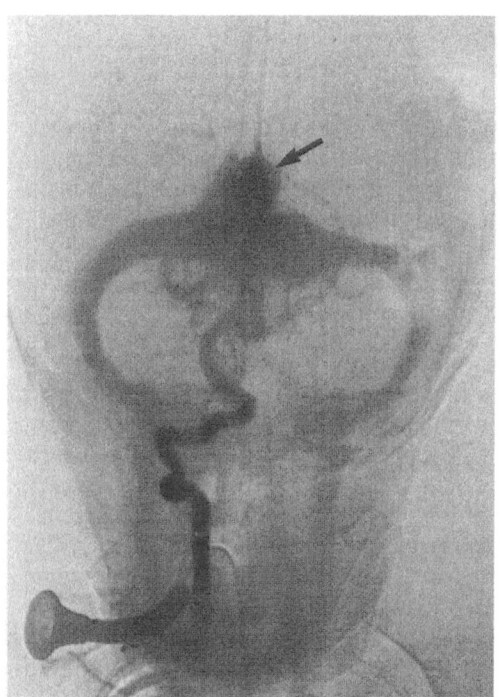
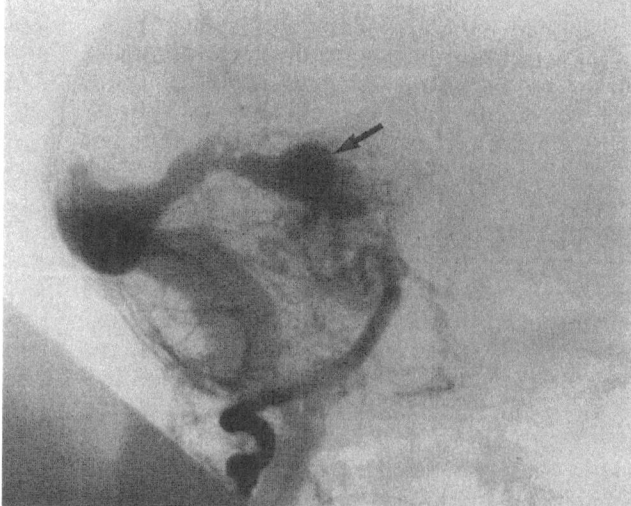

Fig. 6.32. Vertebral angiogram, (**a**) frontal and (**b**) lateral projections showing typical aneurysmal dilatation of the vein of Galen (*arrows*) with drainage into a dilated straight sinus. Abnormal angiomatous vessels are also seen around the posterior thalamus.

toms of macrocrania, subarachnoid haemorrhage or seizures will predominate. In the age group two to fifteen years, the symptoms are essentially neurological with headache, syncope, seizures and subarachnoid haemorrhage (Diebler et al. 1981).

Radiology

Plain skull films occasionally reveal rim or ring calcification in the pineal region.

On CT, the aneurysm of the vein of Galen appears as a hyperdense vascular mass situated posterosuperiorly to the third ventricle. Hydrocephalus resulting from compression of the third ventricle or aqueduct by the malformation is easily demonstrated. Calcification may be seen in the wall of the malformation although this is rare in infancy, but occurs in up to 50% of cases in adolescence (Mori 1985). CT will also readily disclose thrombosis or calcification within the malformation itself.

Ultrasound has been used to detect the abnormality in utero and in the newborn baby (Cubberley et al. 1982).

In early cases, angiographic evaluation is essential for demonstrating the feeding arteries and the venous drainage and if a direct surgical assault is being considered, then bilateral carotid angiography will be required in addition to the conventional vertebral study.

Neonatal Vascular Disease

Neonates of less than about 34 weeks gestational age are at risk from *periventricular haemorrhage*, which arises mainly from the germinal matrix at the head of the caudate nucleus. Four grades are defined (Papile 1978); Grade 1, subependymal haemorrhage; Grade 2, intraventricular haemorrhage without ventricular dilatation, and Grade 3, intraventricular haemorrhage with ventricular dilatation; Grade 4, involving parenchymal haemorrhage (Fig. 6.33). The delicacy of the germinal matrix capillary bed and incompletely developed cerebrovascular autoregulation are thought to be contributary factors.

Cerebral ischaemia in the immature neonate is manifest by periventricular leucomalacia (PVL), since the periventricular white matter is the watershed zone between cortical and central vascular territories. White matter necrosis may ensue and ultimately lead to cystic change. Cranial ultrasonography is the examination of choice in the premature neonate since the conditions described can be readily assessed and, because the equipment is portable, serial examinations can be undertaken easily.

In the mature neonate, hypoxia may lead to border zone infarction similar to that found in adults or, if very severe, diffuse cerebral involve-

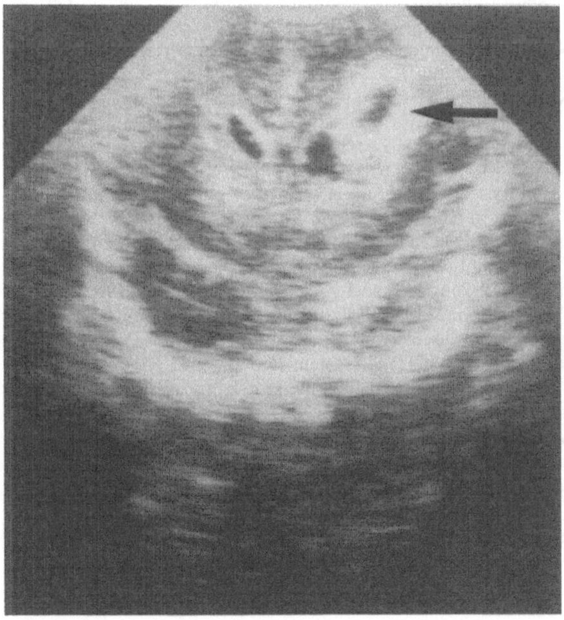

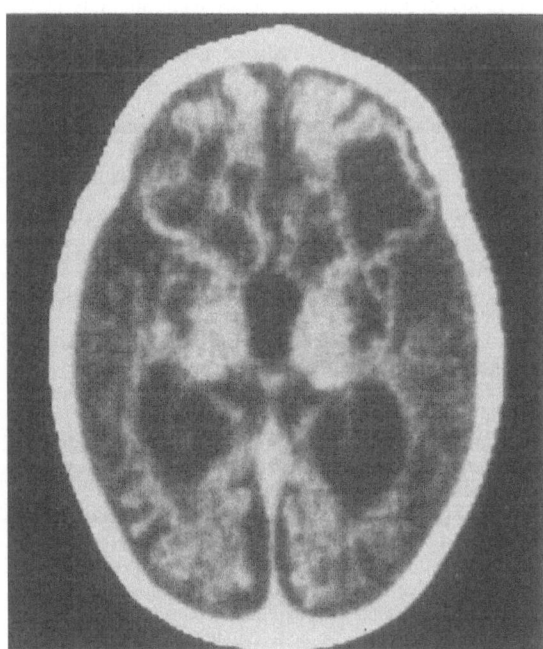

Fig. 6.33. Transcranial ultrasound. Intraparenchymal haemorrhage (*arrow*) manifest as an echogenic region adjacent to a frontal horn.

Fig. 6.34. Cranial CT. Cystic encephalopathy in a mature neonate.

ment. Necrosis may then be correspondingly severe and lead to widespread cystic replacement of both grey and white matter (Fig. 6.34). CT is the preferred examination in term neonates with suspected asphyxia since it is more sensitive to the parenchymal changes encountered than ultrasound (Flodmark 1987).

There are obvious practical difficulties in performing neonatal MRI scans but it has been used to assess normal and abnormal myelination and may be of some value in the prediction of developmental delay (Dietrich et al. 1988).

References

Albright AL, Guthkelch AN, Packer RJ, Price RA, Rourke LB (1986) Prognostic factors in paediatric brain-stem gliomas. Neurosurg 65: 751–755

Al-Mefty O, Hassounah M, Weaver P, Sakati N, Jinkins JR, Fox JL (1985) Microsurgery for giant craniopharyngioma in children. Neurosurgery 17: 585–595

Altman N, Fitz CR, Chuang S, Harwood-Nash D, Cotter C, Armstrong D (1985) Radiological characteristics of primitive neuroectodermal tumours in children. AJNR 6: 15–18

Byrd SE, Harwood-Nash DC, Fitz CR, Rogovitz DM (1978) Computed tomography in the evaluation of encephaloceles in infants and children. Comput Assist Tomogr 2: 81–87

Cabezudo JM, Vaquero J, Garcia-de-Sola R, Lenda G, Nombela L, Bravo G (1981) Craniopharyngioma. Surg Neurol 15: 422–427

Camins MB, Cravioto HM, Epstein F et al. (1980) Medulloblastoma: an ultrastructural study – evidence of astrocytic and neuronal differentation. Neurosurgery 6: 398–411

Cubberley DA, Jaffe RB, Nixon GW (1982) Sonographic demonstration of galenic arteriovenous malformations in the neonate. AJNR 3: 435–439

Diebler C, Dulac O (1987) Pediatric neurology and neuroradiology. Cerebral and cranial diseases. Springer, Berlin, Heidelberg, New York

Diebler C, Dulac O, Renier D, Ernest C, Lalande G (1981) Aneurysms of the vein of Galen in infants aged 2–15 months. Diagnosis and natural evolution. Neuroradiology 21: 185–197

Dietrich RB, Bradley WG, Zaragoza E et al. (1988) MR evaluation of early myelination patterns in normal and developmentally delayed infants. AJNR 9: 69–76

Epstein F (1985) A staging system for brain stem gliomas. Cancer 56: 1804–1806

Epstein F, McCleary EL (1986) Intrinsic brain stem tumours of childhood: surgical indications. Neurosurg 64: 11–15

Farwell JR, Dohrmann GJ, Flannery JT (1977) Central nervous system tumors in children. Cancer 40: 3123–3132

Fletcher WA, Imes RK, Hoyt WF (1986) Chiasmal gliomas: appearance and long-term changes demonstrated by computerized tomography. J Neurosurg 65: 154–159

Flodmark O (1987) The neonatal brain. In: A categorical course in diagnostic radiology (neuroradiology). 73rd Scientific Assembly of the Radiological Society of North America

Gjerris F, Klinken L (1978) Long-term prognosis in children with benign cerebellar astrocytoma. J Neurosurg 49: 179–184

Gomez MR, Whitten CS, Nolke K, Berstein H, Meyers JS (1963) Aneurysmal malformation of the great vein of Galen causing heart failure in early infancy. Pediatrics 31: 400–411

Heafner MD, Schut L, Packer RJ, Bruce DA, Bilaniuk LT,

Sutton LN (1985) Discrepancy between computed tomography and magnetic resonance imaging in a case of medulloblastoma. Neurosurgery 17: 487–489

Heinz ER, Drayer BP, Haenggeli CA, Pointer MJ, Crumrine P (1979) Computed tomography in white-matter disease. Radiology 130: 371–738

Huckman MS, Fox JH, Ramsay RG (1977) Computed tomography in the diagnosis of degenerative diseases of the brain. Semin Roentgenol XII: 63–76

Hurst RW, Newman SA, Cail WS (1988) Multifocal intracranial MR abnormalities in neurofibromatosis. AJNR 9: 293–296

Hoffman H J, Becker L, Craven M A (1980) A clinically and pathologically distinct group of benign brain stem gliomas. Neurosurgery 7: 243–248

Jenkin RDT, Boesel C, Ertel I et al. (1987) Brain-stem tumors in childhood: a prospective randomized trial of irradiation with and without adjuvant CCNU, VCR and prednisone. A report of the children's cancer study group. J Neurosurg 66: 227–233

Johnson MA, Pennock JM, Bydder GM et al. (1983) Clinical NMR imaging of the brain in children. AJR 141: 1005–1018

Jooma R, Hayward RD, Grant DN (1984) Intracranial neoplasms during the first year of life: Analysis of one hundred consecutive cases. Neurosurgery 14: 31–41

Klatee EC, Franken EA, Smith JA (1976) The radiographic spectrum in neurofibromatosis. Semin Roentgenol XI, no 1

Lee BCP, Kneelend JB, Walker RW, Posner JB, Cahill PT, Deck MDF (1985) MR imaging of brain stem tumours. AJNR 6: 159–163

Levene MI, Whitelaw A, Dubowitz V et al. (1982) Nuclear magnetic imaging of the brain in children. Br Med J 285: 774–776

Litvak J, Yahr MD, Ranschoff J (1960) Aneurysms of the great vein of Galen and midline cerebral arterio-venous anomalies. J Neurosurg 17: 945–954

McComb JG, Davis RL, Isaacs H Jr (1981) Extraneural metastatic medulloblastoma during childhood. Neurosurgery 9: 548–551

Mori K (1985) Anomalies of the central nervous system. In Neuroradiology and Neurosurgery. Georg Thieme Verlag, Stuttgart, New York

Naidich TP, Zimmerman RA (1984) Primary brain tumors in children. Semin Roentgenol 19: 100–114

North C, Segall HD, Stanley P, Zee C-S, Ahmadi J, McComb JG (1985) Early CT detection of intracranial seeding from medulloblastoma. AJNR 6: 11–13

Nowell MA, Grossman RI, Hackney DB, Zimmerman RA, Goldberg HI, Bilaniuk LT (1988) MR imaging of white matter disease in children. AJR 151: 359–365

O'Brien MS, Schechter MM (1970) Arteriovenous malformation involving the galenic system. AJR 110: 50–55

Packer RJ, Zimmerman RA, Luerssen TG et al. (1985) Brainstem gliomas of childhood: magnetic resonance imaging. Neurology 35: 397–401

Papile LA, Burstein J, Burstein R, Koffler H (1978) Incidence and evolution of subependymal and intraventricular haemorrhage. J Pediatr 92: 529–534

Park TS, Hoffman HJ, Hendrick EB, Humphreys RP, Becker LE (1983) Medulloblastoma: clinical presentation and management. Experience at the Hospital for Sick Children, Toronto, 1950–1980. J Neurosurg 58: 543–552

Patronas NJ, Dwyer AJ, Papathanasiou M, Schiebler ML, Schellinger D (1987) Contributions of magnetic resonance imaging in the evaluation of optic gliomas. Surg Neurol 28: 367–71

Peterman SB, Steiner RE, Bydder GM (1984) Magnetic resonance imaging of intracranial tumours in children and adolescents. AJNR 5: 703–709

Probst FT (1979) The prosencephalies. Morphology, neuro-radiological appearances and differential diagnosis. Springer, Berlin, Heidelberg, New York

Radkowski MA, Naidich TP, Tomita T, Byrd SE, McLone DG (1988) Neonatal brain tumors; CT and MR findings. J Comput Assist Tomogr 12: 10–20

Sanwaya R, McLaurin RL (1981) Dandy–Walker syndrome. Clinical analysis of 23 cases. J Neurosurg 55: 89–98

Savoiardo M, Harwood-Nash D, Tadmor R et al. (1981) Gliomas of the intracranial anterior optic pathways in children. Radiology 138: 601–610

Stern J, Jakobiec FA, Housepain EM (1980) The architecture of optic nerve gliomas with and without neurofibromatosis.

Arch Ophthalmol 98: 505–511

Stroink AR, Hoffman HJ, Hendrick EB, Humphreys RP (1986) Diagnosis and management of paediatric brain-stem gliomas. J Neurosurg 65: 745–750

Tomita T, McLone DG (1983) Spontaneous seeding of medulloblastoma: results of cerebrospinal fluid cytology and arachnoid biopsy from the cisterna magna. Neurosurgery 12: 265–267

Williams AL (1985) Congenital anomalies. In: Williams AL, Haughton VW (eds) Cranial Computed Tomography A comprehensive text. CV Mosby, St Louis, pp 316–349

Zimmerman RA, Bilaniuk LT (1980) CT of primary and secondary craniocerebral neuroblastoma. AJNR 1: 431–434

Chapter 7

The Spine

Nagui M. Antoun

Degenerative Disease of the Lumbar Spine

Disc Disease

Clinicopathological Aspects

Pathological processes of the spine presenting with back pain and sciatica constitute both a major health problem and an economic burden. The findings of a narrowed disc space, gas within a disc and osteophyte formation constitute the rather vague but encompassing term of "spondylosis". This has a prevalence of between 60% and 80% in patients above the age of 50 years but there is no clear correlation with symptomatology (Quinet and Hadler 1979; Wood and Badley 1987). Clearly complete radiological investigations are not required for the great majority of these patients and following the first attack of severe low back pain with or without sciatica only 15% will undergo radiological studies (Butt 1989).

Clinical examination alone is inadequate and when correlated with myelographic and surgical findings its accuracy in identifying the correct disc level is approximately 50% (Edgar and Park 1974). Proper treatment therefore relies on the radiological identification of the structural abnormality responsible for the symptoms (Kortelainen et al. 1985).

More than 90% of disc herniations occur at L4/5 and L5/S1 levels (Bosacco and Berman 1983) and most acute herniations occur in a posterolateral direction which is where the posterior longitudinal ligament is thinnest (Fig. 7.1). Between leaving the main dural sac and exiting through the intervertebral foramina, the lumbar roots lie in the lateral recess. The root exiting at the level of the herniated disc is usually spared. For example, the

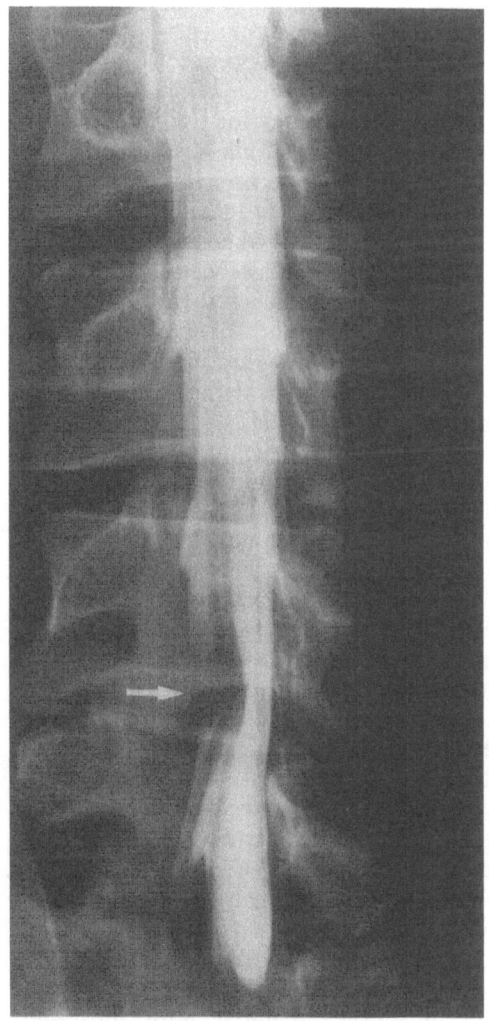

Fig. 7.1. Radiculogram. Extradural impression due to a posterolateral L4/5 disc herniation (*arrow*). (P.B.)

159

L5 root sheath separates from the main dural sac just above the L4/5 disc and leaves the spinal canal below the L5 pedicle. The L5 root is therefore usually affected by disc herniation at L4/5. Exceptions to this occur in the event of a migrating fragment or the, rather uncommon, extreme-lateral disc herniation which usually compromises the exiting nerve root at the same level (i.e. herniation of the L5/S1 disc causes L5 radiculopathy (Firooznia et al. 1984)).

Massive herniation can obviously involve more than one nerve root and a disturbance of autonomic function with paralysis of the bladder and bowel may accompany the large midline disc herniation. The accurate identification of a sequestrated disc fragment is important as its localising signs and symptoms may be atypical or misleading. It is also one of the main contraindications for the use of chymopapain. Moreover, for the complete removal of the sequestrated fragment the neurosurgeon may require to alter his surgical approach (Masaryk et al. 1988).

Spontaneous regression or complete disappearance of the herniated nucleus pulposus has been documented which coincides with improvement of the presenting radicular symptoms following conservative treatment (Teplick and Haskin 1985). This suggests that either the nuclear material retracts back into the annulus or there are mechanisms for active absorption of the herniated fragment (Lindblom and Hultqvist 1950). The prevalence is not known exactly and may be more common than anticipated.

Early intradiscal derangement prior to any overt change in disc height or annular bulge can now be detected by magnetic resonance imaging (MRI). Apart from the potential clinical benefit in identifying these vulnerable discs, their role in the pathogenesis of low back pain remains an interesting speculation (McCarron et al. 1987).

The nucleus pulposus consists of 85%–90% water (Modic et al. 1988a). The nucleus lies just behind the central part of the disc and the annulus is thinnest, and therefore weakest, posteriorly. With ageing the cartilage end plate becomes thinner, more hyalinised and can show fissuring. There is loss of the hydrostatic properties of the disc with an overall reduction of hydration of both annulus and nucleus to 70% of normal. Radial rupture of the annulus often occurs early in the process of degeneration. The annulus may then fragment which predisposes to degeneration and subsequent herniation of nuclear material both into and through the annulus (Modic et al. 1988a). The biochemical changes and state of hydration with ageing and onset of degeneration can be depicted as well

as assessed quantitatively by MRI (Jenkins et al. 1985; Isherwood et al. 1986).

Bulging of the Annulus

The diagnosis of bulging annulus is made when computed tomography (CT) demonstrates generalised expansion of the disc beyond the margins of the adjacent vertebral endplates (Fig. 7.2). A few bulging discs retain the posterior midline concavity that characterises the normal lumbar disc (Williams et al. 1982). The myelographic differentiation from disc herniation depends on the smooth, rounded symmetrical deformity of the theca which does not extend beyond the disc level and is never angular. An additional criterion is the lack of swelling of the nerve root (Kieffer et al. 1982).

Bulging of the annulus is unlikely to cause nerve root compression and is believed to be the result of desiccation of the nucleus pulposus and loss of elasticity of the annulus fibrosus. In these cases, however, CT underestimates the severity of the degenerative changes within the nucleus and annulus. There is a close association between bulging of the annulus and the presence of a radial tear of the annulus fibrosus. In cadaveric cryomicrotome studies it is rare to find a bulging annulus without radial tear which suggests the primary role of the annulus tear in disc degeneration (Yu et al. 1988).

Disc Herniation

There are unfortunately no precise definitions regarding the nomenclature of disc herniations in

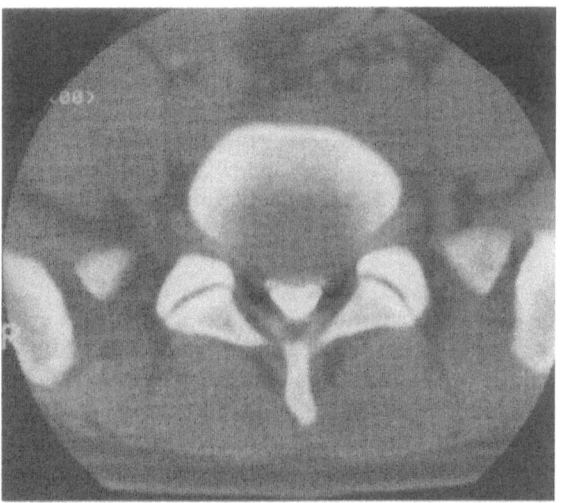

Fig. 7.2. CT myelogram. Annular bulge.

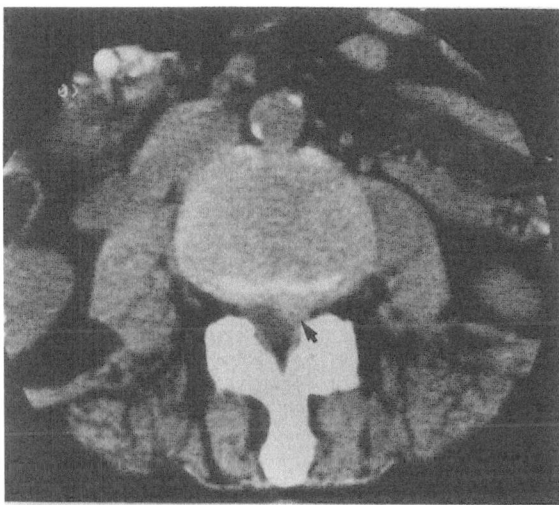

Fig. 7.3. Axial CT. Posterolateral lumbar disc herniation (*arrow*).

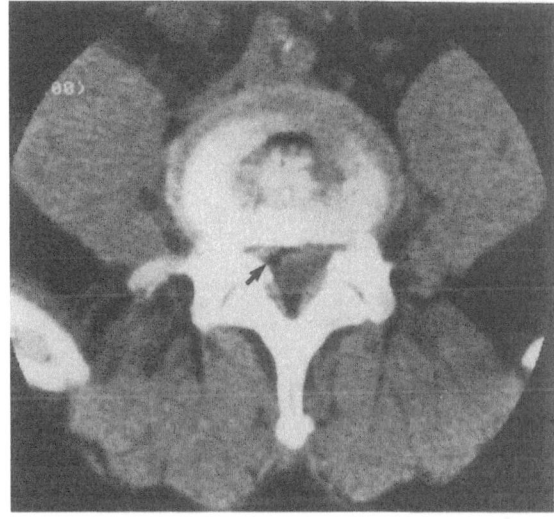

Fig. 7.4. Axial CT. Gas in a herniated lumbar disc (*arrow*).

either the radiological or neurosurgical literature. Focal disc *bulge*, *protrusion* and *prolapse* are terms used interchangeably and perhaps only express a subjective assessment of the degree of herniation. Common to each is that the nuclear material remains within the confines of the outermost fibres of the annulus fibrosus. In disc *extrusion* the annulus develops a complete tear through which the disc material passes and comes to lie under the posterior longitudinal ligament or lateral to it. Once extruded nuclear material is no longer contiguous with the remaining disc and lies in the canal it may travel caudally or cephalad but is still confined by the posterior longitudinal ligament. This is then called *sequestrated* herniation (MacNab 1977; Teplick and Haskin 1983; Masaryk et al. 1988).

Posterolateral/Central Herniation. The majority of disc herniations are directed posterolaterally due to the restriction imparted by the posterior longitudinal ligament. However, central herniations are not uncommon and constitute approximately 30% of all herniations (Fries at al. 1982).

The herniated lumbar disc is readily detected on CT by differences in attenuation between the disc and the contents of the lumbar canal (Fig. 7.3). The epidural fat acts as a natural contrast outlining the theca, back of the vertebra and the annulus fibrosus. Disc herniation often results in asymmetry and displacement of the epidural fat and nerve roots (which may be enlarged by oedema) or indentation of the theca (Williams et al. 1980; Isherwood and Antoun 1987).

The herniated disc may contain calcification (4%) or gas ("vacuum phenomenon" Fig. 7.4). The differ-

entiation between a calcified disc and any associated osteophytes can be difficult even during surgical exploration (Penning et al. 1986). A false negative CT diagnosis can result from missing the large relatively high density herniated disc which almost fills the canal (Fries et al. 1982) (Fig. 7.5). The herniated disc may also be isodense with the canal contents (mostly in patients with canal stenosis where there is a decrease in the amount of CSF (Dixon 1986a)). A migrating nuclear fragment may also be mistaken for an extradural neoplasm.

MRI is very sensitive in the detection of early degenerative disc change (Yu et al. 1989). This is shown as heterogeneous decrease or loss of signal intensity on a T2-weighted sequence (Fig. 7.6). In a study of 101 discs in 36 patients with low back

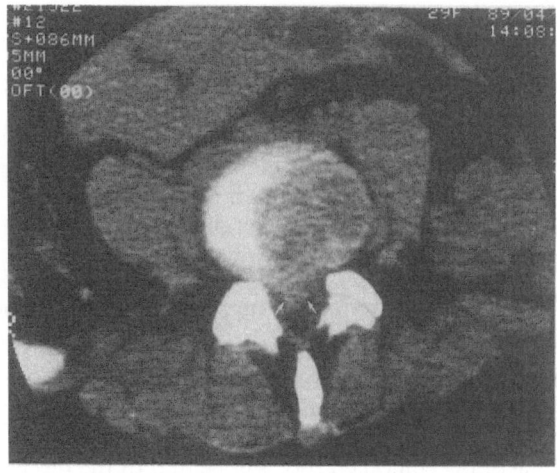

Fig. 7.5. Axial CT. Large lumber disc herniation (*arrows*).

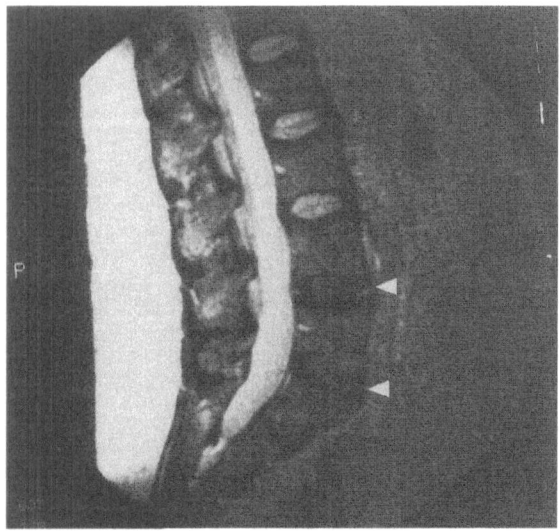

Fig. 7.6. Sagittal MRI (T2-weighted image). There is diminished signal return from the lower two lumber discs indicating degeneration (*arrowheads*).

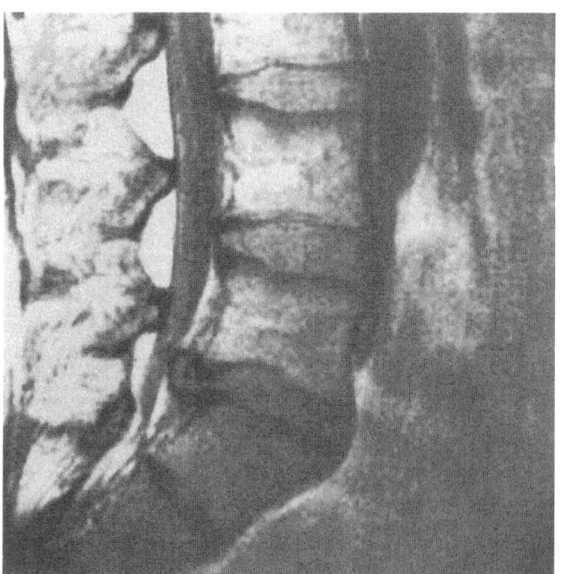

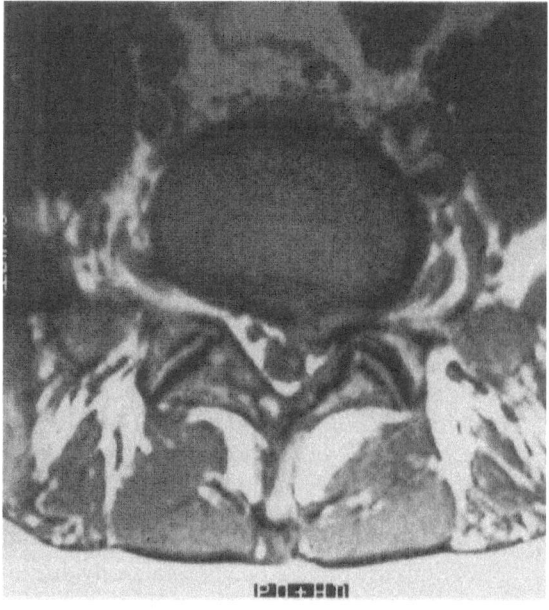

Fig. 7.7. Sagittal (**a**) and axial (**b**) MRI (T1 weighted images). L5/S1 disc herniation.

pain MRI was 99% accurate in predicting their normality or abnormality as determined by discography (Schneiderman et al. 1987).

MRI is as accurate as CT and myelography in the diagnosis of lumbar disc herniation (Fig. 7.7). The focal nature of the disc protrusion, which is the main feature differentiating annular bulge from disc herniation, is not well assessed on sagittal views and necessitates axial images in the manner of CT scanning (Edelman et al. 1985).

Lateral/Foraminal Herniation. Lateral disc herniation, both foraminal or extraforaminal which occurs laterally to the nerve root sheath, has a reported incidence of up to 10% of all herniations (Fig. 7.8). It affects a slightly older age group, the clinical picture is varied and there may be no abnormal neurological findings. Degenerative disease at the L4/5 disc is more likely to result in this type of lesion than at the L5/S1 level. Considering the anatomical location of the herniated fragments, the L4 nerve root is therefore most often affected (Kornberg 1986). As the laterally herniated fragment does not exert any pressure on the exiting nerve sheaths, myelography is often falsely negative in these patients (Mikhael 1983; Nelson and Gold 1983). The foraminal "mass" of a conjoined root (Fig. 7.9) may lead to the erroneous CT diagnosis of a lateral disc herniation. Examination of serial sections will resolve the issue and the attenuation value of the conjoined root will be that of the theca rather than disc (Helms et al. 1982). Indeed CT,

with its capability of resolving density differences especially in the presence of adequate epidural/foraminal fat, is currently the non-invasive examination of choice. The diagnosis, however, can be difficult especially in the presence of fibrosis or severe canal stenosis. If the condition is suspected clinically and CT is inconclusive, discography which then may be followed by CT, can often secure the diagnosis (Jackson and Glah 1987). It is likely that MRI will become the preferred method of

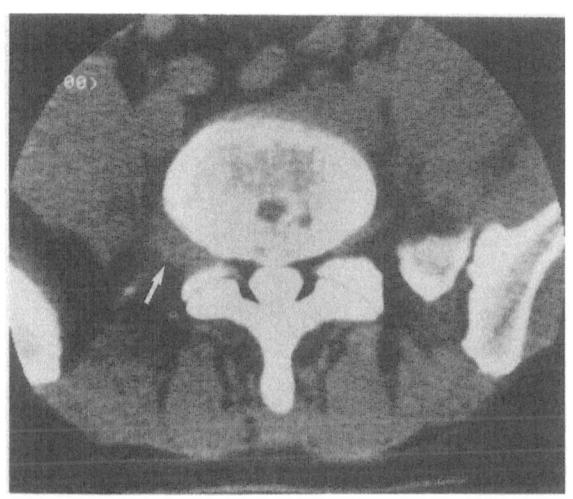

Fig. 7.8. Axial CT. Lateral L5/S1 disc herniation (*arrow*).

examination in this condition since it is accurate, non-invasive and does not rely on ionising radiation.

Sequestrated/Migrating Discs. A sequestrated or free disc fragment is recognised by its polypoid shape seen at some distance from the disc of origin (Fig. 7.10). A normal posterior disc margin does not exclude a free disc fragment (Williams et al. 1983) and approximately one-third of disc fragments are found at surgery to have migrated. The term "migratory" is used when a disc fragment migrates either upwards to lie at the entrance or within the intervertebral foramen, or downwards to the lower part of the lateral recess. Superior (cephalad) migration was found to be more common by Fries et al. (1982) whereas the reverse is documented by

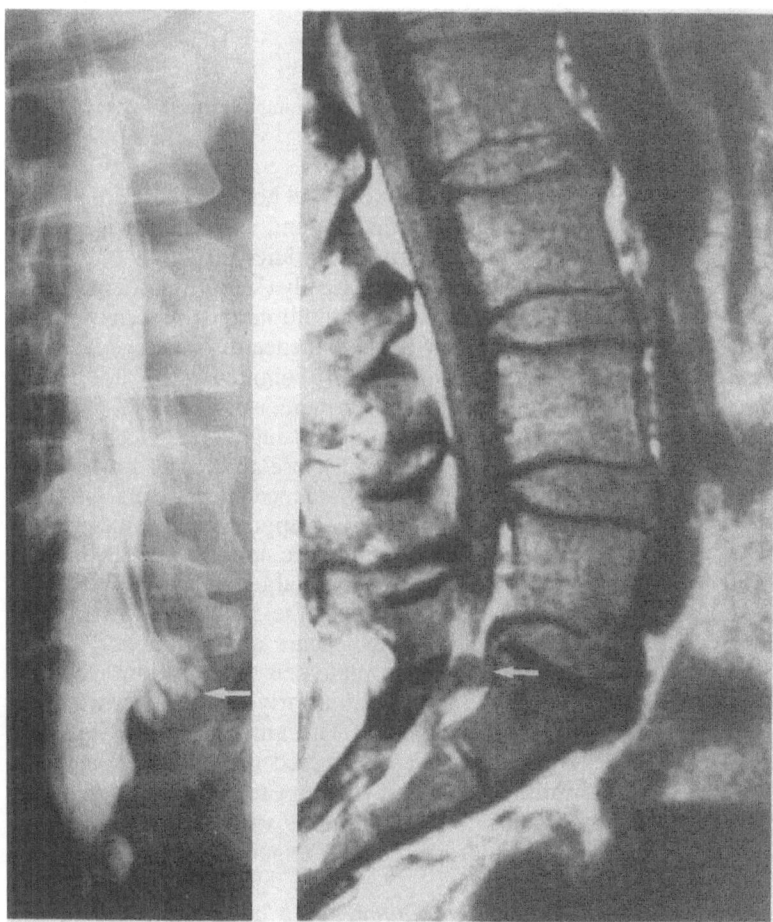

7.9   7.10

Fig. 7.9. Radiculogram. Conjoined L5 and S1 roots (*arrow*).

Fig. 7.10. Sagittal MRI (T1 weighted image). Migratory L5/S1 disc herniation (*arrow*).

others (Williams et al. 1983; Krausé et al. 1986a). Combined cephalad and caudal migration can also occur.

Intradural Disc Herniation. Intradural disc herniation is very rare with a reported incidence of only 0.13% of all herniations (Graves et al. 1986). More than 90% of these occur in the lumbar spine and then mostly at L4/5 interspace. Only 6% are found in the cervical spine (Eisenberg et al. 1986) and very few in the thoracic region.

A firm attachment between the vertebral dura and posterior longitudinal ligament is thought to play an important role. This can occur as a result of several mechanisms including long-standing degenerative or inflammatory change of the disc, minor trauma, surgery and developmental anatomic variation (Graves et al. 1986). The cerebrospinal fluid protein in these cases is consistently raised even in the absence of a block.

The intradural mass found on myelography could easily be misinterpreted as a neurinoma or meningioma especially when the extradural component of the disc is not visualised. On CT myelography the disc material shows as an irregular or lobular intradural mass (Hodge et al. 1978). MRI shows clearly the abnormal signal from the disc and the connection between the disc to the intradural lesion (Holtas et al. 1987).

Intravertebral Herniation: The "Schmorl's Node". In some patients the vertebral end-plate cartilage may be partially deficient, probably corresponding to sites of previous embryonal vessels, and this may lead to the common finding of disc material

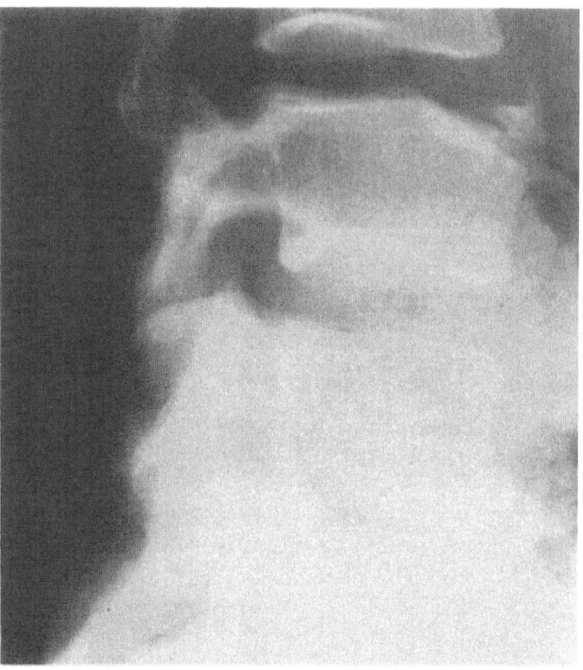

Fig. 7.12. Lateral radiograph. Limbus vertebra (see text).

herniating to the vertebral bodies. These are known as "Schmorl's nodes" and have a prevalence of 40% in post-mortem studies although only 14% are detected radiologically (Vernon-Roberts 1987). They can be single or multiple and are seen in young individuals with no evidence of disc degeneration. They are also seen commonly in adolescent kyphosis or "Scheuermann's disease".

CT sections going through or adjacent to the end plate typically disclose an area of low density surrounded by a well-defined sclerotic margin (Fig. 7.11). This characteristic appearance should prevent any confusion with lytic lesions and Schmorl's nodes are readily identifiable on sagittal MRI sections. Very occasionally the disc herniation through the vertebral body occurs at the junction of the cartilaginous end plate and the bony rim isolating a bony fragment anteriorly. This is known as a "limbus vertebra". The anterosuperior vertebral margin is always involved (Fig. 7.12). The plain radiographic and CT appearances are typical and should not be confused with a fracture or an inflammatory process (Yagan 1984).

Anterior Herniation. Disc herniation beyond the lateral margin of the pedicles can be considered as anterior (Fig. 7.13). The exact incidence and possible clinical implications are not clearly determined. A recent retrospective study reported an incidence of up to 29% of peripheral disc herniations (Jinkins

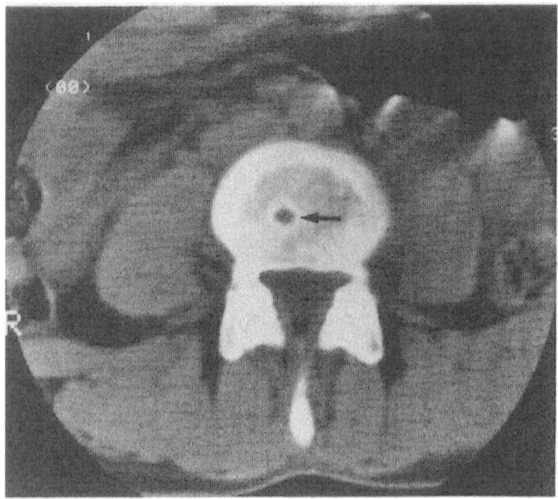

Fig. 7.11. Axial CT. Schmorl's node (*arrow*).

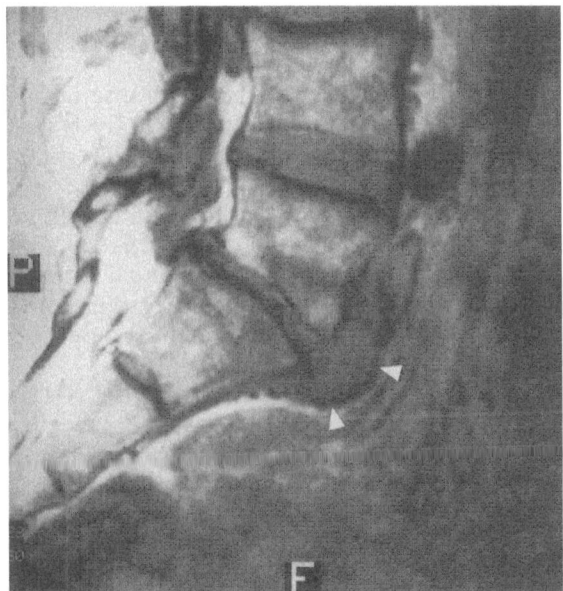

Fig. 7.13. Sagittal MRI (T1 weighted image). Anterior L5/S1 disc herniation (*arrowheads*).

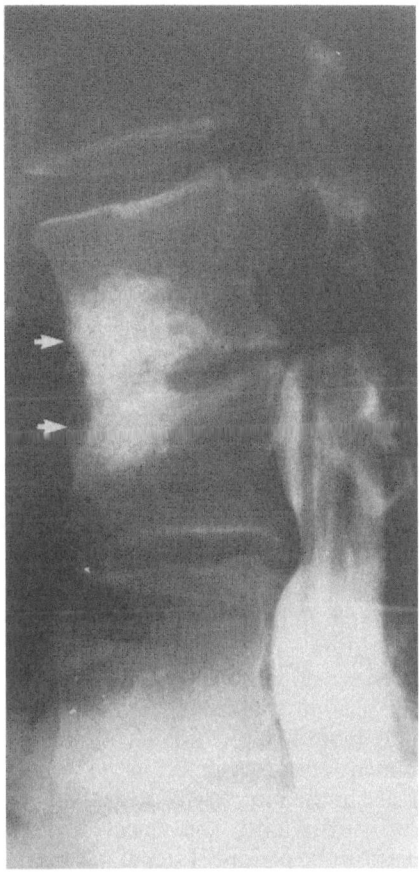

Fig. 7.14. Myelogram. Discogenic vertebral sclerosis (*arrowheads*). (P.B.)

et al. 1989). Such herniation is believed to be implicated in local and referred pain as well as in autonomic reflex dysfunction resulting in alterations of the viscerosomatic tone.

Discogenic Vertebral Sclerosis. Areas of bony sclerosis adjacent to degenerated discs observed on plain films are known as discogenic vertebral sclerosis (Fig. 7.14). Similarly marrow changes have been documented on MRI images on both sides of up to 20% of degenerated discs, which may represent a reparative response to injury (Fig. 7.15) (Modic et al. 1988b; Sobel et al. 1987).

It is important not to confuse this benign incidental finding with infectious spondylitis or metastatic disease.

Chemonucleolysis. Chymopapain chemonucleolysis is a percutaneous method of treatment of lumbar disc herniation (Smith 1964). The enzyme (2.5 ml) is injected into the nucleus pulposus under local anaesthesia and fluoroscopic control. It has a biochemical effect with enzymic hydrolysis of the mucopolysaccharide part of the nucleus pulposus. Careful selection of patients on the basis of objective clinical and radiographic evidence of nerve root compression by disc material, relatively preserved pre-injection disc height and possibly a large uptake of contrast material by the herniated fragment during CT discography ensures a better response (Gentry et al. 1985a; Edwards et al. 1987). The

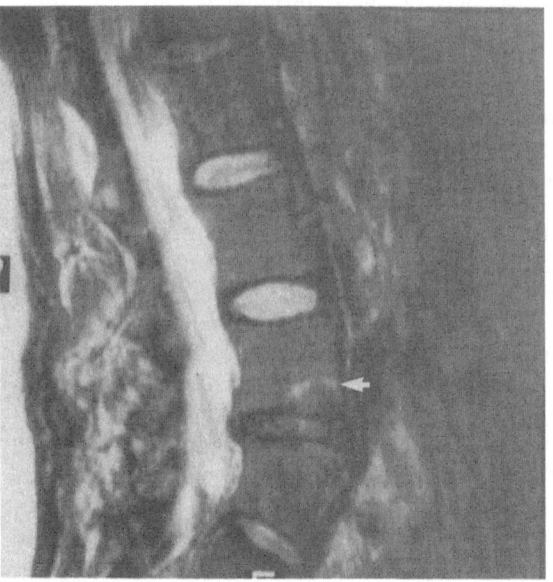

Fig. 7.15. Sagittal MRI (T2 weighted image). Discogenic vertebral sclerosis (*arrow*).

presence of sequestrated disc fragments or other concurrent causes of nerve root compression like lateral recess or central canal stenosis should first be excluded. The effectiveness of the treatment in the properly selected patient is claimed to be similar to that of surgery (Fraser 1982; Javid et al. 1983) but further diagnostic evaluation may be necessary for those patients who fail to respond to treatment. Identification and understanding of the post chemonucleolysis CT and MRI changes are therefore essential.

In a study by Gentry et al. (1985b), six weeks following therapy, 12.5% of patients showed an interspace gas collection and 8.3% had a slight reduction in size of the herniated disc. Of those improving clinically, at six months follow-up 23% had an interspace gas collection and only 59% had a decrease in the size of the herniated disc. Disc space narrowing at follow-up was noted in 50% of patients at six weeks and 72.5% of patients at six months. A decrease in MR signal and decrease in height of the disc seem to be present in all patients after chemonucleation regardless of clinical outcome (Huckman et al. 1987). The post-chemonucleation scan in those cases with a successful outcome is more likely to show a decrease in one or both dimensions of the defect in the thecal sac and an increase in the intensity of the signal of vertebral bodies surrounding the injected disc space. The increase in the peridiscal signal has been attributed to scarring or inflammation resulting from the procedure. Early improvement has been noted in the absence of a decrease in the size of the herniated disc but with a decrease in the disc height. It has therefore been postulated that the "shortened" disc reduces the tension on the nerve root accounting for the early relief without a decrease in the size of the herniation (Spencer et al. 1983; Gentry et al. 1985b).

Osteophytes

The precise pathogenesis and clinical significance of anterior osteophytes remain controversial. Two types have been described, the more common "claw" osteophytes and the less common but more significant "traction" osteophytes which are thought to indicate spinal instability (MacNab 1971). Traction spurs arise 3–4 mm from the discovertebral junction. Claw osteophytes originate at the vertebral margins. A recent radiographic–pathological correlation suggested that both types may coexist and indeed may represent different stages of the same pathological process (Pate et al. 1988). However, in a study by Quinnell and Stockdale (1982) a discographically normal disc

was demonstrated in only 11% in association with traction-type osteophytes as compared with 43% of claw-type osteophytes.

Apart from their association with disc disease, osteophytes are significant when they project posteriorly or posterolaterally to impinge on the central canal or lateral recesses.

Degenerative osteophytes, however, should not be confused with syndesmophytes which result from inflammatory change. Occurring most often in association with ankylosing spondylitis, they arise at the discovertebral junction and are orientated vertically.

Diffuse, idiopathic, skeletal hyperostosis (DISH) (Forestier's disease) may also have a degenerative basis and affects vertebral bodies and ligaments with flowing new bone formation (Jones et al. 1988).

The Vacuum Phenomenon

Gas collections in intervertebral discs and apophyseal joints are commonly demonstrated by CT (25% of patients scanned for back pain). The degenerate disc permits excessive mobility which creates a space ("the vacuum") (Knutsson 1942). This is then filled by an effusion of nitrogen from surrounding fluid (Ford et al. 1977).

Gas within the canal, in the extradural space, is much less common and is usually associated with the vacuum phenomenon in the disc (Gulati et al. 1981; Austin et al. 1981; Yetkin et al. 1986). Its direct relation to symptoms is speculative (Gebarski et al. 1984). Gas can be misinterpreted for calcification on MRI if CT or plain radiography are overlooked.

Apophyseal Joint Disease

The apophyseal (facet) joints are true synovial joints and are subject to the same processes of degenerative change as other synovial joints. These changes can obviously impair the mechanical function of the spine as well as cause back pain (Hukins 1987).

Each facet is covered by a 2–4 mm thick layer of hyaline cartilage. The joint capsule which is lined by synovial membrane is attached to the osteocartilaginous junction. It is reinforced and thickened by the lateral attachment of the ligamentum flavum. The joint and surrounding ligaments are richly innervated by branches from the posterior primary ramus, which also has cutaneous and muscular branches. A constant ascending branch results in overlapping innervations (Pederson et al. 1956; Mooney 1987). The facet joints are more sagittally orientated in the upper lumbar region but assume

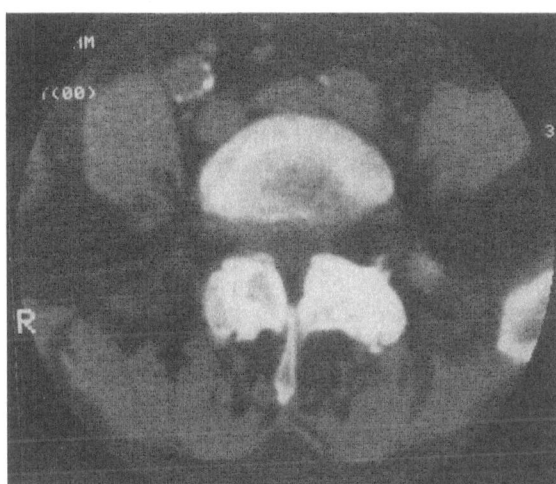

Fig. 7.16. Axial CT. "Tropism". Note the asymmetrical orientation of the facet joints.

a more coronal orientation caudally. As the facet joints resist about 16% of the compressive forces in the upright position (Hukins 1987), degenerative changes are regularly observed even in the absence of disc disease (Ketonen and Gyldensted 1986).

It is natural to assume that asymmetry in the orientation of the facet joints (*tropism*) would tend to focus stress and accelerate local degeneration (Fig. 7.16). Anomalies of orientation of these joints can alter the torsional forces to which the disc is subjected and accordingly this can be a contributory factor in the development of disc herniation (Farfan et al. 1970; Malmivaara et al. 1986; Kier 1988). Conversely primary degenerative changes of the disc and consequent loss of disc height (craniocaudal subluxation) and excessive movement force the malalignment of facet joints and permit secondary osteoarthritic change to occur (Modic et al. 1988a).

Facet disease has been found in between 65% and 76% of patients with back pain both with and without sciatica (Carrera et al. 1980; Ketonen and Gyldensted 1986). Although these changes can be incidental and asymptomatic, they may cause low back and sciatic pain which is indistinguishable from that due to a herniated disc (Carrera et al. 1980; Mooney and Robertson 1976). In some patients this can be explained on the basis of referred pain and appears to respond satisfactorily to intra-articular facet block (Carrera et al. 1980), but further studies are needed (Raymond and Dumas 1984). The hypertrophy of facets and osteophyte formation can, by encroachment, result in canal stenosis which is usually foraminal in type (see below) (Grenier et al. 1987).

Canal Stenosis

Stenotic lesions of the spine can affect the central canal, its lateral recesses or both. The resulting syndromes of intermittent claudication of the cauda equina and radicular pain are well documented (Sarpyener 1945; Verbiest 1954; Blau and Logue 1961, 1978; Schatzker and Pennal 1968).

Aetiology

Stenosis is well recognised in certain rare *congenital* disorders, e.g. achondroplasia. There is also a large, undefined group of people with a *developmental* degree of stenosis who are totally asymptomatic. These individuals are naturally susceptible to the more common *acquired* forms of degenerative canal stenosis. It is commonly accepted that the majority of cases of spinal stenosis are due to a *combination* of a developmentally narrow canal and degenerative lesions (Verbiest 1976; McIvor and Kirkaldy-Willis 1976; Epstein et al. 1977; Postachinni et al. 1980). Other forms of acquired canal stenosis include spondylolysis with or without listhesis, post-traumatic and postsurgical stenosis. Paget's disease, acromegaly and osteoporosis with vertebral collapse can also result in stenosis.

Degenerative Stenosis

Degenerative stenosis affects an older age group than lumbar disc herniations. Stenosis of the lateral canal due to bony overgrowth is recognised as the commonest cause of sciatica above the age of 50 years (Stockley et al. 1988). Men are more commonly affected than women and the onset is often insidious with symptoms of long duration. The sensory and motor dysfunction can be worse on walking or standing. Although neurological examination is usually normal at rest, the syndrome of neurogenic claudication of the cauda equina can usually be differentiated clinically from peripheral vascular claudication.

Central Canal Stenosis. There is often a reduction in the midline sagittal diameter of the bony canal which points towards developmental factors as a basic abnormality (Larsen and Smith 1980a, b). However, bulging of the annulus (generalised or focal), hypertrophy of the apophyseal joints, enlargement of the ligamentum flavum and osteophyte formation are usually also present to contribute to the encroachment on the dural sac and roots within it.

Lateral Recess and Foraminal Stenosis. The lateral recess is bordered laterally by the pedicle and posteriorly by the superior articular facet. The posterolateral surface of the vertebral body and the intervertebral disc form its anterior boundary. The nerve root exits through the foramen immediately below the pedicle. Outgrowth of the inferior facet tends to cause constriction of the central canal, whereas degenerative changes of the superior facet usually produce narrowing of the lateral recess and exit foramen. Facet hypertrophy was found to be the sole cause of root entrapment in 36% of cases in the series of Stockley et al. (1988) but entrapment can also be caused by a combination of a posterolateral vertebral body osteophyte and a bulging disc (Postachini et al. 1980).

Myelography. Myelography usually shows characteristic changes with anterior and posterolateral impressions of the contrast column which result in waist-like constrictions and segmentation. Sometimes myelographic "block" is encountered especially at L3/4 and L4/5 where the canal is usually narrowest (Roberson et al. 1973; McIvor and Kirkaldy-Willis 1976). Apart from the invasiveness of the procedure and possible technical difficulty in performing the examination, the major drawback of myelography is its lack of sensitivity in detecting stenosis of the lateral recesses (Euinton et al. 1986; Stockley et al. 1988).

Computed Tomography. CT is particularly suitable for the investigation of suspected canal stenosis (Fig. 7.17). It provides accurate linear and area measurements of the bony canal and shows the relative contribution of bony and soft tissue elements (Fig. 7.18) (Chafetz and Genant 1983; Isherwood and Antoun 1987). Thickening and buckling of the ligamentum flavum clearly depicted by CT is often a significant contributory factor in compromising the dural sac (Stollman et al. 1987). The absence of epidural fat in stenotic segments is helpful in deciding if clinically significant canal stenosis is present (Dorwart et al. 1983). Its amount has been demonstrated to relate to the anteroposterior diameter of the canal and the cross-sectional area of the theca (Dixon 1986a).

CT is more sensitive than myelography in the diagnosis of both lateral recess and foraminal stenosis (Modic et al. 1986a; Stockley et al. 1988), and is particularly valuable in severe cases where myelographic "block" might be anticipated.

MRI. MRI confers similar advantages to CT and certainly provides comparable information when surface coils are used to improve resolution (Fig. 7.19) (Edelman et al. 1985; Modic et al. 1986a). However, its multiplanar imaging facility permits the elegant display of lateral recess and exit foramina in the sagittal and coronal planes. Moreover MRI is more sensitive than CT at demonstrating disc degeneration (Schnebel et al. 1989).

Quantitative Assessment of the Lumbar Spinal Canal. An anteroposterior diameter (AP) of the lumbar canal of less than 10–12 mm and a cross-sectional area of 1.45 cm² or less are considered indicative of stenosis (Lee at al. 1978; Ullrich et al. 1980; Crouzet et al. 1983). The AP diameter of the lateral recess is measured at the point where the

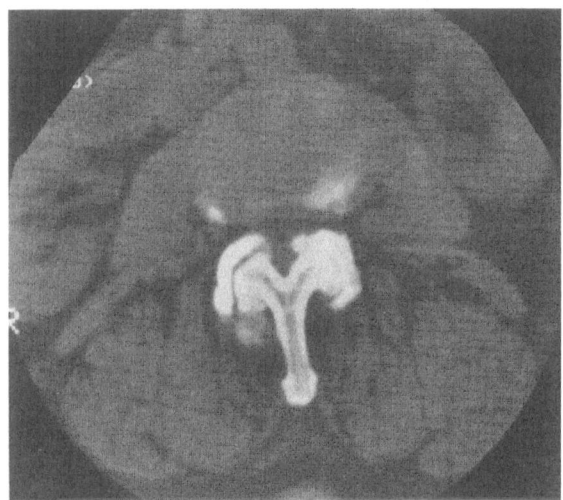

Fig. 7.17. Axial CT. Lumbar canal stenosis.

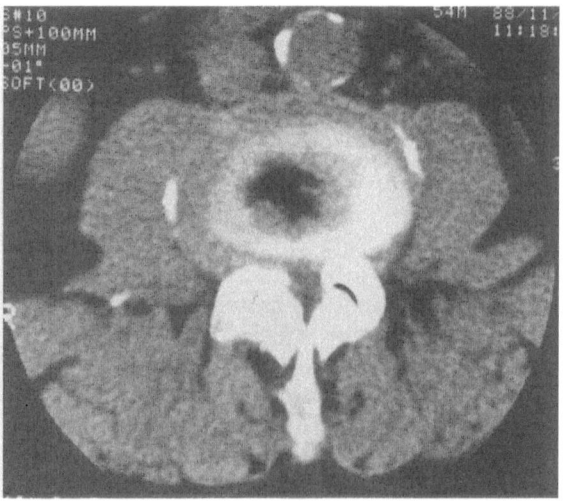

Fig. 7.18. Axial CT. Lumbar canal stenosis with gas in both the disc and facet joint.

Spondylolisthesis and Spondylolysis

Spondylolisthesis is readily identifiable on plain lateral radiographs by the loss of alignment of the vertebral bodies. Bradford (1979) divided the condition into five different aetiological groups. The commonest types are the 'isthmic or spondylolytic" and the "degenerative". The others are very rare and relate to trauma (fractures at sites other than the pars), bone pathology such as Paget's disease and metastases and bone dysplasias including Marfan's syndrome and neurofibromatosis.

Of the nearly 400 patients with spondylolisthesis in the series of Teplick et al. (1986) 53.5% were spondylolytic, 41% degenerative and 3.8% demonstrated reverse spondylolisthesis (retrolisthesis: see below).

Isthmic Spondylolisthesis and Spondylolysis Without Listhesis

Isthmic spondylolisthesis and spondylolysis without listhesis result from a defect in the pars interarticularis, although in 13% the pars is elongated but intact (Oakley and Carty 1984). The exact aetiology of the pars defect is still controversial but the current consensus favours an acquired lesion, most probably an established non-union of a stress fracture originating at some time between infancy and early adult life. In some cases the fracture is acute and preceded by a history of trauma. Spontaneous healing of spondylolytic defects has been reported and callus is present in a number of cases (Wiltse et al. 1975).

Spondylolysis has an overall incidence of 6% (rising to 50% in the Eskimo population) and involves the L5 vertebra in more than 95% of cases (Grogan et al. 1982; Oakley and Carty 1984; Teplick et al. 1986). The occurrence of spina bifida in this group of patients is 6–10 times higher than its incidence in the normal population of 6% (Blackburne and Velikas 1977; Oakley and Carty 1984). The preponderance of spondylolysis at the lumbosacral level and the association with spina bifida suggests that gravity, lordosis, the transition from mobility to fixity and local ligamentous inadequacy are all aetiological factors (Eisenstein 1978).

Although spondylolysis with resultant listhesis can be asymptomatic, the majority present with backache and more than 50% have radicular symptoms (Hanley and Levy 1989). This may be due to the tethering effect on the L5 root due to listhesis.

It is only in the absence of listhesis that oblique radiographs can be useful where a defect in the pars can be seen as a breach in the "Scottie dog's neck".

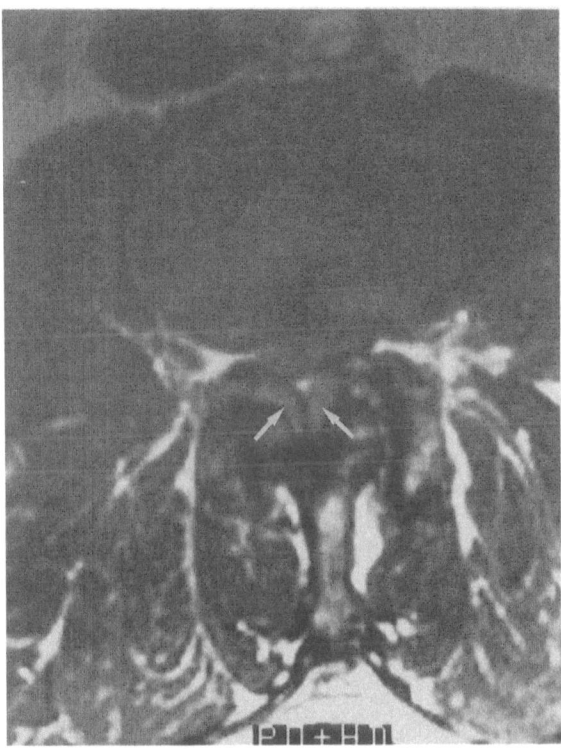

Fig. 7.19. Axial MRI (T1 weighted image). Lumbar canal stenosis. Note the prominent contribution from the ligamentum flavum (*arrows*).

nerve exits. Measurements of 5 mm or more rule out the possibility of stenosis although a normal recess may measure as little as 3 mm (Ciric et al. 1980; Chafetz and Genant 1983). In the lumbar region the normal ligamentum flavum can measure up to 4–6 mm in thickness (Dorwart et al. 1983; Stollman et al. 1987). The size of the dural canal is postulated to be a more reliable measure of canal stenosis (Schnostrom et al. 1985) which is indicated by an area of less than 100 mm². The possibility of a complete spinal block should be entertained when the area of the theca is 50 mm² or less (Dixon 1986a). It must be emphasised, however, that all these are minimum measurements and can only serve as guidelines especially since the range of normal values is rather wide.

In less extreme cases, which are nevertheless clinically significant, the qualitative assessment of the experienced radiologist of the shape of the canal and of the different components contributing to its narrowing is perhaps more valuable especially when correlated with clinical findings. In addition, the accuracy and reproducibility of any measurements, particularly of small areas, are open to random and systematic errors which must be considered carefully (Checkley et al. 1984; Beers et al. 1985).

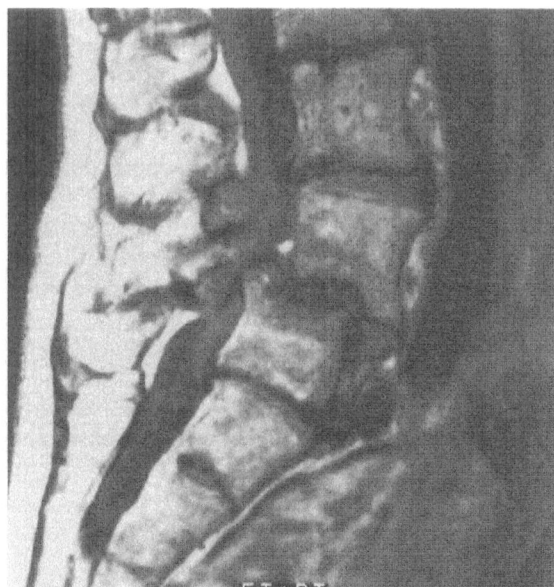

Fig. 7.20. Sagittal MRI (T1 weighted image). Degenerative spondylolisthesis.

Degenerative Spondylolisthesis

Degenerative spondylolisthesis occurs mainly at the L4/5 discal level and is seldom seen before the age of 50 (Fitzgerald and Newman 1976; Teplick et al. 1986). The pars interarticularis is intact but due to the severe degenerative change involving the facet joints, which is a constant and predominant feature, the entire vertebral body with its posterior elements

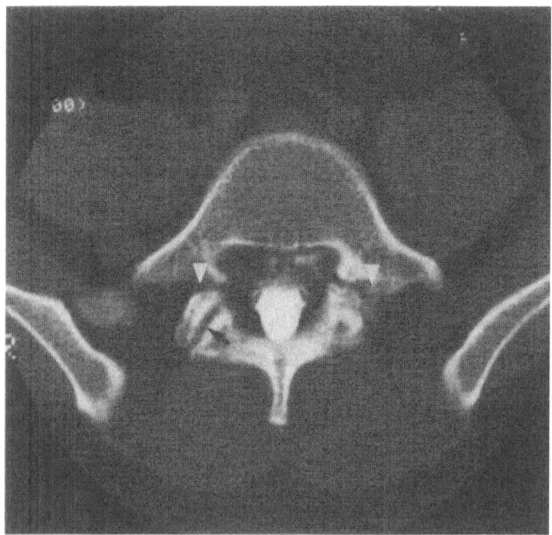

Fig. 7.21. CT myelogram. Spondylolysis. Note the defects (*arrowheads*) and the facet joint (*arrow*).

slips forward (Fig. 7.20). The degree of the slip is usually mild but there is a high incidence of the vacuum phenomenon in the disc and facet joints.

CT demonstrates the tendency of the facet joints to be sagittally rather than horizontally orientated. The superior facet of the caudal vertebra is laterally and posteriorly displaced while the inferior facet of the cephalad vertebra is situated rather anteriorly.

Because of the relative lack of signficant degenerative change in adjacent facet joints Teplick et al. (1986) suggest that the degenerative change may be the result, rather than the cause, of the development of listhesis and that the sagittally orientated facets are the primary aetiological factor.

Retrolisthesis (Reverse Spondylolisthesis)

Retrolisthesis, a rather uncommon form of listhesis, usually involves the L3/4 or L2/3 levels. Degenerative facet joint disease is seldom prominent (Teplick et al. 1986).

Imaging

On the lateral view of the plain radiograph the defect in the pars can be seen in all cases in which listhesis has occurred.

CT scanning is particularly suited for the detection of spondylolysis and is more sensitive than plain radiography (Fig. 7.21) (Teplick et al. 1986). Assessing contiguous slices allows identification and comparison of the defect with adjacent facet joints. The defect has usually a dense irregular margin with occasional bone fragmentation. It is more horizontally orientated and its location above the level of the foramina results in the characteristic "incomplete bony ring sign". Unilateral defects are rare. The posterior projection of the soft tissue of the annulus gives the specific appearance of the "pseudo bulging disc" which typically extends into the neural foramina. The spinal canal also assumes a particular contour resembling an inverted pear with an increase in its AP diameter. The thecal sac is elongated.

A high incidence of neural foraminal stenosis has been reported (Buirski and Watt 1987). There may also be an abnormal disc (usually manifest as an annular bulge and less often, focal herniation) above the level of the defect.

Spondylolysis is suggested on sagittal MR images when there is an interruption of the marrow signal and cortical margins of the pars (best shown on T1 weighted images) (Fig. 7.22). The sagittal view allows the separation of the defect from the joint space since its orientation is perpendicular to the facets (Grenier et al. 1989). Although MRI detects

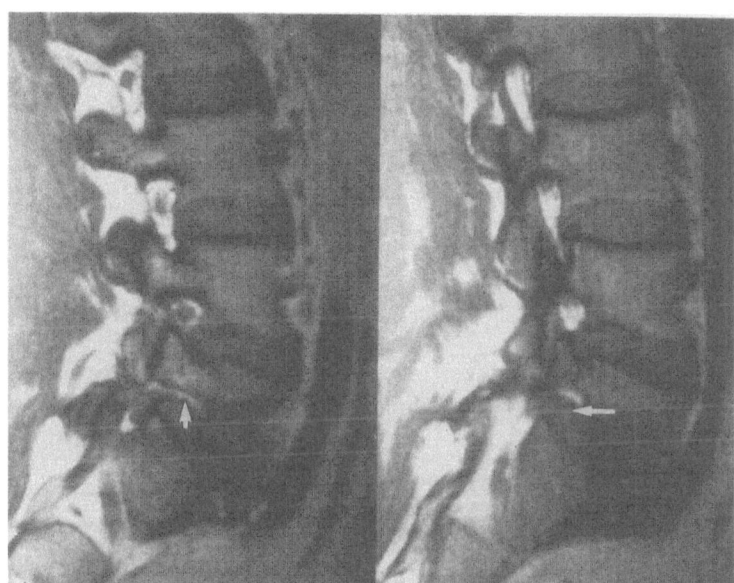

Fig. 7.22. Sagittal MRI (T1 weighted image). Spondylolisthesis of L5 on S1 with spondylolysis. Note the pars defect (*small arrow*) and the pseudobulging of the lumbosacral disc (*large arrow*).

all defects in the pars, the incidence of false-positive interpretation can be high (Johnson et al. 1989). Transaxial imaging, however, is confirmatory with findings almost similar to CT. Neural foraminal stenosis and concurrent disc herniation are readily detected.

The Postoperative Lumbar Spine and the "Failed Back Syndrome"

By far the commonest cause of poor post-surgical response is failure to recognise, or to treat adequately, lateral recess stenosis of the lumbar spine with the resultant nerve irritation and compression (Burton et al. 1981). This may be exacerbated by the upward migration of the superior facet secondary to loss of disc height following discectomy (Ross et al. 1988). Other common causes are recurrent or residual disc herniation, scar formation and adhesive arachnoiditis.

In the immediate postoperative period, however, it is important to recognise, haemorrhage, infection and pseudomeningocele and other fluid collections as causes of continuing symptoms (Ross et al. 1988; Stolke et al. 1989).

"Scar Versus Disc"

Most patients do not benefit from the surgical removal of scars since usually a vicious circle is created with the formation of additional scarring (Teplick and Haskin 1983; Schubiger and Valvanis 1982). The differentiation of disc and hypertrophied scar may not be possible clinically or even following myelography. The unenhanced CT scan is successful in making such a distinction in only 43% of cases (Bundschuh et al. 1988).

Scar formation appears to be very common in scans of asymptomatic postoperative patients (Teplick and Haskin 1983). It is appreciable in 40% of cases and tends to occur on the side of laminectomy (or lateral canal if facetectomy was done). The dural sac retracts towards the soft tissue which contours to the shape of the sac without compressing it. Recurrent discs tend to be continuous with the annulus and produce deformity and displacement of dural sac or root. The density of the disc is also higher than that of scar tissue. An increase in size over serial scans strongly favours a disc recurrence (Teplick and Haskin 1983).

Only when the nature of an extradural mass is uncertain should intravenous contrast enhancement be necessary. Scar tissue shows contrast enhancement (Schubiger and Valvanis 1982) which does not appear to be related to the age of the scar (Fig. 7.23). Contrary to popular belief, scars are very vascular as demonstrated by histological sections (Teplick and Haskin 1984; Ross et al. 1988). A disc herniation remains unenhanced although a rim of enhancing scar tissue posterior to the recurrent disc is characteristic (Fig. 7.24). In fact the vast majority of recurrent discs in patients who underwent re-operation were associated with some scar formation (Bundschuh et al. 1988; Hueftle et al. 1988).

Contrast-enhanced CT and MRI have comparable accuracy of approximately 85% (Teplick and Haskin 1985; Dixon and Bannon 1987; Bund-

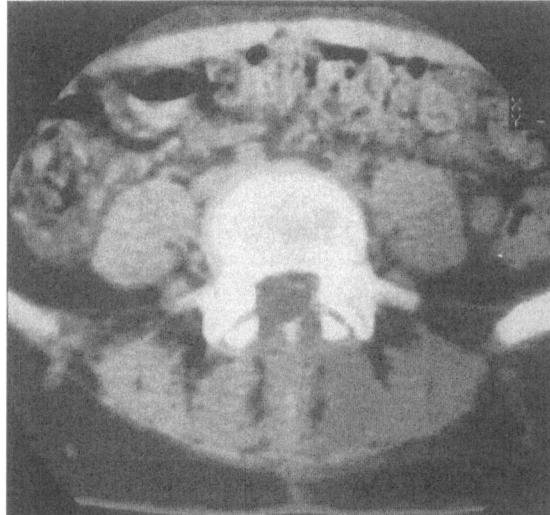

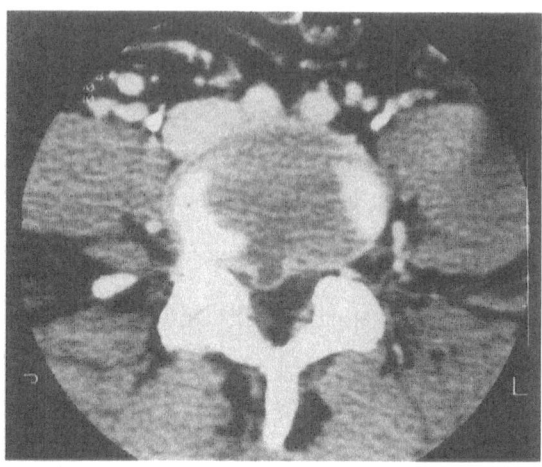

Fig. 7.24. Axial CT after IV contrast. A recurrent lumbar disc herniation is shown with an enhancing rim of scar tissue. (P.B.)

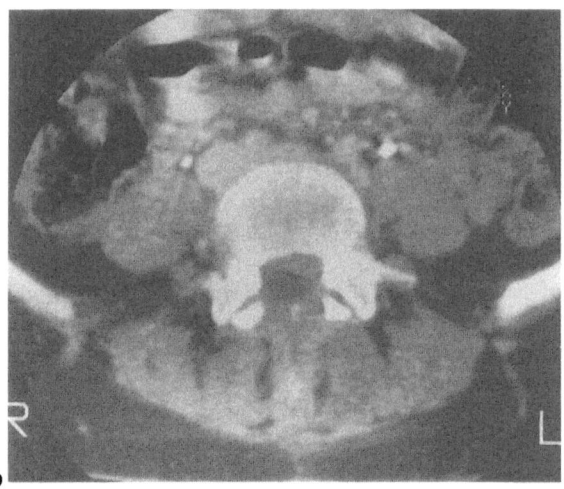

Fig. 7.23. Axial CT before (**a**) and after (**b**) IV contrast. Enhancing scar tissue invests the theca.

schuh et al. 1988). MRI criteria are also dependent on configuration, epidural location, mass effect and signal intensity. Scars as well as free fragments tend to be hyperintense on T2 weighted images (Bundschuh et al. 1988). The use of gadolinium DTPA with T1 weighted spin echo sequences appears to be highly accurate in separating epidural fibrosis from disc herniation (Hueftle et al. 1988).

It is of interest that delayed post-contrast scanning (at 30 minutes after injection) both with CT (iodinated contrast) and MRI (gadolinium DTPA) will show enhancement of both disc material and scar (De Santis et al. 1984; Hueftle et al. 1988; Ross et al. 1989). A nerve root engulfed in scar may show as a "filling defect", but analysis of contiguous sections should distinguish it from a disc fragment.

It is most likely that with the continuing technical improvement in MRI gadolinium will be reserved for a minority of difficult cases (Frocrain et al. 1989).

Pseudomeningocele

Pseudomeningocele formation is a rare surgical complication with an incidence of 0.1% (Schumacher et al. 1988). In a CT study of 400 patients following disc surgery 2% demonstrated this complication (Teplick et al. 1983). This is caused by a dural tear at surgery which can occur in 2%–5% of cases (Stolke et al. 1989). A distinction should be made between this and simple posterior bulging of the intact dura through the laminectomy defect.

Although pseudomeningoceles are asymptomatic in most cases, radicular symptoms can occur as a result of pressure which present in the first few weeks after surgery or years later (Fig. 7.25). These symptoms are often posture-related being worse on standing erect due to the pressure changes within the cyst. Communication between dura and cyst, if it exists, can only be demonstrated by water-soluble myelography; cyst opacification may be demonstrated either immediately or after an interval of some hours.

Arachnoiditis

Minor changes of arachnoiditis are best demonstrated by myelography (Fig. 7.26). In the diagnosis of moderate to severe cases, there is excellent correlation between conventional myelography, MRI and CT myelography (Ross et al. 1987c).

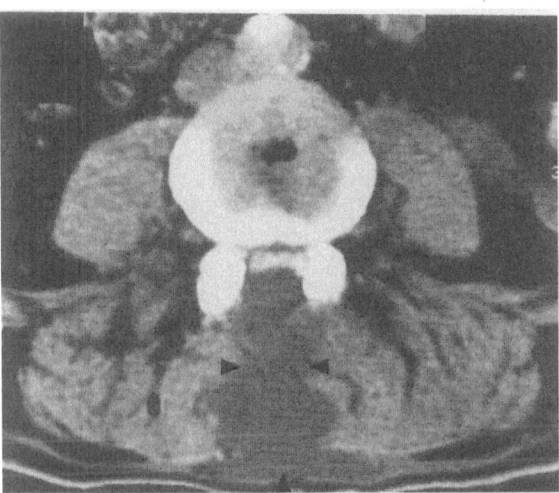

Fig. 7.25. CT myelogram. Pseudomeningocele (*arrowheads*) causing thecal compression.

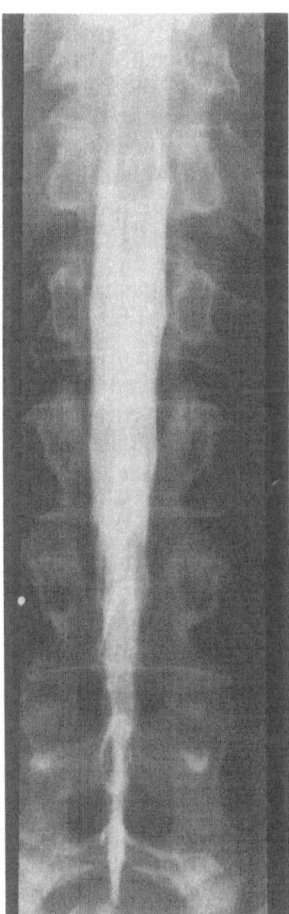

Fig. 7.26. Myelogram. Arachnoiditis. There is tapering of the lower thecal sac and absence of contrast filling the nerve root sheaths.

Spinal arachnoiditis may be a cause of persistent symptoms in between 6% and 16% of postoperative patients (Burton et al. 1981). The clinical diagnosis is difficult because it has no distinct symptom complex. The unpredictable occurrence of arachnoiditis mainly stems from the often multifactorial basis of its aetiology. The combination of a disc lesion, free blood in CSF, oily contrast and auto-immune factors appear to interact to produce arachnoiditis (Burton et al. 1981).

Roots adhere together to form a conglomeration centrally within the sac or are peripherally adherent to the meninges (empty sac appearance). In severe forms there is a soft tissue mass replacing the subarachnoid space leading to myelographic "block" with the distal subarachnoid space, assuming irregular "candle dripping" appearance.

Degenerative Disease of the Cervical Spine

Clinicopathological Aspects

Herniation of a cervical disc usually presents in young or middle-aged adults with features of acute nerve root compression. There is usually a good correlation between the level of the herniated disc as demonstrated radiologically and the clinical picture (Krausé et al. 1986b). Posterolateral herniation is usual and central herniation resulting in cord compression is rare except as a consequence of a hyperextension injury (Hawkins 1984). Acute soft disc herniations can also occur in the presence of cervical spondylosis.

Cervical spondylosis resulting from intervertebral disc and facet joint degeneration is a more common cause of morbidity. It presents with myelopathy, radiculopathy or a combination of both. In view of the high prevalence of plain radiographic changes of spondylosis (85% of those aged 60 or more according to Heller et al. (1983)) more specific imaging is required to exclude the less common causes of myelopathy such as tumour, syringohydromyelia or demyelination.

The underlying pathological changes involved in disc degeneration are similar to those in the lumbar region with the exception that herniation of disc fragments is less common. The annular bulge initiates the formation of osteophytic spurs or bars which in turn encroach upon the cord and nerve roots. The neural canal may be compromised by osteophytes arising at the uncovertebral joint and uncinate process projecting posterolaterally and from the facet joint which forms the posterior boundary of the foramen. The nerve root exiting from the foramen craniad to the corresponding vertebra occupies the lower portion of that foramen whilst its upper part is occupied by fat and epidural veins. Spondylotic changes tend to occur at the most mobile cervical segments (C5/6 and C6/7) and also adjacent to fused vertebrae. Trauma may also precipitate cervical degenerative disease.

Imaging Techniques

Plain Radiographs

There is no clear correlation between symptoms and plain radiographic findings of cervical spondylosis. Plain films are nevertheless valuable to identify alternative pathology such as infection or malignancy.

Myelography

Water-soluble contrast medium can be introduced into the subarachnoid space either via the lumbar route or by direct cervical puncture. The technique is thus invasive and requires hospital admission. It may be technically unsatisfactory if there is loss of the normal cervical lordosis, so that contrast cannot be pooled in sufficient amount in the neck, or if the patient is unable to maintain a prone position with extended neck because of pain (Fon and Sage 1984). Compression of the subarachnoid space may be exaggerated by excessive buckling of the ligamentum flavum in the prone position and may even result in partial myelographic block (Sobel et al. 1984). Recognition of the normal cervical enlargement and pseudo-expansion of cord due to a compressive extrinsic lesion is important to avoid a false-negative diagnosis of an intrinsic cord lesion.

CT

Calcified encroachment upon the canal is clearly demonstrable on plain CT but the cord and nerve roots may not be discernible in the lower cervical spine. The paucity of epidural fat does not normally permit identification of soft disc herniation (Scotti et al. 1983) but discs may sometimes be outlined by the displaced, enhancing epidural veins during intravenous contrast infusion using thin sections (Krausé et al. 1986b; Russell et al. 1984).

CT myelography is a more reliable technique which can either follow conventional myelography or be undertaken on an outpatient basis with the introduction of small doses of contrast medium introduced via lumbar puncture (Zinreich et al. 1988).

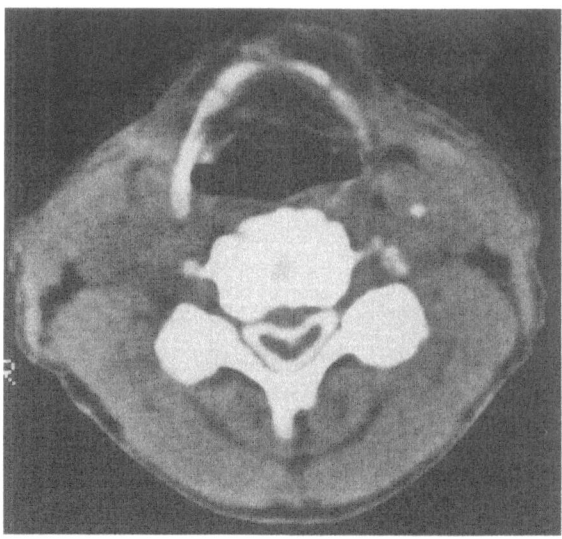

Fig. 7.27. CT myelogram. Central cervical disc protrusion causing cord compression.

In cervical myelopathy the shape of the cord in axial section can be easily seen and the distinction drawn between cord atrophy and reversible cord compression. If the size of the subarachnoid space around the small flattened cord is relatively wide atrophy is suspected and the damage may be irreversible. A cord which is deformed and moulded to the shape of the narrowed subarachnoid space is likely to respond better to surgical decompression (Yu et al. 1986; Penning et al. 1986) (Fig. 7.27). In some cases delayed CT in patients with myelopathy has demonstrated contrast within the cord in patterns suggestive either of cavitation (near to the level of decompression) and myelomalacia (distant from the level of compression (Jinkins et al. 1986)). This may go some way to explain the discrepancies which can exist between the level of maximal compression, the variable neurological signs and the failure to respond to decompressive surgery which are sometimes encountered.

CT can also detect small amounts of contrast media which pass craniad to a partial obstruction so avoiding a second, high cervical injection of contrast. It may also allow the salvage of a poor quality conventional study. Sections of 5 mm are appropriate which facilitate the examination of the entire length of the cervical cord should this be necessary.

In cervical radiculopathy, CT is an invaluable adjunct to myelography. Bony spurs and calcified or soft discs can be shown and their sites determined (Figs 7.28 and 7.29) (Amundsen 1981; Cronquist and Brismar 1981; Landman et al. 1984; Modic et al. 1986b). Narrow (1–2 mm) sections are required

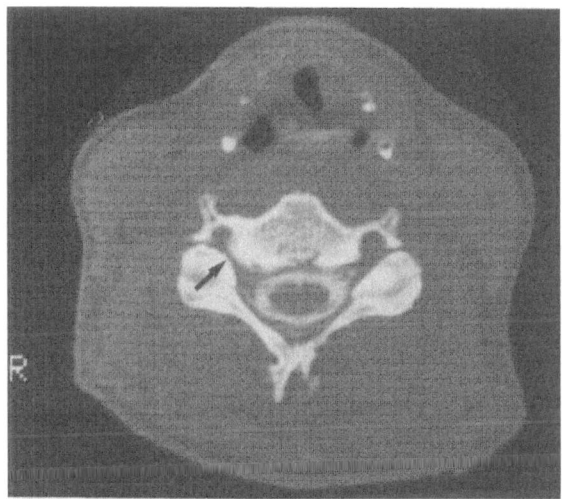

Fig. 7.28. CT myelogram. Osteophytic narrowing of a right cervical exit foramen (*arrow*). (P.B.)

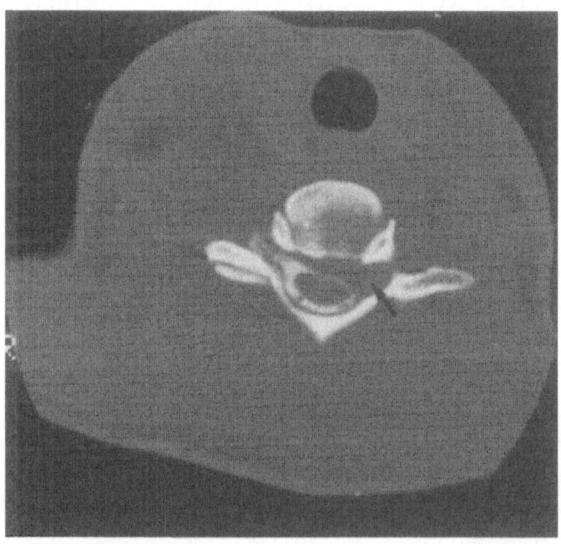

Fig. 7.29. CT myelogram. Posterolateral cervical disc herniation (*arrow*). (P.B.)

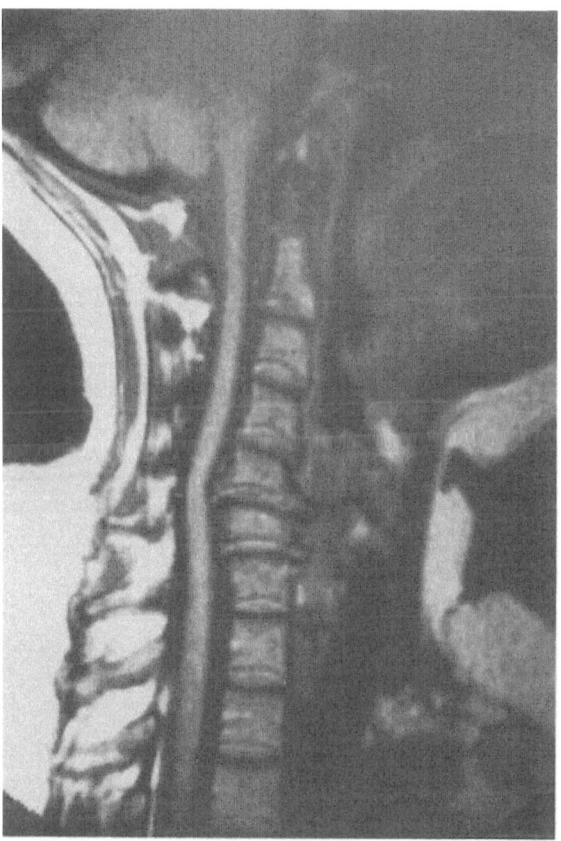

Fig. 7.30. Sagittal MRI (T1 weighted image). Cervical osteophytic disc – bars causing cord compression.

to examine the exit foramina adequately and the examination must necessarily be tailored on the basis of clinical features and the conventional myelographic findings.

MRI

The sagittal MRI T1-weighted sequence remains the most commonly performed and is very useful in patients with cervical myelopathy (Fig. 7.30) (Flannigan 1987; Czervionke et al. 1988; Czervionke and Daniels 1988), but has not yet supplanted CT myelography as the examination of

choice in the cervical radiculopathy – at least in the United Kingdom (Figs 7.31 and 7.32).

Quantitative Assessment (Spinal Canal and Cord Measurements)

The mean anteroposterior (AP) diameter of the spinal canal as seen at myelography is 17 mm (range 12–22 mm) at C3–7 and that of the cord 8–10 mm. Compression of the cord is likely to occur when the canal diameter is reduced to 10 mm or below (Maurice-Williams 1981). The average cord width is 11 mm with a maximum of 13 mm opposite C5 (cervical enlargement) (Lamont et al. 1981). The cord is elliptical in shape as seen on post-myelography CT at all levels but is normally slightly flattened at C4 and C5. Its minimum sagittal diameter is at C4/5 level (6 mm ± 1.5), whilst the transverse diameter is maximum at this level (11.8 mm ± 2.7) (Thijssen et al. 1979).

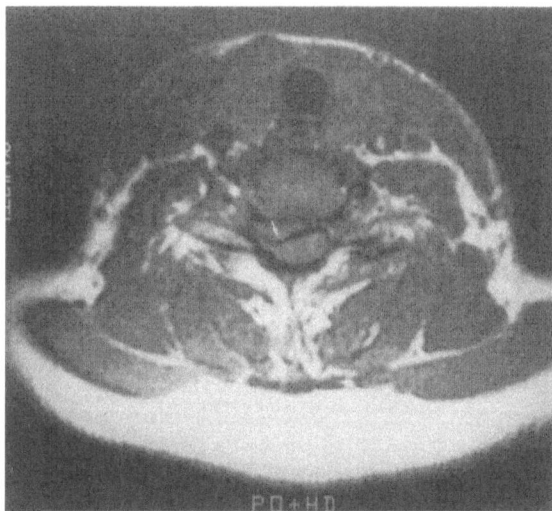

Fig. 7.31. Axial MRI (T1 weighted image). Posterolateral cervical disc herniation (*arrow*).

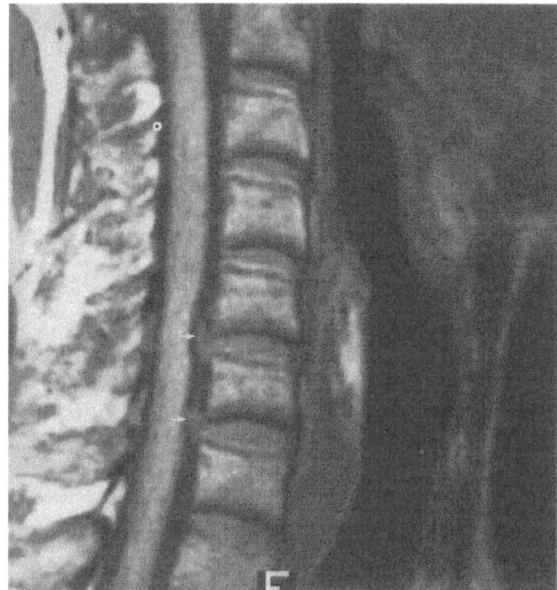

Fig. 7.32. Sagittal MRI (T1 weighted image). Cervical disc herniations impressing the spinal cord (*arrows*).

Degenerative Disease of the Thoracic Spine

Thoracic Disc Herniation

Symptomatic herniation of the thoracic disc is an uncommon condition with a reported incidence of approximately one per million of population per year and surgery for the condition comprises only

0.52% of all disc operations (Love and Shorn 1965; Alberico et al. 1986). Seventy-five per cent of thoracic herniations occur below T8. The true prevalence of thoracic disc herniation is almost certainly much higher than previously realised but the precise clinical significance remains to be established (Ryan et al. 1988; Williams et al. 1989).

Plain radiography is of limited value in suggesting the diagnosis because although calcification in thoracic disc is not uncommon (McAllister and Sage 1976), there is poor correlation between calcification and actual herniation (Goldberg et al. 1988).

Water-soluble myelography reveals extradural compression of the theca but the changes can be subtle and easily missed (Arce and Dohrmann 1985). Plain CT will demonstrate a calcified disc impinging on the spinal canal but intrathecal contrast is required in most cases for the delineation of the prolapsed disc and its relationship to spinal cord and theca (Fig. 7.33). MRI appears to be the most reliable technique currently available (Fig. 7.34). In a study by Ross et al. (1987a), only 9 out of 14 (65%) herniated thoracic discs detected by MRI were demonstrated by myelography.

MRI images obtained after gadolinium DTPA show areas of enhancement adjacent to the protruded thoracic disc, both above and below it. These were found to correspond to engorged dilated epidural veins at surgery (Parizel et al. 1989b).

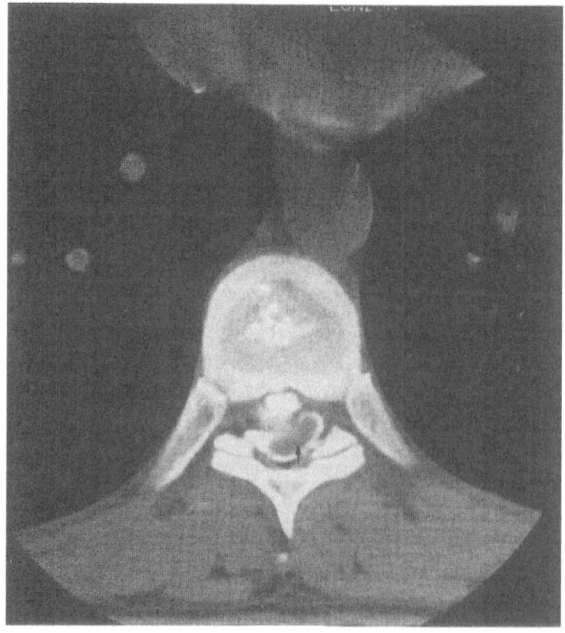

Fig. 7.33. CT myelogram. Large calcified thoracic disc herniation causing cord compression (the cord is *arrowed*). (P.B.)

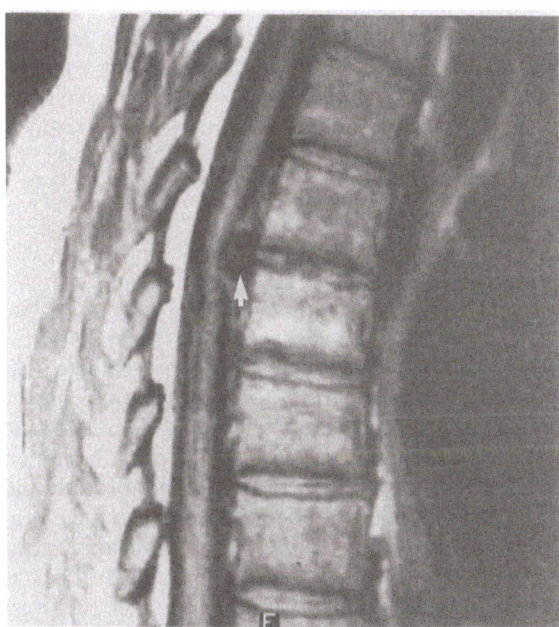

Fig. 7.34. Sagittal MRI (T1 weighted image). Thoracic disc protrusion (*arrow*).

Thoracic Vertebral Stenosis

Thoracic vertebral stenosis is an uncommon and not well recognised cause of myelopathy. Complaints of claudication with back pain or less commonly flaccid or spastic parapareses are the usual presenting features. A reduction in the AP diameter of the canal is not well appreciated on plain radio-

graphs. Myelography may misleadingly suggest a herniated thoracic disc or demonstrate a complete "block". CT is very helpful in demonstrating the true dimensions of the canal, the thickened laminae and the conformation of the facet joints (Yamamoto et al. 1988; Ungersböck et al. 1987). These features may also be demonstrated with MRI (Fig. 7.35).

Ossification of Posterior Longitudinal Ligament (OPLL)

Ossification of PLL is a well recognised cause of cervical canal stenosis and myelopathy (Fig. 7.36) (Minagi and Gronner 1969). Once known as the "Japanese disease", it is found in other races but much less commonly (Jones et al. 1988). It is most common in the cervical region (Murakami et al. 1982; Nose et al. 1987). Although ossification can be seen on plain films, CT myelography is invaluable for diagnosis and preoperative planning (Harsh et al. 1987; Klara and McDonnell 1986). The ossification takes nodular, sessile or rod-like

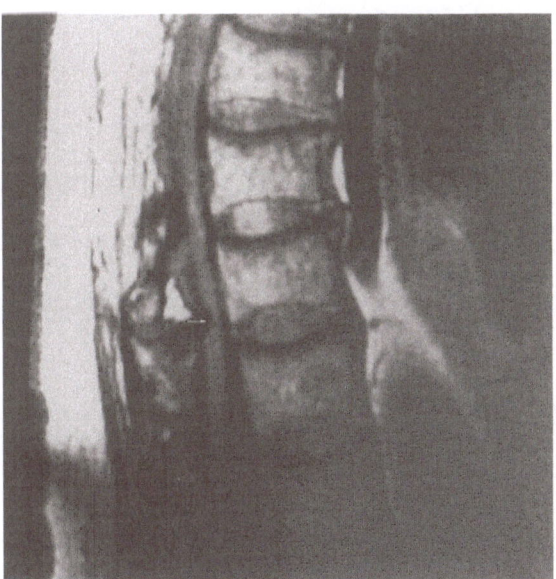

Fig. 7.35. Sagittal MRI (T1 weighted image). Thoracic canal stenosis (*arrow*).

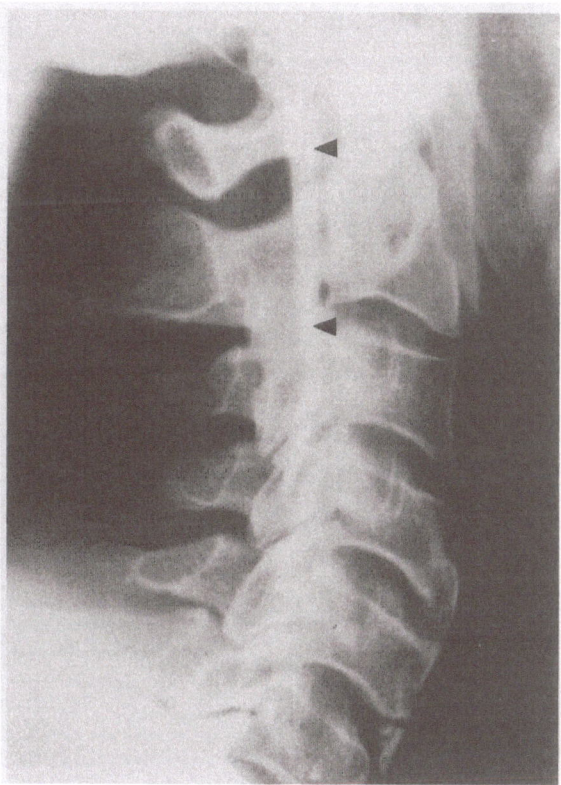

Fig. 7.36. Lateral cervical radiograph. Ossification of the posterior longitudinal ligament (*arrowheads*).

configuration and can cause considerable spinal cord and canal compression although probably in only a minority of cases since there appears to be a high prevalence in autopsy studies (Jones et al. 1988). Its exact aetiology is not known (Alenghat et al. 1982).

The Rheumatoid Cervical Spine

CT myelography utilising narrow axial sections and sagittal and coronal reformatting has been of great value in demonstrating the craniocervical osseous anatomy, erosion of the dens and the distribution of pannus in patients with a compressive myelopathy due to rheumatoid disease (Fig. 7.37) (Stevens et al. 1986).

MRI is in many ways more suitable than CT and is increasingly coming to the fore as the examination of choice because of its non-invasive nature and its multiplanar imaging facility (Fig. 7.38). It is also possible to image with the neck in flexion and in extension which provides some functional infor-

mation when there is vertebral instability – notably atlantoaxial subluxation. Bony detail is less well shown but this can be compensated for by plain films which in combination with MRI constitute the preferred method of examination (Larsson et al. 1989).

Spinal Tumours

Imaging Techniques

Water-soluble contrast myelography has been the traditional investigation for visualisation of the spinal cord and proximal nerve roots. The classical patterns of cord expansion or displacement and the configuration of the contrast-filled theca should allow the distinction to be made between the extradural, intradural extramedullary and the intramedullary lesion. A survey of the entire theca is usually possible which is important since the presence of multiple lesions may influence patient management.

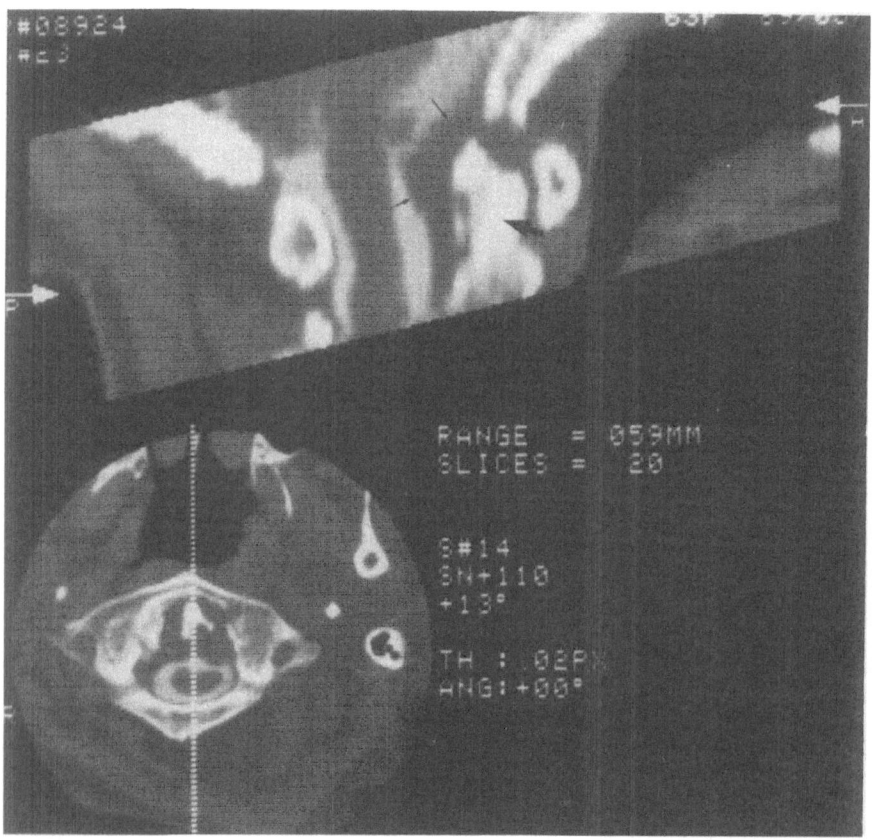

Fig. 7.37. CT myelogram (sagittal reformat). Rheumatoid disease. The dens is eroded (*large arrow*) and invested with pannus (*small arrows*). (P.B.)

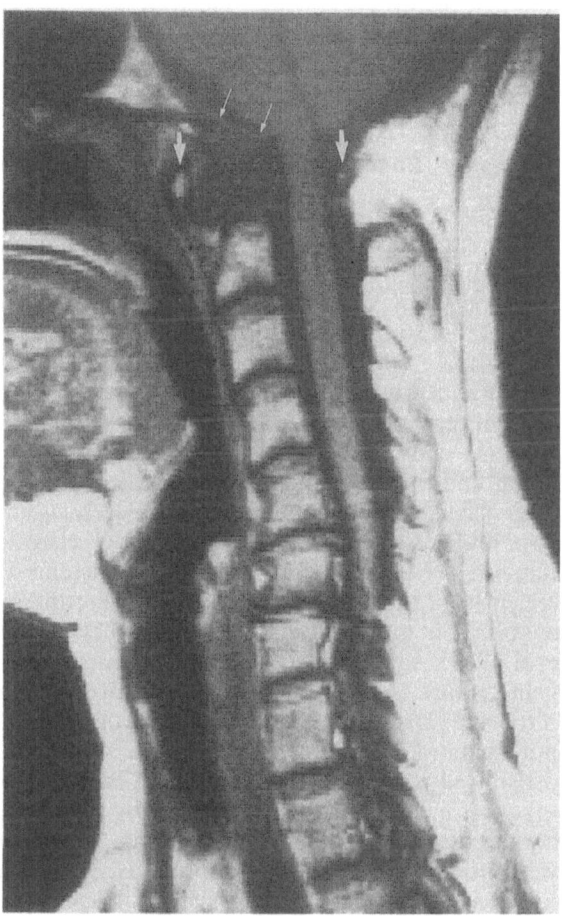

Fig. 7.38. Sagittal MRI (T1 weighted image). Rheumatoid disease. There is a atlantoaxial subluxation (*large arrows*) with dens erosion. Pannus impresses the cervicomedullary junction (*small arrows*). (P.B.)

In cases of myelographic "block" the upper level of the obstructing lesion will not be shown. It is usual in some centres to inject isotonic saline in an attempt to overcome the obstruction and to undertake postmyelography CT either with or without the saline "chaser" since small amounts of contrast medium may cross an obstruction spontaneously given time. It may, nevertheless, occasionally be necessary to introduce contrast medium by cisternal or lateral cervical routes. Neurological deterioration in cases of myelographic block has been reported following diagnostic lumber puncture in 14% of patients (Hollis et al. 1986).

CT will show the extraspinal extent of spinal tumours and can be used to direct a percutaneous biopsy. The nature of the bone destruction is also well shown which is important if a planned decompressive procedure might result in instability. Most intraspinal tumours show enhancement on CT following intravenous contrast (Lapointe et al. 1986). This helps to delineate the extent of the tumour and to separate its cystic and solid components. Both ependymomas and astrocytomas have similar enhancement characteristics and haemangioblastomas enhance consistently because of their very vascular nature.

MRI appears to be sensitive in detecting these lesions by virtue of the change in cord contour (best seen on T1 weighted images) and abnormal signal intensity that is often demonstrated (T2 weighted images).

MRI and postmyelography CT are equally sensitive in the evaluation of intramedullary and epidural disease including any bone involvement (Beltran et al. 1987; Smoker et al. 1987). MRI can not only characterise lesions seen on radionuclide bone scans but can also show early lesions when the scan is (falsely) negative (Colman et al. 1988; Sarpel et al. 1987). All metastases exhibit a low signal on T1 weighted images against a background of high signal marrow fat. Focal fatty replacement of haemopoietic marrow is a common, normal phenomenon and should not be confused with metastases (Hajek et al. 1987). Gadolinium DTPA allows the detection of small low-contrast lesions and often reveals lesions which are not apparent on unenhanced MRI (Bydder et al. 1985; Dillon et al. 1989). The distinction between solid tumour and adjacent cysts as well as tumour recurrence and postirradiation or postsurgical changes is also possible with MRI (Slaskey et al. 1987).

Bone Tumours

Benign Tumours

Primary bony tumours of the spine are rare. They usually present with pain which may be accompanied by a scoliosis. Neurological symptoms are uncommon but this clinical scenario necessitates an isotope bone scan.

Osteoid osteomas (Janin et al. 1981; Swank and Barnes 1987), *osteoblastomas* and *aneurysmal bone cysts* (Beabout et al. 1979) may all occur in the spine. Vertebra plana is a classical manifestation of *eosinophil granuloma* in children.

Haemangiomas occur in the middle decades of life. They are usually asymptomatic and involve the lower dorsal or upper lumbar regions, although they are well known occasionally to give rise to extradural haematomas (McAllister et al. 1975). Plain films have characteristic parallel linear streaks in a vertebral body with an overall increased density. These typical changes are also seen on CT

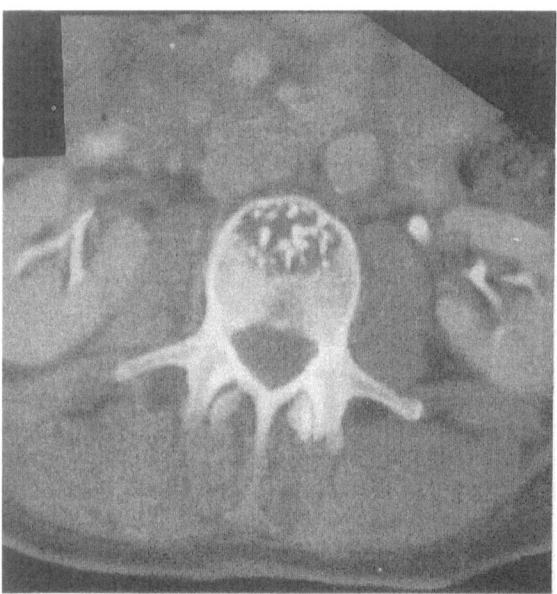

Fig. 7.39. Axial CT. Haemangioma of bone.

and MR pictures (Fig. 7.39). The transaxial images show a stippled pattern which on MRI appears as increased signal on T1 and T2 images (Ross et al. 1987b).

Malignant Bone Tumours

Chordoma. Chordoma is a rare tumour which seldom metastasises. Arising from the remnants of the primitive notochord it occurs mostly in the sacrococcygeal or spheno-occipital areas. Only 15% of these tumours are located in the spinal canal (Firooznia et al. 1986) where the lumbar region is more frequently involved than either the dorsal and cervical regions.

Spinal chordomas usually originate in the vertebral bodies (90%) and have both osteolytic and osteoblastic components (Fig. 7.40). Purely osteolytic and less frequently predominantly sclerotic tumours are also seen. Amorphous calcification is seen in 40% and areas of low attenuation are apparent on CT in more than half of the tumours (Meyer et al. 1984). A paraspinal soft tissue mass is a prominent feature in 60% of patients (de Bruïne and Kroon 1988) and intervertebral disc involvement is not uncommon, making differentiation from spinal osteomyelitis difficult. MRI appears to be as accurate as CT in detecting the tumour and suggesting the correct diagnosis. Chondroid chordoma, a variant with more cartilage and better prognosis, shows a lower signal intensity on T2 weighted images than the typical chordoma (Sze et al. 1988b).

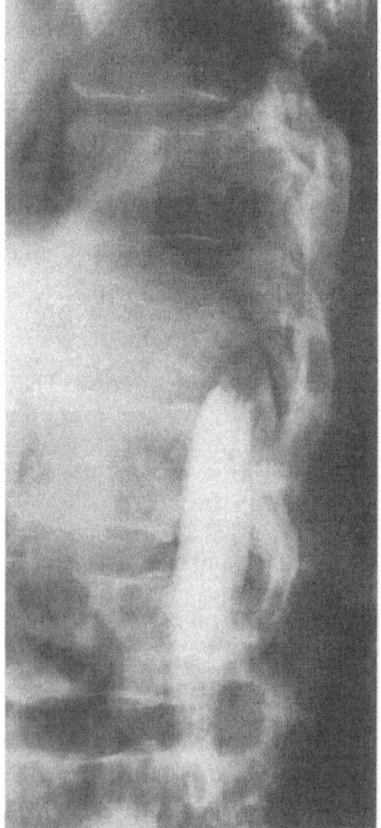

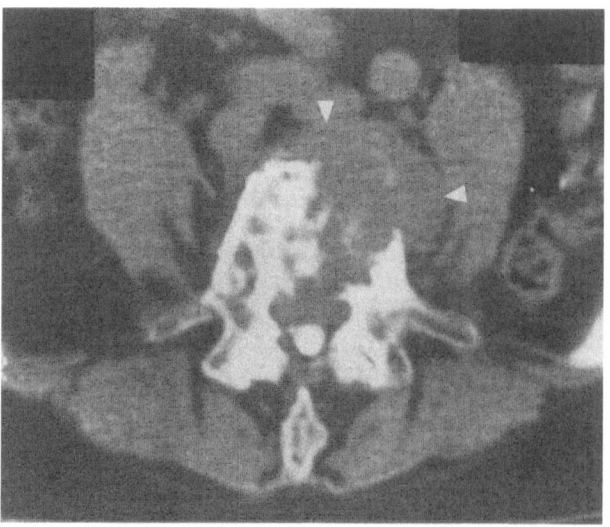

a   **b**

Fig. 7.40. Myelogram (**a**) and CT myelogram (**b**). Extradural block and vertebral destruction due to a spinal chordoma. CT reveals the extraspinal extension (*arrowheads*).

Myeloma (*Plasmacytoma*). Plasmacytoma is a solitary lesion which may precede the development of multiple myeloma and is usually found in males over the age of 50 years. The lesion is typically lytic and expansile and involves the vertebral body. Multiple lesions may be difficult to distinguish from metastases, but in myeloma the soft tissue mass is usually more prominent and the pedicles are less often involved at an early stage. An isotope bone scan is usually abnormal in patients with related pain and partial vertebral collapse. In tumours with exclusively osteoclastic activity the bone scan may remain normal even with extensive plain film changes (Patton and Woolfenden 1977). The spine is involved in two-thirds of patients with myeloma.

The lytic areas are seen on CT as areas of cortical destruction and the soft tissue involvement is also clearly demonstrated. Spinal cord compression on CT is better shown using intrathecal contrast whereas MRI reveals cord compression directly (Zimmerman and Bilaniuk 1988).

Lymphoma. Osteolytic lesions with anterior vertebral erosion and vertebral body collapse are common in lymphomas. There is a tendency to osteosclerosis (Fig. 7.41). The ivory type of sclerotic vertebra is seen in both Hodgkin and non-Hodgkin lymphomas. The extent of the paraspinal soft tissue involvement and epidural extension are clearly demonstrated by both CT and MRI.

Tumours of the Spinal Cord, the Nerve Roots and Their Coverings

Primary Tumours

Neurinomas. Neurinomas are the commonest spinal tumours, constituting about one-third of all non-metastatic tumours. The majority are intradural and extramedullary and only 15% are in the extra-dural space with an additional 15% seen as dumb-bell tumours (with both intra- and extradural elements). Unlike meningiomas there is no clear sex predilection. They are distributed evenly along the spine and in the cervical region they tend to be "hour-glass" shaped (Boisserie-Lacroix et al. 1987). Plain films are likely to show widening of the neural foramen or bony erosion of the pedicle or lamina but to elucidate the full extent of the well-defined soft tissue lesion CT or MRI scans are needed. The lesion is usually hypodense on CT and shows enhancement following intravenous contrast injection. As neurinomas tend to arise from the posterior sensory root, the cord is usually displaced anteriorly and to the opposite side which can clearly be demonstrated by MRI without the need for intrathecal

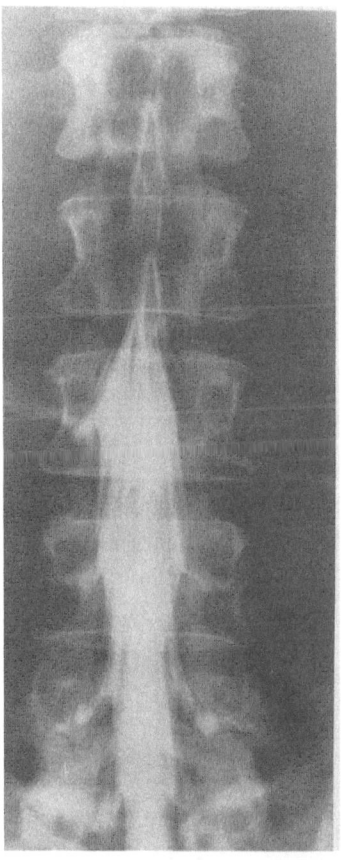

Fig. 7.41. Myelogram. Lymphoma. There is an extradural block, constricting the upper end of the contrast column. Note the sclerotic L1 vertebra and the absence of bone destruction.

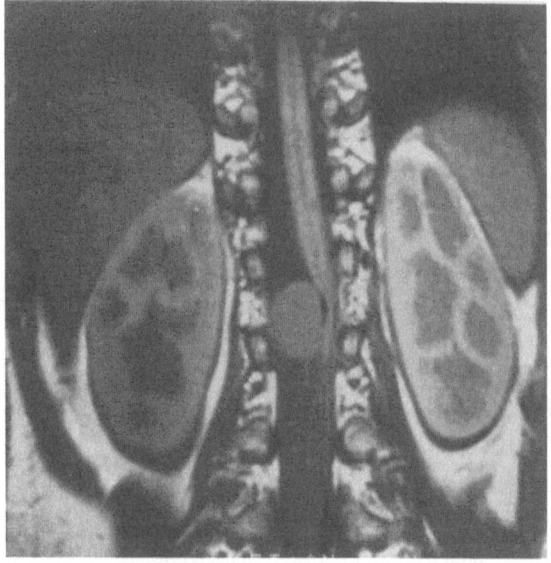

Fig. 7.42. Coronal MRI (T1 weighted image). Neurinoma displacing and compressing the spinal cord.

contrast (Fig. 7.42) (Zimmerman and Bilaniuk 1988).

Meningiomas. Meningiomas are the next most common spinal tumours after neurinomas. The vast majority are intradural and affect females much more commonly than males (8:1). They tend to occur in the fifth and sixth decades of life. Between 70% and 90% are seen in the thoracic region (Fig. 7.43). Calcification is common but best detected by CT (Fig. 7.44). Bony erosion is not as common as with neurinomas. When a meningioma is suspected clinically and MRI is not available, it is best to begin the investigation with myelography since clinical localisation is usually poor (Boisserie-Lacroix et al. 1987).

Intrinsic Tumours of the Cord. In excess of 90% of cord tumours are either ependymomas (two-thirds) or astrocytomas (one-third). Other tumours include

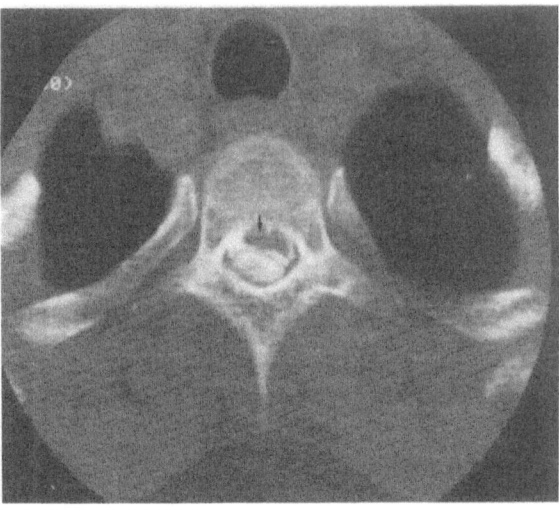

Fig. 7.44. CT myelogram. Meningioma. The spinal cord (*arrow*) is displaced anteriorly and compressed by the posteriorly sited intradural tumour whose relative hyperdensity is due to psammomatous calcification. (P.B.)

oligodendrogliomas and haemangioblastomas. Ependymomas are the commonest tumours of the lower cord, conus and filum terminale (60%). Otherwise the tumour types are distributed evenly throughout the length of the cord. Usually benign, ependymomas grow slowly and involve several segments before becoming symptomatic (Fig. 7.45). Tumours involving the filum appear to be extramedullary. They are rarely extradural but may then

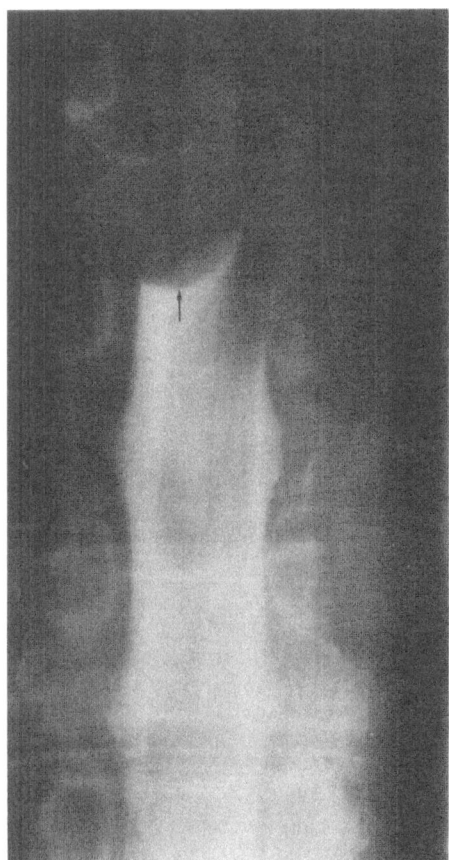

Fig. 7.43. Myelogram. Meningioma. The spinal cord is displaced by the tumour, the lower border of which is outlined by contrast (*arrow*). This is the typical appearance at myelography of an intradural, extramedullary lesion.

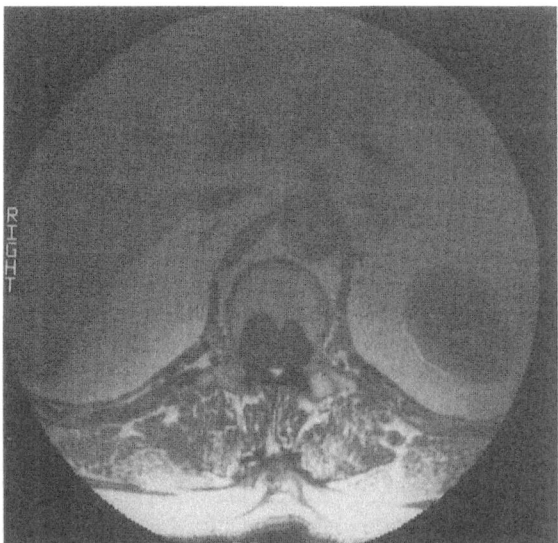

Fig. 7.45. Axial MRI (T1 weighted image). Ependymoma of the lumbar spine with bone erosion. The scalloped appearance of the bone erosion is typical of a slowly growing lesion and may also be found with neurinomas.

form a presacral or dorsal sacrococcygeal mass or cause marked bone destruction (Seigel et al. 1982).

Astrocytomas are more common in children and are found mostly in the cervical region and then the majority are well differentiated, grades I and II, and very few are aggressive (Epstein and Wisoff 1987); Cohen et al. 1989). Cysts can occur within an intramedullary tumour which is surrounded by abnormal glial elements and containing haemorrhagic or xanthochromic fluid. More often though cysts are rostral or caudal to the tumour and are not part of it (Goy et al. 1986).

Myelography shows fusiform expansion of the spinal cord and when followed by CT the cord contour is clearly seen. Opacification of intramedullary cysts can on rare occasions be demonstrated on immediate or delayed scans following myelography. The distinction between syringohydromyelia and cystic or even solid intramedullary tumour can be problematic. It is known that not all syrinx cavities take up contrast and conversely cystic neoplasms and myelomalacia may accumulate contrast on delayed scans (Kan et al. 1983). Focal plain film changes (if present) and irregular rather than smooth expansion of the cord contour favour the diagnosis of tumour. By using the presence of distinct cyst margins and a uniform intensity of signal of the cyst contents similar to that of CSF as criteria. MRI can diagnose a syrinx cavity with an accuracy of 88% (Williams et al. 1987).

Confident differentiation between tumour, a cyst whose contents have a high protein content, or gliosis of the cord can be made following gadolinium DTPA (Slasky et al. 1987). Intravenous gadolinium should always be given if an apparent syringiohydromyelia is not associated with tonsillar descent (Fig. 7.46). Cord swelling can also be seen as a consequence of a myelitis (Fig. 7.47a) and plaques of demyelination may be demonstrated on T2 weighted MR images of the spinal cord (Fig. 7.47b) (Merine et al. 1987).

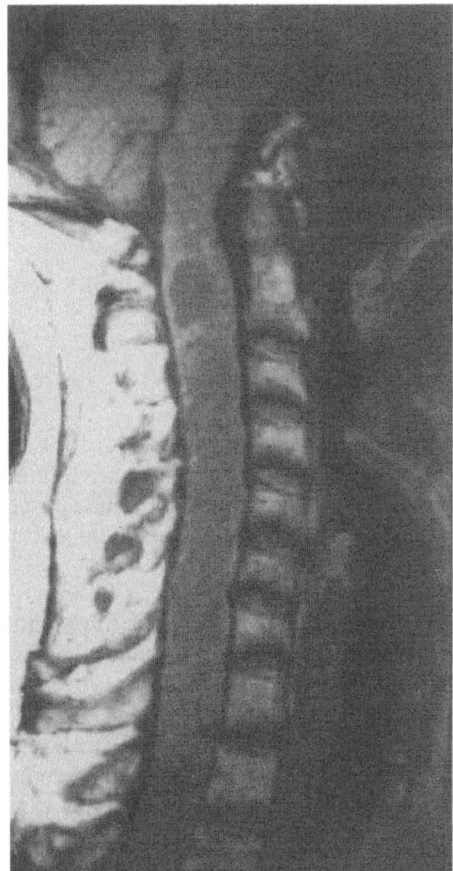 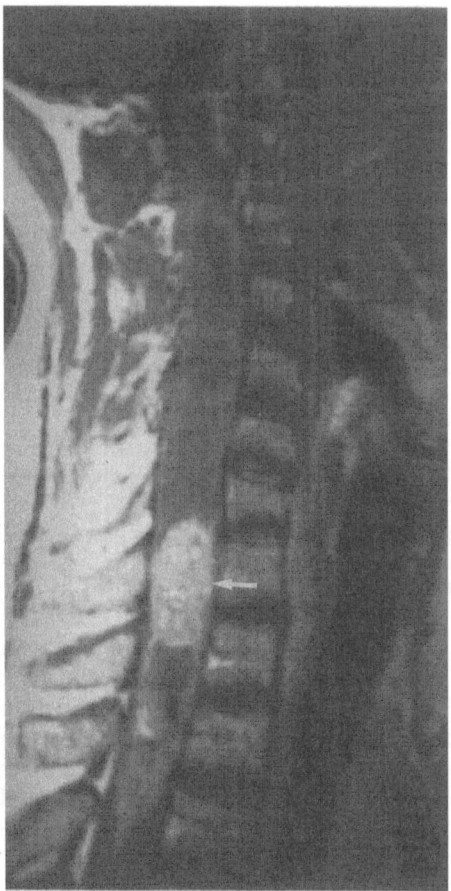

a b

Fig. 7.46. Sagittal MRI (T1 weighted images) before (**a**) and after (**b**) intravenous gadolinium. Cervical ependymoma (*arrow*) with associated tumoral syrinx.

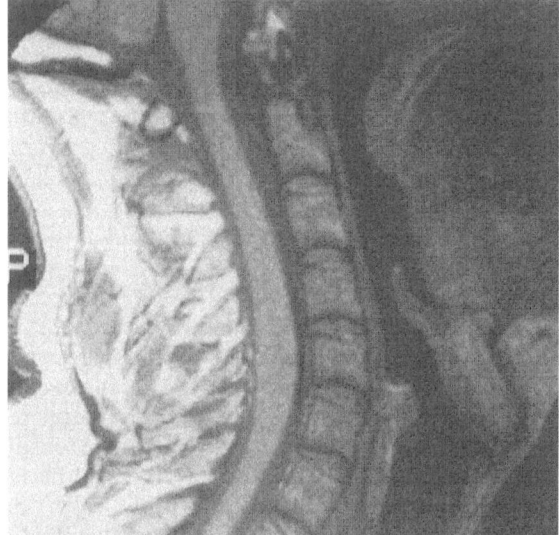

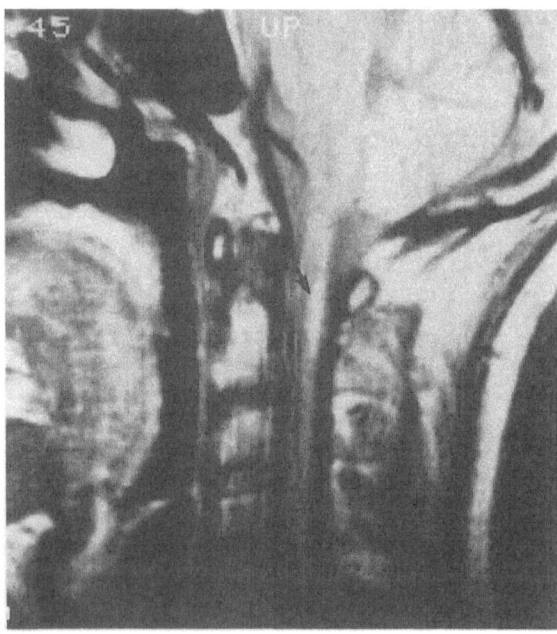

Fig. 7.47. (a) Sagittal MRI (T1 weighted image). Swollen cervical cord due to a transverse myelitis. **(b)** Sagittal MRI (T2 weighted image). Multiple sclerosis showing a high signal plaque within the spinal cord (*arrow*).

Haemangioblastomas. Spinal haemangioblastomas are rare and most occur in patients with von Hippel–Lindau disease. More than 60% are associated with a syrinx cavity (Kaffenberger et al. 1988). Prominent vascular impressions may be demonstrated by myelography (Fig. 7.48) and the tumours show intense enhancement on CT following intravenous contrast administration.

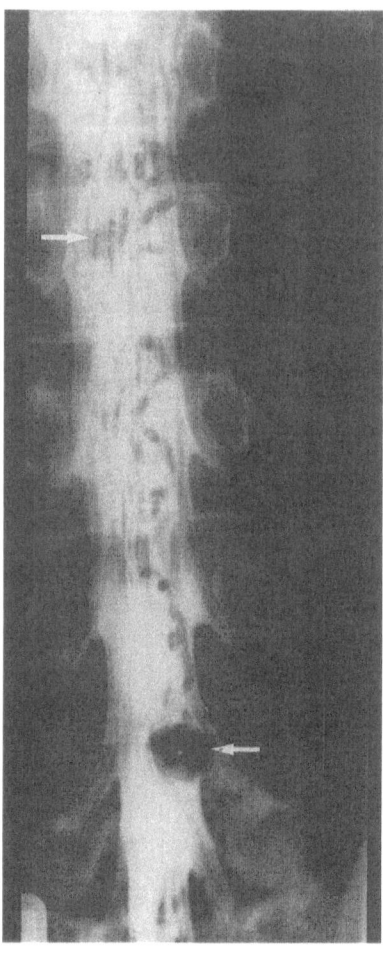

Fig. 7.48. Myelogram. Haemangioblastomata (*arrows*). Note the prominent associated vascularity.

Metastatic Disease of the Spine

Spinal cord compression occurs in 5%–10% of patients with cancer. The vast majority are related to extradural, primarily vertebral, metastases. Intradural involvement whether intra- or extramedullary is rare.

Intramedullary Metastases. At least 1% of patients with non-neurogenic primary tumours develop intramedullary metastases (Chason et al. 1963; Edelson et al. 1972). Carcinoma of the lung followed by carcinoma of the breast appear to be the commonest primary tumours and the thoracic cord is usually affected (Post et al. 1987). The route of spread is believed to be mainly haematogenous although leptomeningeal involvement can also lead to invasion of the cord. Intracranial tumours like medulloblastomas, ependymomas and gliomas commonly seed via the cerebrospinal fluid pathways. Spinal cord metastases from medulloblastoma are reported in 12.5%–43% of cases (Park et al. 1983; Deutsch and Reigal 1980). Many lesions are asymptomatic and myelograms fail to disclose an abnormality in about 40% of cases of intramedullary metastases from non-neurogenic primary tumours (Post et al. 1987).

Intradural Extramedullary Metastases. Metastatic seeding from intracranial tumours such as medulloblastoma, ependymoma and pinealoma is well recognised and influences both the management and prognosis (Fig. 7.49) (Post et al. 1987). Seeding from intracranial metastases from primary tumours originating outside the neuraxis is much less common. Again cerebrospinal fluid pathways provide the most likely route of spread in these cases especially when the intracranial lesions are adjacent to the subarachnoid spaces. Intracranial metastases from bronchial and renal cell carcinomas and melanoma are known to seed (Barloon et al. 1987).

Arachnoid leukaemic infiltration is reported with a surprisingly high incidence at autopsy but it is rarely apparent clinically (McAllister and O'Leary 1987). The imaging appearances are those of thickened roots of the cauda equina (Fig. 7.50). CSF cytology is often helpful in making diagnosis as this is a rather non-specific finding and can be seen in lymphoma, lung, breast and gastric carcinomas. Root thickening can also be a manifestation of neurofibromatosis, hypertrophic interstitial neuropathy (Dejerine and Sottas type) and sarcoidosis (Isherwood and Antoun 1984; McAllister and O'Leary 1987).

The diagnosis of drop metastases is usually made by myelography supplemented by postmyelogram CT. They appear as discrete spherical nodules attached to the nerve roots or spinal cord (Zimmerman and Bilanuik 1988). Unenhanced MRI is often disappointing. The higher water content of these metastases imaged against a "background" of highly proteinaceous CSF makes their detection difficult (Sze et al. 1988a). However gadolinium-enhanced MRI matches the sensitivity of myelography supplemented with CT.

Extradural Metastases. The majority of spinal metastases are located in the vertebrae and in the extradural space (O'Carroll and Witcombe 1979). Lesions are often multiple and result from haematogenous spread. The thoracic spine is most commonly affected.

The extradural space is involved mostly by disruption of the vertebral cortex or by direct spread from paraspinal masses (Fig. 7.51). Lymphoma is

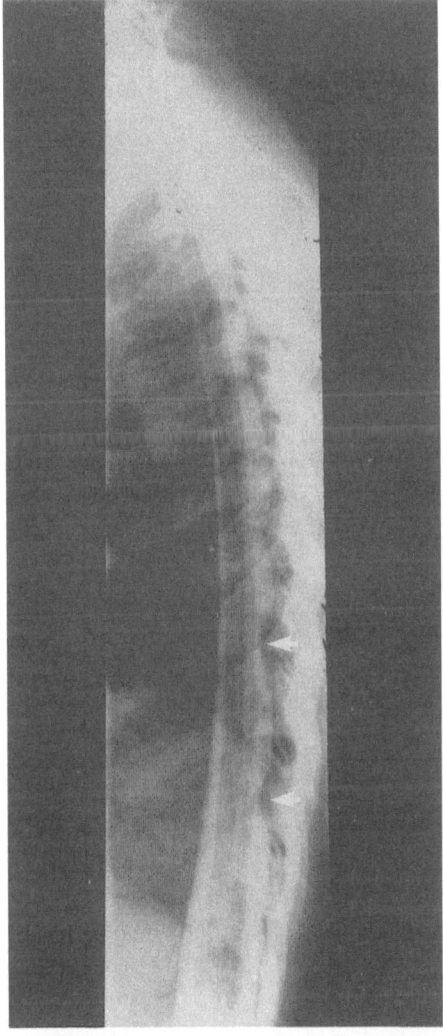

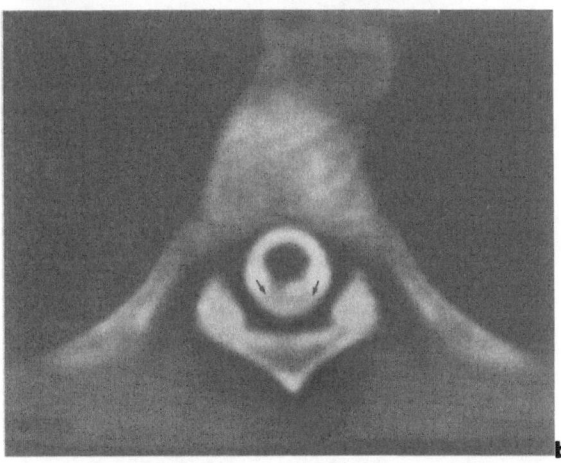

Fig. 7.49. Myelogram (**a**) and CT myelogram (**b**). Intradural seeds from a medulloblastoma. The posterior impressions on the contrast column (*arrows*) suggest extradural type compression. CT reveals the true intradural location (*arrows*).

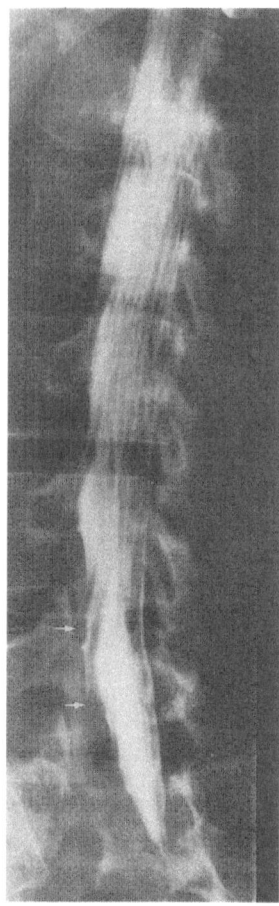

Fig. 7.50. Radiculogram. Leukaemia. There is subtle thickening of the nerve roots due to their infiltration (*arrows*).

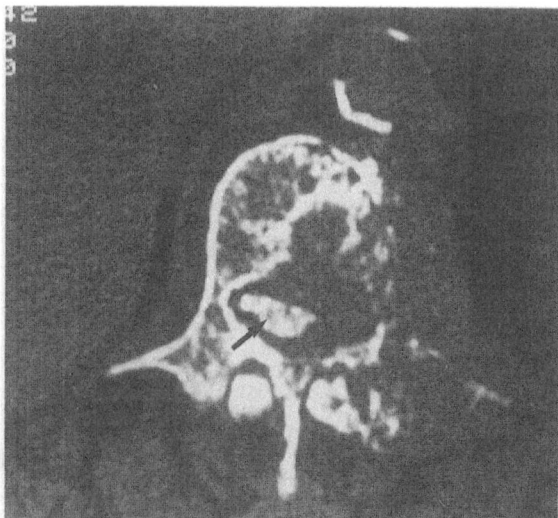

Fig. 7.51. CT myelogram. Metastatic carcinoma of the breast. The *arrow* indicates the contrast-filled theca. (P.B.)

well recognised to spread through the intervertebral foramina often with no associated bony destruction. The intervertebral disc is relatively resistant to the spread of tumour and the presence of vertebral destruction in the absence of significant disc alteration is a reliable indicator of tumour whereas vertebral destruction and involvement of intervertebral disc space suggest infection (Resnick and Niwayama 1978). Discal destruction can nevertheless result from tumour in a minority of instances (Meyer et al 1984; Firooznia et al. 1976). Tumours also tend to be characterised by involvement of the posterior elements, but the distinction of tumour from infection may sometimes be difficult to make.

Tumours in the Paediatric Group

Intramedullary ependymomas and astrocytomas constitute one-third of all non-development spinal tumours in children. Primary and secondary neuroblastoma and sarcoma are the commonest epidural

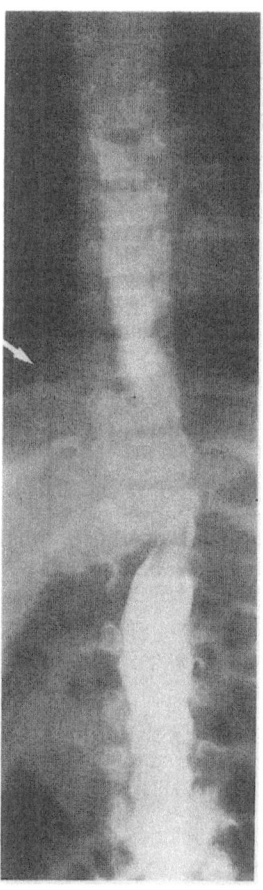

Fig. 7.52. Myelogram. Neuroblastoma. The partial extradural-type block is associated with a paraspinal mass (*arrowheads*) containing flecks of calcification. The lower ribs are also splayed on the affected side.

tumours. The cord is compressed in neuroblastoma by direct extension from the primary tumour in paraspinal ganglia, from nodal metastases or by a vertebral metastasis (Banna and Gryspeerdt 1971) (Fig. 7.52).

Syringohydromyelia and the Chiari Malformations

Cystic Cord Lesions

Syringohydromyelia is characterised by the presence of a longitudinal, fluid-filled cavity within the spinal cord. The differentiation between *syringomyelia* in which the cavity is lined by glial cells and *hydromyelia* where the dilated central canal is lined by ependyma is difficult to make in the majority of instances and, in any case, of dubious significance clinically (Williams 1986). The combined term of *syringohydromelia* is therefore preferred. Extension of the cavity into the medulla is termed syringobulbia and occurs in approximately 10% of cases of syringohydromelia (Lee et al. 1985; Valentini et al. 1986).

Conditions associated with syrinx formation include the Chiari malformations (vide infra), spinal tumours (both intra- and extramedullary (Castillo et al. 1987)) arachnoiditis, irradiation and trauma. Between one-third and one-half of cases of syringohydromyelia have no identifiable associations (Gillespie et al. 1986).

The Chiari Malformations

Herniation of the lower part of the cerebellum through the foramen magnum is the commonest abnormality associated with syringohydromyelia. The cerebellar tonsils are usually well formed and the foramen of Magendie is usually patent. This is known as the *Chiari Type I* herniation or malformation (Fig. 7.53). It is associated with a variety of segmental craniovertebral junction abnormalities including basilar impression (25%) assimilation of the atlas into the occiput (10%), the Klippel–Feil anomaly (10%) and incomplete ossification of the ring of the atlas (5%) (Byrd et al. 1988). In this Chiari type I malformation syringohydromyelia occurs in 60%–70% of cases and hydrocephalus in 25%.

The *Chiari type II* malformation (Fig. 7.54) is a complex developmental anomaly affecting the calvarium, dura and hindbrain. In addition to hydrocephalus, a meningomyelocele is nearly always present. The small cerebellum and brainstem may be caudally displaced through the enlarged foramen

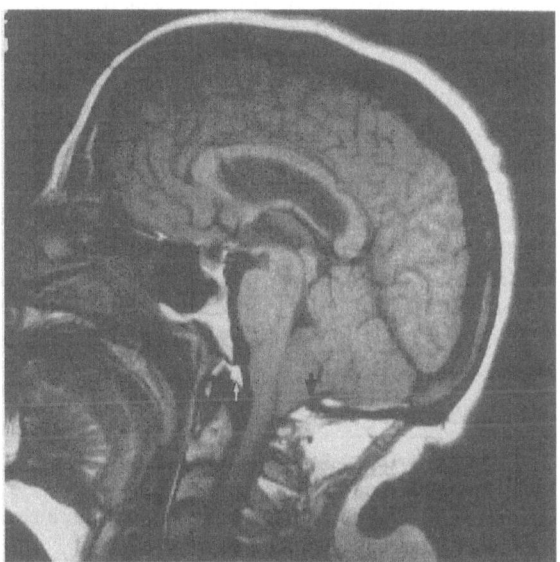

Fig. 7.53. Sagittal MRI (T1 weighted image). Chiari type I malformation. There is tonsillar descent below the level of the foramen magnum, the anterior margin of which is denoted on MRI by the fat pad above the dens (*white arrow*). The posterior margin is shown by the *black arrow*.

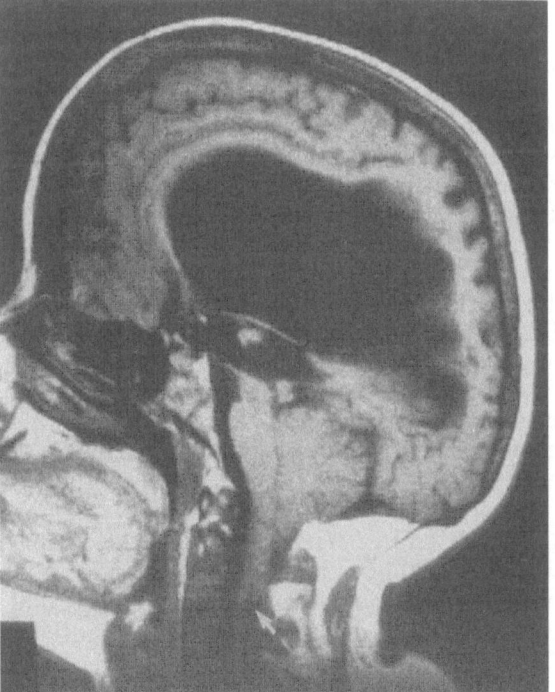

Fig. 7.54. Sagittal MRI (T1 weighted image). Chiari II malformation. There is hydrocephalus with tonsillar and brainstem descent below the level of the foramen magnum. Note the cervicomedullary "kink" (*arrow*). (P.B.)

magnum (Wolpert et al. 1987). Associations exist with syringohydromyelia, diastematomyelia and diplomyelia.

It is important to realise that there are many grades of severity in the Chiari malformation ranging from severe infantile forms associated with gross skeletal abnormalities to those in which the only abnormality may be some degree of cerebellar tonsillar displacement (Mohr et al. 1977). In many instances the division into Chiari type I and type II is somewhat unrealistic, hence the preferred term of "hindbrain herniation" (Williams 1986).

Syringohydromyelia

Diagnostic Imaging

Prior to CT a direct demonstration of the syrinx cavity could only be achieved by cyst puncture and injection of contrast medium ("endo-myelography"). Indirect evidence was provided by the "collapsing cord" sign first described during air myelography (Logue 1971). This is due to the syrinx partially emptying when the patient is moved from the prone to the supine position.

Plain CT occasionally reveals a cavity within an enlarged cervical cord but intrathecal contrast is normally required (Forbes and Isherwood 1978; Bonafe et al. 1980; Pullicino et al. 1979). MRI is currently the examination of choice in the identification of intramedullary cavities.

Myelography. The diagnosis with conventional water-soluble contrast myelography depends on finding a smoothly enlarged cord (Fig. 7.55). However, in approximately one-third to one-half of cases, the cord can be either normal or reduced in size due to atrophy (Bonafé et al. 1980; Lee et al. 1985). This may result in a falsely negative examination, especially if a supine lateral view to discover any tonsillar ectopia is omitted. The presence of a cavity can also be suspected if there is localised or diffuse change in cord size, especially when the change is influenced by the patient's position (Kan et al. 1983).

Computer Assisted Myelography. CT myelography with reformatting in both the coronal and sagittal planes provides important information regarding cord morphology and the presence of an associated Chiari malformation (DiChiro and Schellinger 1976; Forbes and Isherwood 1978). A collapsed cord with flat ventral borders (Bonafé et al. 1980), especially if its shape is position dependent, suggests a cavity (Resjo et al. 1979) but more important is the demonstration of contrast medium within this

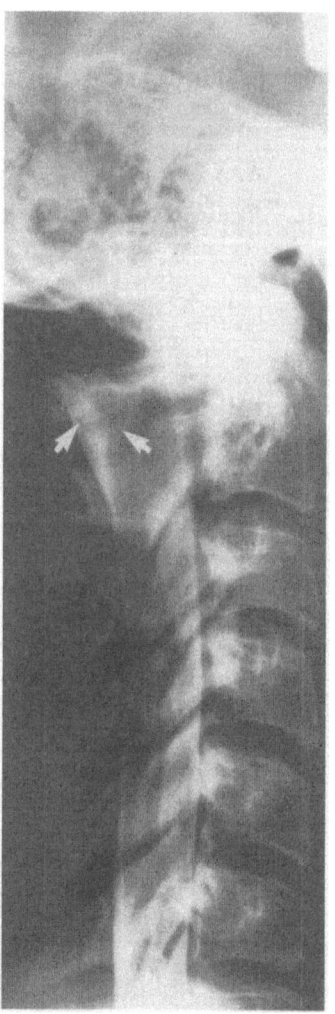

Fig. 7.55. Cervical myelogram (supine lateral projection). Syringomyelia. The cervical cord is smoothly enlarged. Note the tonsillar descent (*arrows*).

cavity on delayed scans. Only two-thirds of cord cavities will opacify between 4–8 hours, after administration of intrathecal contrast (Fig. 7.56) and a further delay (between 12 and 24 hours) will reveal most, if not all, cavities (Li and Chui 1987). Opacification of a cavity does not necessarily imply communication with the ventricular system and may occur by transneural extracellular passage of contrast medium.

MRI. The sagittal MRI T1 weighted sequence usually provides the most useful information. Surface coils and thin sections are essential (Fig. 7.57). T2 weighted images can be useful to demonstrate intra-cavitary fluid turbulence and movement (signal void). It is not certain, however, whether this is a manifestation of potential expan-

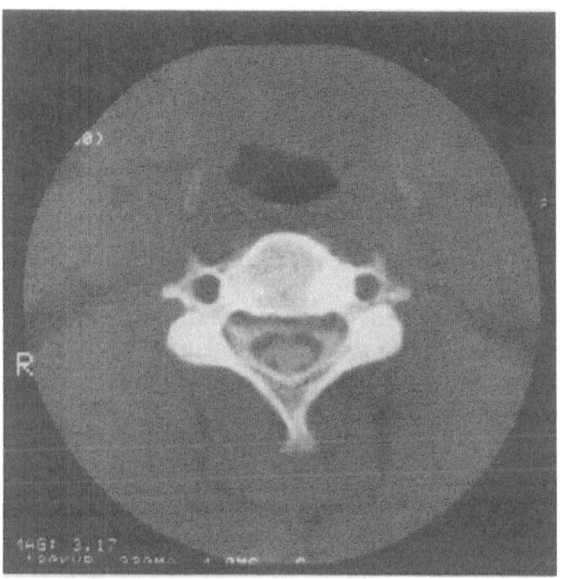

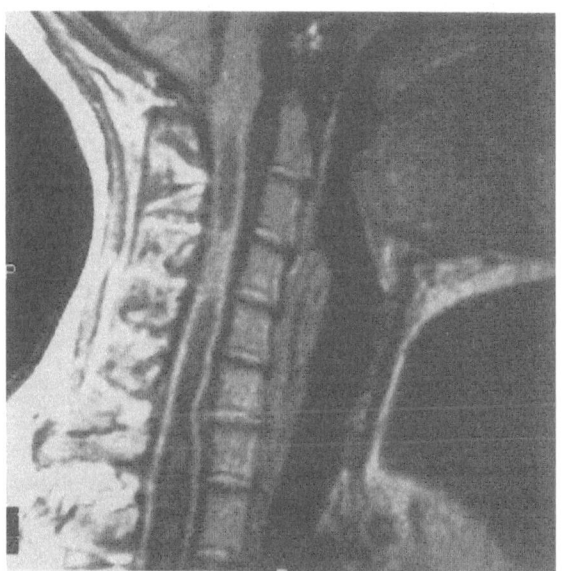

Fig. 7.56. CT myelogram. Syringomyelia. Contrast medium is seen within the syrinx cavity.

sion of the syrinx (Castillo et al. 1987). Table 7.1 summarises the important distinguishing features with MRI between tumoral cysts and syringohydromyelia.

Spinal Dysraphism

Definitions

Spinal dysraphism denotes a group of congenital spinal anomalies caused by defective or incomplete fusion of midline bony, neural and mesenchymal structures which is normally achieved by the fifth embryonal week. The simplest form of dysraphism is *spina bifida occulta* which has a prevalence of 17%–23% in the normal population (James and Lassman 1972; Boone et al. 1985; Fidas et al. 1987). It is regarded as a normal variant and is commoner in men and in the younger age groups. Such defects are commonest in the first and second sacral segments and a defect in the fifth lumbar vertebra is very rare (0.1%) (Fidas et al. 1987). Clinically significant varieties can be classified into two main groups (a) *spina bifida aperta (cystica) and (b) occult spinal dysraphism* (primary tethered cord syndrome).

Spina Bifida Aperta (Cystica)

This implies posterior protrusion through a bony defect of one or all elements normally found within

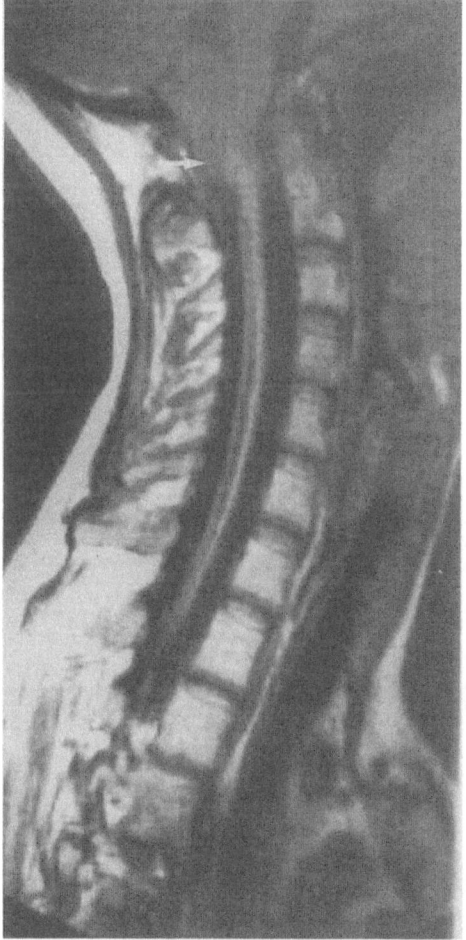

Fig. 7.57. Sagittal MRI (T1 weighted image). Syringomyelia: **a** with enlargement of the cord, **b** within an atrophic cord. Note the tonsillar descent (*arrow*).

Table 7.1. Distinguishing features between tumoral cysts and syringohydromyelia

	Syrinx	Tumour cavity
Clinical aspects		
Age at onset	>15 years	<15 years
Duration of symptoms	>1 year	<1 year
Chiari malformation	50%–80%	Very rare; coincidental if present
Cord		
Size	30%–50% enlarged	>90% enlarged
Contour	Regular	Irregular
Cavity Edge	Sharply defined	Not sharply defined
Signal intensity (T1)	Low signal (CSF-like)	Low signal (but not as low as CSF)
Signal homogeneity(T1)	Homogeneous	Inhomogeneous
T2 signal	↑In 33% Benign gliosis around syrinx cavity	↑In all
Flow void (pulsatile fluid shift)	80% (↓in signal on T2)	20% incidence in any associated syrinx but not in the tumour cavity
Gd DTPA enhancement	Nil	Marked

Data from Slasky et al. (1987), Sherman et al. (1987), Gillespie et al. (1986), Aubin et al. (1981) and Valk and Kaiser (1986).

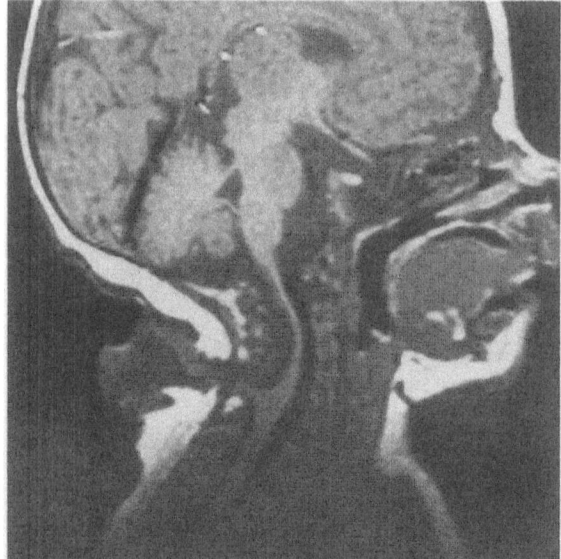

Fig. 7.58. Sagittal MRI (T1 weighted image). Cervical myelomeningocele.

the spinal canal. The simplest and most common form is *meningocele*, which is a simple meningeal sac containing no neural tissue.

A *myelocele* or *myelomeningocele* (Fig. 7. 58) is more serious and less common. Nearly 90% of patients with myelomeningocele have a Chiari type II malformation and 90%–95% also have hydrocephalus (Fitz 1982). Syringohydromyelia is present in 40% (Samuelsson et al. 1987) and diastematomyelia in 30%–45% of patients. There is no indication for detailed neuroradiological investigation of the newborn. Surgical repair of the myelocele and myelomeningocele is undertaken in the early neonatal period along with ventricular shunting for adequate control of hydrocephalus.

Occult Spinal Dysraphism (Tethered Cord Syndrome)

Clinicopathological Aspects

The majority of patients present in childhood or early adult life. The onset of symptoms may be related to periods of rapid growth, but in general the delayed onset of symptoms suggest the importance of secondary factors such as ischaemia due to traction or repeated minor trauma as well as direct damage to the cord by fibrous or bony bands (Guthkelch 1974; Merx et al. 1989).

In almost all patients there is spina bifida and the conus is abnormally low in position and held dorsally due to one or more tethering lesions (Fig. 7.59). As the conus attains its adult level of L1/2 at some time during the first few months of life (Harwood-Nash 1981; Wilson and Prince 1989), tethering is diagnosed when the cord is below the level of the second lumbar vertebra and when the conus fails to move anteriorly when the patient is screened in the prone position during myelography (Scatliff et al. 1989).

The most common tethering lesions, in descending order of frequency, are a lipoma of the conus and filum, a thickened (tight) filum terminale, diastematomyelia and myelomingocele (Raghavan et al. 1989; Scatliff et al. 1989). Other congenital lesions such as neurenteric cysts (always associated with vertebral body dysplasia), intraspinal dermoid/epidermoid, teratoma and arteriovenous malformation are also rarely encountered (Harwood-Nash 1981).

Lipomas

Lipomas are by far the commonest tethering lesions (Raghavan et al. 1989). They can be totally intradural, often infiltrating the conus, adjacent nerve

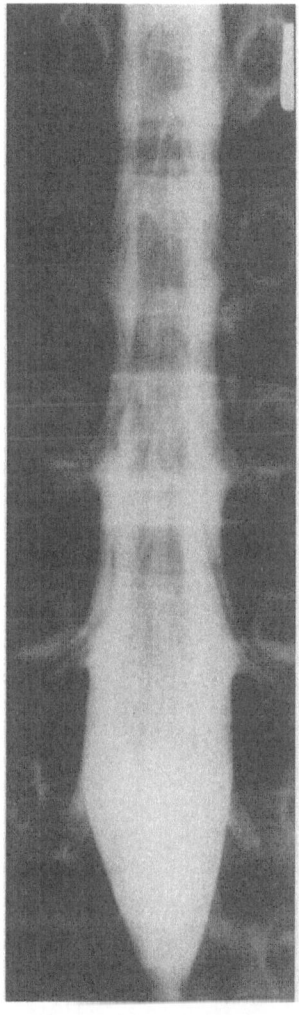

Fig. 7.59. Myelogram. Abnormally low spinal cord.

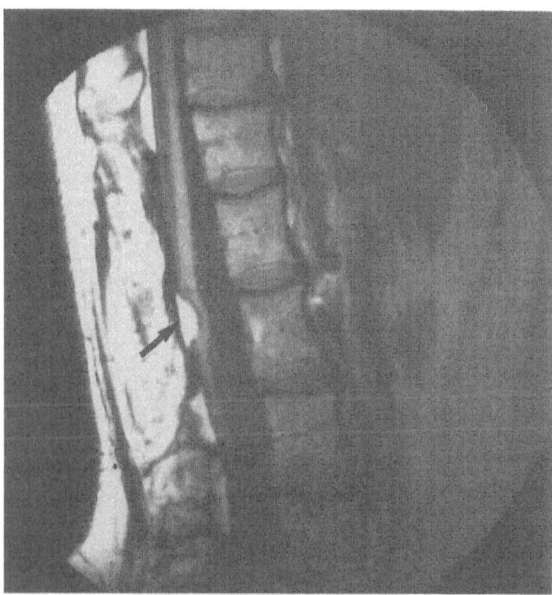

Fig. 7.60. Sagittal MRI (T1 weighted image). Low tethered cord associated with a lipoma (*arrow*).

roots and the filum terminale (Altman and Altman 1987) (Figs 7.60 and 7.61). Extradural extension is not uncommon and lipomas may reach the subcutaneous tissues to present as a skin mass.

The term "lipomyeloschisis" is applied when the incompletely closed end of cord is embedded in the lipoma with no clear identifiable interface (Merx et al. 1989).

Conversely, a subdural lipoma is rare in the absence of dysraphism (1% of all spinal cord tumours). The thoracic and cervicothoracic regions are most commonly affected. With high cervical lesions extension into the posterior fossa may be encountered (Fan et al. 1989). Almost invariably the lipomas are dorsal to the cord and result in its anterior displacement and compression (Giuffre 1966).

Diastematomyelia

Diastematomyelia is the presence of a cleft within the spinal cord resulting in two hemicords, which usually extend over a limited number of segments (Fig. 7.62). Below the level of the defect, which lies in the majority (85%) of cases between the 9th thoracic and first sacral levels, the hemicords unite in 90% of cases to form one cord (Hilal et al. 1974). The hemicords are usually unequal with the smaller being associated with a small extremity (Scatliff et al. 1989). The canal is invariably widened at the site of the split cord. The dura and arachnoid may be duplicated with an osteocartilaginous or fibrous spur penetrating typically the lower part of the intradural cleft. Less commonly the cord is split within the intact dural sleeve (Harwood-Nash 1981; Merx et al. 1989).

Scatliff et al. (1989) found a "hairy patch" on the skin at the level of the spur in 8 patients out of 25 with diastematomyelia.

Plain films are nearly always abnormal but the bony spur may be difficult to detect (Fitz 1982).

Scoliosis is common, occurring in between 60% and 70% of patients. Of patients with congenital scoliosis 18% have occult spinal dysraphism with diastematomyelia as the commonest abnormality (McMaster 1984), but there is no association between idiopathic scoliosis (where there is no congenital bony abnormality) and dysraphism.

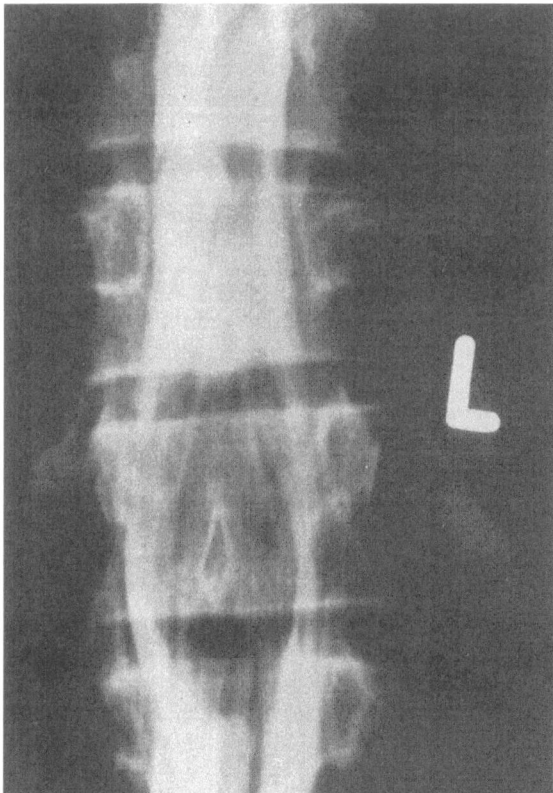

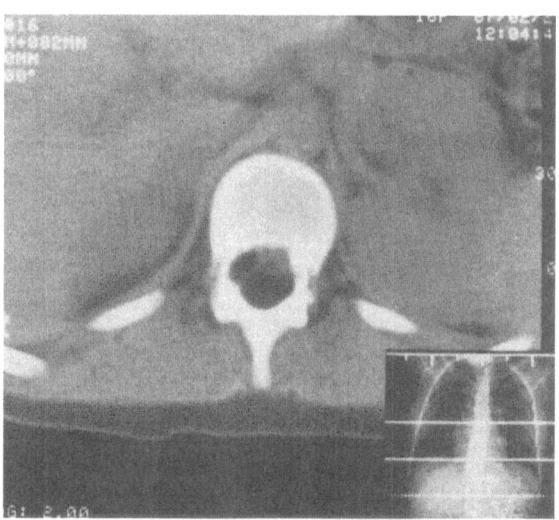

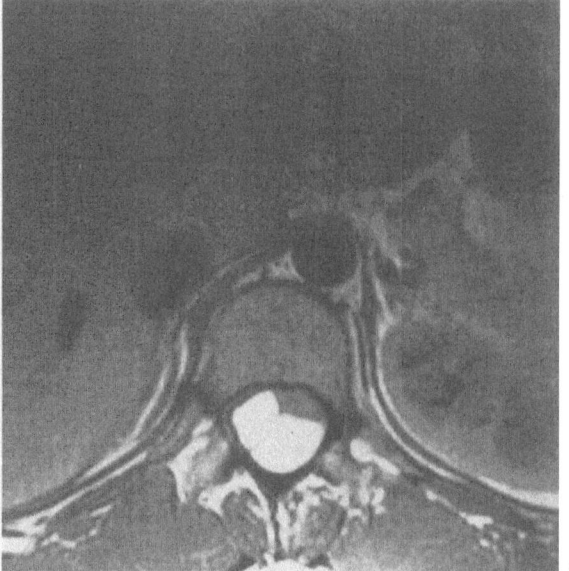

Fig. 7.61. Myelogram (**a**), CT myelogram (**b**) and axial MRI (T1 weighted image) (**c**). Intradural lipoma. On CT the fatty tumour is low in attenuation contrasting with the high signal return with MRI. Fat characteristically returns a high signal on both T1 and T2 weighted images.

Tight Filum Terminale

A pathological filum is short and measures more than 2 mm in thickness at the lumbosacral level (Harwood-Nash 1981). It is attached to the periosteum of the neural arches of the sacrum and thus holds the conus in a low position (Merx et al. 1989). The dura is usually widened and a lipoma, or less commonly a dermoid, may be attached to its distal end.

Split Notochord Syndrome and Arachnoid Cysts

Split notochord syndrome is a consequence of a persisting embryonal communication between gut and dorsal skin. Isolated diverticula, duplications and neurenteric cysts may be found (Burrows and Sutcliffe 1968). As the bowel migrates inferiorly the spinal abnormality is usually located in the thoracic or lower cervical regions. Usually associated with anterior spina bifida, the enteric-lined cysts can be in the prevertebral, postvertebral or intracanalicular compartments. The spinal cord is usually displaced posteriorly and there may be an association with diastematomyelia.

Arachnoid cysts are different from neurenteric cysts (Nabors et al. 1988). They are rare, intra- or extradural diverticula of the subarachnoid space and communicate with the latter through a narrow neck (Kendall et al. 1982; Alvisi et al. 1987).

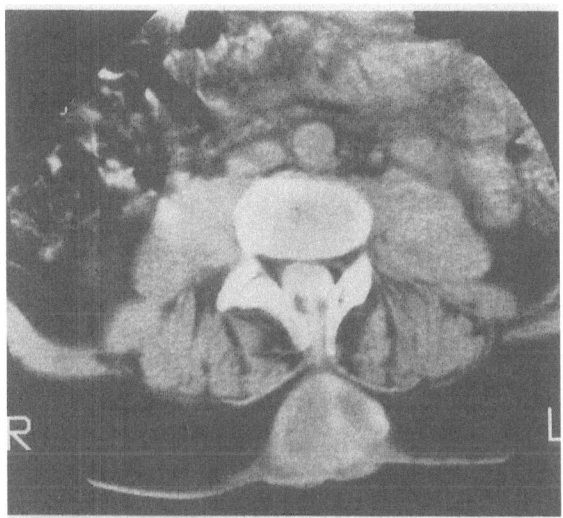

Fig. 7.62. CT myelogram. Diastematomyelia associated with a neural arch defect and meningocele.

Although of congenital origin they are not associated with any spinal dysraphic lesions. They grow slowly perhaps through a valvular action (Kendall et al. 1982). Mostly situated behind the cord in the cervical and dorsal regions, they fill with intrathecal contrast medium only in the supine position. Filling may also be delayed. Neurological symptoms are produced by compression of the cord and nerve roots (Cloward 1968). Pain may result from bone erosion which is seen in all symptomatic cases.

Imaging in Dysraphism

Plain radiography is highly sensitive and clearly demonstrates the osseous defects, scoliosis and bony spurs which accompany dysraphism. Normal radiographs, however, do not exclude a significant dysraphic cord abnormality and more specific investigations should be pursued in the light of clinical suspicion.

Until recently water-soluble myelography and CT had been most sensitive and reliable techniques when used in combination (Resjo et al. 1979). The paramedian approach for the lumbar puncture is advised to avoid possible damage to a low-positioned cord and it can also be anticipated that the cord will be at the convex side of scoliosis (Merx et al. 1989). Myelography has the advantage of screening the entire spine quickly and that an abnormal spinal curvature poses little difficulty. CT should then be performed at the suspicious abnormal areas (Petterson et al. 1982). Recent studies have demonstrated that the sensitivity of MRI compares favourably with CT myelography (Han et al.

1985; Barnes et al. 1986). Multiplanar acquisitions are usually necessary for more complete delineation of the dysraphic myelopathy. Both CT and MRI have the capability of displaying the full extent of any extradural component of the dysraphic abnormality. However, MRI has the additional advantage of detecting any intramedullary abnormalities such as cavities or myelomalacia (Davis et al. 1988; Raghavan et al. 1989).

Spinal Angiomas

Angiomatous malformations of the spine are divided into dural (or epidural) and intradural types. Although this classification is based on anatomical criteria related to location of the nidus, they are likely to be different aetiologically (acquired vs. congenital) and there are also distinctive features in the clinical presentation, response to treatment and prognosis.

A dural arteriovenous fistula is by definition situated on the outer surface of the dura or of a dural extension of a nerve root sheath and is supplied by a dural branch of intercostal or lumbar artery. It drains intrathecally via a medullary vein (occasionally two) retrogradely to the coronal plexus (Kendall and Logue 1977).

Dural malformations are the commonest type and the vast majority are "low flow" lesions. Commoner in men, they usually present in an older age group with steadily progressive paresis (Symon et al. 1984). The symptoms are often exaggerated by exercise. The nidus is situated in 96% of cases in the lower thoracic or lumbar region (Rosenblum et al. 1987). It is often difficult angiographically to be certain whether the dilated vessels are situated just on the outer or also the inner dural surface but the nidus is usually projected outside the confines of the spinal cord (Symon et al. 1984).

The intradural malformations, supplied by medullary arteries, are subdivided further into direct "arteriovenous fistulae" some of which are intramedullary and the "glomus" and "juvenile" intramedullary types. The diagnosis is often suspected clinically when a patient of a younger age group (less than 30) presents acutely with spinal subarachnoid haemorrhage. The majority of the intradural lesions are "high flow" and involve the cervical as well as the thoracic segments. There is a high incidence (44%) of associated arterial or venous saccular aneurysms (Rosenblum et al. 1987). As with dural malformations the venous drainage is effected via the coronal venous plexus. It is assumed that the slow neurological deterioration is due to ischaemic hypoxia or oedema result-

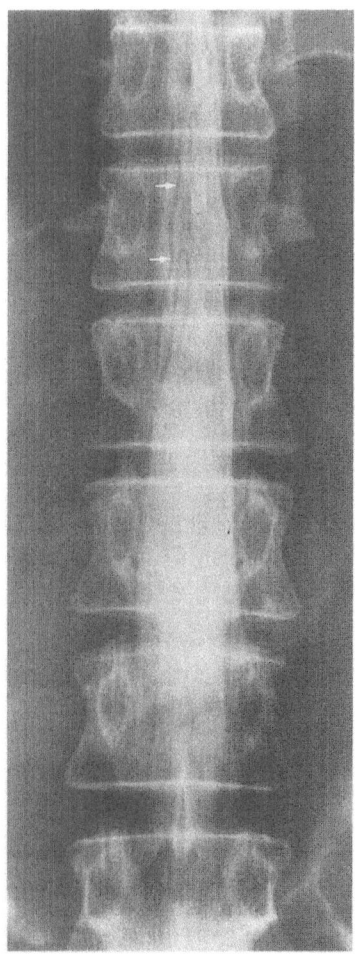

Fig. 7.63. Myelogram. Angioma of the conus. Vessels appear as serpiginous filling defects (*arrows*).

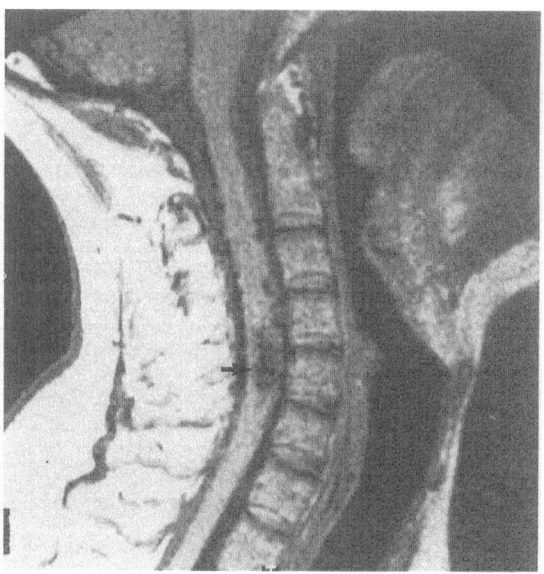

Fig. 7.64. Sagittal MRI (T1 weighted image). Cervical intra-medullary angioma (*arrow*). Vessels are seen superiorly as rounded "signal voids".

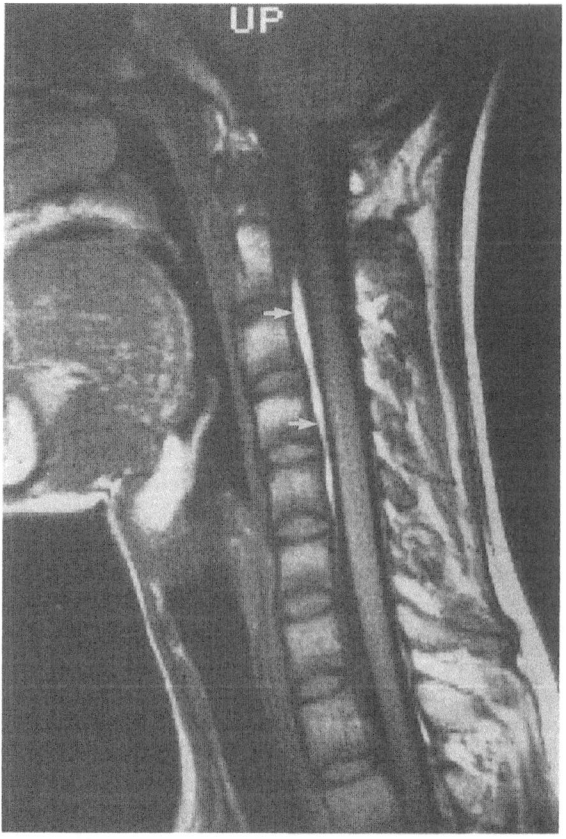

Fig. 7.65. Sagittal MRI (T1 weighted image). Cervical extradural haematoma (*arrow*). (By courtesy of P. Hudgson, Newcastle.)

ing from the high venous pressure in both types of lesions. In almost all cases of vascular malformations the dilated and tortuous coronal venous plexus is seen on myelography, particularly the supine radiographs. It is often impossible to differentiate on myelography between dural and intra-dural lesions or accurately to localise the site of the nidus (Fig. 7.63). Difficulties in diagnosis arise when there is cord enlargement with dilated vessels evident on myelography making intramedullary tumours or haemorrhage and oedema indistinguishable.

MRI particularly utilising gradient echo sequences is sensitive in detecting these vascular malformations and in determining the intra-medullary component of the arteriovenous malformation (Fig. 7.64). The differentiation between nidus, haemorrhage and tumour can be readily made (Minami et al. 1988).

Selective angiography, however, remains the procedure of choice for accurate assessment prior to any therapeutic attempt whether by surgery (Symon et al. 1984; Rosenblum et al. 1987) or percutaneous embolisation (Doppman et al. 1971; Horton et al. 1986).

Spinal Epidural Haematoma

An epidural haematoma is a rare but important cause of spinal cord compression. The majority of cases seem to be spontaneous although minor trauma is implicated in some cases. Other recognised associations include anticoagulant therapy, vertebral haemangioma, lumbar puncture and epidural anaesthesia. The diagnosis can be made with CT (Williams and Nelson 1987) but MRI is the preferred investigation (Fig. 7.65) (Rothfus et al. 1987).

References

Alberico AM, Sahni KS, Hall JA, Young HF (1986) High thoracic disc herniation. Neurosurgery 19:449–451

Alenghat JP, Hallett M, Kido DK (1982) Spinal cord compression in diffuse idiopathic skeletal hyperostosis. Radiology 142:119–120

Altman NR, Altman DH (1987) MR imaging of spinal dysraphism. AJNR 8:533–538

Alvisi C, Cerisoli M, Giulioni M, Guerra L (1987) Long term results of surgically treated congenital intradural spinal arachnoid cysts. J Neurosurg 67:333–335

Amundsen P (1981) Cervical myelography with metrizamide: Seven years' experience. Radiologe 21:282–287

Arce CA, Dohrmann GJ (1985) Thoracic disc herniation: improved diagnosis with computed tomography screening and review of literature. Surg Neurol 23:356–361

Aubin ML, Vignaud J, Jardin C, Bar D (1981) Computed tomography in 75 clinical cases of syringomyelia. AJNR 2:199–204

Austin RM, Bankoff MS, Carter BI (1981) Gas collections in the spinal canal on computed tomography. J Comput Assist Tomogr 5:522–524

Banna M, Gryspeerdt GL (1971) Intraspinal tumours in children (excluding dysraphism). Clin Radiol 22:17–32

Barloon TJ, Yuh WTC, Yang CJC, Schultz DH (1987) Spinal subarachnoid tumour seeding from intracranial metastasis: MR findings. J Comput Assist Tomogr 11:242–244

Barnes PD, Lester PD, Yamanashi WS, Prince JR (1986) MRI in infants and children with spinal dysraphism. AJR 147:339–346

Beabout JW, McLeod RA, Dahlin DC (1979) Benign tumours. Semin Roentgenol XIV:33–43

Beers GJ, Carter AP, Leiter BE, Tilak SP, Shah RR (1985) Interobserver discrepancies in distance measurements from lumbar spine CT scans. AJR 144:395–398

Beltran J, Noto AM, Chakeres DW, Christoforidis AJ (1987) Tumours of the osseous spine: Staging with MR imaging versus CT. Radiology 162:565–569

Blackburne JS, Velikas EP (1977) Spondylolisthesis in children and adolescents. J Bone Joint Surg 59B:490–494

Blau JN, Logue V (1961) Intermittent claudication of the cauda equina. Lancet i:1080–1086

Blau JN, Logue V (1978) The natural history of intermittent claudication of the cauda equina. A long-term follow-up study. Brain 101:211–222

Boisserie-Lacroix M, Kien P, Caille JM (1987) Imaging of intradural extramedullary tumours: neurinomas and meningiomas. J Neuroradiol 14:66–81

Bonafé A, Manelfe C, Espagno J, Guiraud B, Rascol A (1980) Evaluation of syringomyelia with metrizamide computed tomographic myelography. J Comput Assist Tomogr 4:797–802

Boone D, Parsons D, Lachmann SM, Sherwood T (1985) Spina bifida occulta: lesion or anomaly? Clin Radiol 36:159–161

Bosacco SJ, Berman AT (1983) Surgical management of lumbar disease. Radiol Clin North Am 21:377–393

Bradford DS (1979) Spondylolysis and spondylolisthesis. Curr Pract Orthop Surg 8:12–37

Buirski G, Watt I (1987) Computed tomography (HRCT) of spondylytic spondylolisthesis. Clin Radiol 38:553 (Abs)

Bundschuh CV, Modic MT, Ross JS, Masaryk TJ, Bohlman H (1988) Epidural fibrosis and recurrent disk herniation in the lumbar spine: MR imaging assessment. AJR 150:923–932

Burrows FGO, Sutcliffe J (1968) The split notochord syndrome. Br J Radiol 41:844–847

Burton CV, Kirkaldy-Willis WH, Yong-Hing K, Heithoff KB (1981) Causes of failure of surgery on the lumbar spine. Clin Orthop 157:191–199

Butt, WP (1989) Radiology for back pain. Clin Radiol 40:6–10

Bydder GM, Brown J, Niendorf HP, Young IR (1985) Enhancement of cervical intraspinal tumours in MR imaging with intravenous Gadolinium-DTPA. J Comput Assist Tomogr 9:847–851

Byrd SE (1988) Disorders of midline structures: Holoprosencephaly, absence of corpus callosum and chiari malformations. Semin US CT MR 9:201–215

Carrera GF, Haughton VM, Syvertsen A, Williams AL (1980) Computed tomography of the lumbar facet joints. Radiology 134:145–148

Castillo M, Quencer RM, Green BA, Montalvo BM (1987) Syringomyelia as a consequence of compressive extramedullary lesions: Postoperative clinical and radiological manifestations. AJNR 8: 973–978

Chafetz N, Genant HK (1983) Computed tomography of the spine. Orthop Clin North Am 14:147–169

Chason JL, Walker FB, Landers JW (1963) Metastatic carcinoma in the central nervous system and dorsal root ganglia. Cancer 16:781–787

Checkley DR, Zhu XP, Antoun NM, Chen SZ, Isherwood I (1984) An investigation into the problems of attenuation and area measurements made from CT images of pulmonary nodules. J Comput Assist Tomogr 8:237–243

Ciric I, Mikhael MA, Tarkington JA, Vick NA (1980) The lateral recess syndrome. J Neurosurg 53:433–443

Cloward RB (1968) Congenital spinal extradual cysts: Case report with review of literature. Ann Surg 168:851–864

Cohen AR, Wisoff JH, Allen JC, Epstein F (1989) Malignant astrocytomas of the spinal cord. J Neurosurg 70:50–54

Colman LK, Porter BA, Redmond III J et al. (1988) Early diagnosis of spinal metastases by CT and MR. J Comput Assist Tomogr 12: 423–426

Cronqvist S, Brismar J (1981) Cervical myelography with metrizamide. Acta Radiol [Diagn] (Stockh) 21:282–287

Crouzet G, Vasdev A, Chirossel JP (1983) Computerized tomography in sciaticas due to lumbar degenerative lesions (disc herniation/spondylosis, narrow lumbar canal). J Neuroradiol 10: 325–344

Czervionke LF, Daniels DL (1988) Cervical spine anatomy

and pathologic processes: Application of new MR imaging techniques. Radiol Clin North Am 26:921–948

Czervionke LF, Daniels DL, Ho PSP et al. (1988) Cervical neural foramina: Correlative anatomic and MR imaging study. Radiology 169: 753–759

Davis PC, Hoffman JC, Ball TI et al. (1988) Spinal abnormalities in pediatric patients: MR imaging findings compared with clinical, myelographic and surgical findings. Radiology 166:679–685

De Bruïne FT, Kroon HM (1988) Spinal chordoma: Radiologic features in 14 cases. AJR 150:861–863

De Santis M, Crisi G, Folchivici F (1984) Late contrast enhancement in the CT diagnosis of herniated lumbar disk. Neuroradiology 26:303–307

Deutsch M, Reigel DH (1980) The value of myelography in the management of childhood medulloblastoma. Cancer 45:2194–2197

DiChiro G, Schellinger D (1976) Computed tomography of spinal cord after lumbar intrathecal introduction of metrizamide (computer assisted myelography). Radiology 120:101–104

Dillon WP, Norman D, Newton TH, Bolla K, Mark A (1989) Intradural spinal cord lesions: Gd-DTPA-enhanced MR imaging. Radiology 170:229–237

Dixon AK (1986a) Computed tomography of the lumbar spine. In: Steiner RE, Sherwood T (eds) Recent advances in radiology and medical imaging, vol 8. Churchill Livingstone, Edinburgh, pp 25–43

Dixon AK (1986b) Who has most epidural fat? Information from computed tomography. BrJ Radiol 59:475–480

Dixon AK, Bannon R (1987) Computed tomography of the post operative lumbar spine: the need for, and optimal dose of, intravenous contrast medium. Br J Radiol 60: 215–222

Doppman JL, Di Chiro G, Ommaya AK (1971) Percutaneous embolisation of spinal cord arteriovenous malformations. J Neurosurg 34:48–55

Dorwart RH, Vogler JB, Helms CA (1983) Spinal stenosis. Radiol Clin North Am 21:301–325

Edelman R, Shoukimas G, Stark D et al. (1985) High resolution surface-coil imaging of lumbar disk disease. AJR 144:1123–1129

Edelson RN, Deck MP, Posner JB (1972) Intramedullary spinal cord metastases: clinical and radiographic findings in nine cases. Neurology 22:1222–1231

Edgar MA, Park WM (1974) Induced pain patterns on passive straight leg raising. J Bone Joint Surg 56B:658–667

Edwards WC, Orme TJ, Orr-Edwards G (1987) CT discography: Prognostic value in the selection of patients for chemonucleolysis. Spine 12:792–795

Eisenberg RA, Bremer AM, Northup HM (1986) Intradural herniated cervical disk: A case report and review of the literature. AJNR 7:492–494

Eisenstein S (1978) Spondylolysis: A skeletal investigation of two population groups. J Bone Joint Surg 60B:488–494

Epstein BS, Epstein JA, Jones MD (1977) Lumbar spinal stenosis. Radiol Clin North Am 15:277–240

Epstein F, Wisoff J (1987) Intra-axial tumors of the cervicomedullary junction. J Neurosurg 67:483–487

Euinton HA, Locke TJ, Barrington NA, Getty CJM, Davies GK (1985) Is water soluble radiculography accurate in predicting the level of bone entrapment of lumbosacral nerve roots? J Bone Joint Surg 67B:499

Fan CJ, Veerapen RJ, Tan CT (1989) Case report: Subdural spinal lipoma with posterior fossa extension. Clin Radiol 40:91–94

Farfan HF, Cossette JW, Robertson HG, Wells RVR, Kraus H (1970) The effects of fusion on the lumbar intervertebral joints: The role of fusion in the production of disc degeneration. J Bone Joint Surg 52A:468–497

Fidas A, MacDonald HL, Elton RA, Wild SR, Chisholm GD, Scott R (1987) Prevalence and patterns of spina bifida occulta in 2707 normal adults. Clin Radiol 38:537–542

Firooznia H, Pinto RS, Lin JP, Baruch HH, Zansner J (1976) Chordoma: Radiographic evaluation of 20 cases. AJR 127:797–805

Firooznia H, Benjamin V, Kricheff I, Rafii M, Golimbu C (1984) CT of lumbar spine disk herniation: Correlation with surgical findings. AJR 142:587–592

Firooznia H, Golimbu C, Rafii M, Reede DL, Kricheff I, Bjorkengren A (1986) Computed tomography of spinal chordomas. J Comput Assist Tomogr 10:45–50

Fitz CR (1982) Midline anomalies of the brain and spine. Radiol Clin North Am 20:95–104

Fitzgerald JW, Newman PH (1976) Degenerative spondylolisthesis. J Bone Joint Surg 58B:184–192

Flannigan BD, Lufkin RB, McGlade C et al. (1987) MR imaging of the cervical spine: Neurovascular anatomy. AJNR 8:27–32

Fon GT, Sage MR (1984) Computed tomography in cervical disc disease when myelography is unsatisfactory. Clin Radiol 35:47–50

Forbes WStC, Isherwood I (1978) Computed tomography in syringomyelia and the associated Arnold–Chiari type I malformation. Neuroradiology 15:73–78

Ford LT, Gilula LA, Murphy WA, Gado MN (1977) Analysis of gas in vacuum lumbar disc. AJR 128:1056–1057

Fraser RD (1982) Chymopapain for the treatment of intervertebral disk herniation: A preliminary report of a double blind study. Spine 7:608–612

Fries JW, Abodeely DA, Vijungco JG, Yeager VL, Gaffey WR (1982) Computed tomography of herniated and extruded nucleus pulposus. J Comput Assist Tomogr 6:874–887

Frocrain L, Duvauferrier R, Husson JL, Noel J, Ramee A, Pawlotsky J (1989) Recurrent postoperative sciatica: Evaluation with MR imaging and enhanced CT. Radiology 170:531–533

Gebarski S, Maynard FW, Gabrielsen KO, Knake JE, Latack JT, Hoff JT (1984) Post traumatic progressive myelopathy. Radiology 157:379–385

Gentry LR, Strother CM, Turski PA, Javid MJ, Sackett JF (1985a) Chymopapain chemonucleolysis: Correlation of diagnostic radiographic factors and clinical outcome. AJNR 6:311–320

Gentry LR, Turski PA, Strother CM, Javid MJ, Sackett JF (1985b) Chymopapain chemonucleolysis: CT changes after treatment. AJNR 6:321–329

Gillespie JE, Jenkins JPR, Metcalfe RA, Isherwood I (1986) Magnetic resonance imaging in syringomyelia. Acta Radiol [Suppl] 369:239–369

Giuffre R (1966) Intradural spinal lipomas: Review of the literature (99 cases) and report of an additional case. Acta Neurochir (Wien) 14:69–95

Goldberg AL, Rothfus WE, Deeb ZL, Khoury MB, Daffner RH (1988) Thoracic disc herniation versus spinal metastases: Optimizing diagnosis with magnetic resonance imaging. Skeletal Radiol 17:423–426

Goy AMC, Pinto RS, Raghavendra BN, Epstein FJ, Kricheff II (1986) Intramedullary spinal cord tumours: MR imaging with emphasis on associated cysts. Radiology 161:381–386

Graves VB, Finney HL, Mailander J (1986) Intradural lumbar disk herniation. AJNR 7:495–497

Grenier N, Kressel HY, Schiebler ML, Grossman RI, Dalinka MK (1987) Normal and degenerative posterior spinal structures: MR imaging. Radiology 165:517–525

Grenier N, Kressel HY, Schiebler ML, Grossman RI (1989) Isthmic spondylolysis of the lumbar spine: MR imaging at 1.5T. Radiology 170:489–493

Grogan JP, Hemminghytt S, Williams AL, Carrera GF, Haughton VM (1982) Spondylolysis studied with computed tomography. Radiology 145:737–742

Gulati AN, Weinstein R, Studdard E (1981) CT scan of the spine for herniated discs. Neuroradiology 22:57–60

Guthkelch AN (1974) Diastematomyelia with median septum. Brain 97:729–742

Hajek PC, Baker LL, Goobar JE et al. (1987) Focal fat deposition in axial bone marrow: MR characteristics. Radiology 162:245–249

Han JS, Benson JE, Kaufman B et al. (1985) Demonstration of diastematomyelia and associated abnormalities with MR imaging. AJNR 6:215–219

Hanley FN, Levy JA (1989) Surgical treatment of isthmic lumbosacral spondylolisthesis – Analysis of variables influencing results. Spine 14:48–50

Harsh GR, Sypert GW, Weinstein PR, Ross D, Wilson C (1987) Cervical spine stenosis secondary to ossification of the posterior longitudinal ligament. J Neurosurg 67:349–357

Harwood-Nash DC (1981) Computed tomography of the paediatric spine: A protocol for the 1980s. Radiol Clin North Am. 19:479–494

Hawkins TD (1984) The abnormal spine. In: du Boulay GH (ed) A textbook of radiological diagnosis, vol I. HK Lewis, London, pp 455–509

Heller CA, Staney P, Lewis-Jones BC, Heller RF (1983) Value of X-ray examination of the cervical spine. Br Med J 287:1276–1278

Helms CA, Dorwart RH, Gray M (1982) The CT appearance of conjoined nerve roots and differentiation from a herniated nucleus pulposus. Radiology 144:803–807

Hilal SK, Marton D, Pollack E (1974) Diastematomyelia in children: Radiographic study of 34 cases. Radiology 112: 609–621

Hodge CJ, Binet EF, Kieffer SA (1978) Intradural herniation of lumbar intervertebral discs. Spine 3:346–350

Hollis PH, Malis LI, Zapulla RA (1986) Neurological deterioration after lumbar puncture below complete spinal subarachnoid block. J Neurosurg 64:253–256

Holtås S, Nordström C-H, Larson E-M, Pettersson H (1987) MR imaging of intradural disk herniation. J Comput Assist Tomogr 11:353–356

Horton JA, Latchaw RE, Gold LHA, Pang D (1986) Embolisation of intramedullary arteriovenous malformations of the spinal cord. AJNR 7:113–118

Huckman MS, Clark JW, McNeill TW et al. (1987) Chemonucleation and changes observed on lumbar MR scan: Preliminary report. AJNR 8:1–4

Hueftle MF, Modic MT, Ross JS et al. (1988) Lumbar spine post operative MR imaging with Gd-DTPA. Radiology 167:817–824

Hukins DWL (1987) Properties of spinal materials. In: Jayson MIV (ed) The lumbar spine and back pain, 3rd edn. Churchill Livingstone, Edinburgh, pp 138–160

Isherwood I, Antoun NM (1984) Computed tomography of the spine. In: du Boulay GH (ed) A textbook of radiological diagnosis, vol I. HK Lewis, London, pp 581–601

Isherwood I, Antoun N (1987) CT scanning in the assessment of lumbar spine problems. In: Jayson MIV (ed) The lumbar spine and back pain. Churchill Livingstone, Edinburgh, pp 269–285

Isherwood I, Prendergast DJ, Hickey DS, Jenkins JPR (1986) Quantitative analysis of intervertebral disc structure. Acta Radiol [Suppl] 369:492–495

Jackson RP, Glah JJ (1987) Foraminal and extraforaminal lumbar disc herniation: diagnosis and treatment. Spine 12:577–585

James CCM, Lassman LP (1972) Spinal dysraphism: Spina bifida occulta. Butterworths, London, pp 82–96

Janin Y, Epstein JA, Carras R, Khan A (1981) Osteoid osteoma and osteoblastomas of the spine. Neurosurgery 8:31–38

Javid MJ, Nordby EJ, Ford LT (1983) Safety and efficacy of chymopapain (chymodiactin) in herniated nucleus pulposus with sciatica: Results of a randomised double-blind trial. JAMA 249:2489–2494

Jenkins JPR, Hickey DS, Zhu XP, Machin M, Isherwood I (1985) MR imaging of the intervertebral disc: A quantitative study. Br J Radiol 58:705–709

Jinkins JR, Bashir R, Al-Mefty O, Al-Kawi MZ, Fox JL (1986) Cystic necrosis of the spinal cord in compressive cervical myelopathy: Demonstration by iopamidol CT myelography. AJR 147:767–775

Jinkins JR, Wiltemore AJ, Bradley WG (1989) The anatomic basis of vertebrogenic pain and the autonomic syndrome associated with lumbar disk extrusion. AJNR 10:219–231

Johnson DW, Farnum GN, Latchow RE, Erba SM (1989) MR imaging of the pars interarticularis. AJR 152:327–332

Jones MD, Pais MJ, Omiya B (1988) Bony overgrowths and abnormal calcifications about the spine. Radio Clin North Am 26:1213–1234

Kaffenberger DA, Shah CP, Murtagh FR, Wilson CA, Silbiger M (1988) MR imaging of spinal cord haemangioblastoma associated with syringomyelia. J Comput Assist Tomogr 12:495–498

Kan S, Fox AJ, Viñuela F, Debrun G (1983) Spinal cord size in syringomyelia: Change with position on metrizamide myelography. Radiology 146:409–414

Kendall BE, Logue V (1977) Spinal epidural angiomatous malformations draining into intrathecal veins. Neuroradiology 13:181–189

Kendall BE, Valentine AR, Keis B (1982) Spinal arachnoid cysts: Clinical and radiological correlation with prognosis. Neuroradiology 22:225–234

Ketonen L, Gyldensted C (1986) Lumbar disc disease evaluated by myelography and postmyelography spinal computed tomography. Neuroradiology 28:144–149

Kieffer SA, Sherry RG, Wellenstein DE, King RB (1982) Bulging lumbar intervertebral disk: Myelographic differentiation from herniated disk with nerve root compression. AJNR 3:51–58

Kier EL (1988) Some developmental and evolutionary aspects of the lumbosacral spine. In: Gouaze A, Salamon G (eds). Brain anatomy and magnetic resonance imaging. Springer, Berlin, Heidelberg, New York, pp 116–139

Klara PM, McDonnell DE (1986) Ossification of the posterior longitudinal ligament in Caucasians. Diagnosis and surgical intervention. Neurosurgery 19:212–217

Knutsson F (1942) The vacuum phenomenon in the intervertebral discs. Acta Radiol 23:173–179

Kornberg M (1986) Extreme lateral lumber disc herniation: Clinical syndrome and computed tomography recognition. Spine 12:586–589

Kortelainen P, Puranen J, Koiristo E, Lahde S (1985) Symptoms and signs of sciatica and their relation to the localisation of the lumbar disc herniation. Spine 10:88–92

Krausé D, Maitrot D, Veillon F et al. (1986a) Migratory lumbar disc herniation, computerized tomography and surgery. J Neuroradiol 13:39–52

Krausé D, Woerly B, Drapé JL et al. (1986b) Soft cervical disc herniations. Acta Radiol [Suppl] 369:236–238

Lamont AC, Zachary J, Sheldon PWE (1981) Cervical cord size in metrizamide myelography. Clin Radiol 31:409–412

Landman JA, Hoffman Jr JC, Braun IF, Barrow DL (1984) Value of computed tomographic myelography in the recognition of cervical herniated disk. AJNR 5:391–394

Lapointe JS, Graeb DA, Nugent RA, Robertson WD (1986) Value of intravenous contrast enhancement in the CT evaluation of intraspinal tumour. AJR 146:103–107

Larsen JL, Smith D (1980a) Size of the subarachnoid space in stenosis of the lumbar canal. Acta Radiol [Diagn] 21:627–632

Larsen JL, Smith D (1980b) Vertebral body size in lumbar canal stenosis. Acta Radiol [Diagn] 21:785–788

Larsson EM, Holtas S, Zygmunt S (1989) Pre- and postoperative MR imaging of the craniocervical junction in rheumatoid arthritis. AJNR 10:89–94

Lee BCP, Kazam E, Newman AD (1978) Computed tomography of the spine and cord. Radiology 128:95–102

Lee BCP, Zimmerman RD, Manning JJ, Deck MDF (1985) MR imaging of syringomyelia and hydromyelia. AJNR 6:221–228

Li KC, Chui MC (1987) Conventional and CT metrizamide myelography in Arnold–Chiari I malformation and syringomyelia. AJNR 8:11–17

Lindblom K, Hultqvist G (1950) Absorption of protruded disc material. J Bone Joint Surg 32A:557–560

Logue V (1971) Syringomyelia: A radiodiagnostic and radiotherapeutic saga. Clin Radiol 22:2–16

Love JG, Shorn VG (1965) Thoracic disc protrusion. JAMA 191:627–631

Macnab I (1971) The traction spur. J Bone Joint Surg 53A:663–670

Macnab I (1977) Backache. Williams and Wilkins, Baltimore

Malmivaara A, Videman T, Euosma E, Troup JDG (1986) Facet joint orientation, facet and costovertebral joint osteoarthrosis, disc degeneration, vertebral body osteoporosis and Schmorl's nodes in thoracolumbar junctional region of cadaveric spines. Spine 12:458–463

Masaryk TJ, Ross JS, Modic MT, Boumphrey F, Bohlman H, Wilber G (1988) High resolution MR imaging of sequestrated lumbar intervertebral disks. AJR 150:1155–1162

Maurice-Williams RS (1981) Spinal degenerative disease. John Wright, Bristol

McAllister MD, O'Leary DH (1987) CT myelography of subarachnoid leukemic infiltration of the lumbar thecal sac and lumbar nerve roots. AJNR 8:568–569

McAllister VL, Sage MR (1976) The radiology of thoracic disc protrusion. Clin Radiol 27:291–299

McAllister VL, Kendall BE, Bull JWD (1975) Symptomatic vertebral haemangiomas. Brain 98:71–80

McCarron RF, Wimpee MW, Hudkins PG, Laros GS (1987) The inflammatory effect of nucleus pulposus. A possible element in the pathogenesis of low back pain. Spine 12:760–764

McIvor GWD, Kirkaldy-Willis WH (1976) Pathological and myelographic changes in the major types of lumbar canal stenosis. Clin Orthop 115:72–76

McMaster MJ (1984) Occult intraspinal anomalies and congenital scoliosis. J Bone Joint Surg 66A:588–601

Merine D, Wang H, Kumar AJ, Ziureich SJ, Rosenbaum AE (1987) CT myelography and MR imaging of acute transverse myelitis. J Comput Assist Tomogr 11:606–608

Merx JL, Bakker-Niezen SH, Thijssen HOM, Waeder HAD (1989) The tethered spinal cord syndrome: a correlation of radiological features and preoperative findings in 30 patients. Neuroradiology 31: 63–70

Meyer JE, Lepke RA, Lindfors KK et al. (1984) Chordomas: Their CT appearance in the cervical, thoracic and lumbar spine. Radiology 153:693–696

Mikhael MA (1983) High resolution computed tomography in the diagnosis of laterally herniated lumbar discs. Comput Radiol 7:161–166

Minagi H, Gronner AT (1969) Calcification of the posterior longitudinal ligament. A cause of cervical myelopathy. AJR 105:365–369

Minami S, Sagoh T, Nishimura K et al. (1988) Spinal arteriovenous malformation: MR imaging. Radiology 169:109–115

Modic MT, Masaryk T, Bounphrey F, Goormastic M, Bell G (1986a) Lumber herniated disk disease and canal stenosis: Prospective evaluation by surface coil MR, CT and myelography. AJR 147:757–765

Modic MT, Masaryk TJ, Mulopulos GP, Bundschuh C, Han JS, Bohlman H (1986b) Cervical radiculopathy: prospective evaluation with surface coil MR imaging, CT with metrizamide and metrizamide myelography. Radiology 161:753–759

Modic MT, Masaryk TJ, Ross JS, Carta J (1988a) Imaging of degenerative disk disease. Radiology 168:177–186

Modic MT, Steinberg P, Ross JS, Masaryk TJ, Carta J (1988b) Degenerative disk disease: Assessment of changes in vertebral body marrow with MR imaging. Radiology 166:193–199

Mohr PD, Strang FA, Sambrook MA, Boddie HG (1977) The clinical and surgical features in 40 patients with primary cerebellar ectopia (adult Chiari malformation). QJ Med [New Series] 46:85–96

Mooney V, (1987) Facet joint sydrome. In: Jayson MIV (ed) The lumbar spine and back pain, 3rd edn. Churchill Livingstone, Edinburgh

Mooney V, Robertson J (1976) The facet syndrome. Clin Orthop 115:149–156

Murakami J, Russell WJ, Hayabuchi N, Kimura S (1982) Computed tomography of posterior longitudinal ligament ossification: Its appearance and diagnostic value with special reference to thoracic lesions. J Comput Assist Tomogr 6:41–50

Nabors M, Patt G, Byrd E et al. (1988) Updated assessment and current classification of spinal meningeal cysts. J Neurosurg 68:366–377

Nelson MJ, Gold LHA (1983) CT evaluation of intervertebral foramina lesions with normal or non-diagnostic myelograms. Report of ten cases. Comput Radiol 7:155–160

Nose T, Egashira T, Enomoto T, Maki Y (1987) Ossification of the posterior longitudinal ligament: a clinico-radiological study of 74 cases. J Neurol Neurosurg Psychiatry 50:321–326

Oakley RH, Carty H (1984) Review of spondylolisthesis and spondylolysis in paediatric practice. Br J Radiol 57:877–885

O'Carroll MP, Witcombe JB (1979) Primary disorders of bone with 'spinal block'. Clin Radiol 30:399–406

Parizel PM, Balériaux D, Rodesch G et al. (1989a) Gd-DTPA-enhanced MR imaging of spinal tumours. AJNR 10:249–258

Parizel PM, Rodesch G, Baleriaux D et al. (1989b) Gd-DTPA-enhanced MR in thoracic disc herniation. Neuroradiology 31:75–79

Park TS, Hoffman HJ, Hendrick EB, Humphreys RP, Becker LE (1983) Medulloblastoma: clinical presentation and management. Experience at the Hospital for Sick Children Toronto 1950–1980. J Neurosurg 58:543–552

Pate D, Goobar J, Resnick D, Haghighi P, Sartoris D, Pathria MN (1988) Traction osteophytes of the lumbar spine: Radiographic–pathologic correlation. Radiology 166:843–846

Patton DD, Woolfenden JM (1977) Radionuclide bone scanning in discitis of the spine. Radiol Clin North Am 15:177–201

Pedersen HE, Blunk CFJ, Gardner E (1956) The anatomy of lumbosacral posterior rami and meningeal branches of spinal nerves (sinu-vertebral nerves). J Bone Joint Surg 38A:377–391

Penning L, Wilmink JT, Van Woerden HHF, Knol E (1986) CT myelographic findings in degenerative disorders of the cervical spine: Clinical significance. AJNR 7:119–127

Petterson H, Harwood-Nash DCF, Fitz OR, Chuang HS, Armstrong E (1982) Conventional metrizamide myelography (MM) and computed tomographic metrizamide myelography (CTMM) in scoliosis. Radiology 142:111–114

Post MJD, Quencer RM, Green BA et al (1987) Intramedullary spina cord metastases, mainly of non-neurogenic origin. AJNR 8:339–346

Postacchini F, Pezzeri G, Montanaro A, Natali G (1980) Computed tomography in lumbar stenosis. J Bone Joint Surg 62B:78–82

Pullicino P, du Boulay GH, Kendall BE (1979) Xenon enhancement for computed tomography of the spinal cord. Neuroradiology 18:63–66

Quinnell RC, Stockdale HR (1982) The significance of osteophytes on lumbar vertebral bodies in relation to discographic findings. Clin Radiol 33:197–203

Quinnet RJ, Hadler NM (1979) Diagnosis and treatment of backache. Semin Arthritis Rheum 8:261–287

Raghavan N, Barkovich AJ, Edwards M, Norman D (1989) MR imaging in the tethered spinal cord syndrome. AJNR 10:27–36

Raymond J, Dumas JM (1984) Intra articular facet block: Diagnostic test or therapeutic procedure? Radiology 151:333–336

Resjo IM, Harwood-Nash DC, Fitz CR, Chuang S (1979) Computed tomographic metrizamide myelography in syringohydromyelia. Radiology 131:405–407

Resnick D, Niwayama G (1978) Intervertebral disc abnormalities associated with vertebral metastasis: observations in patients and cadavers with prostatic cancer. Invest Radiol 13:182–190

Roberson GH, Llewellyn HJ, Taveras JM (1973) The narrow lumbar spinal canal syndrome. Radiology 107:89–97

Rosenblum B, Oldfield E, Doppman J, DiChiro G (1987) Spinal arteriovenous malformations: a comparison of dural arteriovenous fistulas and intradural AVMs in 81 patients. J Neurosurg 67:795–802

Ross JS, Perez-Reyes N, Masaryk TJ, Bohlman H, Modic M (1987a) Thoracic disk herniation: MR imaging. Radiology 165:511–515

Ross JS, Masaryk TJ, Modic MT, Carter J, Mapstone T, Dengel FH (1987b) Vertebral haemangiomas: MR imaging. Radiology 165:165–169

Ross JS, Masaryk TJ, Modic M et al. (1987c) MR imaging of lumbar arachnoiditis. AJR 149:1025–1032

Ross JS, Modic MT, Masaryk TJ, Hueftle MG (1988) The post operative lumbar spine. Semin Roentgenol 23:125–136

Ross JS, Delamater R, Hueftle MG et al. (1989) Gadolinium-DTPA-enhanced MR imaging of the post operative lumbar spine: Time course and mechanism of enhancement. AJNR 10:37–46

Rothfus WE, Chedid MK, L-Deeb Z, Abla A, Maroon J, Sherman R (1987) MR imaging in the diagnosis of spontaneous spinal epidural haematomas. J Comput Assist Tomogr 11:851–854

Russell EJ, D'Angelo CM, Zimmerman RD, Czervionke LF, Huckman MS (1984) Cervical disk herniation: CT demonstration after contrast enhancement. Radiology 152:703–712

Ryan RW, Lally JF, Kozic Z (1988) Asymptomatic calcified herniated thoracic disks: CT recognition. AJNR 9:363–366

Samuelsson L, Bergström K, Thuomas K-Å, Hemmingsson A, Wallensten R (1987) MR imaging of syringohydromyelia and Chiari malformation in myelomeningocele patients with scoliosis. AJNR 8:539–546

Sarpel S, Sarpel G, Yu C et al. (1987) Early diagnosis of spinal epidural metastasis by magnetic resonance imaging. Cancer 59:1112–1116

Sarpyener MA (1945) Congenital stricture of the spinal canal. J Bone Joint Surg 27B:70–79

Scatliff JH, Kendall BE, Kingsley DP, Britton J, Grant DN, Hayward RD (1989) Closed spinal dysraphism: Analysis of clinical, radiological and surgical findings in 104 consecutive patients. AJNR 10:269–277

Schatzker J, Pennal G (1968) Spinal stenosis: A case of cauda equina compression. J Bone Joint Surg 50B:606–618

Schnebel B, Kingston S, Watkins R, Dillin W (1989) Comparison of MRI to contrast CT in the diagnosis of spinal stenosis. Spine 14:332–337

Schneiderman G, Flannigan B, Kingston S, Thomas J, Dillin WH, Watkins RG (1987) Magnetic resonance imaging in the diagnosis of disc degeneration: correlation with discography. Spine: 12:276–281

Schonstrom NS, Bolender NF, Spengler DM (1985) The pathomorphology of spinal stenosis as seen on CT scans of the lumbar spine. Spine 10:806–811

Schubiger O, Valvanis A (1982) CT differentiation between recurrent disc herniation and post operative scar formation: The value of contrast enhancement. Neuroradiology 22: 251–254

Schumacher H-W, Wassman H, Podlinski C (1988) Pseudomeningocele of the lumbar spine. Surg Neurol 29:77–78

Scotti G, Scialfa G, Pieralli E, Boccardi E, Valsecchi F, Tonon C (1983) Myelopathy and radiculopathy due to cervical spondylosis: myelographic–CT correlations. AJNR 4:601–603

Seigel RS, Williams AG, Metler FA, Wicks JD (1982) Intraspinal, extradural ependymoma. J Comput Assist Tomogr 6:189–192

Sherman J, Barkovich AJ, Citrin CM (1987) The MR appearances of syringomyelia. New observations. AJR 148:381–391

Slasky BS, Bydder GM, Niendorf P, Young IR (1987) MR imaging with Gadolinium-DTPA in the differentiation of tumor, syrinx and cyst of the spinal cord. J Comput Assist Tomogr 11:845–850

Smith L (1964) Enzyme dissolution of the nucleus pulposus in humans. JAMA 187:137–140

Smoker WR, Godersky JC, Knutzon RK, Keyes WD, Norman D, Bergman W (1987) The role of MR imaging in evaluating metastatic spinal disease. AJNR 8:901–908

Sobel DF, Barkovich AJ, Munderloh SH (1984) Metrizamide myelography and postmyelographic computed tomography: Comparative adequacy in the cervical spine. AJNR 5:385–390

Sobel DF, Zyroff J, Thorne RP (1987) Diskogenic vertebral sclerosis: MR imaging. J Comput Assist Tomogr 11:855–858

Spencer DL, Irwin GS, Miller JAA (1983) Anatomy and significance of fixation of the nerve roots in sciatica. Spine 8:672–679

Stevens JM, Kendall BE, Crockard HA (1986) The spinal cord in rheumatoid arthritis with clinical myelopathy. J Neurol Neurosurg Psychiatry 49:140–151

Stockley I, Getty CJM, Dixon AK, Glaves I, Euinton HA, Barrington NA (1988) Lumbar lateral canal entrapment: clinical, radiographic and computed tomographic findings. Clin Radiol 39:144–149

Stolke D, Sollman WP, Seifert V (1989) Intra and post operative complications in lumbar disc surgery. Spine 14:56–59

Stollman S, Pinto R, Benjamin V, Kricheff I (1987) Radiologic imagining of symptomatic ligamentum flavum thickening with and without ossification. AJNR 8:991–994

Swank SM, Barnes RA (1987) Osteoid osteoma in a vertebral body. Spine 12:602–605

Symon L, Kuyama H, Kendall B (1984) Dural arteriovenous malformations of the spine – clinical features and surgical results in 55 cases. J Neurosurg 60:238–247

Sze G, Abramson A, Krol G et al. (1988a) Gadolinium-DTPA in the evaluation of intradural extramedullary spinal disease. AJNR 9:153–163

Sze G, Michanco III LS, Brant-Zawadzki MN et al. (1988b) Chordomas: MR imaging. Radiology 166:187–191

Teplick JG, Haskin ME (1983) CT and lumbar disc herniation. Radiol Clin North Am 21:259–288

Teplick JG, Haskin ME (1984) Intravenous contrast enhanced CT of the post operative lumber spine. AJNR 5:373–383

Teplick JG, Haskin ME (1985) Spontaneous regression of herniated nucleus pulposus. AJNR 6:331–335

Teplick JG, Peyster RG, Teplick SK, Goodman LR, Haskin ME (1983) CT identification of post laminectomy pseudomeningocele. AJNR 4:179–182

Teplick JG, Laffey PA, Berman A, Haskin ME (1986) Diagnosis and evaluation of spondylolisthesis and/or spondylolysis on axial CT. AJNR 7:479–491

Thijssen HOM, Keyser A, Horstink MWM, Meijer E (1979) Morphology of the cervical spinal cord on computed tomography. Neuroradiology 18:57–62

Ullrich CG, Binet EF, Sanecki MG, Kieffer SA (1980) Quantitative assessment of the lumbar spinal canal by computed tomography. Radiology 134:137–143

Ungersbock K, Perneezky A, Korn A (1987) Thoracic vertebrostenosis combined with thoracic disc herniation. Spine 12:612–615

Valentini MC, Bracchi M, Gaidolfi E, Savoiardo M (1986) Radiologic demonstration of syringobulbia. Acta Radiol [Suppl] 365:245–247

Valk J, Kaiser M (1986) Magnetic resonance imaging in the differentation of spinal cord tumours and hydromyelia. Acta Radiol [Suppl] 365:242–244

Verbiest H (1954) A radicular syndrome from developmental narrowing of the lumbar vertebral canal. J Bone Joint Surg 36B:230–237

Verbiest H (1976) Fallacies of the present definition, nomenclature and classification of the stenoses of the lumbar vertebral canal. Spine 1:217–225

Vernon-Roberts B (1987) Pathology of intervertebral discs and apophyseal joints. In: Jayson MIV (ed) The lumbar spine and back pain, 3rd edn. Churchill Livingstone, Edinburgh, pp 37–55

Williams AL, Haughton VM, Syvertsen A (1980) Computed tomography in the diagnosis of herniated nucleus pulposus. Radiology 135:95–99

Williams AL, Haughton VM, Meyer GA, Ho KC (1982) Computed tomographic appearance of the bulging annulus. Radiology 142:403–408

Williams AL, Haughton VM, Daniels DL, Grogan JP (1983) Differential CT diagnosis of extruded nucleus pulposus. Radiology 148:141–148

Williams AL, Haughton VM, Pojunas KW, Danields DL, Kilgore DP (1987) Differentiation of intramedullary neoplasms and cysts by MR. AJNR 8:527–532

Williams B (1986) Progress in syringomyelia. Neurol Res 8:130–145

Williams MP, Cherryman GR, Husband JE (1989) Significance of thoracic disc herniation demonstrated by MR imaging. J Comput Assist Tomogr 13:211–214

Williams C, Nelson M (1987) The varied computed tomographic appearance of acute spinal epidural haematoma. Clin Radiol 38: 363–365

Wilson DA, Prince JR (1989) MR imaging determination of the location of the normal conus medullaris throughout childhood. AJNR 10: 259–262

Wiltse LL, Widell EH Jr, Jackson DW (1975) Fatigue fracture: The basic lesion in isthmic spondylolisthesis. J Bone Joint Surg 57A:17–22

Wolpert SM, Anderson M, Scott RM, Kwan ES, Runge VM (1987) Chiari II malformation: MR imaging evaluation. AJNR 8:783–792

Wood PH, Badley EM (1987) Epidemiology of back pain. In: Jayson MIV (ed) The spine and pack pain, 3rd edn, Churchill Livingstone, Edinburgh, pp 1–36

Yagan R (1984) CT diagnosis of limbus vertebra. J Comput Assist Tomogr 8:149–151

Yamamoto I, Matsumae M, Ikeda A, Shibuya N, Sato O, Nakamura K (1988) Thoracic spinal stenosis: Experience with seven cases. J Neurosurg 68:37–40

Yetkin Z, Chintapalli K, Daniels DL, Haughton VN (1986) Gas in spinal articulations. Neuroradiology 28: 150–153

Yu S, Haughton VM, Sether LA, Wagner M (1988) Annulus fibrosus in bulging intervertebral discs. Radiology 169:761–763

Yu S, Haughton VM, Sether LA, Ho K-C, Wagner M (1989) Criteria for classifying normal and degenerated lumbar intervertebral disks. Radiology 170:523–526

Yu YL, du Boulay GH, Stevens JM, Kendall BE (1986) Computed tomography in cervical spondylotic myelopathy and radiculopathy: visualisation of structures, myelographic comparison, cord measurements and clinical utility. Neuroradiology 28:221–236

Zimmerman RA, Bilaniuk LT (1988) Imaging of tumours of the spinal canal and cord. Radiol Clin North Am 26:965–1008

Zinreich SJ, Waugh H, Updike ML et al. (1988) CT myelography for outpatients. Radiology 157:387–390

Chapter 8

Imaging the Orbit

Glyn A. S. Lloyd

Plain X-ray films of the skull and computed tomography (CT), augmented by magnetic resonance imaging (MRI), are currently the dominant radiological investigations of the orbit and the majority of patients presenting with exophthalmos can be fully evaluated by these techniques alone.

Plain Film Changes

Alterations in the general radiographic density of the orbit are dependent on a decrease or increase of the soft tissue contents; thus, in the presence of a space-occupying lesion causing proptosis, oedema of the soft tissue or ecchymosis, a decrease in orbital translucence is to be expected. Conversely, enophthalmos resulting from a decrease in the contents of the orbit, will produce a slight hypertranslucency. These changes in the soft tissue density of the orbit are of little practical diagnostic significance and simply reflect a change which is obvious clinically.

Alterations in the size of the orbit are a common accompaniment of long-standing orbital pathology. *Decrease in size* may occur after early enucleation of the eye before the orbit has reached adult size; it may also be seen in congenital microphthalmos and anophthalmos. *Enlargement* is normally the result of raised intraorbital pressure producing changes in the orbit analogous to those seen in the calvarium in raised intracranial pressure. Any growing tumour may produce these X-ray changes if sufficient time has elapsed, but the response of the orbit to a space-occupying lesion is more rapid in a child than an adult and, whilst orbital enlargement usually denotes a benign lesion of long standing, this rule is not applicable to children.

Invasion and erosion of the walls of the orbit may take the form of *osseous destruction* and is then usually due to a malignant primary or secondary neoplasm. Rarely it may be due to an infective process such as tuberculosis. A local indentation of the orbital wall with clear-cut edges is characteristic of a benign tumour such as a dermoid cyst or epidermoid. Increased bone density or hyperostosis in the orbit may occur in a number of conditions, principally a pterional or sphenoid ridge *meningioma*, but it may also be due to osteoblastic *metastases, fibrous dysplasia, Paget's disease* and *osteitis* associated with chronic sinus infection.

Calcification within the soft tissues of the orbit is uncommon. Within the globe it may be present in the lens in *senile cataract*, and ossification may occur in the vitreous and choroid as a result of degenerative changes following injury or infection. Finely stippled calcification may be demonstrable in cases of *retinoblastoma*, and Taybi (1956) has reported macroscopic global calcification in 14 of 22 children with *retrolental fibroplasia*. Calcinosis oculi has also been reported in *hyperparathyroidism* (Heath 1962). Calcification in the retro-orbital structures may be seen in *meningioma* of the optic nerve. This may take the shape of calcification within the sheath of the optic nerve, or a finely stippled calcification may be present in the tumour mass, usually located towards the apex of the orbit. The identification of phleboliths in the orbit is an important observation in the differential diagnosis of patients presenting with proptosis and indicates the presence of abnormal veins in the orbit and a venous malformation.

Changes in the optic foramina and in the sphenoidal fissure may also indicate the presence of an intraorbital lesion. This is described elsewhere (see below).

CT and MRI

Direct coronal scanning is necessary for the adequate demonstration of orbital pathology. With CT, reformats should be reserved for sagittal or oblique sections. With MRI such sections can be obtained directly. In this technique the best quality scans of the orbit are obtained by using a specially designed surface coil which fits over the eyes like a pair of goggles. The purpose of this is to bring the receiving coil for the magnetic resonance signal as close as possible to the object to be imaged, thus producing as strong a signal as possible with the minimal amount of signal "noise", which may seriously degrade the image.

The role of magnetic resonance in orbital diagnosis is currently directed more towards tissue recognition than the identification of structural abnormality and mass lesions. These can be readily demonstrated by CT. Direct three-plane imaging is a feature of magnetic resonance tomography and provides the opportunity to use three different pulse sequences, i.e. a different pulse sequence for each plane – axial, coronal and sagittal. Multislice T_1 and T_2 weighted spin echo sequences are used, which may be combined with an inversion recovery sequence. These will provide optimum information concerning the spin-characteristics of any pathological tissue. An additional short inversion recovery sequence (STIR) scan may be useful. In this the pulse sequence is timed so that no signal from fat is received. Eliminating the strong fat signal from the orbit may provide improved delineation of tumours and other pathology.

Differential Diagnosis of Orbital Mass Lesions by CT

There are three ways in which a differential diagnosis of orbital space-occupying lesions may be achieved:

1. By showing the site of origin of the lesion, for example the optic nerve.
2. By the shape and density of the lesion (CT morphology.)
3. By consideration of the attenuation values before and after intravenous contrast injection.

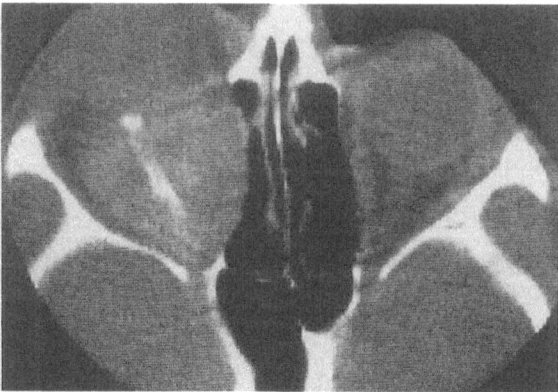

Fig. 8.1. Axial CT. Linear calcification in an optic sheath meningioma.

Optic nerve tumours, whether glioma or meningioma, may be identified when the optic nerve is shown to be enlarged in both axial and coronal section. Further differentiation may be arrived at by consideration of the age of the patient: most optic nerve sheath meningiomas occur in the elderly and middle-aged, whereas optic nerve glioma is a disease of childhood and young adults. The presence of calcification in the tumour shown by CT, indicates a meningioma (Fig. 8.1); optic canal enlargement is the rule in gliomas and is only seen in a minority of sheath meningiomas.

A diagnostic feature of the sheath meningiomas is the presence of "tramline" enhancement after intravenous contrast or sometimes shown as calcification (Fig. 8.1). There is no specific shape of

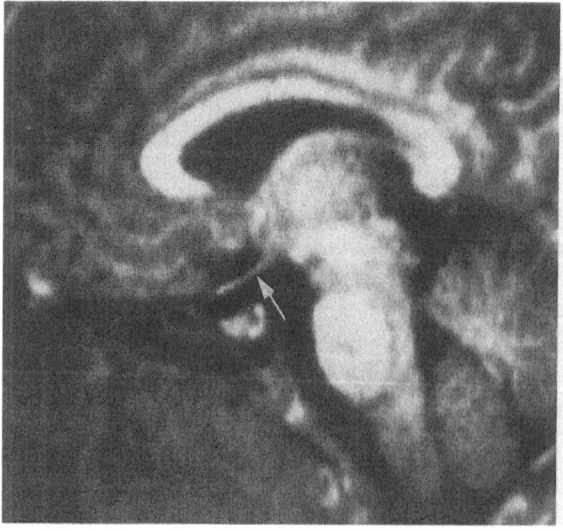

Fig. 8.2. Cranial MRI showing the optic chiasm in the sagittal plane.

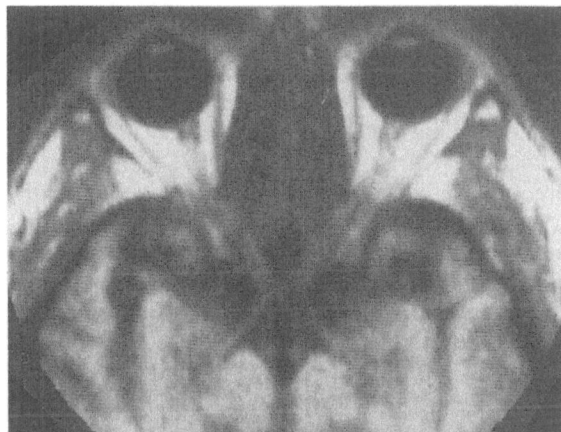

Fig. 8.3. Cranial MRI showing the optic chiasm in axial plane.

the optic nerve enlargement which can identify one or other of these tumours; but a smooth "figure of eight" outline is likely to represent a glioma in the ratio of approximately 8 : 1. The role of magnetic resonance in the management of these tumours, especially the gliomas, is to show intracranial extension and involvement of the optic chiasm. The latter is optimally demonstrated by this technique (Figs. 8.2 and 8.3).

Benign encapsulated tumours can be readily identified by CT by their shape and even density. The commonest tumour in this group is a cavernous haemangioma (Fig. 8.4). This gives a rounded contour sometimes almost circular in outline and is almost invariably intraconal in location. Another tumour which may be indistinguishable on CT from a cavernous haemangioma is a neurinoma; in general these are larger than the cavernous haemangiomas, but it is usually not necessary to make a differentiation between the two tumours since the treatment is the same in either case: namely, excision by lateral orbitotomy. Another lesion which may present as a clearly defined rounded mass is an orbital varix.

When these encapsulated tumours grow to a large size they may fill almost the whole of the intraconal space but even the largest will invariably leave some translucence on the scan at the orbital apex, a point of differentiation from infiltrative processes in the muscle cone. The commonest of these is a granuloma or pseudotumour which may be distinguished from the clearly defined tumours described above by their ill-defined edge and heterogeneous density, often involving the extraocular musculature. The other common lesions which may show an infiltrative process in the orbit are lymphomas and metastases. Although an absolute distinction between these lesions and the pseudotumour group is not always possible on CT the characteristic distribution of the lesion in the orbit may suggest the diagnosis prior to biopsy (see below).

Contrast medium. The injection of contrast medium for orbital CT scanning is no longer a routine procedure. If possible, postcontrast scans to show tissue enhancement are to be avoided since the injection of contrast converts what is essentially a noninvasive procedure into one which carries a similar morbidity and mortality to intravenous urography. The possibility of tissue recognition in the orbit by the behaviour of the attenuation values pre- and postcontrast injection is severely limited, and since most patients with proven mass lesions will have either a biopsy or surgical excision of the lesion, contrast injection is seldom justified. Thus, for orbital scanning contrast medium should be used to show up doubtful space-occupying lesions in better detail and when intracranial spread is suspected. If a clearly defined lesion is shown on the unenhanced scans injection is usually unnecessary. One condition can, however, be diagnosed on the evidence of the attenuation values but without contrast enhancement: approximately two-thirds of dermoid cysts in the orbit show areas of negative attenuation due to the presence of fat or oil in the tumour (Fig. 8.5).

Contrast Studies of the Orbit

In addition to plain radiography and CT scan, two angiographic methods of investigation of the orbit may be required in some patients.

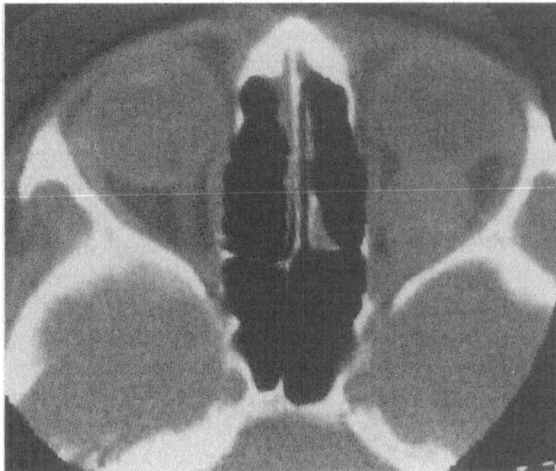

Fig. 8.4. Axial CT. Cavernous haemangioma.

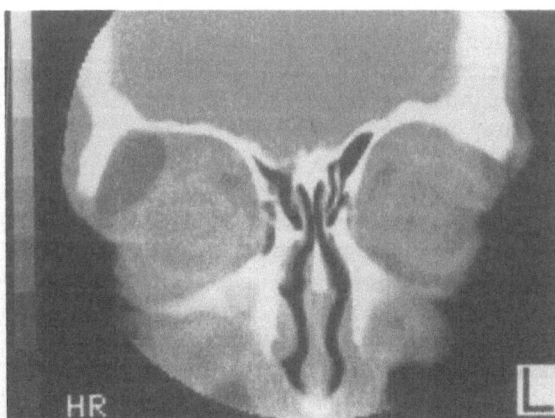

Fig. 8.5. Coronal CT. Orbital dermoid cyst. There is an area of negative attenuation in the superotemporal quadrant of the orbit.

Carotid Arteriography

CT has rendered carotid angiography unnecessary for the routine investigation of unilateral exophthalmos and has taken over the role of angiography in the exclusion of intracranial lesions causing proptosis. This investigation should therefore only be carried out on selected patients, principally those with suspected vascular anomalies, either in the orbit or middle fossa; for example a dural arteriovenous malformation or infraclinoid aneurysm. In the orbit it should be remembered that approximately 25% of space-occupying lesions may be classified as vascular anomalies and these are by their nature best demonstrated by angiography, by venography in the case of a venous malformation and by arteriography when there is an arteriovenous shunt. Arteriography may also be needed to define the blood supply to a vascular tumour in the orbit prior to surgery (Lloyd 1969).
Diagnosis. Orbital tumours may be shown by carotid angiography in three ways (Lloyd 1975):

1. By displacement of vessels.
2. By the demonstration of a pathological circulation.
3. By the deformation of the choroid crescent.

Orbital Phlebography

The method normally used is that described by Vritsios (1961). The injection of contrast is made into a frontal vein or main tributary. Immediately prior to injection a rubber band is placed around the forehead at the hairline, to prevent reflux of contrast medium over the scalp, and the facial veins also need to be occluded either by a compression bandage or by finger pressure applied by the patient (Lloyd 1975).

Between 10 and 12 ml of Conray 280 or equivalent contrast medium is used to make the injection and films are taken after delivery of 5 ml and immediately prior to the end of the injection. A preliminary control film is also obtained for subtraction studies. Both orbital venous systems normally fill provided sufficient contrast medium is used and this is an advantage of the frontal vein approach since minor degrees of displacement of the veins on the abnormal side may be detected by comparison with the opposite, normal side. In over 90% of patients frontal venography can be performed without anaesthesia and on an outpatient basis. In children, and in adults with difficult veins, in whom venepuncture has failed initially, a general anaesthetic may be required.

Diagnosis. A tumour or other space-occupying lesion in the orbit may be demonstrated by venography in three ways: (a) it may cause displacement of veins; (b) it may obstruct the venous system in the orbit; or (c) it may be revealed by the presence of a pathological venous circulation. These changes are often found in combination, but the type of change indicates to a very great extent the likely pathology present; displacement is usually caused by a benign tumour, obstruction by an inflammatory or malignant process and pathological veins by a venous malformation.

Congenital Disease

Cyclopia, anophthalmos, microphthalmos and buphthalmos are anomalies of the globe which are rarely seen but which may have a secondary effect on the bony orbit. The first three of these may be associated with problems in forebrain differentiation, i.e. holoprosencephaly. This means an arrest in the cleavage of the prosencephalon of the cerebral hemispheres, so that the frontal poles of the frontal lobes do not develop. The most severe deformity in this group is cyclopia in which there is only a solitary median eye present. Anophthalmos strictly defined means complete absence of the eye, but in fact histological studies usually reveal some form of rudimentary eye and in some cases a cystic mass may replace the unformed globe. Primary clinical anophthalmos, which is the most common type, is due to failure of development of the optic anlage. It occurs sporadically and is often bilateral. In these patients the failure of growth of the eye results in underdevelopment of the bony orbit with overgrowth of the paranasal sinuses (Fig. 8.6).

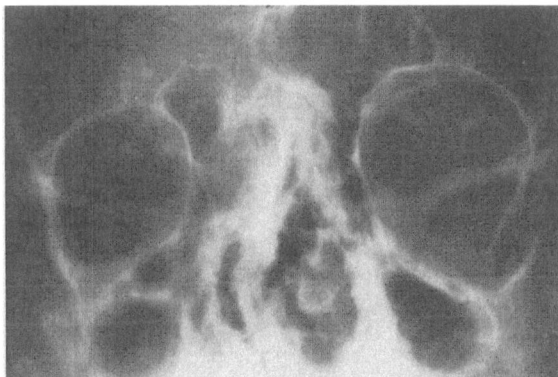

Fig. 8.6. Bilateral congenital anophthalmos. Both orbits are smaller than normal and there is overpneumatisation of the paranasal sinuses.

Microphthalmos is the term used to denote a variety of abnormalities of the globe when it is smaller than normal. Pure microphthalmos or nanophthalmos is a small but otherwise normal eye. Buphthalmos denotes enlargement of the globe and is seen as an hereditary disorder of the drainage system of the anterior chamber causing glaucoma and enlargement of the eyeball; it may be associated with neurofibromatosis.

Hypertelorism is a widening of the distance between the eyes with increase in the interpupillary measurement, and shows radiologically as an increase in the distance between the medial walls of the orbits on postero-anterior projections. It was originally described by Greig (1924) as ocular hypertelorism or greater breadth between the eyes without other associated abnormalities. Since then the condition has been reported with a variety of other anomalies and Beck and McCarthy (1986) list 107 conditions associated with increased distance between the eyes.

An important group of conditions which may be associated with hypertelorism are the frontal, ethmoidal or sphenoidal meningo-encephaloceles. These may be grouped according to their anatomical site into occipital, sincipital, and basal. The latter two are of interest to the ophthalmologist. In the naso-orbital sincipital encephalomeningocele there is a defect in the suture line between the frontal lacrimal and ethmoid bones with herniation of the meninges and sometimes brain into the orbit causing a protuberance at the inner canthus of the eye. The basal cerebral hernias are those which occur through the cribriform plate or through the sphenoid bone, the herniation appearing in the nasal cavity, nasopharynx, sphenoid sinus or posterior orbit. Pollock et al. (1968) described the clinical and radiological features of eight patients with

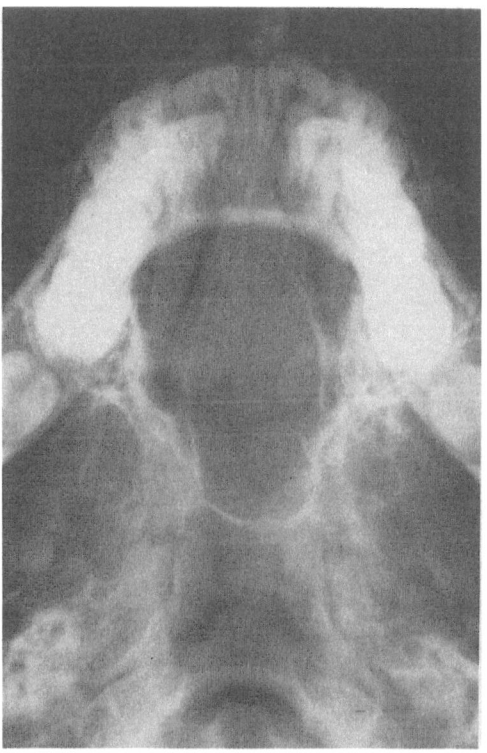

Fig. 8.7. Skull base view showing the bone defect of a spheno-ethmoidal encephalocele.

basal encephaloceles – five transsphenoidal and three transethmoidal. Two clinical findings suggest a basal encephalocele: a facial deformity with hypertelorism, and a midline soft tissue mass in the nose or epipharyngeal space. In the sphenoid variety a defect in the base of the skull can be shown on plain axial views (Fig. 8.7), but in the transethmoidal variety some form of tomography is needed for their demonstration. Lusk and Dunn (1986) have recorded the findings on MRI of a 19-month-old child who was shown at surgery to have an anterior cranial fossa encephalocele. In this instance magnetic resonance proved superior to CT scan in its ability to distinguish brain from normal tissues in the nose. An example of an encephalocele demonstrated by magnetic resonance is shown in Fig. 8.8.

Spheno-orbital encephalocoeles involve the posterior orbit and they are commonly associated with neurofibromatosis producing the "bare" orbit sign of this condition.

The term hypotelorism refers to an abnormal shortening of the distance between the eyes and orbits accompanied by an ethmoid labyrinth that is narrower than normal. It has been reported to occur in several syndromes and is associated with holo-

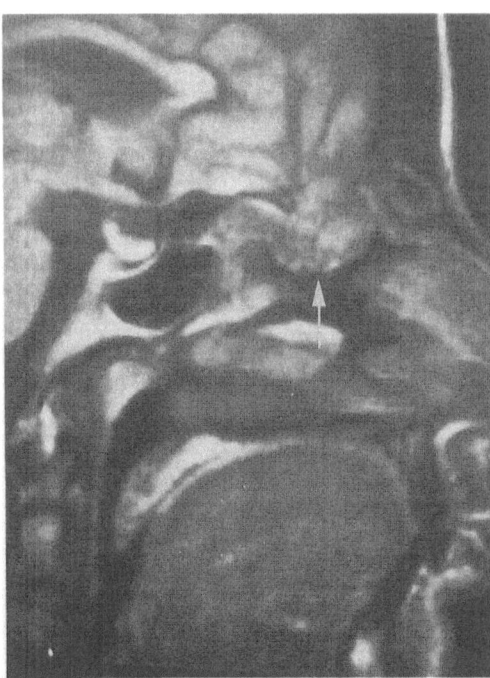

Fig. 8.8. Cranial MRI (sagittal section). Anterior ethmoid encephalocele (*arrow*).

prosencephaly. Becker and McCarthy (1986) list 16 syndromes associated with orbital hypotelorism.

Fractures

The orbit is involved in the majority of bony injuries to the facial skeleton, and very often the secondary effect on the eye and orbital soft tissue contents is a prominent feature both of the initial clinical signs and late disability.

Fractures of the Middle Third of the Facial Skeleton

Isolated fractures of the maxillary antrum may involve the infraorbital margin, whereas the whole of the floor of the orbit and lateral orbital wall may be disrupted in a malar or tripod fracture. This occurs as the result of laterally disposed violence to the facial bones. The force of the blow causes the malar bone to be displaced downwards, inwards and posteriorly, with a hinge movement and slight separation at the frontomalar suture. This is accompanied by a fracture of the zygomatic arch with little or no displacement. At the same time separation occurs at the junction of the medial third

and lateral two-thirds of the inferior orbital rim, usually with depression of the outer fragment. Sometimes this is also associated with disruption of the orbital floor. If the force is moderate the body of the malar bone is left intact, but in a more severe injury this bone is comminuted and may become impacted into the maxillary antrum. With severe degrees of impaction there is nearly always a comminution of the orbital floor, with prolapse of the orbital contents into the maxillary antrum.

Le Fort Injuries

The orbits may be involved in severe fractures of the facial bones, usually sustained during a road accident. Le Fort described anatomical lines of weakness in the facial skeleton, and his name has been given to the fractures which follow these lines. In a Le Fort II injury the line of fracture runs across the nasal bones, extending on both sides across the frontal process of the maxilla, and across the nasolacrimal canal (Fig. 8.9). From this point the line of weakness (or fracture) traverses the floor of the orbit, crossing the lower orbital margin in the region of the maxillozygomatic suture, eventually involving the lateral wall of the maxillary antrum and pterygoid laminae. This type of fracture is produced by force applied to the middle level of the facial skeleton from an anteroposterior direction, or sometimes from a lateral direction. Force applied to the facial bones from a superior direction will result in a local fracture of the nasal and ethmoid bones if the momentum is small, or a high level Le Fort type III fracture when the impact is severe. The line of fracture starts at the upper part of the nasal bones close to the frontonasal suture. In some cases the dislocation of the nasal bones at this site results in disruption of the cribriform plate of the ethmoid, and fracture of the floor of the anterior fossa. From its midline point of origin, the fracture runs through the medial wall of the orbit in the neighbourhood of the frontomaxillary suture, crossing the lacrimal bone and medial orbital wall and extending backwards to the inferior orbital fissure. At this point the line of fracture bifurcates, one component running upwards and forwards to terminate in the lateral wall of the orbit immediately below the frontomalar suture, while the lower component of the fracture runs downwards and backwards from the pterygomaxillary fissure to involve the roots of the pterygoid laminae. In this injury, therefore, there is a virtual separation or partial separation of the facial bones from the cranium above the zygomatic arch, the force of the trauma causing the entire middle third of the facial skeleton to hinge backwards through the ethmoid labyrinth.

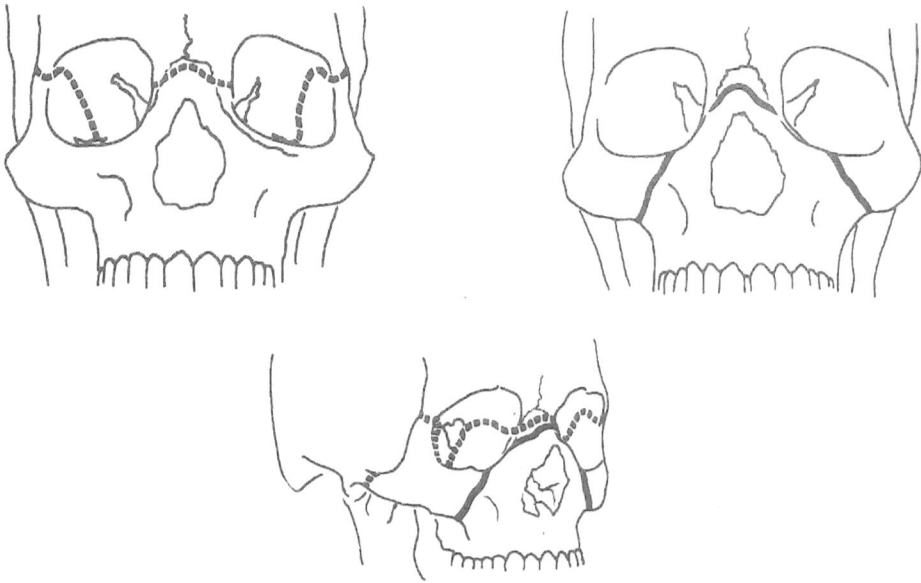

Fig. 8.9. Line drawing of the Le Fort injuries, which affect the orbit. The continuous line represents a Le Fort II fracture, the interrupted line a Le Fort III.

Blow-Out Fractures

Blow-out fractures are classically caused by violent contact with a round hard object such as a cricket ball, hurling ball or baseball, but the vast majority are the result of a blow in the eye from a closed fist. According to Smith and Regan (1957), the mechanism of injury is as follows: part of the impact of the blow is absorbed by the orbital rim, which remains intact, but the force of the blow causes a backward displacement of the eye and an increase in intraorbital pressure, with a resultant fracture of the orbital floor or medial wall, decompressing the orbit and causing a herniation of orbital soft tissues into the maxillary antrum or ethmoid cells. The adjacent extraocular muscles may be impeded as a result of this herniation producing an impairment of ocular mobility and diplopia. The inferior rectus, inferior oblique, or more rarely the medial rectus muscle may be involved. It is the impairment of muscle function which constitutes the particular gravity of a blow-out fracture. Early surgical intervention may be required to release the trapped muscle and restore free movement of the globe. Unless this is done the diplopia will persist. Clinically, vertical diplopia is the most important feature and may be accompanied by paraesthesia or anaesthesia of the cheek and upper lip, in the distribution of the infraorbital nerve, which may be involved in the fracture.

The characteristic radiological appearance is that of a small, soft-tissue shadow in the roof of the maxillary antrum, due to the herniated soft tissues from the orbit; this is associated with a depressed bony fragment, which is nearly always visible on plain radiograph at the fracture site. Sometimes oblique views are necessary to show a depressed fragment convincingly or it may be best shown on a lateral film, but the projection which consistently shows these fractures, even when only minimal changes are present, is the nose–chin or occipito-oral view of the orbits (Fig. 8.10). Tomography in the coronal plane may confirm the fracture but is not usually needed to make the diagnosis.

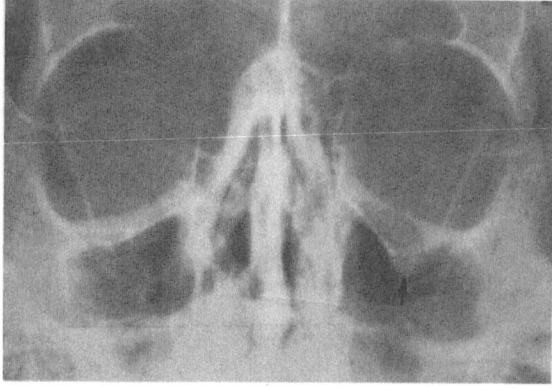

Fig. 8.10. Typical blow-out fracture shown on plain radiograph, with depressed fragment of bone and herniation of the soft tissues through the antral roof (*arrow*).

CT can be used as a substitute for conventional tomography in the demonstration of blow-out fractures. CT has the advantage of showing not only the site of fracture, but also the state of the rectus muscles; and it is possible to show herniation of the extraocular muscles. However, herniation of the medial or inferior rectus muscles does not imply that the muscle action is impeded and conversely the absence of herniation does not necessarily mean that there is no entrapment. The explanation for this has been given by Korneef (1982). Anatomical studies have shown that in the normal orbit there is a series of fibrous connective tissue septa which join the periorbita to the rectus muscle sheaths and the tendinous ring connecting them. Frequently it is the entrapment of these connective tissue elements which causes the muscle dysfunction without the muscle being displaced. Entrapment of the connective tissue septa in an orbital blow-out fracture may cause a downward drag on the medial or lateral rectus muscle via the tendinous ring which joins them to the inferior rectus muscle (Fig. 8.11). This change can be detected on CT scan as a downward displacement of the medial rectus muscle (Fig. 8.12) and, when present, may indicate the need for surgical intervention to release the trapped muscle. Another feature which can be shown on CT is the presence of fibrous adhesions within the antrum (Fig. 8.13), which clearly need to be dealt with if restoration of a normal orbital floor is to be achieved surgically.

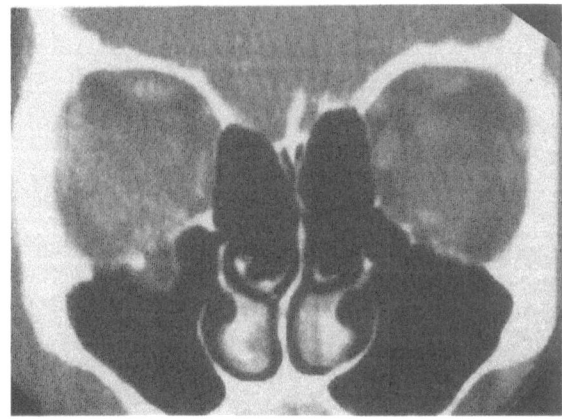

Fig. 8.12. Coronal CT. Blow-out fracture associated with displacement of the medial rectus inferiorly by the "drag" on the tendinous ring connecting the rectus muscles.

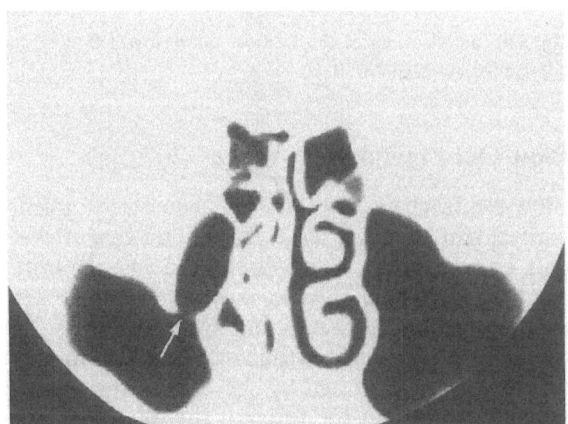

Fig. 8.13. Coronal CT scan. Orbital blow-out fracture. An adhesion to the medial antral wall is shown.

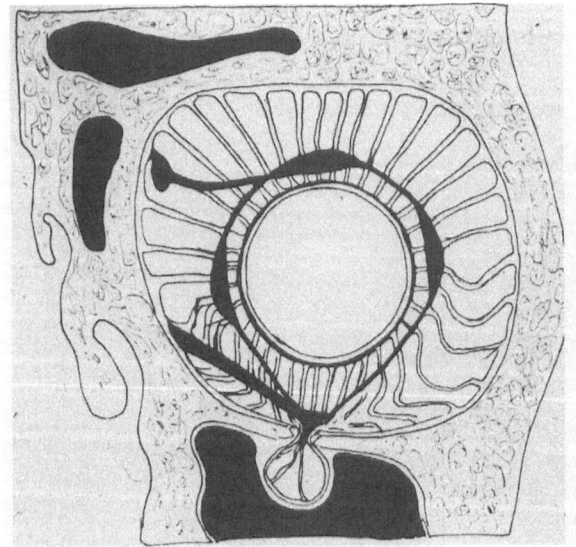

Fig. 8.11. Schematic representation of an antral blow-out fracture showing connective tissue entrapment and secondary "drag" on the medial rectus muscle.

Tumours of the Orbit

Orbital Meningioma

Meningioma in the orbit may occur as a primary tumour or it may be present as the secondary extension of a growth originating in the anterior or middle fossa of the skull.

Primary intraorbital meningioma may be classified as: (a) extradural, arising within the orbit remote from the optic nerve; (b) sheath meningioma, arising from clusters of arachnoid cap cells found in the meningeal sheath covering the optic nerve. The sheath meningiomas may be further subdivided into intracanalicular or foraminal tumours, and tumours arising from the retrobulbar part of the optic nerve. True intracanalicular tumours are, however, a great rarity and the majority of these

so-called foraminal meningiomas are in fact extensions of intracranial tumours. The retrobulbar
sheath meningiomas occur predominantly in
middle-aged women. Characteristically they give
little sign of their presence on plain radiographs,
but may show minor variations in the size of the
optic canal or calcification in the tumour (Fig. 8.1).
The radiological diagnosis is based on the computed
tomography findings. Visual deterioration in the
middle-aged or elderly patient with obvious optic
nerve enlargement on CT and minimal or no
enlargement of the optic canal is characteristic of a
sheath meningioma. Primary extradural meningiomas in the orbit usually present with proptosis
before compressing the optic nerve. The majority
of these show some plain X-ray evidence of their
presence such as localised or generalised orbital
enlargement, hyperostosis of the orbital walls, or
changes in the adjacent sinuses.

Pneumosinus Dilatans

When meningiomas arise in close proximity to the
superomedial wall of the orbit they may provoke
the condition known as pneumosinus dilatans. This
consists of an abnormal dilatation of the paranasal
air sinuses containing air only and lined by
normal epithelium. The condition is most commonly observed when it affects the sphenoid sinus as
a response to a local meningioma of the tuberculum

sellae or planum sphenoidale but it may also be seen
in the walls of the orbit formed by the paranasal air
sinuses. The importance of recognising this condition is in alerting the radiologist to the possible
presence of an occult meningioma requiring soft-
tissue imaging techniques, either computed tomography or magnetic resonance (Fig. 8.14a and b).

Secondary Meningioma

Secondary meningiomas occur as an extension of a
meningioma arising in the middle fossa of the skull
or less commonly in the anterior fossa. Meningioma
en plaque, affecting the greater and lesser wings of
the sphenoid and taking origin in the region of the
pterion, is the most common variety to affect the
orbit secondarily (Fig. 8.15). In these patients the
cause of the proptosis is the result of a hyperostosis
on the lateral wall and roof of the orbit, provoked
by the meningioma affecting the inner surface of
the greater wing of the sphenoid. The degree of
hyperostosis and its extent is best assessed by tomography, either conventional or computed, particularly in the axial plane; it is often much more
extensive than suspected on plain radiograph.

Dermoids and Epidermoids

These tumours result from sequestration of the
primitive ectoderm in the region of the orbit. Epi-

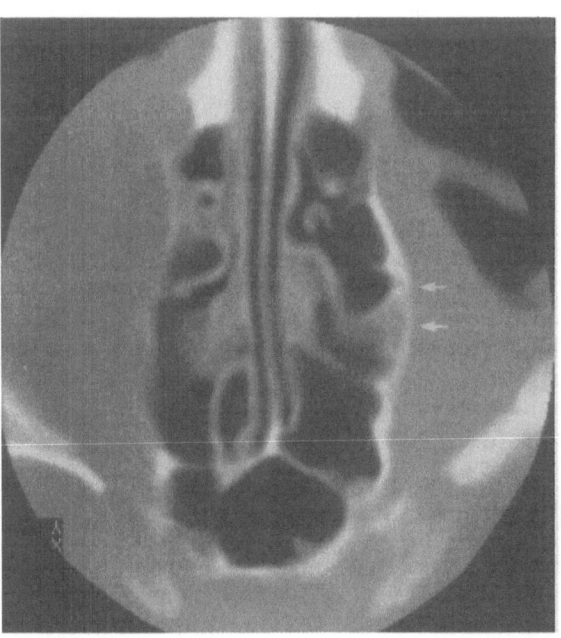
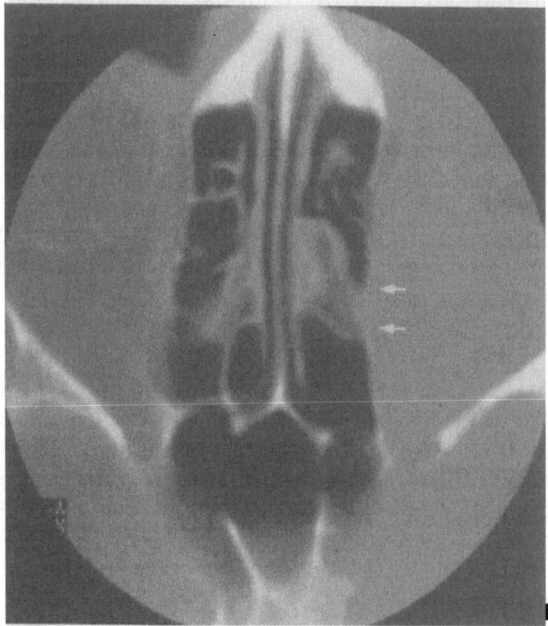

Fig. 8.14. Axial CT. Pneumosinus dilatans due to a recurrent sheath meningioma in the orbit. **a** Initially the presence of the tumour
has caused an inward lowing of the medial orbital wall (*arrows*). **b** Further CT scan after exenteration of the orbit. Residual
meningioma is still present in the orbit and has provoked a hyperostosis of the medial orbital wall with dilatation of the ethmoid
cells locally.

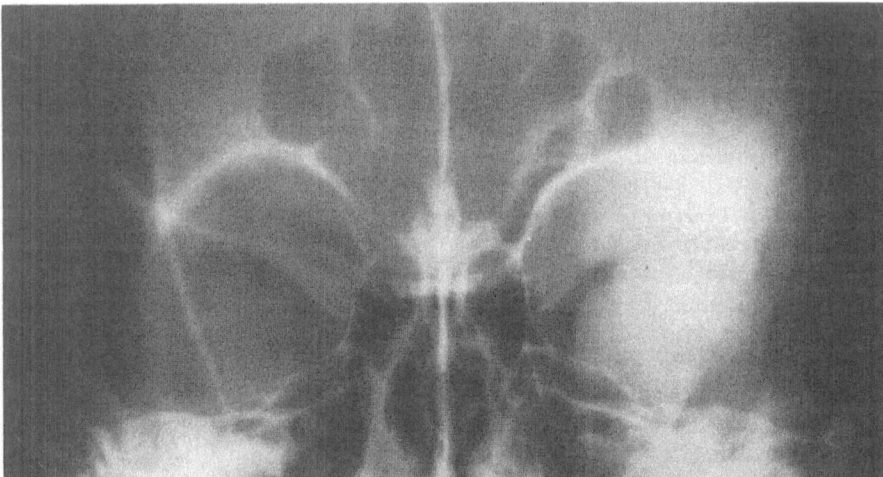

Fig. 8.15. Typical dense hyperostosis affecting the greater and lesser wings of the sphenoid due to meningioma.

dermoids occur when epidermal elements are solely concerned, and a dermoid when the deeper dermal layer is also involved (Pfeiffer and Nicholl 1948). Strict differentiation of the two types of tumour is to a large extent academic and many are of a transitional type, but the dermoids are cystic and may contain oil, sebum, cholesterol and hair, whereas the epidermoids are solid tumours consisting of a mass of desquamated cells containing keratohyaline, encased in a capsule of well-differentiated stratified squamous epithelium. Both may arise in the diploe of the skull and bones of the orbit and in their growth expand both inner and outer tables, thus producing sharply demarcated bone defects on the radiographs, with well-defined and in some cases slightly sclerotic margins. They occur in characteristic locations in the orbit, most commonly in the superolateral quadrant, but they frequently occur in the medial part of the orbital roof, and sometimes in the greater wing of the sphenoid or lateral wall of the orbit, where they produce a very characteristic cyst-like appearance in the bone. Rarely, they may present in the inferior part of the orbit.

Dermoids may give a characteristic appearance on CT scan. The presence of oil or fat produces a localised area of low attenuation in the negative range of the Hounsfield scale. In the author's series this sign has been present in approximately two-thirds of surgically proven dermoids (Fig. 8.5).

The superficially placed periorbital dermoids may also show minor radiographic changes. The most common locality for these tumours is the outer part of the upper eyelid and they may cause a shallow localized indentation on the orbital rim at its superolateral angle.

Rhabdomyosarcoma

Rhabdomyosarcoma of the orbit, although a rare tumour in absolute terms, is nevertheless the most common cause of malignancy in the orbit of children, and the majority of these tumours occur in the first decade of life. Three histological types are recognised: (a) embryonal rhabdomyosarcoma; (b) differentiated rhabdomyosarcoma; and (c) alveolar rhabdomyosarcoma, which is the most malignant variety with an invariably poor prognosis. Clinically the condition presents with exophthalmos with rapid and even alarming progression (Jones, et al. 1966) and this is often accompanied by a superficial swelling in the eyelids, canthi or fornices.

Radiologically these tumours produce progressive enlargement of the orbit and later they may cause bone destruction with extension to extraorbital structures including the temporal fossa and cranial cavity. Enlargement of the orbit may be appreciated on plain radiographs. CT shows a bulky tumour which usually enhances after contrast, frequently occupies an anterior location in the orbit and may extend both intra- and extraconally.

Lymphoma

Both benign and malignant lymphomas occur in the orbit. The so-called benign lymphoma is, however, better termed benign reactive lymphocytic hyperplasia and should be classified as a variety of pseudotumour. However, the histopathology of these tumours gives no indication of the ultimate outcome; a tumour diagnosed benign may later

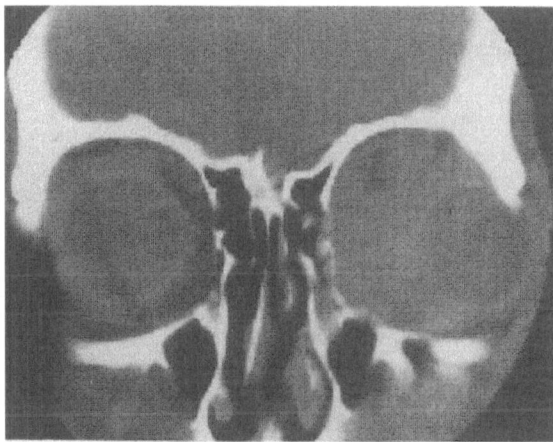

Fig. 8.16. Coronal CT scan. Orbital lymphoma in an elderly patient surrounding the globe anteriorly.

disseminate and, conversely, a histologically malignant tumour may not. Prolonged follow-up is in fact necessary to arrive at a diagnosis of benignity or malignancy. Separation of tumours into monoclonal and polyclonal cell types is also no sure guide to prognosis; a substantial minority of polyclonal tumours disseminate, whereas well-differentiated monoclonal tumours do so rarely.

Lymphomas occur most frequently in the sixth and seventh decade and have an equal sex distribution. They tend to arise outside the muscle cone in the anterior orbit. On plain radiography they seldom show any abnormality. On CT it is not always possible to distinguish a lymphoma in the orbit from other infiltrating processes, such as a pseudotumour or metastasis. However, some clue to the diagnosis may be derived from the location of the mass in the orbit. In a series of 46 histologically proven lymphomas, two-thirds were both anterior and extraconal in location. This gives rise to the characteristic pattern of these tumours: an anterior, palpable mass enveloping the globe (Fig. 8.16) in an elderly patient. Lymphomas arising in the orbit do not, as a rule, involve bone; only one out of the 46 patients showed bone erosion associated with the soft tissue mass.

Metastases

In contradistinction to the lymphomas, metastases commonly involve bone. On plain radiograph the typical appearance is that of an ill-defined osteolysis, often difficult to appreciate, but frequently accompanied by loss of the innominate line on the PA projection. Osteoblastic secondaries occur in the orbit, usually from a breast primary in

women or prostate primary in men, and may be indistinguishable from the hyperostosis provoked by a sphenoidal meningioma. These changes can also be demonstrated on CT scan. In a series of 19 patients with proven metastases, 30% showed bone destruction or sclerosis in addition to a soft tissue mass. Involvement of the extraocular muscles is also a feature of some metastases and a single rectus muscle may be involved without infiltration of other structures.

Lacrimal Gland Tumours

These may be: (a) benign pleomorphic adenoma; (b) carcinomas including adenocarcinoma, adenoid cystic carcinoma and undifferentiated types; and (c) lymphomas.

The prognosis of lacrimal gland tumours depends upon the histology and whether there is extension of the tumour outside the gland capsule. Benign mixed tumours if completely removed with capsule intact have a favourable prognosis, but in contrast the carcinomas, even after total exenteration of the orbit, result in a fatal outcome in almost all cases.

Radiological Features. Plain radiographic changes depend on the histological type of tumour to some extent. In general the mixed cell type of tumour of relatively slow growth and long duration produces more obvious changes in the underlying lacrimal fossa. The most common sign is a local enlargement of the lacrimal fossa without bone invasion. This is seen in approximately 80% of benign mixed tumours, but will also occur in some 50% of carcinomas. Differentiation on plain radiograph is, therefore, not always possible. However, the diagnosis and pathological type may be suggested by a combination of conventional radiography and CT scan. Radiographic signs of malignancy in lacrimal gland tumours include invasion and sclerosis of the adjacent bone of the lacrimal fossa, calcification in the tumour and extension of the mass outside the lacrimal gland area as demonstrated on CT scan. In addition to showing the size and extent of the tumour in the orbit CT may demonstrate calcification (Fig. 8.17), when not revealed by conventional techniques. Bone erosion is also demonstrable at an early stage if high resolution CT is employed (Lloyd 1981).

Neoplastic involvement of the lacrimal gland may also be due to lymphoma. These tumours occur in an older age group than the epithelial tumours and on plain X-ray films show minimal enlargement of the lacrimal fossa in approximately 50% of patients, the rest showing no abnormality. The CT changes are also non-specific with either a simple

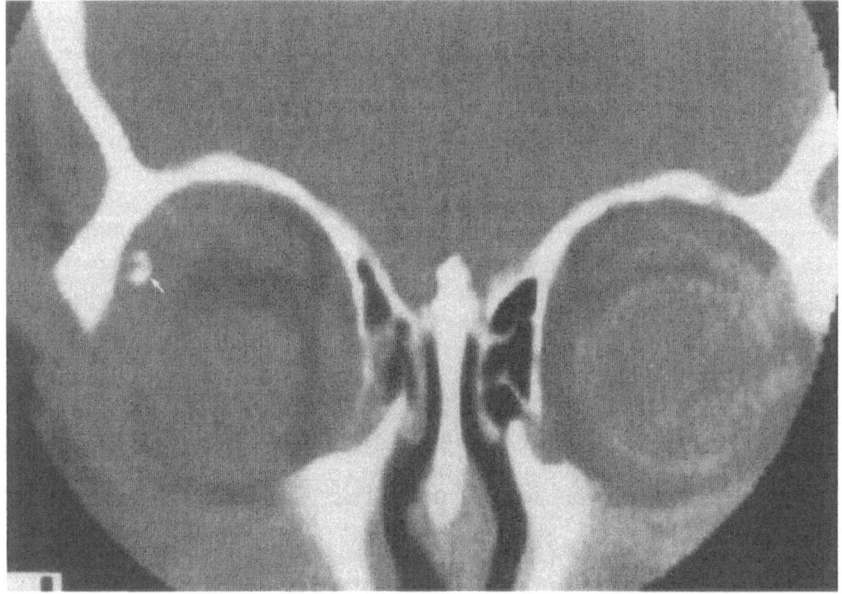

Fig. 8.17. Coronal CT. Calcification in a lacrimal gland carcinoma (*arrow*). The presence of calcification in an epithelial tumour of the lacrimal gland indicates malignancy in over 90% of patients.

enlargement of the lacrimal gland or a more wide-spread change as described above (see section on Lymphoma).

Inflammatory Conditions in the Orbit

Acute Infection

Orbital cellulitis results from acute bacterial infection which in most patients is secondary to sinus infection, usually an ethmoiditis or maxillary antritis. A dental abscess may be the initial cause in some instances. In the author's series two-thirds of patients showed obvious sinus infection on plain X-ray films, and very occasionally gas and a fluid level may be visible within the orbital soft tissues indicating the presence of abscess formation. Computed tomography will also show associated sinus infection with or without fluid levels in the sinuses. It is also useful to distinguish between preseptal cellulitis – a less serious infection – and true orbital cellulitis, when the clinical diagnosis is in doubt (Krohel et al. 1982). In addition to the presence of sinus infection adjacent to the affected orbit, CT may show widening of the extraconal space between the ethmoids and the periorbita due to oedema or abscess formation (Fig. 8.18). In addition, local rectus muscle enlargement due to extension of the inflammatory process may be demonstrated. It is important to localise abscess formation when it is

present. Unequivocal evidence is provided when there is soft tissue gas with or without a fluid level. Ring enhancement after intravenous contrast will also suggest abscess formation.

Chronic Infection: Orbital and Retro-orbital Pseudotumours

The name pseudotumour has been given to a group of cases which are difficult to differentiate clinically from orbital tumours but which on pathological investigation have proved to be of chronic inflamm-

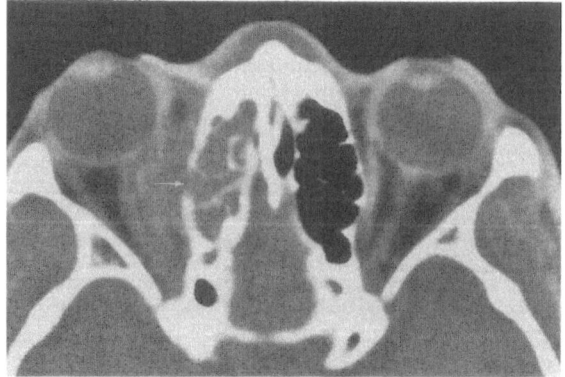

Fig. 8.18. Axial CT. Orbital cellulitis. Ethmoiditis is associated with abscess formation in the orbit and erosion of the medial orbital wall (*arrow*).

atory origin. Pseudotumours of the orbit present a difficult nosological problem as they are a spectrum of different conditions rather than a single entity. They occur throughout the orbit from the region of the lacrimal gland to the orbital apex and present very different signs and symptoms according to their position. Plain X-ray examination seldom shows any significant abnormality in the affected orbit, but some patients with pseudotumours show an associated clouding of the nasal sinuses due to infection or nasal polyposis. One other feature that may occur in the more posteriorly placed granulomas is an enlargement of the sphenoidal fissure. This has been observed in three of our patients and has been recorded by other authors (Lombardi 1967). On orbital venography, pseudotumours may produce a displacement of the venous system in the orbit, but the most characteristic venographic feature is a venous block usually in the second or third part of the superior ophthalmic vein. Positive evidence of the lesion within the orbit is best obtained by CT scan. Characteristically the changes are those of an infiltrative lesion, with an irregular ill-defined edge and variable density.

Analysis of a series of 61 patients with histologically proven pseudotumours showed that they occurred with equal frequency in an anterior or posterior location in the orbit. 28% were associated with enlargement of one or more rectus muscles and 16% were associated with sinus infection. In addition one-third showed a diffuse mass in the orbital apex which is the characteristic location for these inflammatory processes. Although a similar appearance can be demonstrated in some patients

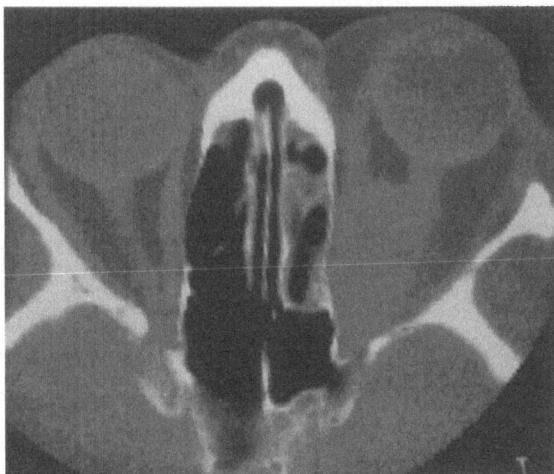

Fig. 8.19. Axial CT. Orbital pseudotumour. There is a non-specific inflammatory process in the muscle cone involving the medial rectus muscle and optic nerve.

with metastases or lymphomas, a painful mass filling the orbital apex with local muscle enlargement (Fig. 8.19) is very suggestive of this condition.

The Tolosa–Hunt Syndrome

Tolosa–Hunt syndrome is characterised by an ophthalmoplegia, usually of rapid onset, and preceded by pain in the back of the orbit and in the distribution of the first division of the trigeminal nerve. In the full condition there is a complete superior orbital fissure syndrome, with involvement of the IIIrd, IVth, Vth and VIth cranial nerves. In some of the patients described by Hunt et al. (1961) there was also optic nerve involvement, although this would imply that the cause in these patients was in the orbital apex rather than the superior orbital fissure. As in the case of pseudotumours in the orbit, the condition usually responds dramatically to steroid therapy and the aetiology is generally considered to be due to a non-specific inflammatory process with the presence of granulation tissue in the superior orbital fissure (Laake 1962) or in the cavernous sinus. In Tolosa's (1954) case, which came to autopsy, granulation tissue was found within the cavernous sinus surrounding the internal carotid artery and causing narrowing of the vessel by extrinsic pressure; adjacent nerve trunks were found to be included in the inflammatory mass. A similar autopsy report has also been described by Levy et al. (1973).

Lesions in the cavernous sinus region which can produce similar signs include intracavernous aneurysm, thrombosis, metastasis and meningioma. CT is the primary investigation and will identify the lesion in many cases, particularly if there is extension into the orbit. However, inflammatory or other lesions confined to the cavernous sinus can be difficult to demonstrate on CT. The X-ray changes which accompany the syndrome may be characteristic, and consist of:

1. Venous obstruction at the superior orbital fissure (Fig. 8.20) or in the cavernous sinus on orbital venography. This is usually not accompanied by any significant displacement of the vein, and it may be possible to demonstrate recanalisation of the superior ophthalmic vein following successful steroid therapy (Lloyd 1972).

2. On carotid angiography a smooth narrowing of the intracavernous segment of the internal carotid artery may be demonstrable (Fig. 8.21). This corresponds to the narrowing, which has been shown at autopsy (see above) to be caused by the extrinsic pressure of granulation tissue in the cavernous sinus.

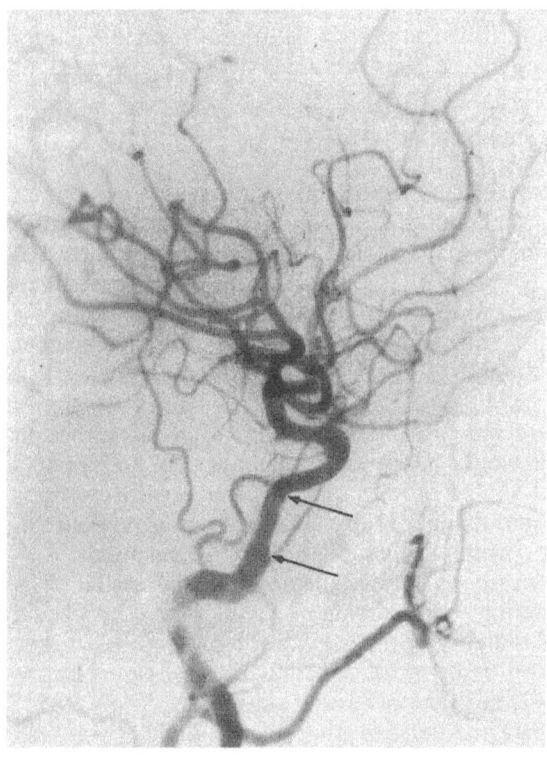

Fig. 8.20. Carotid angiography (lateral projection). Tolosa–Hunt syndrome. Smooth narrowing of the intracavernous segment of the internal carotid artery (*arrows*).

Cholesterol Granuloma

Cholesterol granuloma is a rare condition which is thought to originate from a haemorrhage into the diploe of the frontal bone. It is characterised by the presence of a bone defect in the outer roof of the orbit, the formation of a soft tissue mass below the supraorbital ridge, a characteristic histology and a benign course. The lesion is thought to occur as a reaction to the breakdown products of red blood cells, with the formation of cholesterol crystals, and the development of a foreign body granuloma. The lesion occurs almost exclusively in the supero-temporal quadrant of the orbit involving the adjacent bone, although cases have been known to involve the orbital soft tissues only. The typical radiological picture is that of a clearcut area of osteolysis in the lateral part of the supra-orbital ridge, the frontal bone and orbital roof. A defect in a similar location may be observed in a dermoid cyst, but in the latter the osteolytic area is usually better defined with a slightly sclerotic margin. A distinctive feature of cholesterol granuloma is that it may extend into the diploe of the zygomatic process of the frontal bone as far as the frontomalar suture (Nichols 1956) (Fig. 8.22). This is a sign not seen in dermoids. A further point of distinction is that approximately two-thirds of dermoids will show areas of negative attenuation on CT due to

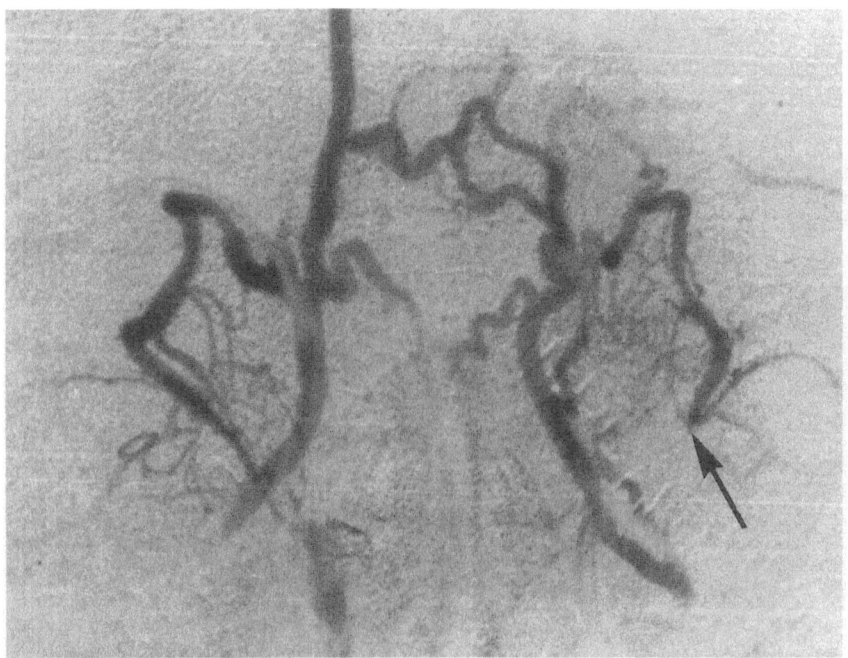

Fig. 8.21. Orbital venogram. Tolosa–Hunt syndrome. Obstruction of the superior ophthalmic vein (*arrow*) immediately anterior to the superior orbital fissure.

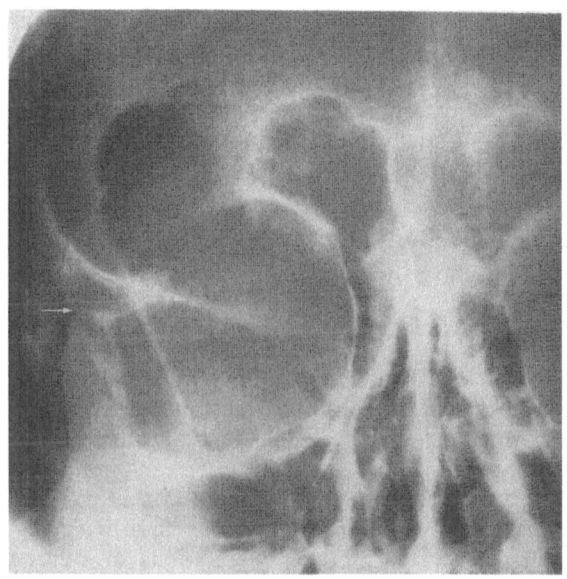

Fig. 8.22. Plain radiograph of a cholesterol granuloma affecting the orbit and frontal bone. There is a sharply demarcated area of osteolysis with extension into the diploe of the zygomatic process down to the front-malar suture (*arrow*).

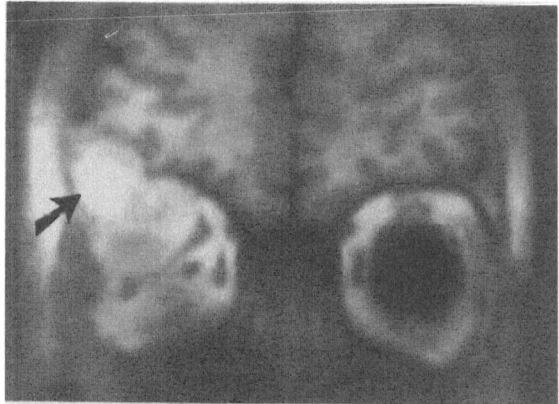

Fig. 8.23. Cranial MRI (coronal section, T1 weighted image). Cholesterol granuloma (*arrow*).

the presence of oil or fat; this has not been observed in cholesterol granuloma.

Although the diagnosis of this condition is invariably made on the plain radiographic appearances, total confirmation may be obtained on magnetic resonance: the presence of cholesterol or the products of haemorrhage has the effect of shortening the T1 relaxation time producing high signal on T1 inversion recovery sequences (Fig. 8.23).

Vascular Anomalies

Vascular anomalies in the orbit may be classified into (a) ophthalmic artery aneurysms; (b) arteriovenous malformations; (c) haemangiomas; (d) venous malformations and (e) blood cysts and haematomas.

Ophthalmic Artery Aneurysm

Saccular aneurysms arising from the intraorbital course of the ophthalmic artery are extremly rare and the majority of ophthalmic artery aneurysms arise from the junction of the internal carotid and ophthalmic arteries: they are usually described as carotid-ophthalmic aneurysms.

Arteriovenous Malformation

The orbit is a relatively uncommon site for an arteriovenous malformation but the condition is being increasingly reported largely because of the use of angiographic techniques. The condition may occur as a congenital anomaly or in some patients following trauma to the anterior orbit. Clinically an orbital arteriovenous malformation presents either as pulsating exophthalmos, sometimes with an audible bruit, or as a simple proptosis; and in the latter instance the need for angiography may not be recognised unless clear evidence of enlarged orbital vessels is present on CT scan. Carotid angiography is the essential investigation to show both the nature of the lesion and its blood supply, which may be derived from both the internal and external carotid circulations.

Haemangioma

Histologically the orbital haemangiomas are divided into (a) capillary and (b) cavernous varieties. Capillary haemangioma is a lesion which occurs in infants. It is often associated with a superficial capillary naevus and it may be demonstrated as a fine vascular network occupying a large part of the orbit on arteriography or a similar diffuse mass on CT scan. Cavernous haemangioma on the other hand is a disease of adults and is seen as a benign encapsulated lesion, which is typically found within the muscle cone giving rise to an axial proptosis. These tumours are well demonstrated prior to orbitotomy by CT scan, the lesion showing as a well-demarcated tumour mass with even density values and a rounded margin (Fig. 8.4). Although CT has made arteriographic studies unnecessary in the investigation of these patients, the most positive evidence of a cavernous haemangioma is provided

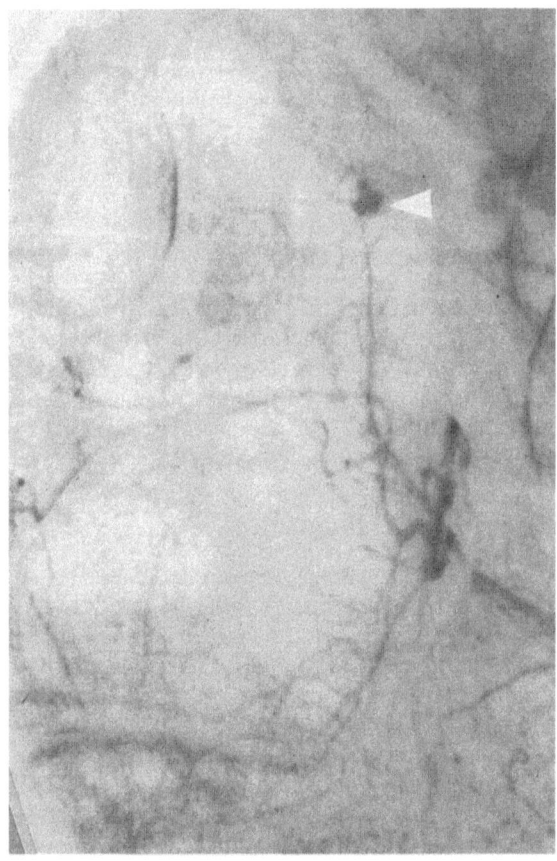

Fig. 8.24. Cavernous haemangioma (lateral subtraction angiogram) showing a venous "pool" (*arrowhead*) fed from a branch of the external carotid artery.

by arteriography: venous "pooling" of contrast in the late arterial phase of the examination, coupled with the demonstration of feeding vessels derived from the external carotid artery via its internal maxillary branch, are pathognomonic features (Fig. 8.24).

Venous Malformations

Patients with orbital varices usually give a history of proptosis dating from birth or early childhood and characteristically the proptosis is provoked or made worse by an increase in venous pressure in the head. Extensive venous malformations may give a characteristic triad of signs on plain radiograph: the orbit may be grossly enlarged and contain one or more phleboliths, and in a minority of patients evidence of venous dilatations may be provided by the presence of multiple indentations or venous "lakes" in the frontal bone over the affected side. On venography they present essentially in two forms: either a local dilatation of an otherwise normal venous system, as it were a venous aneurysm; or a whole series of abnormal venous channels in the orbit largely replacing the normal veins and affecting either the superior ophthalmic vein, the inferior ophthalmic, or both (Fig. 8.25). These are the extremes of abnormality and intermediate types may also be found. To a large extent the CT morphology of venous malformations follows the venographic appearances: there may be a diffuse change often associated with phleboliths (Fig. 8.26) and affecting both the intraconal and extraconal orbit,

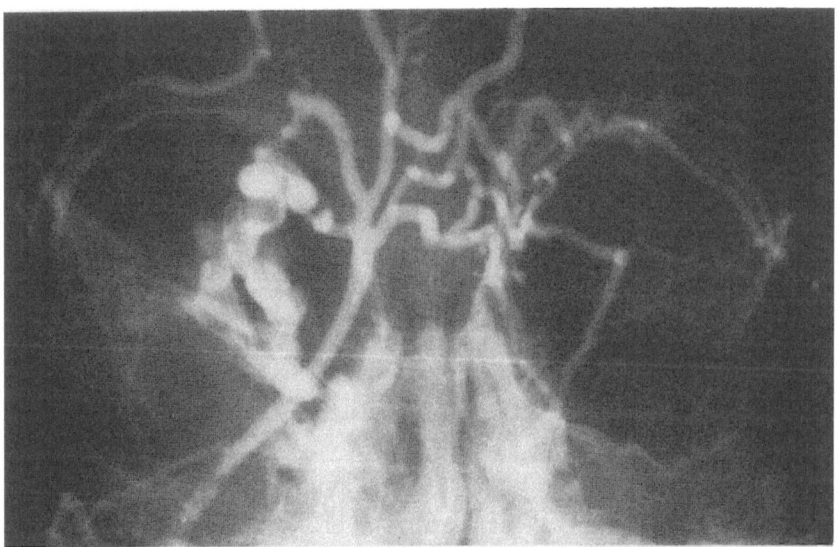

Fig. 8.25. Orbital venogram. Venous malformation in the right orbit. Both the superior and inferior ophthalmic veins are involved.

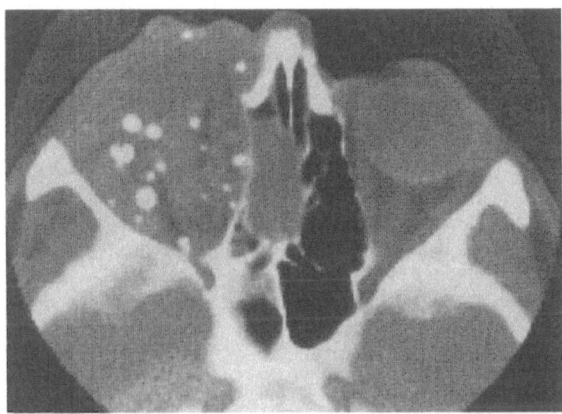

Fig. 8.26. Axial CT. Venous malformation. There is enlargement of the orbit, with multiple phleboliths and obliteration of the normal orbital structures by the dilated veins.

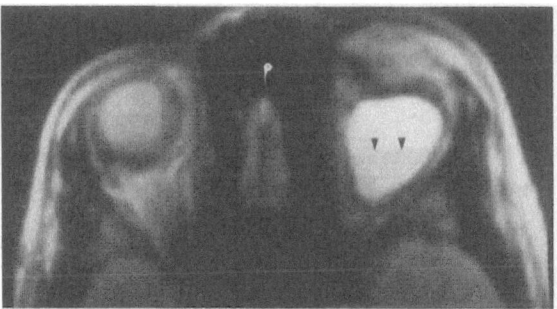

Fig. 8.27. Cranial MRI (axial section, T1 weighted image). Blood cyst in a 7-year-old girl. There is high signal from the haematoma with layering effect (*arrows*).

or they may present as a rounded mass intra- or extraconally. Intermediate forms also exist and a slightly irregular or lobulated intraconal mass may suggest a venous malformation. A clearly defined rounded varix in the muscle cone may present a problem in CT differential diagnosis since it may mimic the commoner intraconal tumours such as haemangioma or neurinoma. When in doubt repeat scans in the prone position may be helpful and will normally show an increase in size of a varix when the head is dependent.

The dilatation of the orbital veins which occurs in caroticocavernous fistula or dural arteriovenous shunt are described as secondary orbital varices since they consist of otherwise normal veins, which simply dilate in response to increased blood flow. A similar effect may be seen when the orbital venous system takes part in the venous drainage of an arteriovenous malformation elsewhere in the middle fossa or in the anterior cranial fossa.

Blood Cysts and Haematomas

Blood cysts in children may present with an acute onset of proptosis, pain, vomiting and diminished visual acuity, or the child may have a painless space-occupying haematoma that evolves over several months and clinically resembles an orbital neoplasm. It is probable that these haematomas are derived from the rupture of pre-existing varices, but in some children there may be an underlying blood dyscrasia. The cysts often have an endothelial lining and have a strong tendency to recur. They are now readily diagnosable by magnetic resonance imaging, producing high signal on T2 weighted spin-echo sequences with a layering effect due to

cellular precipitation within the haematoma (Fig. 8.27).

Dysthyroid Disease

The enlargement of the extraocular muscles which occurs in dysthyroid disease may be clearly demonstrated by computed tomography or magnetic resonance. In dysthyroid patients multiple rectus muscle enlargement is usually present bilaterally. Unilateral enlargement is less common, and single muscle enlargement may also occur in a minority of patients. The expansion tends to affect the belly of the muscle rather than its origin or insertion and this may help to differentiate the condition from a pseudotumour involving muscle or a myositis. When dysthyroid muscle enlargement affects the medial recti it will produce a characteristic indentation on the medial orbital wall (Fig. 8.28). This

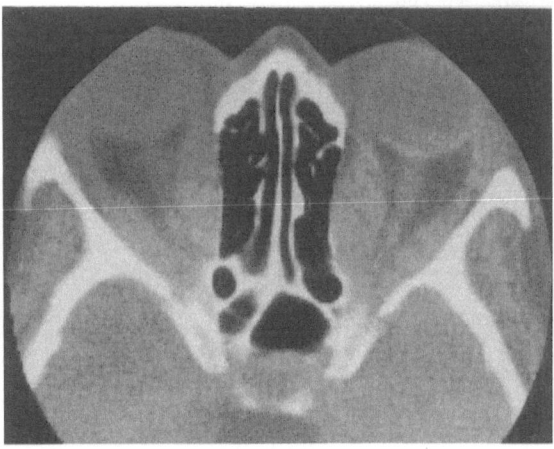

Fig. 8.28. Axial CT. Dysthyroid disease showing typical rectus muscle enlargement and indentation of the medial walls of the orbits.

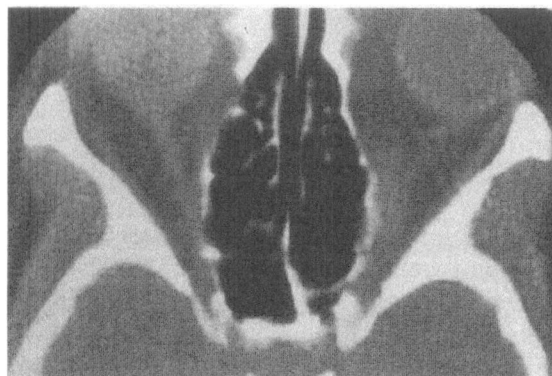

Fig. 8.29. Axial CT. Dysthyroid disease. Second type of change. There is a generalised increase in the fat content of both orbits without rectus muscle enlargement.

indentation tends to persist after regression of muscle enlargement and will remain as evidence that the muscle has been enlarged in the past.

In some dysthyroid patients the fat content of the orbit may increase and this may be the primary cause of the exophthalmos with little or no muscle enlargement (Fig. 8.29). This will produce a different appearance on CT, showing a generalised increase in the orbital fat content, an enlarged intraconal space, forward displacement of the eyeball and sometimes a characteristic angulation of the lateral rectus muscle at the point, where it is held by the lateral check ligaments.

References

Becker MH, McCarthy J G (1986) Congenital abnormalities. Diagnostic imaging in ophthalmology, Springer, Berlin, Heidelberg, New York

Greig D (1924) Hypertelorism. A hitherto undifferentiated congenital deformity. Edinburgh Med J 31: 560–593

Heath P (1962) Calcinosis oculi. Am J Ophthalmol 54: 771–781

Hunt WE, Meagher JM, Lefever JE, Zeman W (1961) Painful ophthalmoplegia: its relation to indolent inflammation of the cavernous sinus. Neurology 11: 56–62

Jones IS, Reese AB, Kraut J (1966) Orbital rhabdomyosarcoma: an analysis of 62 cases. Ophthalmology 61: 721–736

Koornneef L (1982) Current concepts on the management of orbital blow-out fractures. Ann Plast Surg 9: 185–200

Krohel GB, Krauss HR, Winnick J (1982) Orbital abscess. Ophthalmology 89: 492–501

Laake JPW (1962) Superior orbital fissure syndrome. Arch Neurol 7: 289

Levy IS, Wright JE, Lloyd GAS (1973) In: Proceedings of the 2nd International Symposium on Orbital Disorders, Amsterdam. Karger, Basel

Lloyd GAS (1969) A technique for arteriography of the orbit. Br J Radiol 42: 252–255

Lloyd GAS (1972) The localisation of lesions in the orbital apex and cavernous sinus by frontal venography. Br J Radiol 45: 405–414

Lloyd GAS (1975) Radiology of the orbit. WB Saunders, London

Lloyd GAS (1981) Lacrimal gland tumours: the role of CT and conventional radiology. Br J Radiol 54: 1034–1038.

Lombardi G (1967) Radiology in neuro-ophthalmology. Williams and Wilkins, Baltimore

Lusk RP, Dunn VD (1986) Magnetic resonance imaging in encephalocoeles. Ann Otol Rhinol Laryngol 95: 432–433

Nichols JV (1956) Cholesterol containing granuloma of the orbital wall. Am J Ophthalmol 41: 234–247

Pfeiffer RL, Nicholl RJ (1948) Dermoids and epidermoid tumours of the orbit. Arch Ophthalmol 40: 639–664

Pollock JA, Newton TH, Hoyt WF (1968) Transsphenoidal and transethmoidal encephalocoeles. Radiology 90: 443–449

Smith B, Regan WF (1957) Blow out fractures of the orbit: mechanism and correction of the inferior orbital fracture. Am J Ophthalmol 44: 733–739

Taybi H (1956) Ocular calcification and retrolental fibroplasia. AJR 76: 583–593

Tolosa E (1954) Periarteritis of carotid siphon with clinical features of carotid infraclinoid aneurysm. J Neurol Neurosurg Psychiatry 17: 300–302

Vritsios A (1961) Method de phlebographie des veins ophthalmiques, des veins de la face et des vaisseaux superfices du crane. Arch Soc Ophthalmol Grece de Nord 12: 223–227

Chapter 9

The Petrous Bone

Philip L. Anslow

Introduction

High-resolution computed tomography (HRCT) is central to the radiographic study of the petrous bone. The contrast resolution of HRCT more than compensates for its inferior spatial resolution when compared to pluridirectional tomography and the resulting images are clearer and easier to interpret.

Plain radiographic examinations or thick section tomography (zonography) may nevertheless still find a place, for example, in the initial screening of patients with sensorineural deafness where access to CT is limited.

Angiography fulfils a subsidiary role in evaluating suspected vascular lesions or in charting their vascular anatomy prior to surgery.

CT Imaging of the Posterior Fossa

The initial step consists of 4 mm or 5 mm axial sections before and after intravenous contrast medium, using both "soft tissue" and "bone" windows. If there remains doubt about the presence of a small cerebellopontine angle tumour, further thin axial sections (1.5 or 2 mm) can be performed through this region. If on clinical or radiological grounds it becomes necessary to exclude a wholly intracanalicular acoustic tumour, CT gas meatography should be undertaken.

This invasive measure involves the introduction of a small amount of air or carbon dioxide into the subarachnoid space via lumbar puncture (Sortland 1979; Bird et al. 1985). By fairly simple positioning the gas can be made to enter the cerebellopontine (CP) angle cistern and leaving the spinal needle in situ permits both a second attempt if the first fails

and also the examination of the other side if this is clinically indicated. Such additional amounts of air increase the likelihood of headache which may occur in any case due to cerebrospinal fluid (CSF) leak through the dura. The risk of such "low pressure" headache may be minimised by the use of fine bore needles and by encouraging the patient to rest after the procedure. Many centres carry out this study on an outpatient basis although it is becoming less common as magnetic resonance imaging (MRI) becomes the imaging method of choice (Kingsley et al. 1985) (Figs. 9.1 and 9.2).

If a small CP angle mass lesion is identified or if it is uncertain as to whether such a lesion is intra- or extra-axial, positive contrast CT cisternography is occasionally performed (Fig. 9.3). Iodinated contrast medium is introduced usually into the lumbar theca. The patient is then tipped head down so that contrast flows into the basal cisterns and after allowing some time to elapse for the contrast to become evenly mixed with CSF, axial scans are made. Again MRI provides a non-invasive alternative.

CT Imaging of the Petrous Bone

The ability of CT to image bone as well as soft tissue detail is exploited in the examination of the petrous bone. Modern scanners are capable of 1–1.5 mm sections in both coronal and axial planes which lead to an exquisite display of the petrous bone architecture (Swartz 1983; Chakeres et al. 1983). The coronal and axial planes each have their particular advantages but usually a scan in one plane suffices. The main exception to this is the request to exclude a facial neurinoma or an extensive cholesteatoma.

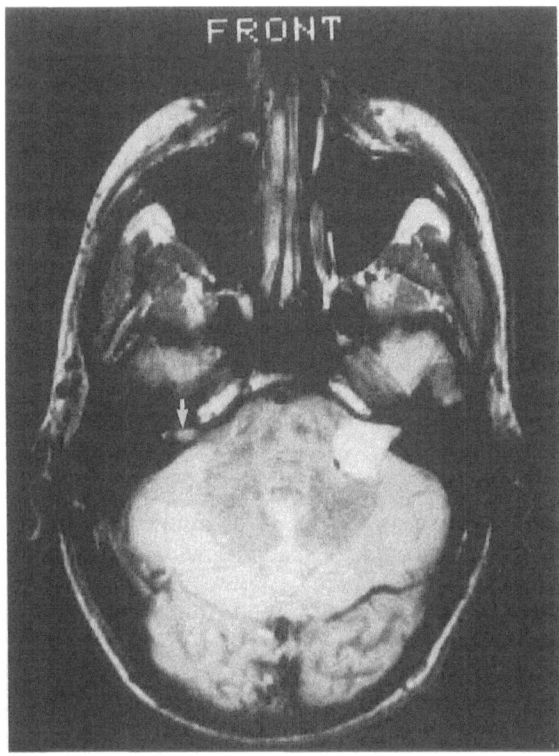

Fig. 9.1. Axial MRI. Right acoustic nerve tumour. The normal seventh and eighth nerve bundle is shown on the left (*arrow*). (P.B.).

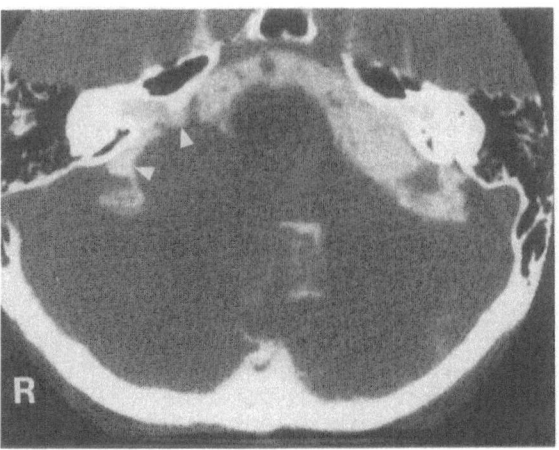

Fig. 9.3. Positive contrast cisternography. Exophytic extension of a cerebellar metastasis into the right CP angle cistern (*arrowheads*). (P.B.).

Anatomy of the Nerves: Acoustic, Facial, Nervus Intermedius

All three nerves originate in nuclei within the brainstem, leaving it at the lower border of the pons. Anteriorly is the facial nerve, posteriorly the acoustic. They pass laterally and slightly anteriorly across the subarachnoid space of the CP angle cistern into the internal auditory meatus (IAM). Within the IAM the various nerves and divisions are arranged as shown in Fig. 9.4. It can be seen that the acoustic

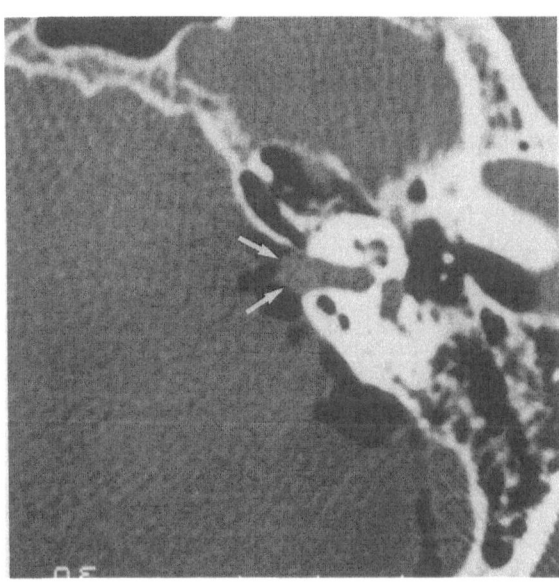

Fig. 9.2. CT gas meatography. A predominantly intracanalicular acoustic neurinoma extends into the cerebellopontine angle cistern (*arrows*).

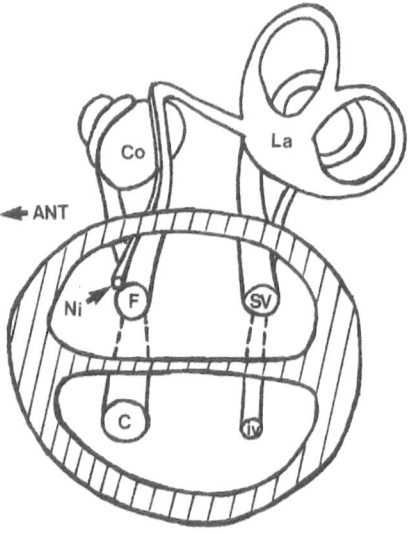

Fig. 9.4. Diagram of the arrangement of the seventh and eighth cranial nerves within the internal auditory canal. Co, cochlea; La, labyrinth; F, facial nerve; Ni, nervus intermedius; SV, superior vestibular nerve; C, cochlear nerve; iv, inferior vestibular nerve.

nerve consists of three main divisions, the cochlear, superior and inferior vestibular nerves, and that the horizontally orientated bony septum, the crista falciformis, separates the four main nerves into two groups. The fibres of the acoustic nerve pass through bony foramina to supply the named structures of the inner ear whilst the facial nerve continues on a complex route.

The facial nerve perforates the bone together with the nervus intermedius. Within its bony canal, the nerve passes forwards and slightly laterally within the dense bone of the labyrinth and it is here that the nerve is particularly vulnerable to traumatic damage from transverse fractures of the petrous bone and from damage secondary to translabyrinthine surgery. The nerve passes forward between the cochlea and the labyrinth to reach an expansion in the bony canal, the geniculate fossa (Fig. 9.5).

The nervus intermedius terminates here on cell bodies which continue forward as the greater superficial petrosal nerve eventually reaching the lacrimal gland via the pterygopalatine ganglion.

Also within the geniculate ganglion are the cell bodies of the sensory fibres of taste (the chorda tympani). The remainder of the ganglion simply consists of nerve fibres passing through it.

Within the geniculate ganglion the facial nerve fibres turn acutely posteriorly (the first genu) and pass horizontally along the medial wall of the middle ear cleft, descending slightly to pass underneath the horizontal semicircular canal, between it

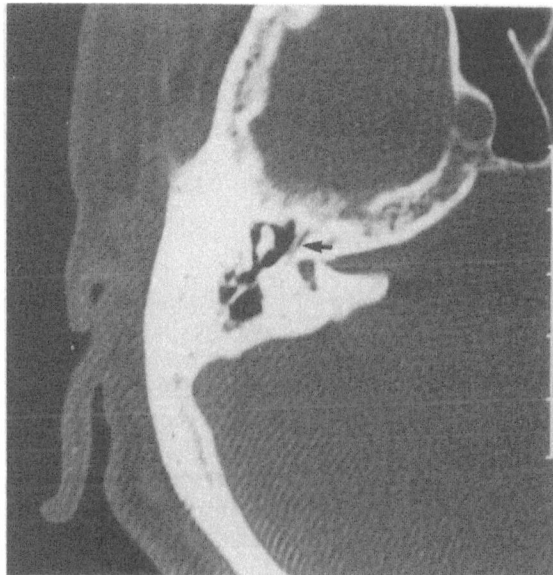

Fig. 9.6. Axial HRCT. The tympanic portion of the facial nerve passes through the middle ear cleft (*arrow*).

and the oval window (Fig. 9.6). Upon reaching the posterior aspect of the cleft, the fibres again turn (the second genu), this time to run vertically through the stylomastoid canal and foramen (Fig. 9.7). The fibres of chorda tympani leave the facial nerve within the stylomastoid canal. Once through the foramen, the nerve passes into the parotid gland where it cannot be demonstrated by CT.

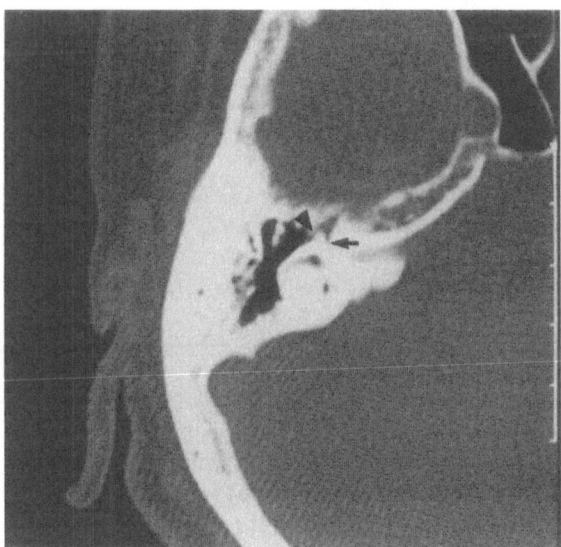

Fig. 9.5. Axial HRCT. The facial nerve sweeps forward in its bony canal towards the geniculate fossa (*arrow*) and the initial portion of the tympanic segment is shown directed posteriorly (*arrowhead*).

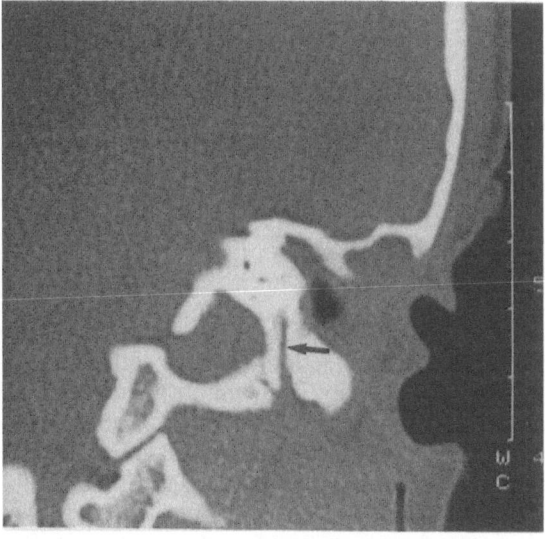

Fig. 9.7. Coronal HRCT. The second genu of the facial nerve and the stylomastoid canal are shown (*arrow*). The patient has had a mastoidectomy.

It can be seen from this account that the facial nerve is exposed within the middle ear cleft to all the various pathologies arising here, separated only by bone which may be deficient or so thin as to be invisible even at maximal resolution.

Acoustic Neurinomas

More correctly known as Schwannomas, these benign tumours of the nerve sheath usually originate as the nerve perforates the meninges at the CP angle. True neurinomas may originate directly from the nerve. Acoustic neurinomas account for 10% of all intracranial tumours and the majority of CP angle lesions. The cardinal presenting feature is of progressive sensorineural deafness which may occasionally be abrupt in onset. There may also be tinnitus or vertigo and as the tumour enlarges the clinical features relating to an expanding posterior fossa mass lesion may supervene.

A major debate continues regarding the protocol for the investigation of patients with suspected acoustic neurinoma. Only 1% or 2% of the patients presenting with isolated sensorineural deafness to an otologic clinic will subsequently turn out to have acoustic tumours and some sort of screening has, therefore, to be undertaken if radiology departments are not to become overburdened by large numbers of unnecessary "normal" investigations. If high quality brainstem evoked response equipment is available this undoubtedly provides the most effective screening test since it will identify with a high degree of accuracy patients likely to have an acoustic tumour. Unfortunately this test is not widely available, at least in the United Kingdom, and radiology will play a major part in the screening process. The protocol for investigation eventually used in any particular unit will depend entirely on the equipment available and whilst the gold standard of gadolinium enhanced MRI may be a counsel of perfection the high cost of MRI and restricted access leaves CT as the major imaging modality for acoustic neurinomas in the United Kingdom.

The hallmark of an acoustic neurinoma on CT is of a CP angle mass lesion isodense with adjacent brain which enhances uniformly with intravenous contrast. The tumour emerges from a widened and eroded IAM although in a proportion of cases there may be no demonstrable bone change. Some acoustic tumours can be of mixed density with irregular enhancement patterns and cystic change is not uncommonly encountered (Fig. 9.8). The differential diagnosis includes meningioma, arachnoid

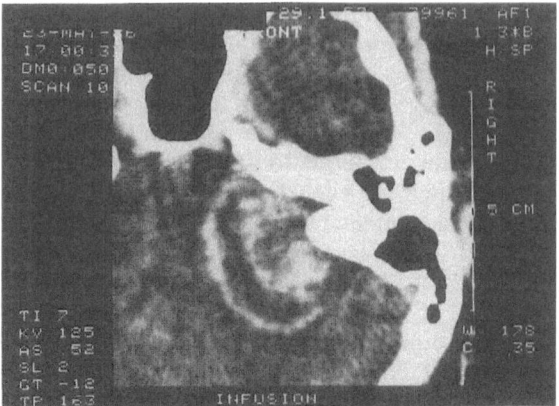

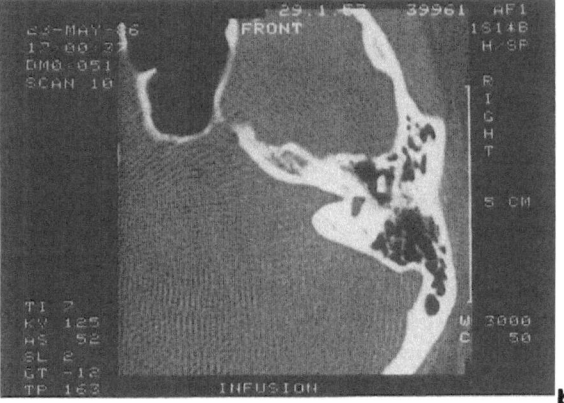

Fig. 9.8. Cranial CT after IV contrast. A mixed attenuation acoustic neuroma (**a**) emerges from a widened, eroded IAM (**b**).

cyst, epidermoid, aneurysm and exophytic extension of an intra-axial mass.

Facial Neurinomas

These usually present with a slowly progressive facial palsy and usually arise near to the geniculate ganglion. The CT demonstration of the entire length of the facial canal will require:

1. Gas meatography to show the intracanalicular portion
2. Axial scans for the labyrinthine portion
3. Sequential coronal scans to show the nerve in cross section as it descends along the middle ear cleft (the tympanic portion)
4. Coronal scans for the stylomastoid canal

An intracanalicular or CP angle facial neurinoma will closely resemble the CT appearances of an acoustic neurinoma although it may additionally expand into the geniculate fossa (Fig. 9.9).

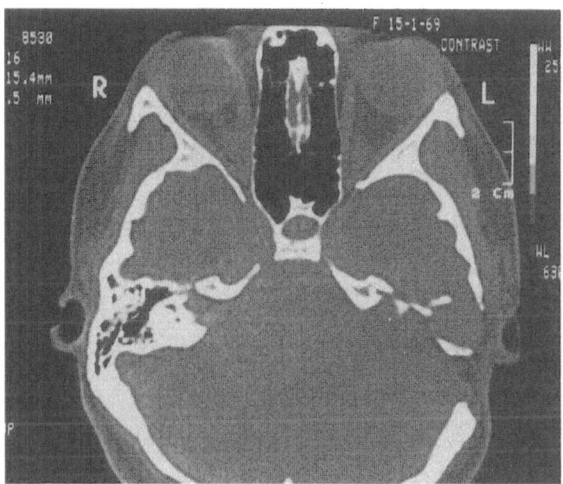

Fig. 9.9. Axial HRCT. Right facial neurinoma. Bone erosion can be seen extending to the geniculate fossa (*arrow*). A left facial neurinoma had been removed previously from this patient with neurofibromatosis. (P.B.)

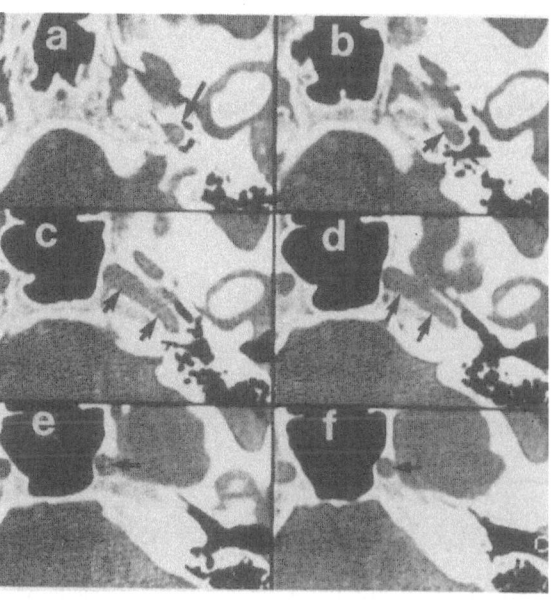

Fig. 9.10. Axial HRCT (**a–f** run inferiorly to superiorly). The course of the carotid canal is shown (*arrows*).

The Inner Ear

Congenital and inherited conditions constitute the most significant group of disorders to affect the labyrinth. Congenital sensorineural hearing loss may result from nerve damage due to intrauterine infection such as maternal rubella or from a structural abnormality. Anomalies of the inner ear may be part of a more widespread skeletal condition such as Crouzon's, Apert's and Hurler's syndromes. Alternatively the findings may not allow such characterisation into eponymous syndromes. This emphasises the main requirement for the radiologist in this situation which is to give an accurate description of the anatomy as seen (Phelps et al. 1975).

Imaging of the Vessels

The Internal Carotid Artery (ICA)

The artery perforates the base of the skull through the carotid canal, entering it vertically. It then turns to run horizontally, anteromedial to the petrous apex where it reaches the inferior aspect of the cavernous sinus. Here it turns for the second time to run vertically towards the carotid siphon (Fig. 9.10). The first turn of the carotid artery is evident as a promontory in the inferior aspect of the middle ear cleft (hypotympanum) from which it is separated only by a thin plate of bone.

Although intrapetrous aneurysms of the ICA have been described (Willinsky et al. 1987) perhaps the most important anomaly of this vessel is the "aberrant carotid artery" which may present as a mass in the hypotympanum. The bony wall encasing the artery is deficient and the vessel bulges upwards and laterally and is seen as a vascular mass in the inferior aspect of the middle ear cleft. It is well shown on axial or coronal CT and this may obviate the need for angiography (Fig. 9.11) (Swartz et al. 1985a, b).

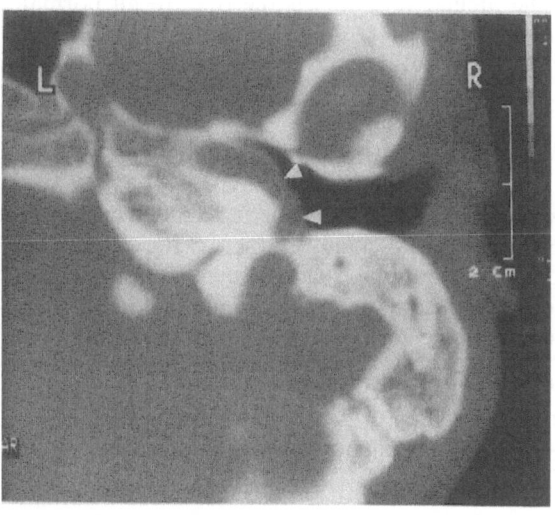

Fig. 9.11. Axial HRCT. Aberrant right carotid artery (*arrowheads*). (By courtesy of Dr. R. Dosseter.)

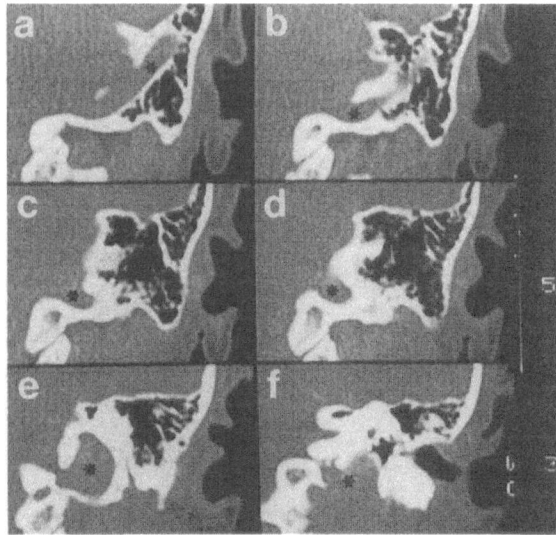

Fig. 9.12. Coronal HRCT (**a–f** run posteriorly to anteriorly). The path of the lateral sinus into the jugular bulb is shown(*).

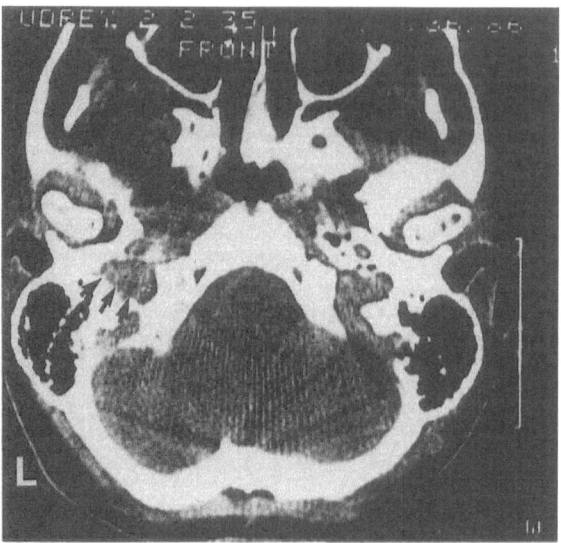

Fig. 9.13. Axial HRCT. Left glomus jugular tumour with loss of the corticated margin of the jugular foramen (*arrows*).

The Internal Jugular Vein and Lateral Sinus

The jugular foramen transmits venous blood from the sigmoid sinus in the posterior fossa into the jugular vein in the neck. It is divided into two parts by a fibrous (or occasionally bony) septum. The smaller compartment contains the glossopharyngeal nerve and the inferior petrosal sinus (which drains the cavernous sinus), whilst the larger contains the jugular bulb and the vagus and accessory cranial nerves. Both the glossopharyngeal and vagus nerves give off small branches which contain glomus formations in their walls.

It is important to realise that variation in the size of the jugular foramina is the rule. In all normal foramina, however, the bony cortex will be well defined (Fig. 9.12).

Glomus Tumours

Paraganglionoma is the generic name given to the slow-growing vascular lesions arising from the glomus formations – clusters of cells comprising the chemoreceptor system. Specific tumours from this class are named after their site or origin, thus:

Carotid body – carotid body tumour
Nodose ganglion of the vagus – glomus vagale
Adventitia of the jugular bulb – glomus jugulare
Cochlea promontory – glomus tympanicum

Glomus tumours are the second commonest tumour of the petrous temporal bone after acoustic neurinomas. These tumours extend by local invasion into the adjacent bone and along vascular channels, through the air cells and bony foramina. Conductive hearing loss can result from middle ear invasion. Destruction of the vestibular apparatus may cause vertigo and tumour vascularity tinnitus. There may also be progressive involvement of the lower cranial nerves.

The key radiological finding is of a highly vascular mass arising within the petrous bone with local bone destruction (Fig. 9.13). The mass may extend into the posterior fossa and into the soft tissue below the skull base along the line of the jugular vein (Duncan et al. 1979; Lo et al. 1984). Internal and external carotid angiography is indicated when every effort must be made to establish the patency of the jugular vein. Angiography may also help to discriminate between glomus tumours and other lesions which must be considered in the presence of a destructive mass centred on the jugular foramen (Hesselink et al. 1981). These include metastasis, myeloma, cholesteatoma, chordoma, chondrosarcoma and neurinoma. Glomus tumours will usually have a major supply from the ascending pharyngeal artery.

The Sound Conducting Structures

External Auditory Canal

The external auditory meatus (EAM) can be divided into two parts: a lateral fibrocartilaginous portion rich in hair and ceruminous glands, and a

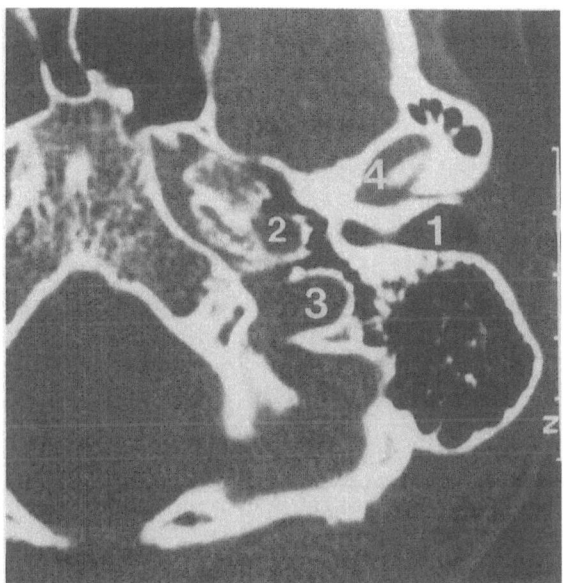

Fig. 9.14. Axial HRCT. The relations of the external auditory meatus. 1 External auditory meatus; 2 carotid canal; 3 jugular foramen; 4 temporomandibular joint.

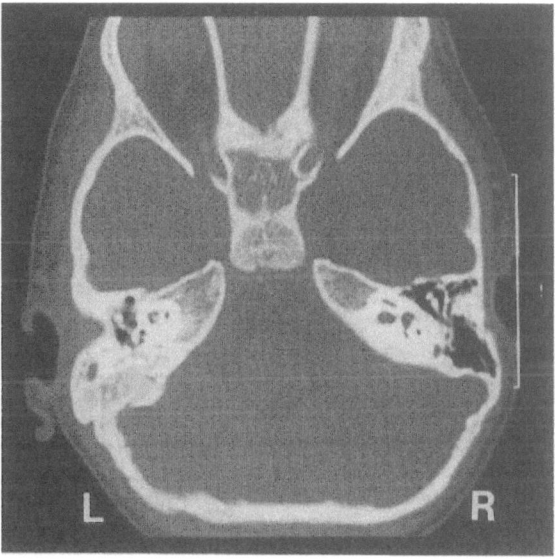

Fig. 9.15. Axial HRCT. Treacher Collins syndrome. The right petrous temporal bone is normal. The left shows atresia of the EAM and a poorly developed middle ear. The inner ear is normal.

medial osseous portion lined with very thin skin deficient in hair and containing only a few ceruminous glands. The skin is closely adherent in both parts of the canal and in the osseous portion in particular, the skin is directly bound to the periosteum of the bone. Lesions within the canal generate considerable tension and pain.

The temporomandibular joint (TMJ) is a close anterior relation and joint dysfunction may cause aural pain (Fig. 9.14).

Atresias of the EAM usually occur in isolation but can be part of named syndromes, e.g. Crouzon's and Treacher Collins syndromes (Fig. 9.15). The canal is narrowed or even obliterated and often angled sharply upwards medially. There may be accompanying abnormalities of the TMJ.

Atresias of the EAM are often accompanied by anomalies of the middle ear cleft. The cleft may be obliterated or there may be an ossicular abnormality involving their fusion into a mass (the atretic plate). In these circumstances the radiologist should ensure that the inner ear is structurally normal prior to surgery and that the course of the facial nerve is established.

Inflammatory processes

Malignant otitis externa should be considered as an osteomyelitis of the EAM occurring particularly in immunocompromised patients and in severe dia-betics. Despite advances in surgical and antibiotic treatment it still carries a high morbidity and mortality. *Pseudomonas aeruginosa* is one of a number of organisms responsible which are often resistant to many antibiotics. Uncontrolled infection will spread inferiorly into the infratemporal region of the skull base, with involvement of the facial nerve. Anterior and posterior extension will involve the TMJ and mastoid respectively. Intracranial extension will lead to abscess, empyema or meningitis.

Axial CT slices will usually be obtained in this condition since the patient will be too unwell to tolerate coronal scanning. Permeative destruction of the bony confines to the EAM will be easily seen and the lumen will be obliterated by a soft tissue mass. This mass can be seen to involve adjacent tissues and the full extent of the lesion can be appreciated (Curtin et al. 1982; Mendelson et al. 1983).

Malignant Neoplasms

All of the cutaneous neoplasms can occur within the external auditory canal, notably squamous and basal cell carcinomas, malignant melanomas and metastatic disease. There is often a history of chronic infection predisposing to malignant degeneration and patients are mostly elderly. CT will assist greatly in assessing the extent of these lesions (Bird et al. 1983).

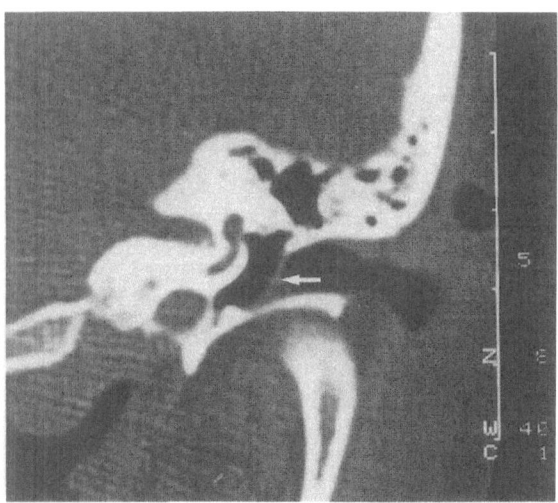

Fig. 9.16. Coronal HRCT. Thickened tympanic membrane (*arrow*).

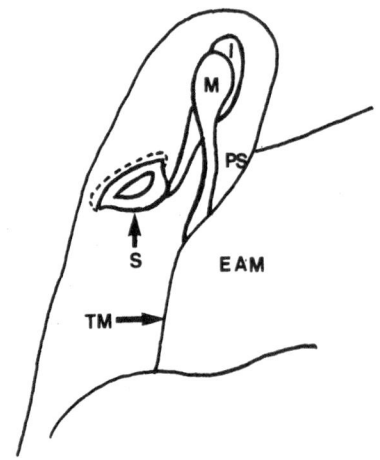

Fig. 9.17. Diagram of the ossicles of the middle ear. EAM, external auditory meatus; TM, tympanic membrane; PS, Prussak's space; S, stapes; M, malleus; I, incus.

Tympanic Membrane

This is an oval membrane consisting of an outer layer, continuous with the skin of the external auditory canal, two layers of fibrous tissue and an inner layer continuous with the mucosa of the middle ear cleft. Part of the membrane, the pars flaccida, is distinguished from the remainder, the pars tensa, in being deficient in the central two layers of fibrous tissue. It is this weakened area of the membrane which is so important in the aetiology of cholesteatoma (see below).

The membrane can nearly always be seen on coronal high resolution scans, but less easily on axial scans. Perforations and retractions of this membrane can be easily appreciated both by the examining clinician and the radiologist, but the radiologist has the additional advantage in being able to see behind the outer surface of the intact membrane. Thus thickening of the membrane and fluid and soft tissue within the cleft can be readily identified (Fig. 9.16).

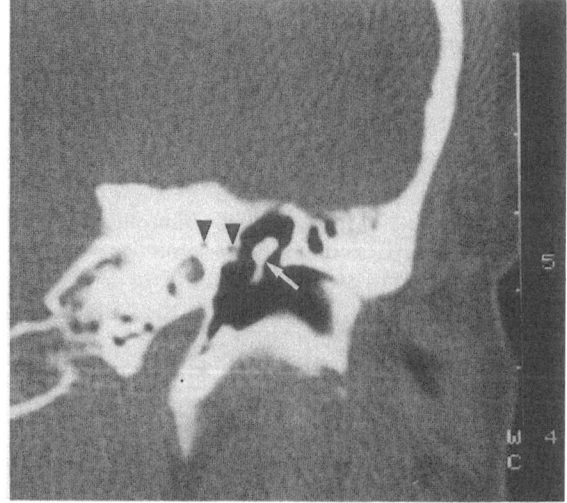

Fig. 9.18. Coronal HRCT (**a**) shows the bodies of the malleus and incus which are inseparable on this scan plan (*arrow*). Note also the facial nerve which is "cut" twice as it passes to and from the geniculate ganglion. It lies above the cochlea and the appearance has been termed "snake's eyes" (*arrowheads*). **b** A more posterior view which shows the long process of the incus (*arrow*). The two crura of the stapes lie in a plane inclined from the horizontal and cannot be identified on coronal scans and only rarely on axial scans.

Middle Ear Cleft and Ossicular System

The middle ear cleft can be best understood if it is thought of as a simple space within the complex of air cells of the petrous bone and mastoid. It is inclined at approximately 30° to the vertical and is somewhat arbitrarily divided into a number of compartments for descriptive purposes; the epitympanum superiorly, the mesotympanum and inferiorly, the hypotympanum.

The ossicles are arranged across the cleft so that the long process of the malleus is embedded in the tympanic membrane and the stape "fits" into the oval window (Fig 9.17 and 9.18). Prussak's space is an important area to observe since it is bounded laterally by the pars flaccida of the tympanic membrane and is thus obliterated early in retractions of this structure. Posteriorly it opens into the epitympanum.

It is thought that the primary process underlying all inflammatory processes in the middle ear is Eustachian tube dysfunction. Inadequate drainage and/or ventilation of the normally air-filled middle ear cleft leads to mucosal oedema, effusions and subsequent infection. The finding of a middle ear effusion in an adult should always raise the possibility of a nasopharyngeal carcinoma obstructing the Eustachian tube orifice.

Infected fluid from the middle ear may pass freely into the mastoid air cells, causing mastoiditis (Fig. 9.19) and infection can subsequently spread:

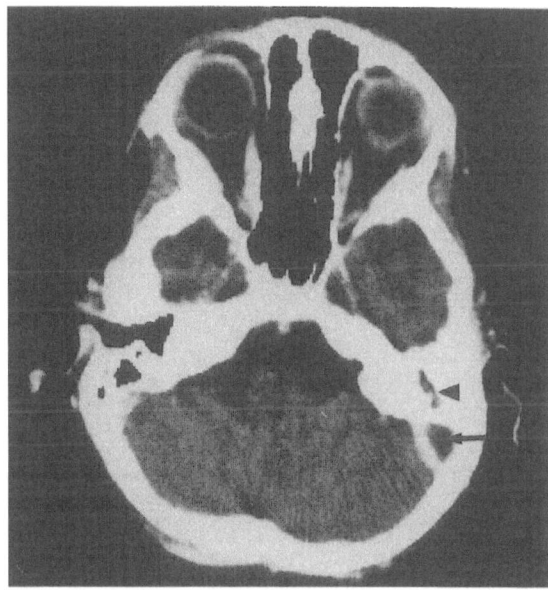

Fig. 9.20. Cranial CT. Lateral sinus thrombosis (*arrow*) associated with a middle ear infection (*arrowhead*).

1. Through the tegmen to the cranial cavity leading to extradural and subdural empyema, meningitis and cerebral abscess
2. Posteriorly to involve the lateral sinus leading to thrombosis, venous infarction of the brain, and hydrocephalus (Fig. 9.20)
3. Medially to the petrous apex (if pneumatised) to cause a chronic infection with irritation of the Vth and VIth cranial nerves

Korner's septum usually presents no difficulty in diagnosis, but if unusually thickened, the surgeon can believe that the medial wall of the antrum has been fully explored, when in fact there remains considerable disease behind it (Fig. 9.21).

Granulation Tissue

In response to chronic irritation, granulation tissue may develop which is usually vascular and bleeds easily. Fresh granulation tissue is very friable. Older tissue will be tougher due to the presence of a variable amount of fibrosis and some tissue will develop a central "cyst" full of cholesterol crystals.

Granulomas will have the same CT attentuation as any other tissue or fluid within the cleft. They can be partially distinguished from fluid in that they do not move when the patient's position is changed, and granulomas can be distinguished from cholesteatomas in that they only rarely destroy bone, whereas bone destruction is the hallmark of cholesteatoma.

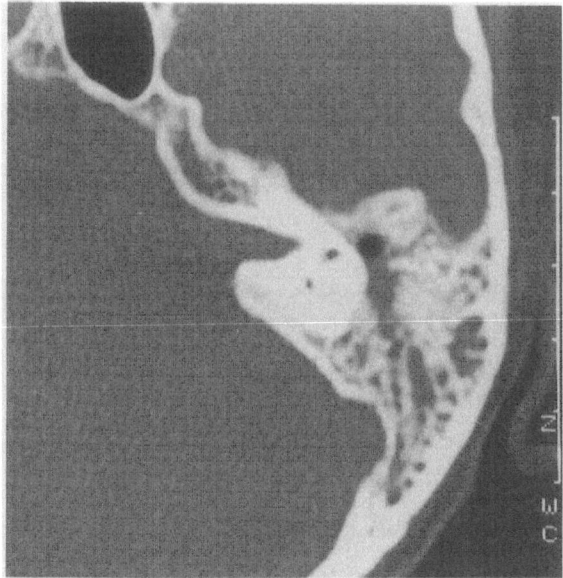

Fig. 9.19. Axial HRCT. Mastoiditis. There is a middle ear effusion and near complete opacification of the cellular mastoid.

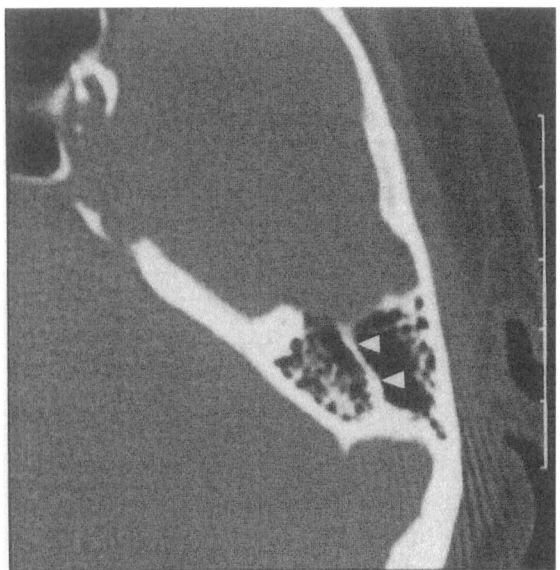

Fig. 9.21. Axial HRCT. Korner's septum (*arrowheads*).

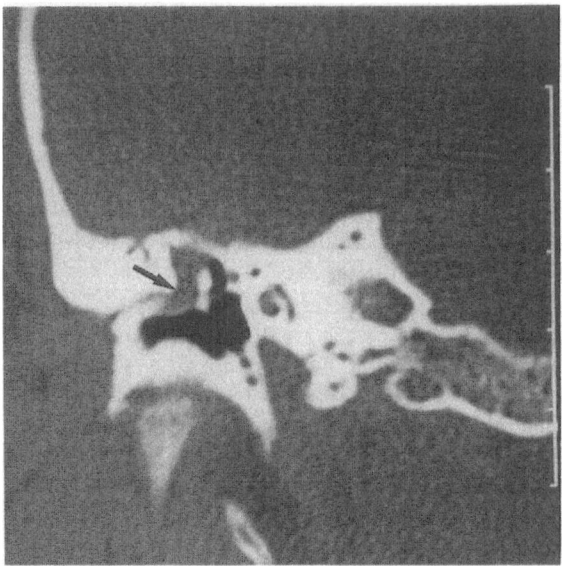

Fig. 9.22. Coronal HRCT. Attic cholesteatoma. Note the erosive blunting of the scutum (*arrow*).

Expansile cystic lesions of the petrous bone may result from giant cholesterol cysts (cholesterol granulomas). They too may have an inflammatory basis and disclose characteristic MRI appearances with increased signal intensity on both T1 and T2 weighted images consistent with chronic haemorrhage. They may thus be distinguished from epidermoid tumours (Griffin et al. 1987; Greenberg et al. 1988).

Cholesteatoma

The initial event in the development of the majority of acquired cholesteatomas is the formation of a retraction pocket in the pars flaccida of the tympanic membrane. This retraction, once again is probably secondary to Eustachian tube dysfunction. As long as the normal desquamative process can continue the retraction pocket can remain stable for many years. Once this normal desquamation is disrupted, the dead keratinised epithelial cells accumulate and the cholesteatoma develops. The lesion will start in Prussak's space and then usually spread posteriorly into the epitympanum (Fig. 9.22). It should be remembered that the clinician will often see only a small retraction pocket whilst the cholesteatoma is spreading extensively within the middle ear cleft.

Destruction of bone is a common finding caused both by pressure erosion and possibly direct enzymatic destruction by collagenases, the ossicles are rapidly destroyed and then later there is destruction of the tegmen. Should the cholesteatoma become

infected (and dead skin is an excellent culture medium) the consequences can be easily appreciated. The possibilities are much as those described under otitis media with the addition of the serious complication of erosion into the labyrinth. This can result in total hearing loss and labyrinthitis (Fig. 9.23) (Swartz 1984; Johnson et al. 1983).

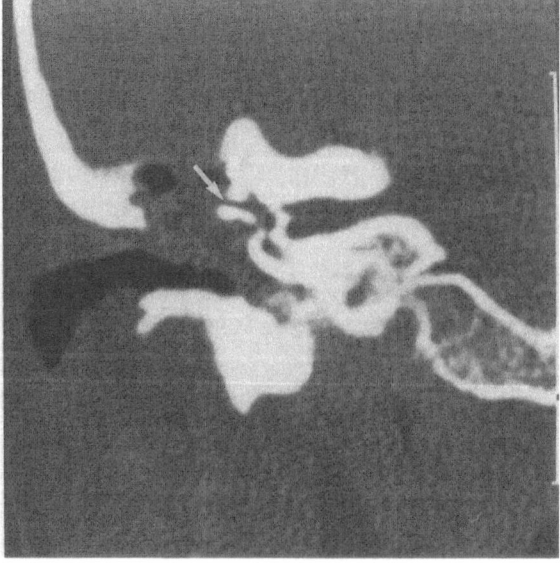

Fig. 9.23. Coronal HRCT. Cholesteatoma with erosion into the labyrinth (*arrow*) and into the middle cranial fossa.

Otospongiosis (Otosclerosis)

In otospongiosis the normal very dense endo-chondral bone is replaced by foci of spongy vascular new bone, which is less dense than the original bone. In the later stages of the disease this new bone becomes more sclerotic. Two types of otosclerosis are described, in one of which the disease is centred on the oval window (the fenestral type), and in the second the disease is more widespread and involves the capsule of the cochlea.

In the fenestral variety the disease presents in the second or third decade of life with tinnitus which may progress to deafness. This occurs when the annular ligament of the stapes becomes involved limiting transmission of sound into the inner ear. In extreme cases the footplate of stapes becomes fused to the oval window. Bony overgrowth around the oval window is seen limiting its aperture. Great care must be made in making this interpretation however since the problems of the partial volume effect make accurate assessment of the oval window difficult, and it is easy to "over-read" CT scans.

In the retrofenestral type, the hearing loss is of the sensorineural type and reflects damage to the cochlea itself. In many patients there are no abnormal radiographic findings.

Some authors have speculated that the investigation has been performed when the active phase of the disease has passed. In other patients areas of demineralisation are seen around the cochlea, representing the formation of spongy new bone.

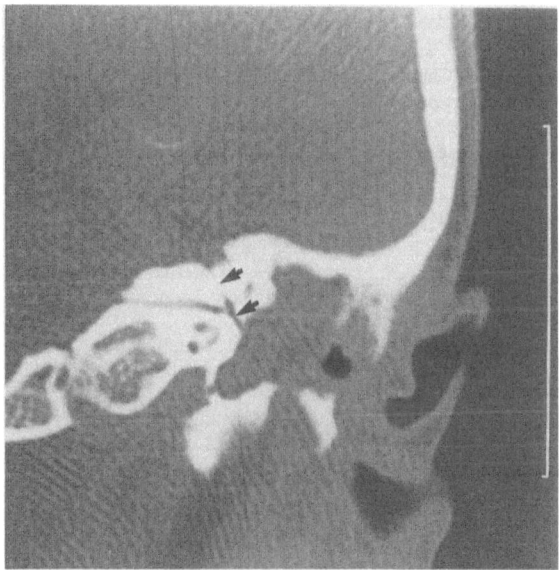

Fig. 9.25. Coronal HRCT. Transverse fracture (*arrows*). The horizontal "defect" is the petromastoid canal.

Trauma

Longitudinal Fractures

These account for 70% of petrous fractures and are caused by a direct blow to the side of the head. The fracture extends along the pyramid towards the apex and will usually involve the external meatus, the tympanic membrane and the middle ear cleft. Ossicular disruption is often found (if sought!), and there is an increased risk of the subsequent development of cholesteatoma due to damage to the tympanic membrane (Fig. 9.24) (Johnson et al. 1984; Avrahami et al. 1988).

Transverse Fractures

These are less common (20%) but much more severe. The petrous component of the fracture is but a small part of the whole fracture which extends from the occiput to the middle cranial fossa and beyond following direct trauma to the back of the head. Damage to the acoustic and facial nerves as they pass within the bone is common, leading to sensorineural hearing loss and facial palsy (Fig. 9.25).

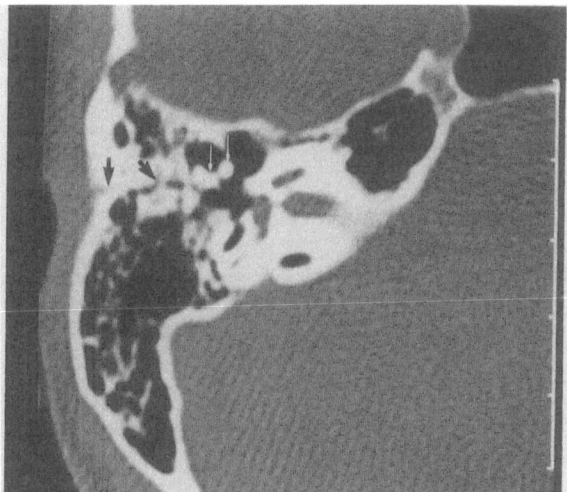

Fig. 9.24. Axial HRCT. Longitudinal fracture with ossicular disruption (the malleus and incus (*white arrows*) no longer lie in close apposition). Part of the complex fracture line is indicated (*black arrows*).

Complex Fractures

These can ramify through the skull base and may be difficult to classify because of their extent.

References

Avrahami E, Chen Z, Solomon A (1988) Modern high resolution computed tomography (CT) diagnosis of longitudinal fractures of the petrous bone. Neuroradiology 30:169–174

Bird CR, Hasso AN, Stewart CD, Hinshaw DB, Thompson JR (1983) Malignant primary neoplasms of the ear and temporal bone studied by high resolution computed tomography. Radiology 149:171–174

Bird CR, Hasso AN, Drayer BP, Hinshaw DB, Thompson JR (1985) The cerebellopontine angle and internal auditory canal: Neurovascular anatomy on gas CT cisternograms. Radiology 154:667–670

Chakeres DW, Spiegal PK (1983) A systematic technique for comprehensive evaluation of the temporal bone by CT. Radiology 146:97–106

Curtin HD, Wolfe P, Pay M (1982) Malignant external otitis: CT evaluation. Radiology 145:383–388

Duncan AW, Lack EE, Deck MF (1979) Radiological evaluation of paragangliomas of the head and neck. Radiology 132:99–105

Greenberg JJ, Oot RF, Wismer GL et al. (1988) Cholesterol granuloma of the petrous apex: MR and CT evaluation. AJNR 9:1205–1214

Griffin C, De La Paz R, Enzmann D (1987) MR and CT correlation of cholesterol cysts of the petrous bone. AJNR 8:825–829

Hesselink JR, Davis KR, Traveras JM (1981) Selective arteriography of glomus jugular tumors: Techniques, normal and pathologic arterial anatomy. AJNR 2:289–297

Johnson DW, Voorhees RL, Lufkin RB, Hanafee W, Canalis R (1983) Cholesteatomas of the temporal bone: Role of CT. Radiology 148:733–737

Johnson DW, Hasso AN, Stewart CD, Thompson JR, Hinshaw DB (1984) Temporal bone trauma: High resolution computed tomographic evaluation. Radiology 151:411–415

Kingsley DPE, Brooks GB, Leung AWL, Johnson MA (1985) Acoustic neuromas: Evaluation by magnetic resonance imaging. AJNR 6:1–5

Lo WWM, Solti-Bohman LG, Lambert PR (1984) High resolution CT in evaluation of glomus tumours of the temporal bone. Radiology 150:737–742

Mendelson DS, Som PM, Mendelson MH, Parisier SC (1983) Malignant external otitis: The role of computed tomography and radio nuclides in evaluation. Radiology 149:745–749

Phelps PD, Lloyd GAS, Sheldon PWE (1975) Deformity of the labyrinth and internal auditory meatus in congenital deafness. Br J Radiol 48:973–978

Sortland O (1979) Computed tomography combined with gas cisternography for the diagnosis of expanding lesions in the cerebellopontine angle. Neuroradiology 18:19–22

Swartz JD (1983) High resolution computed tomography of the middle ear and mastoid, Part I: Normal anatomy including normal variations. Radiology 148:449–454

Swartz JD (1984) Cholesteatomas of the middle ear. Diagnosis, etiology and complications. Radiol Clin North Am 22:15–35

Swartz JD, Faerber EN, Wolfson RJ, Marlowe FI (1984) Fenestral otosclerosis: Significance of pre-operative CT evaluation. Radiology 151:703–707

Swartz JD, Bazarnic ML, Naidich TP, Lowry LD, Doan HT (1985a) Aberrant internal carotid artery lying within the middle ear: High resolution CT diagnosis and differential diagnosis. Neuroradiology 27:322–326

Swartz JD, Mandell DW, Berman SE, Wolfson RJ, Marlow EI, Popky GL (1985b) Cochlear otosclerosis (otospongiosis): CT analysis with audiometric correlation. Radiology 155:147–150

Willinsky R, Lasjaunias P, Pruvost P, Boucherat M (1987) Petrous internal carotid artery aneurysm causing epistaxis: balloon embolisation with preservation of the parent vessel. Neuroradiology 29:570–572

Further Reading

Swartz JD (1986) Imaging of the temporal bone: A text/atlas. Thieme Medical Publishers, New York

Swartz JD (1989) Current imaging approach to the temporal bone. Radiology 171:309–317

Chapter 10

Muscle and the Peripheral Nervous System

Chandra H. Thakkar and Michael Swash

Introduction

Neuromuscular disorders are usually diagnosed by consideration of the results obtained by clinical examination, biochemical studies such as creatine kinase, enzyme determinations in peripheral venous blood, electromyography and nerve conduction velocity measurements, and histopathological examination of the muscle biopsy (Swash and Schwartz 1988). The newer techniques of molecular biology and genetics are beginning to be applied to the diagnosis of specific syndromes, such as Duchenne dystrophy and Becker muscular dystrophy, in which the genetic locus is known (Rowland 1988). Imaging methodologies have only recently been applied to muscles, following the development of computed tomographic (CT) scanning and magnetic resonance imaging (MRI) and their role in diagnosis and management is, as yet, relatively neglected (Bulcke and Baert 1982). However, imaging methodologies have played a fundamental role in the more accurate assessment of other conditions in other bodily systems and it is likely that their application to diseases of muscle and of the peripheral nervous system will be equally valuable.

Clinical examination can provide information as to the muscle bulk, muscle tone, reflex activity, and strength (Swash 1988). With experience this information is highly reliable but the possibility of highly selective involvement of muscles acting around a single joint, for example around the knee, is difficult to assess. The flexor and extensor compartments of the thigh contain many muscles, yet the clinician can only assess strength during the hinge movements of extension and flexion and muscle bulk is particularly difficult to assess in the flexor compartment because of the thickness of the subcutaneous fat in this region of the body in most

persons, particularly those relatively immobilised by weakness. Sophisticated judgements as to asymmetrical involvement are particularly difficult. Indeed, most neuromuscular diseases are regarded by clinicians as causing symmetrical and rather striking proximal muscular weakness; only peripheral neuropathies, and certain rare distal myopathies causing distal weakness. Asymmetrical weakness is usually a feature of disorders affecting individual peripheral nerves or plexuses, such as diabetic neuropathy or pressure neuropathies, or of the inflammatory myopathies such as polymyositis (Swash and Schwartz 1988). It is also a feature of the earlier stages of motor neurone disease (amyotrophic lateral sclerosis) (Swash and Schwartz 1982; Swash and Ingram 1988).

The investigations used in neuromuscular disease tend to be highly selective but cannot be applied to many muscles. For example, needle electromyography has the capacity of assessing several different muscles, given the patient's ability to withstand the multiple skin punctures necessary for the satisfactory performance of the technique, but the method is highly selective and only certain zones within any given muscles are assessed. Muscle biopsy is likely to be applied only to one or at the most two muscles in any given patient. Thus the histopathological changes revealed by the biopsy may not be at all representative of involvement of all the muscles in the body (Van der Walt et al. 1987).

Imaging with modern methodologies offers the possibility of non-invasive image production, using reproducible standardised procedures without undue exposure to ionising or other radiations. Since all the muscles in any given part of the body can be imaged in the plane of section in which the technology is applied the possibility of highly selective involvement of individual muscles or parts of muscles can be considered, thus opening up a new dimension in the investigation of these cases.

Imaging Methodologies

A number of different techniques have been applied to the neuromuscular system. Many of these have been rendered obsolete by computed tomography and magnetic resonance imaging but some, particularly ultrasonography (Heckmatt et al. 1982; Kamala et al. 1985), still have a place, particularly in the assessment of young children. Abnormalities in the spine, e.g. kyphoscoliosis, and in limb bones, especially demineralisation, splaying of the epiphyses and narrowing of the shafts of long bones are common in muscular dystrophies (Walton and Warwick 1954; Wilkins and Gibson 1976). In myotonic dystrophy the sella turcica is small and the skull-vault shows hyperostosis (Caughey 1952), and in the congenital myopathies kyphoscoliosis, a high-arched palate and hip dysplasia or dislocation occur.

Soft Tissue Radiography

Muscular tissues and fat are highly permeable to conventional X-rays but soft tissue radiology has the capacity to detect calcification in muscles, as is found in certain infestations, such as cysticercosis (Fig. 10.1), or trichinosis, in which calcified oocysts occur within muscle, in myositis ossificans and in patients with ectopic calcification due to trauma, focal inflammatory disorders, local infections, or in some patients with hypothyroidism.

Technical improvements, using improved photo development methods (Di Chiro and Nelson 1965; Frantzell and Inglemark 1951) made it possible to demonstrate subcutaneous, intramuscular and subfascial fat, and to improve the delineation of individual muscles. These studies were extended by Palvolgyi (1978) and Palvolgyi and Gallai (1980) who demonstrated relatively selective muscular atrophy in different disorders, including selective atrophy of individual muscles, asymmetry between the two sides, and even lacerations in muscle and tendon from trauma and in the Ehlers–Danlos syndrome (Palvolgyi et al. 1979; Palvolgyi and Balint 1979). These changes are more readily delineated with xeroradiography using either positive or negative mode imaging (Palvolgyi and Pentek 1977; Osterman et al. 1977).

Radioisotope imaging using [99m]technetium pyrophosphate has been used to demonstrate muscle

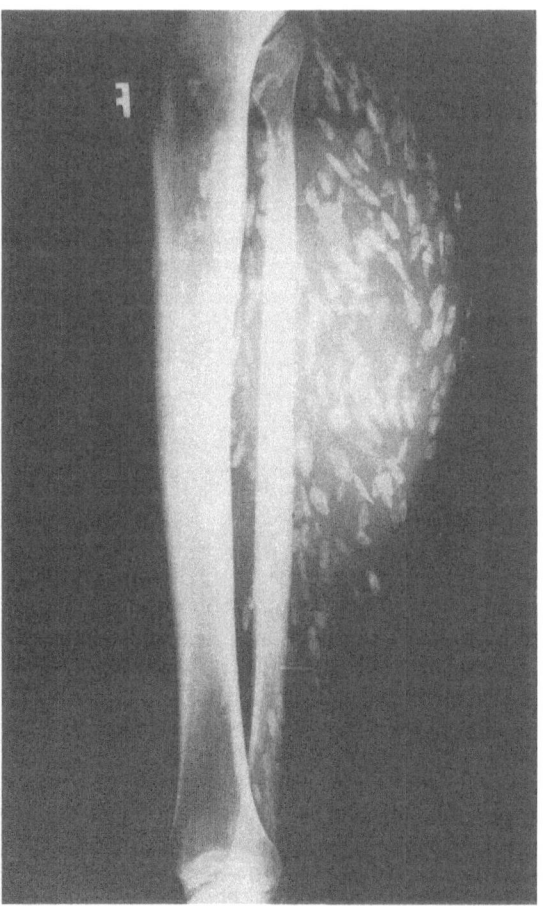

Fig. 10.1. Cysticercosis. The calcified cysts are visible in the calf muscles.

necrosis and inflammation, as in polymyositis (Suzuki et al. 1974; Steinfeld et al. 1977; Swift and Brown 1978) and it has been suggested that this technique might be useful in the management of polymyositis, particularly during the healing phase. In these respects this technique is comparable to thallium scanning in the heart in ischaemic heart disease.

Computed Tomography of Skeletal Muscles

Transverse images of skeletal muscles can be obtained for the limbs, pelvis and trunk using conventional CT scanners, without intravenous contrast, and with most scanners in current use the surface dose is less than 1 mGy per slice.

Bulcke and Baert (1982) have evaluated technical aspects of X-ray CT of the muscular system in some detail and recommend six levels of scanning, through the neck, the pectoral girdle at the subhumeral level, the abdomen at the L3/4 level, the pelvic girdle muscles through the level of the greater trochanters, and lower limb muscles in midthigh, and midcalf slices (Fig. 10.2). The abdominal and pelvic cuts also produce images of the forearm just below the elbow, and of the wrists, respectively. These six slices therefore produce images of proximal, axial and distal muscles and these can be used to assess selective involvement, symmetrical or asymmetrical involvement and proximal versus distal involvement in neuromusclar disorders. The

major muscles used for standing and walking, and for lifting objects with the arms are contained within the images. A slice through the neck musculature is not regularly used but the remainder, i.e. pectoral, abdominal, pelvic, midthigh and midcalf slices, provide a great deal of information that is not otherwise obtainable, either by clinical examination, or by other investigative procedures.

The pectoral slice (Fig. 10.2a) includes images of the *deltoids*, *pectoral* muscles, *trapezii* and *latissimus dorsi* muscles, and of the periscapular muscle groups. The upper part of the thoracic cavity and great vessels are also contained within the image.

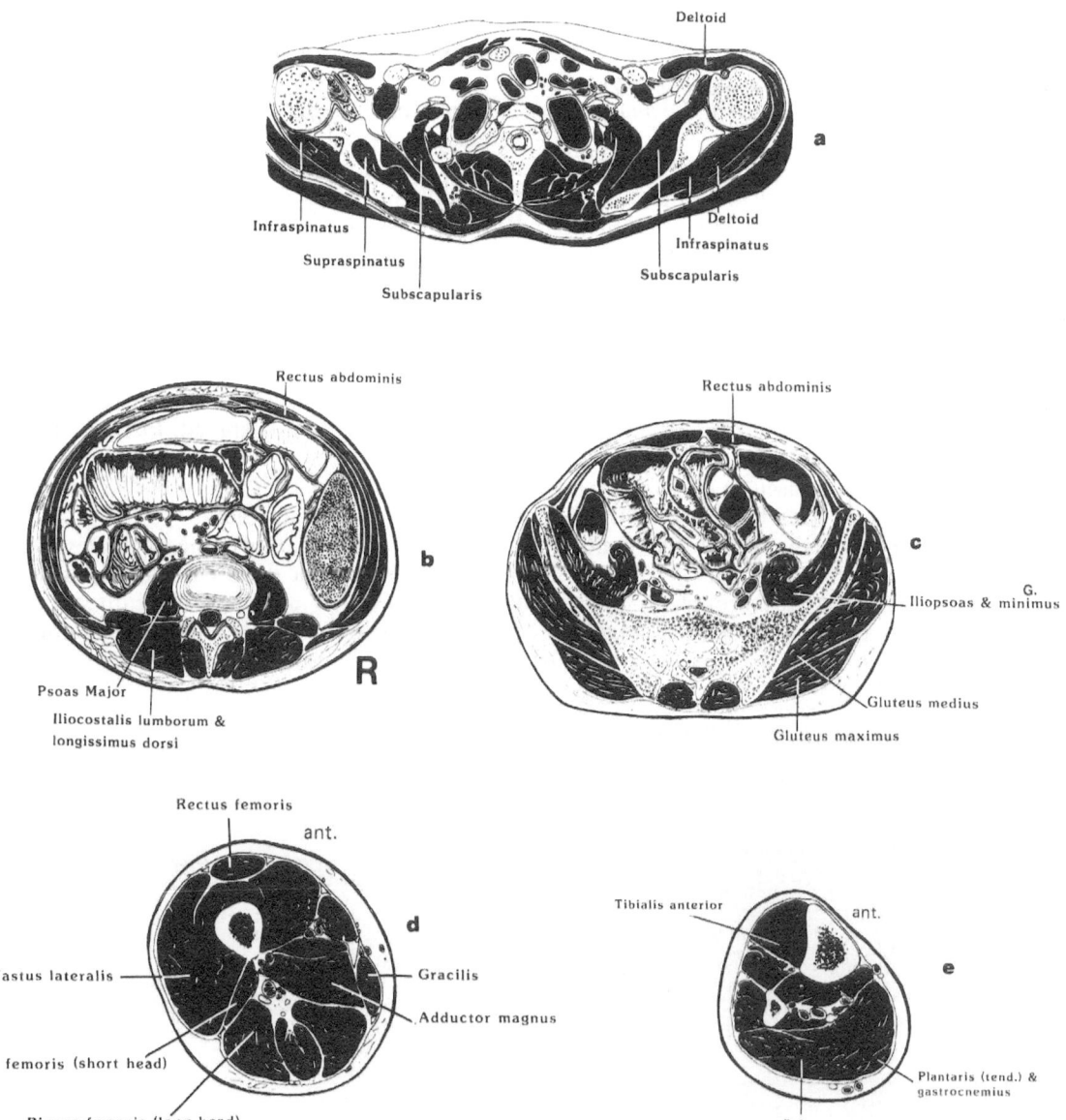

Fig. 10.2. Normal cross-section anatomy at the level of: **a** the pectoral region, **b** the abdomen, **c** the midpelvis, **d** the midthigh, **e** the midcalf.

The abdominal slice, at the L3/4 (Fig. 10.2b) level, visualises the *psoas* muscles, the complex muscle groups making up the *erector spinae* muscles and the internal and external oblique abdominal and transverse abdominal muscles. The *rectus abdominis* muscles are also visualised. The image contains the abdominal aorta, the vertebra, and abdominal viscera. In normal subjects the distinction between the various muscle groups making up the erector spinae muscles is not clear. The pelvic slice (Fig. 10.2c) contains *sartorius, tensor fasciae latae, gluteus medius, gluteus minimus* and *gluteus maximus* muscles together with the *iliopsoas* and *obturator* muscles. The rectum, sacrum and part of the bladder and genital organs are also imaged. A slightly higher slice visualises the gluteus maximus rather better. It is often possible to identify the beginnings of the anterior compartment of the thigh and the *semimembranosus* muscles in the *hamstring* compartment.

The slice through the midthigh (Fig. 10.2d) reveals the rectus femoris and the anterior compartment making up the *quadriceps femoris* muscles. Posterior to the femur, which is itself well visualised, can be seen the *adductor, magnus, gracilis, sartorius,* semimembranosus, semitendinosus and *biceps femoris* muscles, the latter three comprising the muscle groups making up the lateral hamstring groups. In normal subjects delineation of the boundaries of these muscles, making up the flexor and extensor compartments, is often unclear but in the presence of neuromuscular disease these muscles become more clearly delineated. The neurovascular bundle consisting of the femoral arteries and veins and the sciatic nerve can sometimes be made identified. A slice through the midcalf (Fig. 10.2e) reveals the tibia and fibula together with the *tibialis anterior*, extensor digitorum longus and extensor hallucis longus muscles and the peroneus longus muscle in the anterior compartment of the calf. The peroneal and tibialis posterior muscles can also be seen and the soleus and *gastrocnemius* muscles are well visualised. Varicosities in the venous system in the subcutaneous regions can also often be clearly recognised.

In normal muscle groups the boundaries of individual muscles are not easy to define (Fig. 10.3). The range of normal areas and attenuation values in normal muscles in man and woman and the effects of ageing, have not yet been defined (see Bulcke and Baert 1982).

Abnormalities in Muscles Found on CT

The transverse image produced by CT scanning can be used to assess the area of individual muscles and thus the presence of muscular atrophy or hypertrophy occurring as a diffuse or localised process. Right/left asymmetry can be evaluated. The presence of fatty infiltration within individual muscles can be recognised and, in some disorders, a strikingly patchy process of attenuation of the image in individual muscles can be seen representing fibrous tissue or fatty replacement in areas of damaged muscle (Hadar et al. 1983). This patchy loss of attenuation may be widespread, localised to individual muscles, or asymmetrical in homologous muscles on the two sides of the body (Termote et al. 1980; Schwartz et al. 1988).

The relative distribution of these changes is determined not only by the disease process itself, but by the extent, severity, and stage of the disease (Stern et al. 1984; Schwartz et al. 1988). For example, in

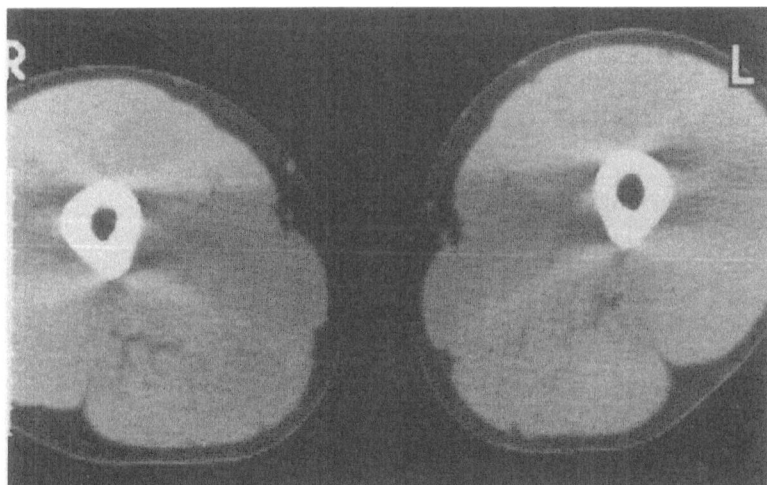

Fig. 10.3. Axial CT mid thigh. Normal study. The boundaries of individual muscles are not clearly defined.

polymyositis changes in healing muscles are not necessarily the same as those in a phase of acute necrosis. In other disorders, such as Duchenne muscular dystrophy, limb girdle muscular dystrophy, spinal muscular atrophy (De Visser and Verbeeten 1985; Schwartz et al. 1988), and myotonic dystrophy, the abnormalities found in skeletal muscles with CT X-ray scanning are strikingly different at different stages in the disorder (Bulcke and Baert 1982). Thus, in Duchenne muscular dystrophy there is considerable loss of muscle tissue in the late stages with marked attenuation of the image (Bulcke et al. 1981; Hawley et al. 1984; Calo et al. 1986). All muscles are involved at this late stage although there is much more severe involvement of axial and proximal muscles than of distal, for example calf, muscles.

The phenomenon of pseudohypertrophy may be seen by an increased bulk with some fatty replacement in affected muscles, such as the calf and pec-

toralis major muscles. The gluteus maximus may similarly be affected by pseudohypertrophy. Even in Duchenne dystrophy, and limb girdle muscular dystrophy, however, individual muscles are involved in a relatively selective manner at different stages in the disease (Fig. 10.4). Thus the gracilis muscle is nearly always relatively spared and there are variable patterns of involvement of the different components of the flexor muscles of the thigh. Although these disorders are classically symmetrical, quite marked asymmetrical involvement, as shown by the degrees of abnormality in homologous muscles, may be seen in the early and intermediate stages (Bulcke and Baert 1982).

Muscular atrophy itself is a process that is determined by the underlying pathological disorder. For example, in motor neurone disease, and in the peripheral neuropathies, there is relatively diffuse involvement of affected muscles. Peripheral neuropathies are usually quite strikingly symmetrical and this is reflected by the CT appearance (Fig. 10.5). In the axonal neuropathies, as in type II hereditary and sensorimotor neuropathy (Charcot–Marie–Tooth syndrome) distal muscles are predominantly affected. In neurogenic disorders of this type muscle bulk gradually diminishes without any markedly patchy change in attenuation values within affected muscles. On the other hand in polymyositis, a disorder which may be asymmetrical and which tends to involve proximal more than distal muscles both clinically and radiologically, there is a patchy loss of attenuation in affected muscles (Fig. 10.6). The quadriceps (Fig. 10.7) is particularly susceptible and changes are often also found in adductor magnus

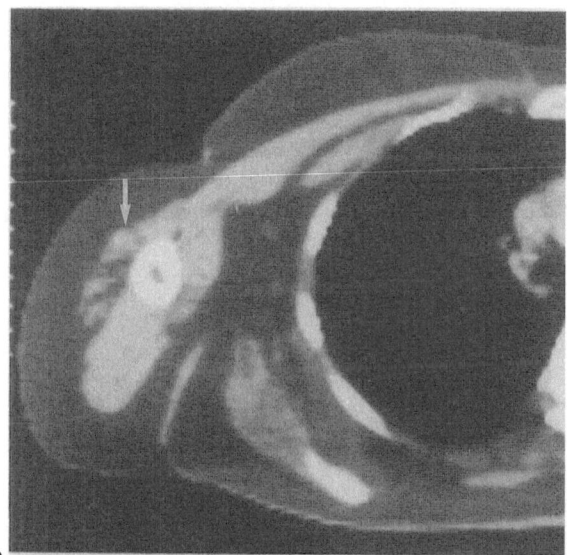

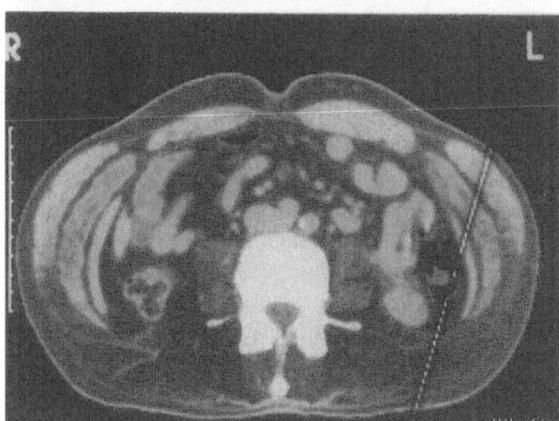

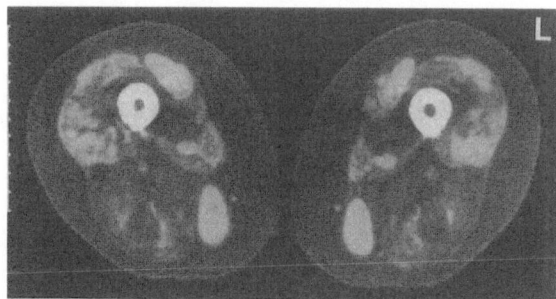

Fig. 10.4. Axial CT. Limb girdle muscular dystrophy. **a** Pectoral region – marked abnormality in the deltoid muscle (*arrow*) with relatively less severe involvement of pectoral and periscapular muscles. **b** Abdomen – diffuse low attenuation is seen in all the posterior spinal muscles with relative sparing of the rectus abdominis and of the lateral abdominal wall musculature. A linear artefact is present. **c** Mid thigh – there is involvement of the quadriceps and flexor compartment muscles with striking sparing of the gracilis muscles. The appearance is bilaterally symmetrical. Fat deposition in the subcutaneous tissues is evident.

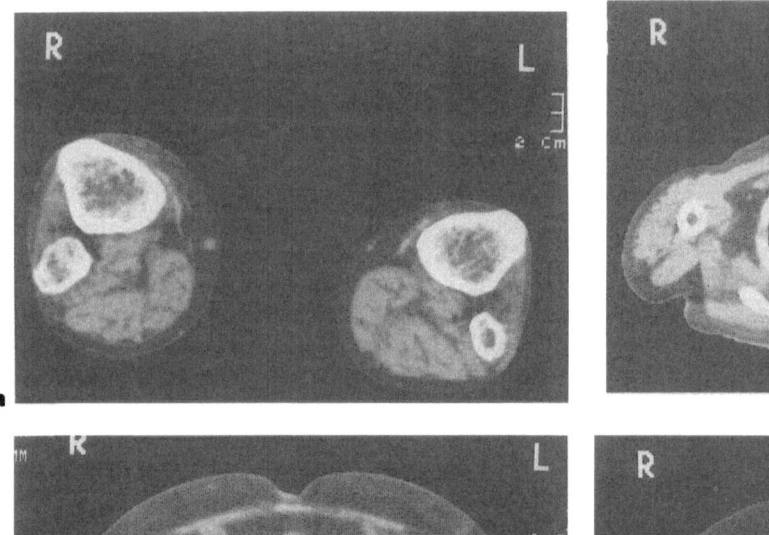

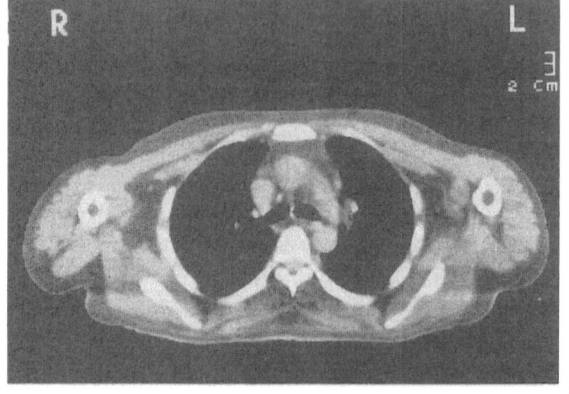

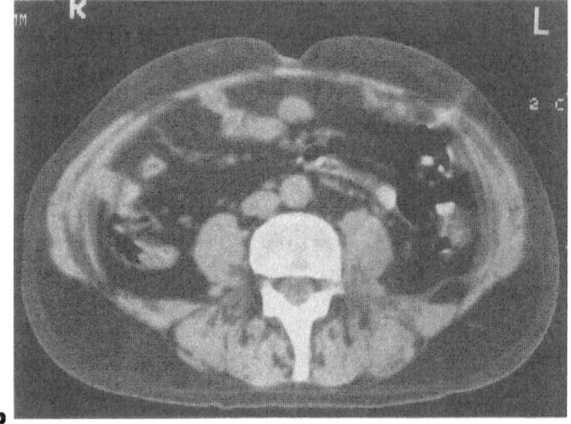

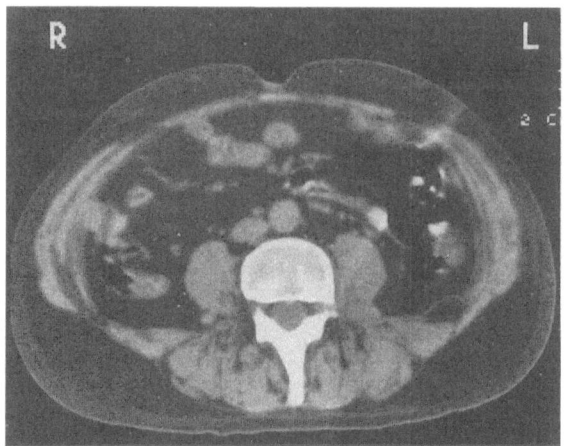

Fig. 10.5. Axial CT. Chronic relapsing Guillain–Barré syndrome. The distal involvement with severe atrophy and the relative sparing of more proximal muscles are shown. The process is symmetrical and the atrophy diffuse. The rectus abdominis muscles are also atrophic. **a** Midcalf; **b** abdomen.

Fig. 10.6. Axial CT. Acute dermatomyositis. **a** Pectoral region: there is atrophy of the deltoid muscle, which shows a characteristically wavy outline. Zones of decreased attenuation can be seen in the paraspinal muscles. At the time of the scan the patient was unable to rise to the sitting position from lying, and was unable to walk. **b** Abdomen: there is low attenuation in the paraspinal muscles with normal psoas muscles. **c** Pelvis: the gluteus medius muscle is atrophic but the gluteus maximus and gluteus minimus are spared.

although the biceps femoris and gracilis muscles may be spared. Axial extensor muscles, particularly the erector spinae muscles, are abnormal but the psoas muscles are relatively less affected. Thus patchy loss of attenuation is followed by an appearance of large zones of fat replacement and, later, by marked atrophy of the muscle as a whole.

In the spinal muscular atrophies (Fig. 10.8) a similar rather patchy process, at first of a pinpoint nature, then coalescing to form large zones of fat replacement, is seen, often strikingly asymmetrical in the earlier stages. This process, as in the muscular dystrophies and inflammatory myopathies, tends to involve proximal and axial muscles more than distal muscles. In myotonic syndromes muscular hypertrophy is characteristic. In myotonic dystrophy, however, there are dystrophic changes in the muscle in addition to the myotonia itself. In the quadriceps femoris Bulcke and Baert (1982) described atrophy beginning in the vastus inter-

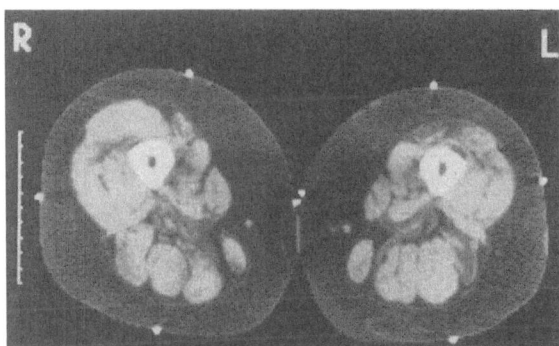

Fig. 10.7. Axial CT. Chronic polymyositis. There is involvement of the left quadriceps muscle with less severe abnormality on the right. The adductor magnus muscles are involved bilaterally. There is marked deposition of adipose tissue in this woman, who had been treated with steroids for some months. The perspex markers are related to sterotaxic EMG electroplacement (see Schwartz et al. 1988).

medius and spreading centrifugally towards the vastus lateralis and vastus medialis, finally involving the rectus femoris. As in the spinal muscular atrophies a "shell-like" appearance of a peripheral rim of relatively preserved muscle tissue may be found in these quadriceps muscles.

The relatively selective involvement of individual muscles within apparently functionally related muscle groups in these different disorders raises fundamental questions concerning the susceptibility of muscles to neurogenic, or dystrophic change and to involvement in polymyositis that require further studies for complete analysis. CT studies have also been used to detect metastatic disease in muscle (Schultz et al. 1986).

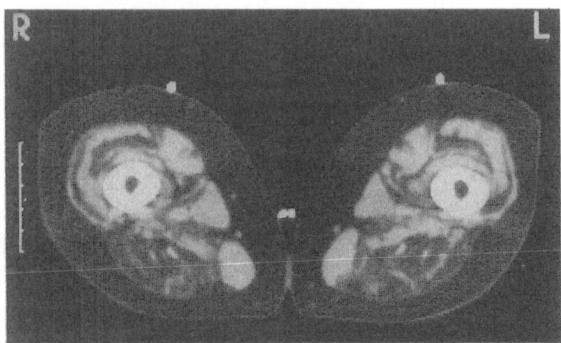

Fig. 10.8. Axial CT. Spinal muscular atrophy (Type 3; Kugelberg Welander disease). This woman was severely disabled but still able to walk unaided although she required help to rise from the sitting position. There is very marked involvement of all the muscles of the thighs apart from the gracilis muscles which are spared. Only a rim of quadriceps tissue remains. The process is symmetrical. Perspex EMG markers (Schwartz et al. 1988) are present on the skin.

Magnetic Resonance Imaging

This technique has not so far been applied in a systematic way to the investigation of neuromuscular disorders (Murphy et al. 1985). There are many theoretical advantages. First, MRI does not use ionising radiation and it is therefore possible to evaluate neuromuscular disorders in serial studies, and to assess women of childbearing age and children without fear of exposure to potentially toxic radiation. Second, MRI more clearly distinguishes between muscle, fat, blood vessels, bone and connective tissues than CT and thus allows the quantification of fatty and fibrous tissue replacement of muscle more accurately (Fig. 10.9). Since bone is of relatively low signal intensity there is no potential problem from partial volume averaging effect between the high attenuation values of bone and the low attenuation values of soft tissues, as with CT. Indeed, the relatively clear delineation of fat in T1 and T2 weighted sequences enables the anatomy of muscles to be very readily demonstrated in MRI studies. It is likely, therefore, that this methodology will have considerable application to neuromuscular disease in the future (Editorial 1988).

CT Evaluation of Plexus and Nerve Lesions

Transverse axial tomography is useful in the evaluation of patients with tumours involving peripheral nerves, the lumbar or brachial plexus, and nerve roots in the spinal canal. It also has a place, combined with water-soluble contrast, myelography and radiculography, in the investigation of patients with spinal lesions.

Malignant infiltration of the brachial plexus can be well visualised (Fig. 10.10) by the presence of a soft tissue shadow encroaching on the paraspinal muscles, entering the intervertebral foramen, and even displacing the spinal cord. This is a particularly common appearance in patients with malignant infiltration of the brachial plexus by breast cancer or lymphoma (Armington et al. 1987). CT scanning of this region can be of great help in the distinction between pain in the arm occurring as a consequence of malignant infiltration of the plexus, and of radiation plexitis. This distinction has important implications for management. Contrast-enhanced scanning techniques are important in assessing the presence of malignant infiltration of these patients.

Avulsion of the brachial plexus, in torsional injuries in which traction forces are applied to the arm, can also be recognised by CT myelography.

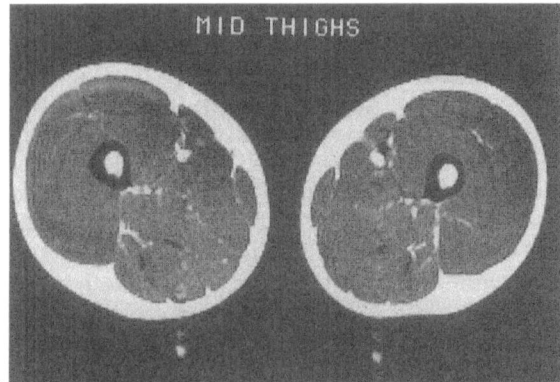

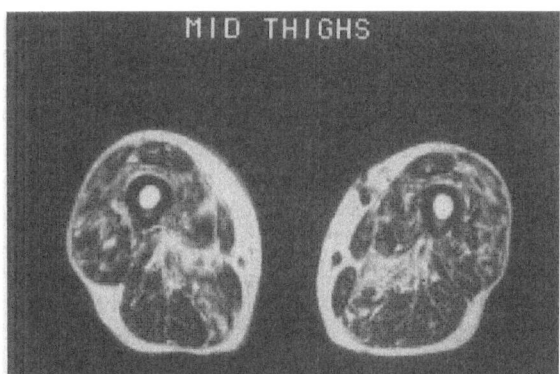

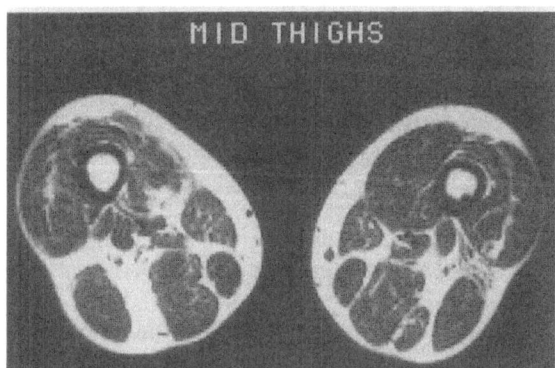

Fig. 10.9. Axial MRI (T1 weighted image), midthigh. The cortex of the femur appears black because of the paucity of protons within bone and the fat content of the bone marrow appears white, since fat returns a high signal on both T1 and T2 weighted sequences. **a** Normal appearances. **b** Polymyositis: patchy and asymmetrical involvement of muscles seen with hyperintense bright areas due to fat deposition. The adductor magnus is most severely involved bilaterally. **c** Limb girdle muscular dystrophy: the semitendinosus on the right is completely "washed out" and is atrophic on the left. The surrounding muscles are also atrophic.

The avulsed root can sometimes be seen indenting the contrast column and in cases in which a false meningomyelocele is formed when the root is torn this may also be filled by the contrast enhanced cerebrospinal fluid (Fig. 10.11). These appearances

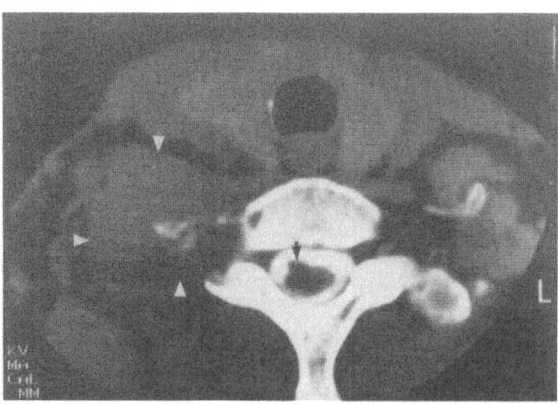

Fig. 10.10. CT myelogram. Metastatic disease with destruction of the adjacent cervical vertebra (*arrowheads*). An intradural deposit is also present (*arrow*). (P.B.)

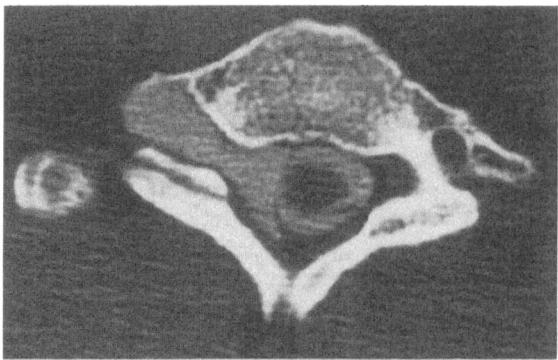

Fig. 10.11. CT myelogram. Brachial plexus avulsion. A post-traumatic meningocele is shown associated with tearing of the root pouch. (P.B.)

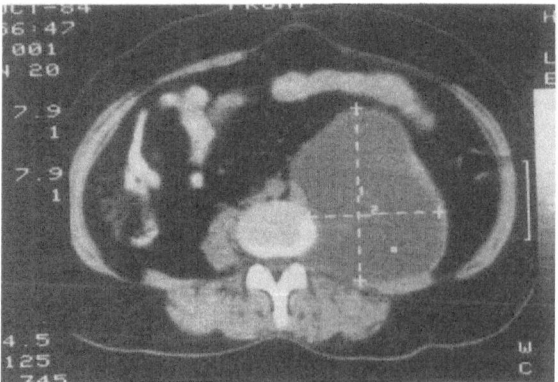

Fig. 10.12. Axial CT. There is a large, left-sided, intra-abdominal neurofibroma extending from its origin in the intervertebral foramen in this lumbar section. the tumour has infiltrated and destroyed the psoas muscle on the left.

have been well described in the literature (Gebarski et al. 1982; Armington et al. 1987; Cobby et al. 1988).

Neurofibromas may rise from the sensory roots in the spinal canal, presenting as extramedullary intradural tumours, often with an extradural component. These lesions are associated with Von Recklinghausen's disease and may be multiple. Similar neurofibromas may arise on the peripheral nerves but these are only rarely demonstrable by CT scanning, although MRI may be more useful in their recognition. Sometimes there is a large intra-abdominal or intrathoracic extension of the tumour (Fig. 10.12).

References

Armington WG, Hornsberg HR, Osborn AG, Sear AR (1987) Radiographic evaluation brachial plexopathy. AJNR 8:361–367

Bulcke JAL, Baert AL (1982) Clinical and radiological aspects of myopathies. Springer, Berlin Heidelberg New York

Bulcke JA, Crolla D, Termote J-L, Palmers Y, Van den Bergh R (1981) Computed tomography of muscle. Muscle Nerve 4:67–72

Calo M, Crisi G, Martinelli C, Colombo A, Schoenhuber R, Gilbertoni M (1986) CT and the diagnosis of myopathies. Neuroradiology 28:53–57

Caughey JE (1952) Radiological changes in skull in dystrophia myotonica. Br Med J i:137–139

Cobby MJD, Leslie IJ, Watt I (1988) Cervical myelography of nerve root avulsion injuries using water soluble contrast media. Br J Radiol 61:673–678

DeVisser M, Verbeeten B (1985) Computed tomography of the skeletal musculature in Becker-type muscular dystrophy and infantile spinal muscular atrophy. Muscle Nerve 8:435–444

Di Chiro G, Nelson KB (1965) Soft tissue radiography of the extremities in neuromuscular disease with histological correlations. Acta Radiol [Diagn] (Stoch) 3:65–88

Editorial (1988) Magnetic resonance imaging of the musculoskeletal system. Lancet i:570

Frantzell A, Inglemark BE (1951) Occurrence and distribution of fat in human muscles at various age levels: a morphological and roentgenologic examination. Upsala Oakoref fork 56:59–87

Gebarski KS, Glazer GM, Gebarski SS (1982) Brachial plexus. Anatomical, radiological, pathological correlations using CT. J Comput Assist Tomogr 6:1058–1063

Hadar H, Gadoth N, Heifetz M (1983) Fatty replacement of lower paraspinal muscles: normal and neuromuscular disorders. AJR 141:895–898

Hawley RJ, Schillinger DM, O'Doherty DS (1984) Computed tomographic patterns of muscles in neuromuscular disease. Arch Neurol 41:383–387

Heckmatt JZ, Leeman S, Dubowitz V (1982) Ultrasonic imaging in the diagnosis of muscle disease. J Pediatr 101:656–660

Kamala D, Suresh S, Githa K (1985) Real-time ultrasonography in neuromuscular problems of children. J Clin Ultrasound 13:465–468

Murphy WA, Totty WG, Carroll JE (1985) MRI of normal and pathologic skeletal muscle. AJR 146:565–574

Osterman FA Jr, Zeman GH, Gopola UVR, Gayler B, Kirk BF, James AEJ (1977) Negative-mode soft tissue xeroradiography. Radiology 124:689–694

Palvolgyi R (1978) Ueber die Roentgenmorphologie der Veranderingen der extremitatenmusculatur. Radiologe 18:469–474

Palvolgyi R, Balint BJ (1979) Radiographic diagnosis of closed muscle and tendon injuries of the upper arm. Arch Orthop Trauma Surg 95:177–180

Palvolgyi R and Gallai R (1980) Use of x-ray techniques to demonstrate selectively increased damage to certain muscles in patients suffering from muscular diseases. ROEFO 133:58–62

Palvolgyi R, Pentek Z (1977) Xeroradiographic demonstration of soft tissues of the extremities. Acta Morphol Acad Sci Hung 25:189–195

Palvolgyi R, Balint BJ, Tozsa L (1979) The Ehlers–Danlos syndrome causing lacerations in tendons and muscles. Arch Orthop Trauma Surg 95:173–176

Rowland LP (1988) Clinical concept of Duchenne muscular dystrophy: The impact of molecular genetics. Brain 111 479–495

Schultz SR, Bree RL, Schwab RE, Raiss G (1986) CT detection of skeletal muscle metastases. J Comput Assist Tomogr 10:81–83

Schwartz MS, Swash M, Ingram D et al. (1988) Patterns of selective involvement in thigh muscles in neuromuscular disease: concordance of CT and single fibre EMG assessment. Muscle Nerve 12:1240–1245

Steinfeld JR, Thorne NA, Kennedy TF (1977) Positive ^{99m}Tc-pyrophosphate bone scan in polymyositis. Radiology 122:168

Stern LM, Candoly DJ, Perret LV, Bolde DW (1984) Progression of muscular dystrophy assessed by computed tomography. Dev Med Child Neurol 26:569–573

Swash M (1988) Hutchison's clinical methods, 19th edn. Baillière-Tindall, London

Swash M, Ingram D (1988) Preclinical and subclinical events in motor neuron disease. J Neurol Neurosurg Psychiatry 51:165–168

Swash M, Schwartz MS (1982) A longitudinal study of changes in motor units in motor neurone disease. J Neurol Sci 56:185–197

Swash M, Schwartz MS (1988) Neuromuscular disease: a practical approach to diagnosis and management, 2nd edn. Springer, Berlin, Heidelberg, New York

Swift TR, Brown M (1978) Tc-99m pyrophosphate labeling in McArdle syndrome. Neur Med 19:295–297

Suzuki Y, Hisada K, Takeda M (1974) Demonstration of myositis ossificans by ^{99m}Tc-pyrophosphate bone scanning. Radiology 111:663–664

Termote JC, Baert A, Crolla D, Palmers Y, Bulcke JA (1980) Computed tomography of the normal and pathological muscular system. Radiology 137:439–444

Van der Walt JD, Swash M, Leake J, Cox EL (1987) The pattern of involvement of adult-onset acid maltase deficiency at autopsy. Muscle Nerve 10:272–281

Walton JN, Warwick CK (1954) Osseous changes in myopathy. Br J Radiol 27:1–15

Wilkins KE, Gibson DA (1976) The patterns of spinal deformity in Duchenne muscular dystrophy. J Bone Joint Surg 58A:24–32

Chapter 11

Isotope Brain Imaging

Neil W. Garvie

Cerebral Scintigraphy

Pathophysiology

The capillaries of the normal brain present a barrier to the free diffusion of water-soluble molecules. However, the abnormal capillary circulation that exists around most cerebral abnormalities – particularly those of an inflammatory or neoplastic nature – are more permeable, and readily permit passage of molecules into the extracellular fluid space, which is greater in such lesions compared to normal brain tissue. This transfer is also aided by pinocytosis, which is not a feature of normal cerebral endothelium. The enhanced transit of water-soluble tracers through the altered blood–brain barrier into cerebral lesions provides the physiological basis underlying cerebral scintigraphy. A number of radiopharmaceuticals have been employed to image the brain in this way, but currently sodium pertechnetate, technetium–DTPA and technetium glucoheptonate are the most important.

Properties of Technetium-99m

Technetium-99m (Tc) is an ideal isotope for diagnostic purposes. With a short half-life of 6 hours, it can be administered to patients in sufficient quantity to enable adequate images, for an acceptable level of total radiation dose. Depending on the study, this dose is, in most cases, equivalent to or less than comparable radiographic techniques. In addition, Tc possesses the advantage of chemical versatility, and can be easily combined with a large number of different molecules, to constitute specific radiopharmaceuticals for imaging the organ systems of the human body. Its principal method of radioactive decay involves the production of a

single gamma ray, of 140 keV, ideally suited for detection by modern gamma cameras. Unlike many radioisotopes, no charged particles, which are intensely destructive to biological tissues, are produced and no radioactive "daughter" products are formed.

Tc is generated as a product from the decay of molybdenum-99. This longer-lived parent isotope is widely available. Tc is removed, as sodium pertechnetate, by saline elution, a process which can be repeated many times during the life of each molybdenum generator.

Pharmaceuticals for Cerebral Scintigraphy

The simplest pharmaceutical, since no further labelling procedure is required, is sodium pertechnetate. This compound is, however, also taken up by the thyroid gland and is partially bound to albumen in the blood-stream, leading to visualisation of vascular structures within the brain, such as the choroid plexi. These side-effects can be reduced by the prior administration of 200 mg of potassium perchlorate orally 1–2 hours before injection of the pertechnetate.

Tc-labelled diethylenetriamine penta-acetic acid (Tc-DTPA) is eliminated rapidly by the kidneys, so that imaging must be performed earlier than with pertechnetate, if a satisfactory count-rate is to be achieved.

Tc-Glucoheptonate has been shown to exhibit greater selective uptake in brain tumours than the other compounds. This may be related to its close chemical similarity to glucose, enhancing absorption through an ability to participate in tumour metabolism (Leveille et al. 1977). Like DTPA, it is cleared from the blood by the kidneys, but, unlike DPTA, it is bound to the renal parenchyma and is not excreted.

Technique

A similar technique is used for each type of radio-pharmaceutical. It is divided into two parts: a flow study (which is optional) and an equilibrium study.

Flow Study

In the flow study, as the compound is injected intravenously, with the patient's head positioned under the gamma camera, a rapid sequence of images – or frames – is taken by the on-line computer system. When cerebral perfusion is to be studied, a vertex view is usually performed. For carotid flow studies, an anterior view is preferable. Images are acquired at a rate of four frames per second, taken over a period of 45 seconds. The flow study can be inspected visually, or analysed mathematically.

By observation alone, an impression of carotid artery flow can be gained. Within the cerebrum, regional or global disturbances in blood flow can be seen and highly vascular tumours such as meningiomas and arteriovenous malformations demonstrated by the presence of early or prolonged venous filling. Non-filling of the relevant dural venous sinus is a reliable guide to the presence of thrombosis (Fig. 11.1). Subdural haematomas, when viewed tangentially, manifest as a crescentic area of absent perfusion, with a hyperperfused rim due to crowding of adjacent cerebral vessels.

Mathematical analysis of the data may be performed to yield the transit time of the compound within the cerebral substance. This is prolonged in patients with restricted perfusion. Transit time images may also be constructed, to provide regional information on the extent of cerebrovascular disease.

The flow study may also be employed to diagnose "brain death", when no entry of radio-pharmaceutical into the brain occurs (Nagle 1980).

There are, however, newer and more sophisticated isotope techniques for studying cerebral blood flow, although this technique is still widely used as a supplement to the information gained from the equilibrium study.

Equilibrium Study

After the flow study, views are obtained to seek areas of abnormal uptake of radiopharmaceutical within the brain. These are usually performed between 1 and 4 hours after injection, to allow the background level of intravascular tracer to subside so that the lesion may be seen with greater contrast. Four views are usually taken (Fig. 11.2), the vertex view being optional.

Equilibrium Study: Abnormal Appearances

The recent advances in new technology available for cerebral imaging have tended to obscure the value of the conventional isotope brain scan.

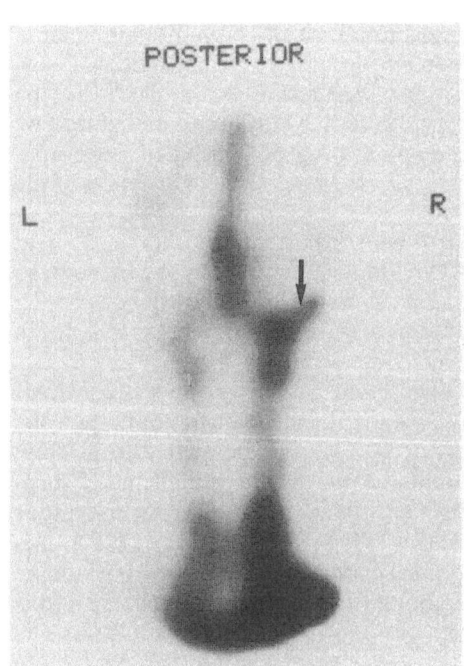

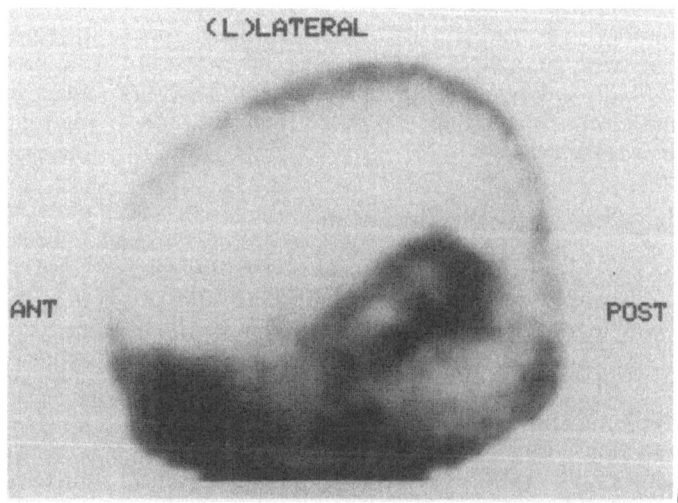

Fig. 11.1. Cerebral scintigram (^{99m}Tc-DTPA). Lateral sinus thrombosis. **a** Posterior view at 2 minutes postinjection showing absence of filling of the left lateral sinus. Compare with the normal right lateral sinus (*arrow*). **b** Lateral view at 3 hours postinjection with intense uptake at the site of thrombosis.

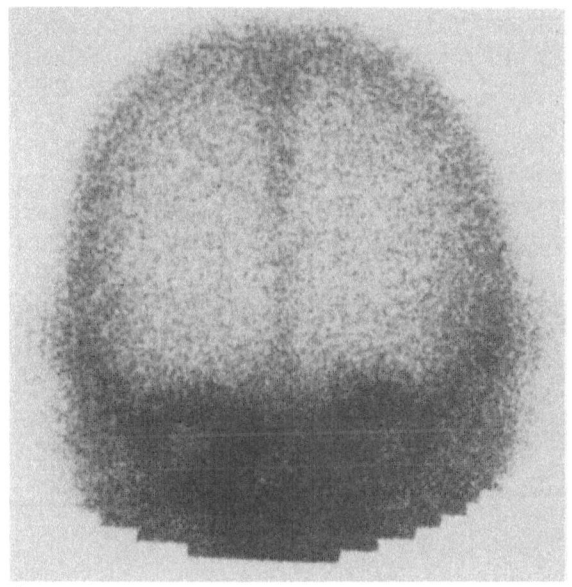

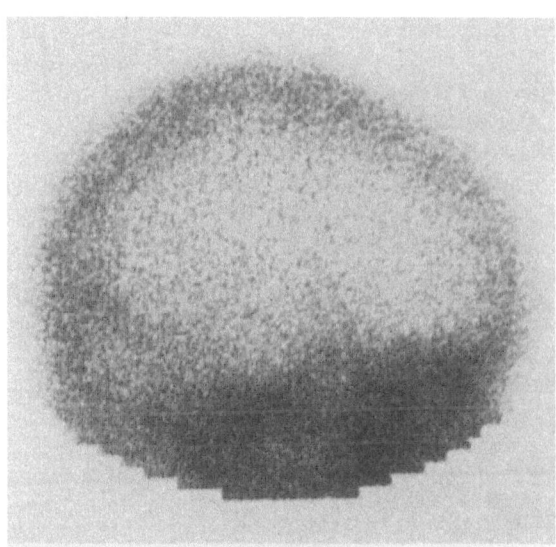

Fig. 11.2. Normal cerebral scintigram (^{99m}Tc-DTPA), 3 hours postinjection. Note the residual activity in the dural venous sinuses. **a** Anterior view; **b** posterior view; **c** lateral view.

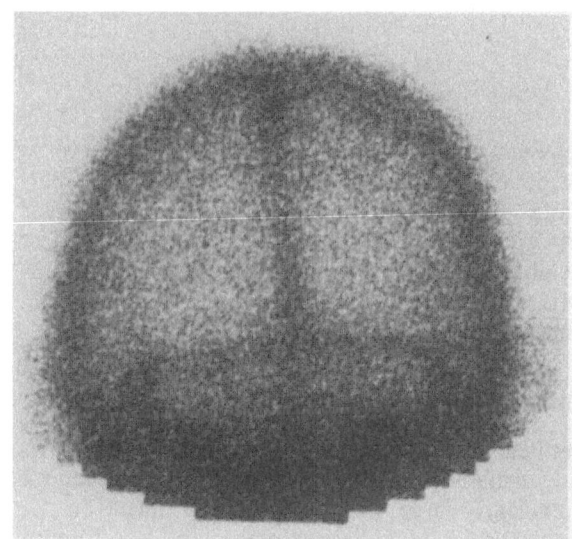

systems, in which the gamma camera(s) can be used in the tomographic or conventional mode. This latter alternative is a particularly flexible arrangement of relatively low cost, especially if an existing computer system is used for image processing.

When simple planar views, as shown in Fig. 11.2, are used for lesion detection, then the greater accuracy of computed tomography (CT) is clearly evident (Du Boulay and Marshall 1975). If, however, isotope tomographic scans, using single photon emission computerised tomography (SPECT) are taken, then the results are comparable to CT (Ell et al. 1980), and a combination of SPECT and conventional CT can further improve diagnostic accuracy (Table 11.1).

There are a number of alternative methods of performing SPECT and this facility is now available in most nuclear medicine departments. Options range from totally dedicated machines to simpler

Table 11.1. Brain imaging: conventional, gamma camera (GC), SPECT, and radiographic transmission tomography, (TCAT) compared

	True-positives		True-negatives	
Carril et al. (1979) Scanner	83/140	59%	363/372	98%
SPECT	107/140	76%	367/372	99%
Hill et al. (1980)				
GC	42/62	68%	133/138	96%
SPECT	48/62	77%	137/138	99%
TCAT	26/35	74%	43/47	91%
Ell et al. (1980)				
SPECT	182/209	87%	37/37	100%
TCAT	196/209	94%	36/37	97%

Diagnosis of subdural haematoma

	Present	Equivocal	Missed	Total	Correct
GC	22	1	2	25	92%
TCAT	13	7 (shift only)	5	25	80%

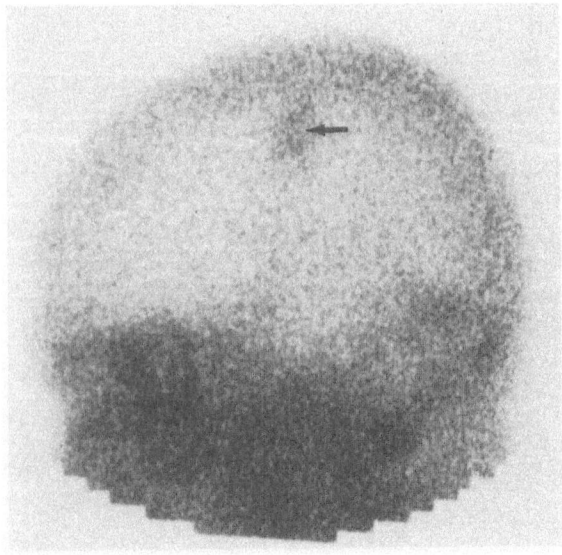

Fig. 11.3. Cerebral scintigram (^{99m}Tc-DTPA), lateral view. Parasagittal meningioma (*arrow*).

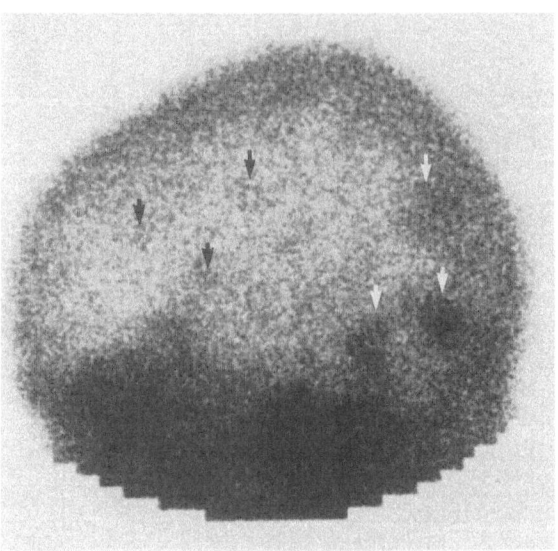

Fig. 11.4. Cerebral scintigram (^{99m}Tc-DTPA), lateral view. Multiple metastases (*arrows*).

Intracranial Tumours

Of all intracranial tumours, the meningioma, due to its high vascularity, is the most easily recognised (Fig. 11.3). It usually presents as a rounded, well-defined area of abnormal uptake, adjacent to a dural surface, although meningioma en-plaque is less easily seen and tangential views are occasionally necessary.

Gliomas vary in their ability to concentrate radiopharmaceuticals, depending upon their size, site, and degree of differentiation. Small low-grade gliomas may be overlooked, particularly if situated close to the skull base, or in the posterior fossa. They show greater pleomorphism than the meningioma, and occasionally uptake is greater at the periphery of the tumour than in the middle, giving a "doughnut" appearance, due to central avascularity or necrosis. Gliomas which are less vascular than normal brain tissue can be difficult to detect.

Because of its position close to the base of the middle cranial fossa, the acoustic neurinoma is difficult to detect on conventional scintigraphy, although SPECT studies are frequently positive.

Since the uptake of a radiopharmaceutical is partly a function of the degree of extracellular fluid present, tumours which are surrounded by substantial oedema are more easily discerned. This is particularly true of cerebral metastases (Fig. 11.4), where the extent of tumour uptake may reflect this phenomenon, rather than actual tumour size. Uptake can, therefore, be used as a guide to management, since these lesions are more likely to respond to dexamethasone. Metastases are perceived scintigraphically as solitary or multiple areas of rounded uptake, similar to the appearances of cerebral abscesses. The number of metastases present, however, is frequently underestimated on the isotope scan, unless SPECT is employed.

Infarction

Immediately after infarction, the equilibrium views are usually negative, although the infarct, if sufficiently large, may be seen as a defect on the flow study. Uptake is maximal at about 7–10 days (Fig. 11.5) and then reduces. Infarcts older than 10 weeks are generally not seen, so that sequential scans show a changing pattern, which is useful in diagnosis. Uptake of isotope is partly dependent on the degree of luxury perfusion around the infarct. Cerebellar or brainstem infarcts are not easily demonstrated, even on SPECT.

Infection

Cerebral abscesses, of the pyogenic or granulomatous type, are readily detected, as rounded areas of increased uptake, occasionally with a "doughnut" appearance. Diffuse inflammatory changes, however, due to encephalitis or meningitis, are less easy to demonstrate, and cerebral scintigraphy should not be employed in this situation.

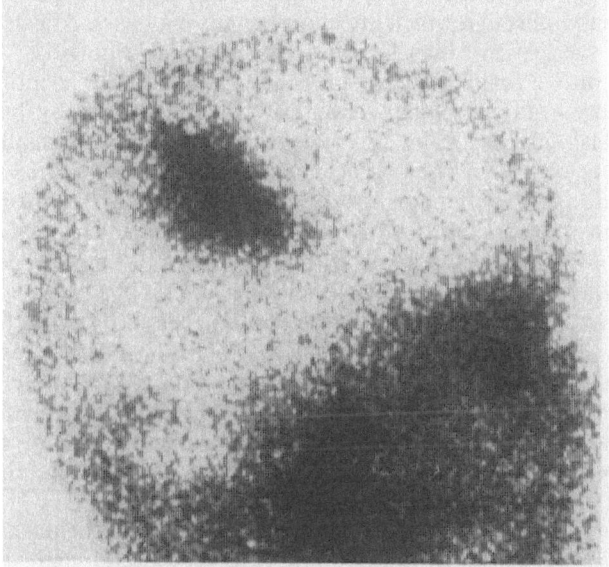

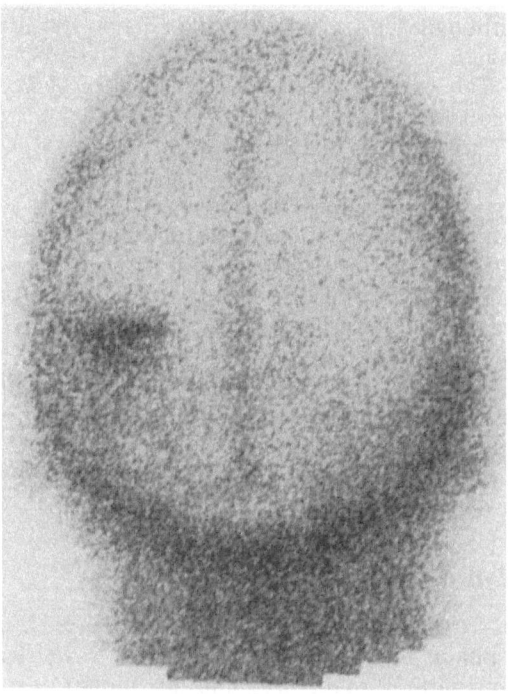

Fig. 11.5. Cerebral scintigram (⁹⁹ᵐTc-DTPA). Parietal infarct, 9 days following a stroke. **a** Lateral view; **b** vertex view.

Trauma

On scintigraphy, cerebral haemorrhage, either "spontaneous" or traumatic, has similar characteristics to infarction. Since it is difficult, therefore, to detect at an early stage, the isotope scan has little to offer the diagnostician. The chronic subdural haematoma is best viewed on the anterior or posterior projections, when it is seen as a lenticulate structure with peripheral uptake. Cerebral scintigraphy, combined with a flow study, is still a valuable test for this condition, which can be overlooked on CT.

Cisternography

Tracer studies can also be used to study the flow of cerebrospinal fluid (CSF). CSF is secreted in the choroid plexi of the ventricular system, and enters the subarachnoid space via foramina in the wall of the fourth ventricle. The majority of the fluid then passes via the basal and cerebral cisterns to rejoin the venous circulation in the superior sagittal sinus, passing through the arachnoid villi. A small portion of the CSF flows around the spinal cord before it passes into the cisternal system.

If a suitable tracer is injected into the lumbar subarachnoid space, it will flow cranially to enter the basal cisterns in a few hours, and the arachnoid villi at 24 hours (Fig. 11.6). Alternatively, the tracer

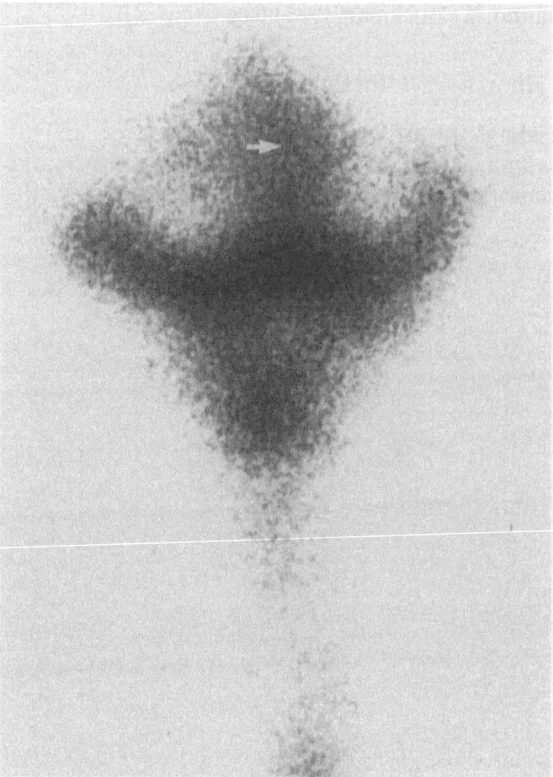

Fig. 11.6. Indium cisternogram (anterior view), normal study. At 8 hours activity is distributed about the brainstem and is entering the superor sagittal sinus (*arrow*).

may be injected directly into the cisterna magna, although this technique has little diagnostic advantage.

The earliest radiopharmaceutical employed in this technique was radio-iodinated human serum albùmen (RISA), labelled with iodine-131. This compound, however, frequently caused severe pyrogenic reactions, and arachnoiditis, and could not be prepared to acceptable pharmaceutical standards for intrathecal use. Radiation dose to the spinal cord was high (particularly if the injection was inadvertently given extrathecally) due to the beta particle emission.

Currently, two pharmaceutical preparations are available – indium-111-DTPA (In-DTPA), and ytterbium-16-DTPA (Yb-DTPA). Both these isotopes have adequate half-lives to permit imaging up to 48 hours.

Hydrocephalus

In communicating "normal"-pressure hydrocephalus, there is reversal of the normal cisternal flow pattern, so that a significant amount of tracer from the subarachnoid space enters the ventricular system (Fig. 11.7). In this way cisternography can detect abnormal CSF flow and assist in making the diagnosis (Huckman 1981) (see Chap. 3).

Rhinorrhoea/Otorrhoea

Leakage of CSF is usually a result of cranial trauma, with rupture of the dural and arachnoid membranes, so that the meninges are directly exposed to the external environment, via a channel through which infectious agents may pass. Affected patients may present with recurrent meningitis.

Small fracture sites may be difficult to identify radiographically, even with CT cisternography, but can be localised by isotopic means. This is especially so when the CSF leak is intermittent.

After packing the nasopharynx or auditory meatus with gauze pledgets, radiopharmaceutical is administered intrathecally. Views of the suspect area may be taken over 3–24 hours, but the localisation of the leak is determined primarily from the activity recorded from the appropriate gauze pack. A small amount of normal activity is present on each pack, due to mucosal secretion, but this should not exceed the activity found in 2 ml of venous blood. In the presence of a fistula, the activity is much higher.

If no abnormal activity is counted on the packs, it is worth obtaining a view of the abdomen, to exclude the diagnosis of rhinorrhoea. If the packs have not been correctly inserted, CSF will trickle into the nasopharynx, and be swallowed into the stomach.

Tests for Shunt Patency

The patency of ventricular shunts can be confirmed by a variety of isotope studies. Injection of ^{111}In-DTPA into the ventricles or shunt cannula, causes rapid visualisation of the patent shunt, and a rise in count over the heart, followed by the appearance of isotope in venous blood samples. In the case of ventriculoperitoneal shunts, counts may be taken over the right hypochondrium.

Cerebral Blood Flow

Cerebral blood flow (CBF) is maintained at a constant level, by autoregulation, and lies between 50 and 60 ml/min per 100 g of brain substance, irrespective of physiological changes in blood pressure. The flow in grey matter is higher (65–85 ml/min per 100 g) than white matter (27–33 ml/min per 100 g). When CBF is reduced, cerebral blood volume (CBV) increases, and there is a rise in oxygen extraction. CBF remains steady between a mean systemic pressure of 140 and 165 mmHg, under normal conditions of arterial pO_2 and pCO_2. When pCO_2 is increased, the pressure–flow relationship becomes linear, so that a rise of 1 mm in the pCO_2 causes a CBF increase of about 3 ml/min per 100 g. Above an arterial pCO_2 of 80 mmHg; no further increase in CBF occurs, since the cerebral vessels are maximally dilated.

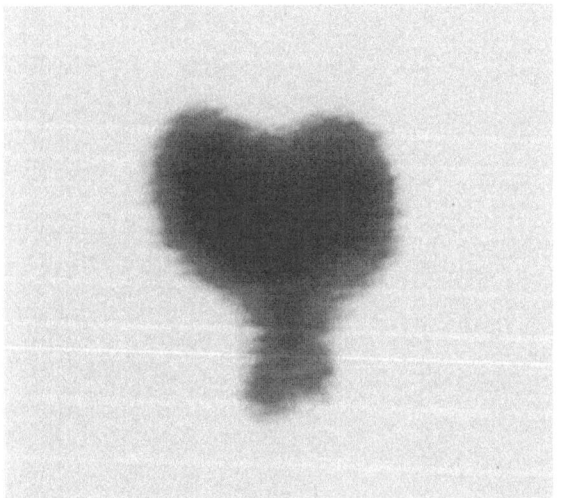

Fig. 11.7. Indium cisternogram (anterior view). Communicating hydrocephalus. Activity is almost exclusively within the ventricles in this study 8 hours after injection of 5 MBq.

In severe cerebrovascular disease, cerebral vaso-dilation is already maximal, and no rise in CBF occurs under hypercapnic conditions. Isotope CBF studies before and after hypercapnia can be used, therefore, to confirm that vasodilation is already maximal, and that the brain is nearing critical ischaemia unless appropriate treatment is given.

At low levels of pCO_2, CBF decreases by 1.5 ml/min/100 g due to vasoconstriction. Below a pCO_2 of 20 mmHg no further constriction occurs, since cerebral hypoxia develops, with the formation of lactic acid which is a potent vasodilator. Physiological control of the cerebral vasodilation is believed to be exerted from the precapillary arterioles, due to a myogenic response mediated by cholinergic sympathetic nerve fibres. Anaesthetics, such as halothane, trichloroethylene, cyclopropane, ether and chloroform reduce CBF by 25%, presumably by direct action on vascular responsiveness.

Breathing oxygen under increased pressure causes vasoconstriction, so that oxygen delivery to the brain is not significantly increased. If CO_2 is added to the inspired O_2, causing vasodilation, dangerously high oxygen levels may be reached, impairing neuronal metabolism and causing death.

Grey matter is responsible for the high cerebral oxygen requirement. This tissue constitutes less than 9% of the total body weight, but uses nearly 20% of the total oxygen consumed by the body (Keele et al. 1982). By contrast, the white matter, being composed of axons similar to peripheral nerves, requires only 3 ml O_2/min, for a brain mass of 1500 g, although it constitutes 60% of this total weight.

The control of CBF is therefore a complex phenomenon, critical for survival. The normal brain can function adequately at a CBF of 20 ml/min per 100 g, but below this level electroencephalographic abnormalities occur and at 15 ml/min per 100 g critical ischaemia is reached which, if sustained, leads to irreversible cellular damage.

CBF Studies Using Non-metabolised Diffusible Tracers

Some chemically inert radioactive tracers have the ability to diffuse freely across the blood–brain barrier and can therefore be used to study cerebral blood flow. The classical substance used is xenon-133, a lipid-soluble gas which may be administered intra-arterially, intravenously, or, most commonly, by direct inhalation. It diffuses rapidly throughout the brain substance, and partitions itself between grey and white matter. After equilibration, the rate of removal (washout) of xenon is proportional to cerebral blood flow. Two components contribute to the washout curve – a slow component, related to white matter perfusion, and an earlier, fast component due to grey matter perfusion. These two phases can be separated mathematically, and the rate constant(s) calculated (λ). These two phases can be extrapolated to yield values in proportion to the grey:white matter flow ratio.

If the partition coefficient (P) for xenon for grey and white matter is substituted, then:

$$\text{Flow/unit weight of tissue} = P \times \lambda$$
$$(\text{ml/min per g})$$

Absolute flow can be measured, if the volume of the tissue is calculated, for example by SPECT.

This type of study provides an adequate method of CBF assessment in the normal cerebrum although it is subject to a number of assumptions. For instance, a recording must be obtained which is representative of the entire cerebrum. Since volume is not known, a detector placed over any part of the cerebrum will not necessarily record a washout curve which is wholly representative. Additionally, the partition coefficient is likely to be affected by disease, since cerebral metabolic activity creates water, altering the lipid/water ratio.

A gamma camera may be used to record the xenon distribution, but more frequently a circumferential array of small probes is placed around the head, to improve counting sensitivity, and to obtain information on regional cerebral flow. Under steady-state conditions SPECT images of regional cerebral blood flow (rCBF) can also be obtained.

Positron Emission Tomography (PET)

When imaging cerebral blood flow, or other aspects of cerebral physiology, tomography is essential in order to obtain accurate regional images of cerebral dysfunction. Two principal techniques exist, one of which, single photon tomography (SPECT) has been briefly discussed. The other technique is positron emission tomography (PET).

Positrons are positively charged electrons, emitted during the decay of certain radionuclides such as oxygen-15, carbon-11, nitrogen-13 and fluorine-18. These isotopes are generally short-lived, and produced by bombardment of a target material by positive particles in a cyclotron. PET is therefore mainly confined to those centres fortunate enough to possess such equipment since, with the majority of these products, decay is so rapid that transport to outlying hospitals is not feasible.

Each positron interacts with a normal electron, resulting in mutual annihilation, and the formation of two equal gamma rays which travel in precisely opposite directions. The patient is scanned between single or multiple pairs of opposed detectors, precisely aligned to detect, by coincidence counting, matching pairs of gamma rays emitted by each annihilation reaction. By rotation of the detectors, the plane of the disintegration can be localised, and tomographic images constructed. This technique differs from SPECT, therefore, in that two gamma ray photons are simultaneously registered, defining the axis along which the source is located.

The positron technique has two other advantages. First, since positron emitters possess short half-lives, the radiation dose to the patient is low and more radioactivity can be administered, to construct clearer images. Second, as mentioned above, positron-emitter radioisotopes exist for carbon, oxygen, nitrogen and the halogen family. These atoms can be incorporated into biological molecules, and can be used to image aspects of cerebral physiology.

Oxygen-15 is a positron-emitting nuclide which has a half-life of 122.5 s, equivalent to that of cerebral metabolic oxidation which it can be used to study. ^{15}O can, also, be used to measure CBF, oxygen extraction and metabolism and blood volume.

Regional Cerebral Blood Volume (rCBV)

A small amount of carbon monoxide labelled with ^{15}O is inhaled (Grubb et al. 1978). The carbon monoxide binds firmly to haemoglobin, and thus constitutes an intravascular marker. At equilibration, after two minutes, the regional radioactivity recorded from the brain is proportional to rCBV (ml/100 g), where

$$rCBV = \frac{Brain\ counts/s\ per\ g \times 100}{Blood\ counts/s\ per\ ml \times R}$$

(R is the ratio of the cerebral haematocrit to the peripheral venous haematocrit and is usually taken as 0.88.)

Tomographic images show differences in the blood-pool distribution, with the well-perfused grey matter seen in contrast against the white matter. Areas of vasodilation secondary to decreased perfusion can be seen. In addition, rCBV images can be used to correct studies using other radiopharmaceuticals, where blood-pool subtraction is necessary in order to visualise uptake within the cerebral substance.   .

Regional Cerebral Blood Flow (rCBF)

^{15}O-labelled water ($H_2{}^{15}O$) can be used to study rCBF. $H_2{}^{15}O$ is a suitable pharmaceutical for this type of study, since it is easily produced, chemically stable, as well as being biologically inert and a natural constituent of body tissue. It is infused by continuous intravenous administration (James et al. 1982) or by inhalation of $C^{15}O_2$ (Baron et al. 1981), whereby the ^{15}O label is transferred to $H_2{}^{15}O$, under the influence of carbonic anhydrase in the lungs. The method assumes that the tracer is freely diffusible across the blood–brain barrier, so that the observed uptake is purely dependent on rCBF. This statement generally holds true, although at high flow rates proportional extraction does reduce, indicating that the process of diffusion requires a finite time which is not attained under high flow conditions. Since the half-life is short, variations in cyclotron supply, or respiratory rate (if the inhalation technique is employed) can lead to alterations in count rate during tomography. rCBF images obtained by this technique are similar, however, to those obtained using other techniques.

Ammonia, labelled with nitrogen-13, has also been used to study rCBF. This agent is incorporated rapidly into glutamate, and its distribution is believed to reflect rCBF, although not in a direct linear fashion. However, alterations in blood–brain pH, glutamine synthetase levels and reduction in the glutamine pool may also affect distribution, so that its application as a rCBF agent in the diseased brain is not yet fully established.

Cerebral Oxygen Metabolism

By using ^{15}O and PET, images of regional cerebral oxygen metabolism ($rCMRO_2$) and regional oxygen extraction fraction (rOEF) can be obtained. There are two inhalation methods: one using a steady-state technique (Subramanian et al. 1978), and the other a short inhalation (Mintun et al. 1984).

The amount of oxygen extracted by the brain depends on the regional extraction (rOEF), and the total supplied, i.e. $rCBF \times P_{art}O_2$. The extracted oxygen is metabolised to water, and excreted via the venous circulation. Thus, at any one time, the $^{15}O_2$ activity in the brain is due to $^{15}O_2$ in the incoming arterial blood, unextracted $^{15}O_2$ in the venous blood, $H_2{}^{15}O$ (water of metabolism) excreted into venous blood, and recirculating $H_2{}^{15}O$ re-entering via the arterial supply.

With the steady-state technique, $C^{15}O$ is used to determine rCBF, and scanning is repeated during inhalation of $^{15}O_2$. rOEF is calculated from the ratio of the counts obtained from each separate pharmaceutical and from the blood concentrations. Correction for the amount of oxygen remaining in the cerebral blood pool can be obtained from the rCBV image, as described earlier. The same data can be used to obtain $rCMRO_2$.

The single inhalation technique uses data derived from a 40 s scan following the brief inhalation of 3000–4000 MBq of $^{15}O_2$, and involve measurement of rCBF with $H_2^{15}O$, and rCBV with $C^{15}O$.

Both measurements involve three separate scans, depicting rCBF, rCBV, and regional cerebral oxygen distribution, and the patient must therefore be kept in a constant position throughout.

Cerebral Glucose Metabolism

Glucose, in the form of 2-deoxy-2-fluoro-D-glucose, can be labelled with fluorine-18, a positron emitter, to form ^{18}F-deoxyglucose (^{18}F-DG), and PET studies can be performed to study cerebral glucose metabolism under different conditions. This compound is phosphorylated by hexokinase, to form ^{18}F-DG-6-phosphate, which is not a suitable substrate for further metabolism, and is therefore trapped in cerebral tissue for sufficient time to perform tomography. Since glucose is not stored in the brain (although it provides 99% of its energy requirements) the uptake of ^{18}F-DG therefore reflects the cerebral glucose utilisation.

A number of experiments have explored the relationship between sensory stimuli, and regional cerebral metabolism. For example, stimulation of one visual field causes increased metabolic activity in the contralateral visual cortex. Unilateral auditory stimulation in control subjects resulted, by contrast, in increased ^{18}F-DG uptake in the right temporal cortex, regardless of the side to which the auditory stimulus was applied, indicating the complexity of the encoding of auditory information (Alani et al. 1981).

Clinical Results Using PET Studies

Studies on normal healthy volunteers have demonstrated that rCBF falls progressively by 5% per decade, after the third decade. This is compensated for, however, by an increase in oxygen extraction (rOER) so that the metabolic rate for oxygen ($rCMRO_2$) is not significantly affected.

In *dementia*, rOER remains constant, and the decline in rCBF is associated with a fall in $rCMRO_2$ to levels of less than 35 ml O_2/100ml/min, from a normal value of 51, in grey matter. White-matter metabolism is equally affected. rCBF measurements, therefore, can be used to measure the decline in cerebral function and metabolism. Since there is

no increase in rOER, there is no support for an ischaemic basis to dementia (Frackowiak et al. 1981).

In *acute infarction*, the decrease in flow is associated with a rise in rOER, which may exceed 70% (Weiss et al. 1982), reflecting the presence of critical ischaemia. After 1–2 days following the onset of stroke, the situation reverses, and there is a rise in rCBF in 95% of cases, to reach a level close to, or above, normal. This is the phase of luxury perfusion, and it is associated with a marked fall in rOER. Attempts to restore cerebral perfusion at this time will therefore be fruitless, since the affected area by then is receiving more blood and oxygen than normal. Indeed, vasodilators may be harmful if they divert blood flow from other critically affected areas. A management scheme which attempts to restore the coupling between flow and metabolism would be more effective. Studies using fluorine-18 labelled glucose have shown that, under hypoxic conditions, glucose metabolism is enhanced, possibly by anaerobic glycolysis (Pulsinelli and Duffy 1979), but that with established stroke after several weeks, this level falls to about 62% of the normal value when flow and metabolism are again matched (Kuhl et al. 1980). Impaired metabolism is seen in areas remote from the site of infarction, reflecting the complex way in which disordered function in one area may depress activity at other sites. These subsidiary areas appear on CT as structurally normal, and therefore PET scanning can provide some insight into the complex neurological disorders that stroke may induce. Similarly, motor and sensory stimulation studies can be used to demonstrate the involvement of intracranial pathways through their effect on glucose metabolism (Reivitch et al. 1979).

^{18}F-DG metabolism has also been used to study *schizophrenia*, where low frontal lobe uptake, reversed by perphenazine, has been found (Farkas et al. 1980). In *epilepsy*, dysfunctional zones have been detected as areas of reduced perfusion and metabolism interictally, which, during the seizure, showed dramatic increases in these parameters to well above normal levels (see Chap. 2 p. 42).

PET Receptor Imaging Agents

A number of positron-emitting neuroreceptor agents have been developed, using both agonists and antagonists. Since specific transport mechanisms are rare, the initial uptake is frequently related to lipid solubility, and the distribution is therefore essentially reflective of rCBF. After an interval of time, to allow dispersal of the unbound neurochemical, the pattern of uptake is more characteristic of receptor distribution.

A number of fluorine-18 and carbon-11 agents have been prepared as dopamine-receptor agents. For example [^{11}C]3-N-methylspiperone (Wagner et al. 1984), which binds to D_2 dopamine and S_2 serotonin receptors. Other dopamine agents include [^{18}F]fluorodopa (Garnett et al. 1983) and [^{11}C]pimozide (Baron et al. 1983). Analogues of haloperidol, spiroperidol, benzodiazepam and chlorpromazine are also known.

Agents have also been developed which bind onto muscarinic–acetylcholine receptors (Eckleman et al. 1984), serotonin (S1 and S2) receptors (Kloster et al. 1984) and opiate receptors (Frost et al. 1984). Monoamine oxidase distribution has also been charted using ^{11}C-labelled N-I-N dimethyl-phenylethylamine (Inoue et al. 1984). Work is currently in progress to investigate Parkinson's disease, Huntington's chorea and schizophrenia, but little is yet known concerning the role of these agents here.

Single Photon Emission Computerised Tomography (SPECT)

Unlike PET scanning, SPECT is available in most Nuclear Medicine Departments, and recent developments in radiopharmaceutical research have made sectional images of cerebral physiology available at a cost comparable to CT scans. These agents use radioisotopes which are readily available in Western Europe and the United States, such as iodine-123 and technetium-99m in the forms of N-isopropyl-p[^{123}I]iodamphetamine (IMP) (Winchell et al. 1980a, b), and hydroxy [^{123}I]iodobenzyl propyldiamine (HIPDM) (Kung et al. 1983) and most recently hydroxymethylpropylene amineoxime (HMPAO), labelled with ^{99m}Tc.

The use of simple single-photon gamma emitters for cerebral tomography imposes a number of requirements. The radiopharmaceutical should be unaffected by its passage through the lungs, should be extracted rapidly in high concentration by the brain tissue, and should be retained unaltered in the brain for a duration sufficient to allow the study to be performed. With a single rotating gamma camera, this interval measures 30–60 minutes.

HMPAO: Pharmacochemistry and Biological Distribution

This lipophilic low-molecular-weight complex is able to cross the blood–brain barrier. The molecules lose their lipophilicity in brain due to the lower pH

of cerebral parenchyma compared with blood and remain effectively fixed. After intravenous administration, 5% of this agent is taken up by the brain of which 86% remains 24 hours after injection, providing a tracer substance of adequate stability and selective uptake for SPECT studies.

The whole body dose for a standard adult administration of 500 MBq is low, approximately 2 milli sieverts (mSv) with a dose of 4 mSv to the brain. The maximal dose is received by the lachrymal glands (35 mSv) (Ell et al. 1987). In addition to a low radiation dose, animal experiments and clinical use have failed to demonstrate any toxic effects related to the use of this neutral substance.

Comparisons of HMPAO images with other methods of assessing rCBF have shown a close correlation in human subjects (Andersen et al. 1987).

HMPAO: Normal Cerebral Appearance

HMPAO is taken up predominantly in grey matter, in relation to rCBF. In addition to demonstration of the cerebral cortex, the cerebellum, thalamus and basal ganglia are well shown (Fig. 11.8). Difficulties in positioning the patient can be overcome by the use of oblique reconstruction, to obtain true transaxial slices. Although many studies are now performed using a single rotating conventional gamma camera, speed of acquisition can be increased using two opposing detector systems, or a custom-built multidetector array.

OPPOSITE PAGE ▶

Cerebral HMPAO studies. Yellow/red, normal perfusion; blue/black, diminished/absent perfusion). (By courtesy of Amersham International.)

Fig. 11.8. Normal axial section.

Fig. 11.9. Multi-infarct dementia. Axial section showing multiple perfusion defects.

Fig. 11.10. Alzheimer's disease. Axial section showing symmetrical frontal and temporo-occipital perfusion defect (*arrows*).

Fig. 11.11. Steele–Richardson syndrome. Bifrontal subcortical defects are shown.

Fig. 11.12. Right frontoparietal infarction, parasagittal reconstruction.

Fig. 11.13. a Impaired perfusion of the left frontal area due to internal carotid artery occlusion. b Improvement following surgical revascularisation.

Fig. 11.14. Coronal reconstruction showing a perfusion defect at the site of an epileptogenic focus in the left frontoparietal region (*arrow*).

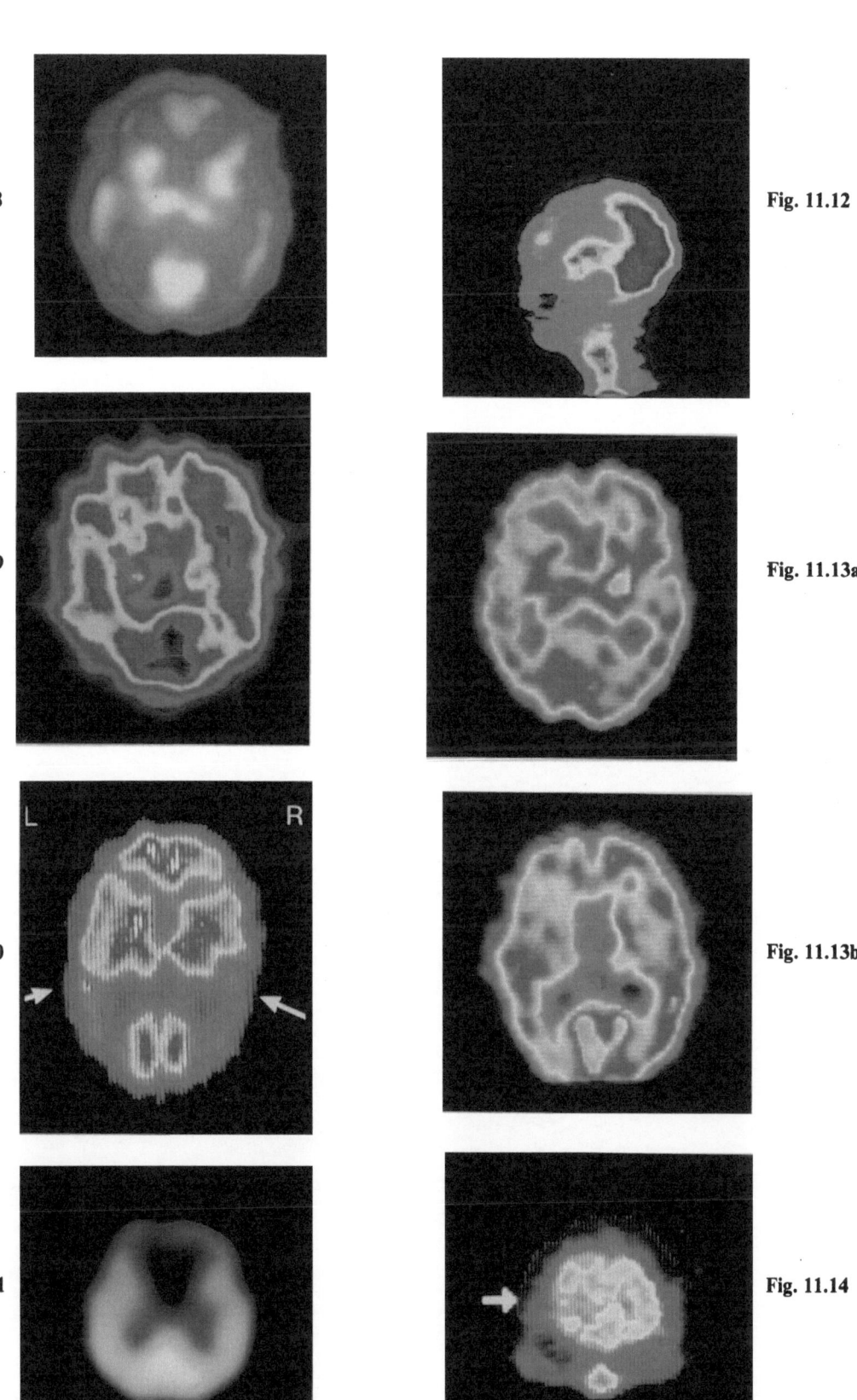

Fig. 11.8

Fig. 11.12

Fig. 11.9

Fig. 11.13a

Fig. 11.10

Fig. 11.13b

Fig. 11.11

Fig. 11.14

HMPAO: In Dementia

About 10% of the adult population over 65 years suffers from dementia, the two commonest types being Alzheimer's disease and multi-infarct dementia, and clinical discrimination between the two disorders may be difficult.

In multi-infarct dementia, multiple small perfusion defects are seen in the cerebral cortex, many of which are not apparent on CT or MRI (Smith et al. 1987) (Fig. 11.9).

In Alzheimer's disease, the pattern is of symmetrical perfusion defects in the frontal, temporoparietal and occipital regions (Fig. 11.10), corresponding to the "watershed" territories of the cerebral arteries.

In the Steele–Richardson syndrome (progressive supranuclear palsy) characteristic subcortical perfusion losses are present in the frontal areas, with preservation of the cortical rim (Fig. 11.11).

HMPAO: In Cerebral Infarction

Following acute infarction, HMPAO shows a perfusion defect corresponding to the site of the lesion, and frequently larger than the abnormality shown by CT. Crossed cerebellar diaschisis is a common feature. Decreased cerebellar activity occurs on the side opposite to a middle cerebral artery territory infarct (Shih et al. 1988). Quantitative comparison of regional cerebral uptake can add statistical significance to the interpretation of the data. Luxury perfusion is a frequent finding in the days following the acute episode. Cerebral infarction may occasionally be silent and lead to a perplexing state of altered behaviour in the patient, for which a number of diagnostic possibilities must be entertained. HMPAO studies in this situation again offer the potential to detect such a lesion, occasionally in circumstances when the CT scan is normal or non-specific.

SPECT studies can be reconstructed in the coronal and sagittal planes, or using a rotating three-dimensional display, for accurate localisation of the site of the lesion (Fig. 11.12).

HMPAO: In Transient Cerebral Ischaemia

Hypoperfused areas are frequently seen using HMPAO in patients suffering transient ischaemic attacks whereas the CT scan is often normal. Similar findings occur with prolonged reversible ischaemic neurological deficit (PRIND), but are slower to reverse. HMPAO can be used to demonstrate areas of prejudiced cerebral blood flow and the cerebral reserve – the ability of the vessels to compensate for low flow rates by vasodilation – can be assessed. This can be achieved by comparing the rCBF image, following HMPAO administration, with the rCBV image, obtained by labelling the blood pool using Tc-pertechnetate and (non-radioactive) stannous pyrophosphate. Alternatively, the HMPAO image can be repeated after acetazolamide, which induces local tissue hypercapnia through an inhibitory effect on carbonic anhydrase. In the first technique, a localised increase in the rCBV/rCBF ratio denotes vasodilation, and in the second technique, absence of change after acetazolamide denotes similar depletion of the cerebral reserve. This may be valuable in the assessment of patients both prior to and following carotid endarterectomy (Fig. 11.13).

HMPAO: In Cerebral Tumours

The role of HMPAO in intracranial tumour detection has not yet been fully assessed, although it is clear that some primary intracerebral tumours (e.g. glioma) are seen as areas of increased uptake, whereas metastases are frequently detected as hypoperfused areas due to local cerebral ischaemia. Such areas are frequently larger than the metastases as demonstrated on the CT scan, and may precede the development of visible oedema.

HMPAO: In Epilepsy

As in the case of [^{123}I]IMP studies, epileptiform foci are seen, in the interictal phase as areas of reduced perfusion. During the ictus, uptake is enhanced to well above normal levels. HMPAO has been used in a number of instances, to localise the dysfunctional area prior to surgery, and to confirm its removal postoperatively. In some patients HMPAO has been able to show the presence of several foci, with a distribution which may render surgery impossible. Given the accepted limitations of CT in detecting epileptogenic lesions, HMPAO is likely to establish itself as a useful diagnostic tool in this situation (Fig. 11.14).

References

Alani A, Reivich M, Greenberg J (1981) Mapping of functional activity in brain with ^{18}F-fluorodeoxyglucose. Semin Nucl Med 11:24–31

Andersen AR, Friberg H, Lassen NA (1987) Serial studies of cerebral blood flow using Tc-HMPAO: A comparison with 133-Xenon. Nucl Med Commun 8:549–557

Baron JC, Steinling M, Tanaka T (1981) Quantitative measurement of CBF, oxygen extraction fraction (OEF) and CMRO$_2$ with the 15–O continuous inhalation technique and positron emission tomography (PET). Experimental evidence and normal values in man. J Cereb Blood Flow Metab 1 [suppl 1:5–6

Baron JC, Comar D, Zarifian E (1983) An in vivo study of the dopaminergic receptors in the brain of man using C-11 pimozide and positron emission tomography. In Magistretti PL (ed) Functional radionuclide imaging of the brain. Raven Press, New York, pp 337–345

Carril JM, MacDonald AF, Dendy PP, Keyes W, Undrill PE, Mallard JR (1979) Cranial scintigraphy. Value of adding emission computed tomographic sections to conventional pertechnetate images. J Nucl Med 20:117–123

Du Boulay GH, Marshall J (1975) Comparison of EMI and radioisotope imaging in neurological disease. Lancet ii:1294–1297

Eckleman WC, Reba RC, Rzeszotarski R (1984) External imaging of cerebral muscarinic acetylcholine receptors. Science 223:291–292

Ell PJ, Deacon JM, Jarritt PH (1980) Atlas of computerised emission tomography. Churchill Livingstone, Edinburgh

Ell PJ, Costa DC, Cullum ID, Jarritt PH, Lui D (eds) (1987) The clinical application of rCBF imaging by SPECT. Amersham International, p 12

Farkas T, Ferris SH, Wold AP (1980) The application of 18-FDG and positron emission tomography in the study of psychiatric conditions. In: Passanean GV, Hawkins RA, Lust WD, Welsh FA (eds) Cerebral metabolism and neurological function. Williams and Wilkins, Baltimore, pp 403–408

Frackowiak RSJ, Pozzelli C, Legg NJ et al. (1981) Regional cerebral oxygen supply and utilisation in dementia. A clinical and physiological study with oxygen-15 and positron tomography. Brain 104:753–778

Frost JJ, Dannals RF, Ravert HT (1984) Imaging opiate receptors with positron emission tomography. J Nucl Med 25:73

Garnett RS, Firnam G, Nahmias C (1983) Dopamine visualised in the basal ganglia of living man. Nature 305:137–138

Grubb RL, Raichle MG, Higgins CS (1978) Measurement of regional cerebral blood volume by emission tomography. Ann Neurol 4:322–328

Hill TC, Lovett RD, McNeil BJ (1980) Observations on the clinical value of emission tomography. J Nucl Med 21:613–616

Huckman MS (1981) Normal pressure hydrocephalus: Evaluation of diagnostic and prognostic tests. AJNR 2: 385–395

Inoue O, Taminaga T, Suzuki K (1984) Development of a new type of radiotracer for in-vivo estimation of brain MAO activity. N-Mmethyl labelled phenethylamine derivatives. In: Fifth International Symposium on Radiopharmaceutical Chemistry, Tokyo, pp 197–199

James SC, Reivich M, Robinson GD (1982) The measurement of cerebral blood flow with positron emission tomography using the continuous infusion of oxygen-15 labelled water. In: Proceedings of the Third World Congress of Nuclear Medicine and Biology, Paris. Pergamon, Oxford, pp 1744–1747

Keele CA, Neil E, Joels N (eds) (1982) Samson Wright's applied physiology, 13th edn. Oxford Medical Publications, Oxford

Kloster G, Hanus J, Vogee R (1984) C-11 mesulergin, a potential agent for mapping the serotonin receptor. Synthesis and animal experiments. In: Fifth International Symposium on Radiopharmaceutical Chemistry, Tokyo, pp 173–174

Kuhl DE, Phelps ME, Kowell AP (1980) Effects of stroke on local cerebral metabolism and perfusion. Mapping by emission computed tomography using 18-FDG and 13-NH$_3$. Ann Neurol 8:47–60

Kung HF, Tramposch KM, Blau M (1983) A new brain perfusion agent, I-123 HIPDM NN[1] trimethyl N[1]2 Hydroxy 3-methyl 5-iodo benzyl 13-propane diamine. J Nucl Med 24:63–72

Leveille J, Pison C, Karakand Y, Lemieux R, Vallieres BJ (1977) Technetium-99m glucoheptonate in brain tumour detection, an important advance in radiotracer techniques. J Nucl Med 18:957–961

Mintun MA, Raichle ME, Markin WRW (1984) Brain oxygen utilisation measured with O-15 radiotracers and positron emission tomography. J Nucl Med 25:177–187

Nagle CE (1980) Use of immediate static scans in combination with radionuclide cerebral angiography as a confirmatory test in the diagnosis of brain death. Clin Nucl Med 5:152–153

Pulsinelli WA, Duffy TE (1979) Local glucose metabolism during controlled hypoxemia in rate. Science NY 204:626–629

Reivitch M, Greenberg J, Alavi A (1979) The use of 18-FDG for mapping functional neural pathways in man. Acta Neurol Scand 60 [Suppl 72]:198–199

Shih WJ, Dekosky S, Coupal JJ, Clark D, Ryo UY, Kung HF (1988) Transtentorial diaschisis in stroke patients demonstrated by I-123 HIPDM Brain imaging (abstract). Radiology 169(P):266

Smith FW, Gemmell HG, Sharp PF (1987) The use of 99m-Tc HMPAO for the diagnosis of dementia. Nucl Med Commun 8:525–533

Subramaniam R, Alpert NM, Hoop B (1978) A model for regional cerebral oxygen distribution during continuous inhalation of 15-O and C-15O$_2$. J Nucl Med 19:48–53

Wagner HN, Burns HD, Dannals RF (1984) Imaging dopamine receptors in the human brain by positron tomography. Science 221:1393–1396

Weiss RJS Bernardi S Frackowiak RSJ (1983) Serial observations on the pathophysiology of acute stroke. Brain 106: 197–222

Winchell HS, Horst WD, Brown L, Oldendorf WH (1980a) N-isopropyl 123-iodoamphetamine. Single pass brain uptake and washout. Binding to brain synaptosomes and localisation in dog and monkey brain. J Nucl Med 21:947–952

Winchell HS, Baldwin RM, Lin TH (1980b) Development of 123-I-labelled amines for brain studies. Localisation of 123-I iodophenyl alkyl amines in rat brain. J Nucl Med 21:940–946

Chapter 12

Contrast Media and the Central Nervous System
Peter Dawson

Introduction

The soft tissues of the body, including those of the central nervous system, are poorly demonstrated on plain X-ray films and the need for agents which would enhance these images was perceived in the very earliest days of radiology (Wallingford 1953; Bull 1961). The story of the development of such agents in fact constitutes a fascinating sub-plot in the history of the subject. The rapid post-war development of neurosurgical techniques was a powerful impetus for further improvements in the potential of neuroradiological imaging and had a significant influence on the development of safer contrast agents (Bull 1961).

Any substance for human administration must be, as far as possible, free from toxic effects, but there is a special dimension to the problem of enhancing central nervous system images which derives from the great sensitivity of neural tissues to chemical agents. A graphic illustration of this is that water-soluble iodinated contrast agents, much used in radiology, are estimated to be some 1400 times as toxic to the neural tissues as to other tissues (Hoppe 1959).

Although gaseous negative contrast media are not entirely benign in the central nervous system, giving rise to a response of pleocytosis and protein and glucose elevation for a period of some 10 days or so, these changes are of apparently little clinical significance and will not be discussed further in this chapter, which will concentrate on the toxic effects of the iodinated positive contrast agents. The most modern of these may be seen as "universal" agents in that they may be used, in principle, with relative safety, in any body compartment. They do, however, have significant neurotoxicity which is worthy of some detailed consideration, not only

because of its obvious relevance to the work of the neuroradiologist, but also because it may play a role in systemic adverse reactions to these agents (Hoppe 1959; Lalli 1980; Lalli and Greenstreet 1981; Shehadi and Toniolo 1980; Ansell et al 1986).

Historical Perspective

Intravascular Contrast Agents

The first quarter of a century of radiology saw much interest in the development of intravascular contrast agents (Bull 1961; Dawson 1987) and a good deal of cadaver angiography was performed to the immeasurable gain of the study of anatomy but all of it with clinically impractical contrast agents (Grainger 1982; Dawson 1987). The first cerebral angiogram on a patient was performed by Egas Moniz (1927) using, first, strontium bromide and, subsequently, 25% solutions of sodium iodide for injection by direct percutaneous carotid puncture. The pain and general toxicity associated with sodium iodide solutions necessitated general anaesthesia and led Moniz, temporarily, down the blind alley of thorotrast, an excellent agent in radiographic terms with virtually no acute toxicity but with, as is now well known, disastrous late sequelae due to its retention in the reticulo-endothelial system and to its α-emitter properties (Thomas et al. 1951; Boyd et al. 1968; Hughes 1953).

The introduction in the late 1920s and early 1930s of, first, mono-iodinated and, subsequently, di-iodinated pyridine compounds gave radiologists a type of agent of significantly lower systemic and organ specific toxicity (Wallingford 1953; French and Blake 1950; Grainger 1982; Broman and Olsson 1984; Dawson 1987), but it was not until the early

1950s that the ionic tri-iodinated benzoic acid derivatives were developed and radiologists were finally provided with compounds of impressively low intravascular toxicity which were very acceptable for cerebral and spinal angiography (Wallingford 1953; Kendall 1964; Grainger 1982; Dawson 1987). However, even these compounds were far from ideal for use in the subarachnoid space where their uncomfortably high neurotoxicity was most obviously manifest. Only in very recent years has a new, though closely related, type of compound been introduced which has remarkably low neurotoxicity and is therefore far more satisfactory for both intravascular and subarachnoid administration. This is the non-ionic type of agent (Dawson 1985, 1987; Dawson et al. 1983), the chemistry of which will be discussed below.

Intrathecal Contrast Agents

Air as a negative contrast agent for the visualisation of the spinal and cerebral subarachnoid spaces was utilised 70 years ago by Dandy (1919, 1925) and air myelography and encephalography soon became important weapons in the neurologist's armoury (Jacobaeus 1921; Dandy 1925; Petrovitch 1981; Rosenbaum and Baker 1984).

It was in 1922, while injecting iodised poppy seed oil into the epidural space for the treatment of sciatica, that Sicard accidentally introduced it into the subarachnoid space (Sicard and Forestier 1922). No ill effects were observed in this patient and the first positive contrast myelogram was thereby achieved. In the next few years Sicard and Forestier reported several hundred patients with varying spinal cord and column pathologies and established the techniques of spinal subarachnoid and intraventricular positive contrast studies (Petrovitch 1981). This radiocontrast agent, "lipiodol", was used for myelography in the USA and Europe until its late toxic effect of adhesive arachnoiditis, which had been recognised as early as 1928, finally made it unacceptable (Howieson 1974; Irastam et al. 1974). Several attempts to modify the basic preparation to reduce its toxicity were tried, such as emulsification, but these only made the situation worse (Jäeger 1950). On the basis of our present knowledge, emulsification might have been expected to produce an increase in toxicity since the emulsification process serves more effectively to present the oily and hydrophobic contrast agent to the neural tissues. Lipiodol was finally replaced by iophendylate (Pantopaque) a mixture of ethyl esters of iodophenylate of an oily nature (Ramsey et al. 1944; Steinhausen et al. 1944; Strain et al; 1946, Strain 1971). Like other agents of its type it was immiscible with the

cerebrospinal fluid, rendering its effective acute neurotoxicity low, but had the radiographic and practical disadvantages of not entering the root sleeves and making them visible. It was associated with various acute and chronic toxic effects (Taren 1960; Mason and Raof 1962; Cristi et al. 1974), including arachnoiditis (Erickson and van Baaren 1953; Feny et al. 1973; Skalpe 1976; Greenberg and Vance 1980; Jones 1980). The late complications were found to be enhanced if the spinal tap was bloody (Haughton et al. 1977). The agent was very slowly absorbed from the central nervous system (CNS) (less than 1 ml per annum) and, therefore, ideally needed to be removed at the end of the procedure. The mechanisms of arachnoiditis have been the subject of much speculation. Agents like Pantopaque increase cerebrospinal fluid (CSF) proteins and induce lymphocytosis suggestive of sterile inflammation but this has not been found to correlate well with the arachnoiditis (Feny et al. 1973).

The first water-soluble agent, sodium iodomethane sulphonic acid (Abrodil), was introduced into neuroradiological practice in Scandinavia (Arnell and Lidstrom 1931). It required spinal anaesthesia and had to be restricted to the lumbosacral region because of its high neurotoxicity, manifest clinically as severe spasms, convulsions and paresis (Arnell and Lidstrom 1931; Lindblom 1947).

Various iodinated "natural" compounds such as amino acids were tried but found to exhibit high neurotoxicity (Lefft and Maclean 1942; Schober 1964). Because they promised better quality images with root sleeve filling, interest was maintained in the possibility of better water-soluble agents but toxicity remained a problem. Meglumine lothalamate, a tri-iodinated benzoic acid (see below) was used and found to be very effective, and better than the similar diatrizoate (Albertson and Doppman 1974), but exhibited, albeit with a lower incidence, similar toxic effects as previous water-soluble compounds (Ahlgren 1972). It was also associated with occasional late arachnoiditis (Kemp 1950).

A dimer of iothalamate, "dimer X", was introduced in an effort to reduce any osmolality component of neurotoxicity (Gonsette 1971; Gonsette and Brucher 1980; Suzuki et al. 1976a, b). It was found to be superior to the iothalamate monomer and achieved general use in Europe with considerable success but its epileptogenic potential in animals and man was soon recognised (Irastam and Sellden 1976; Nishikawa and Yonekawa 1976; Usbeck and Assmann 1977; Kun et al. 1978; Gonsette and Brucher 1980) and, again, arachnoiditis was found to be a not infrequent longer-term complication (Haughton and Ho 1980; Haughton et al. 1978; Irastam and Sellden 1976; Irastam et al. 1974; Skalpe 1976). Aseptic meningitis occurred occasionally (Luce et al. 1951). It was, however, for all its limitations, a reference standard against which the toxicity of the first non-ionic water-soluble contrast agent, metrizamide, was compared on its introduction (Djindjian 1969; Gonsette 1973; Irastam and Sellden 1976). Most recently the second generation non-ionic monomeric agents have been introduced into clinical practice (Dawson et al. 1983; Dawson 1987) and non-ionic dimers have been introduced into clinical trials (Drayer et al. 1984; Muetzel et al. 1984; Dawson and Howell 1986). All the non-ionic agents have exceptional low neurotoxicity, as will be discussed below, and are associated with a very low incidence of acute and chronic effects (Haughton 1976; Hammer and Lackner 1980; Kendall et al 1983; Gabrielson et al. 1984; Lamb 1984; Haughton 1985; Kido et al. 1985; Shaw et al. 1985). They are now the agents of choice for all neuroradiological applications.

Chemistry of the Iodinated Agents

Only the chemistry of the water-soluble agents currently in clinical use will be described. All the modern water-soluble contrast agents are tri-iodinated derivatives of benzoic acid (Fig. 12.1) (Dawson et al. 1983; Dawson 1987). Figure 12.1(a) shows meglumine iothalamate, an ionic monomeric agent which is still used for neuroangiography and was once used as a myelographic medium. Figure 12.1(b) shows the dimeric form of this molecule, meglumine iocarmate (dimer X) which was used for myelography in the 1960s. Figure 12.1(c) is a monoacid dimer, meglumine sodium ioxaglate (Hexabrix), a low osmolality agent developed for angiography but not for intrathecal use. Figure 12.1(d) shows the compound metrizamide, the first generation non-ionic contrast agent which on its introduction revolutionised the practice of myelography. Figure 12.1(e) is a typical representative of the family of second generation non-ionic monomeric agents which are superior even to metrizamide. Figure 12.1(f) is a typical representative of the newest family of agents, the non-ionic dimers which are still undergoing assessment (Drayer et al. 1984; Muetzel et al. 1984; Dawson and Howell 1987).

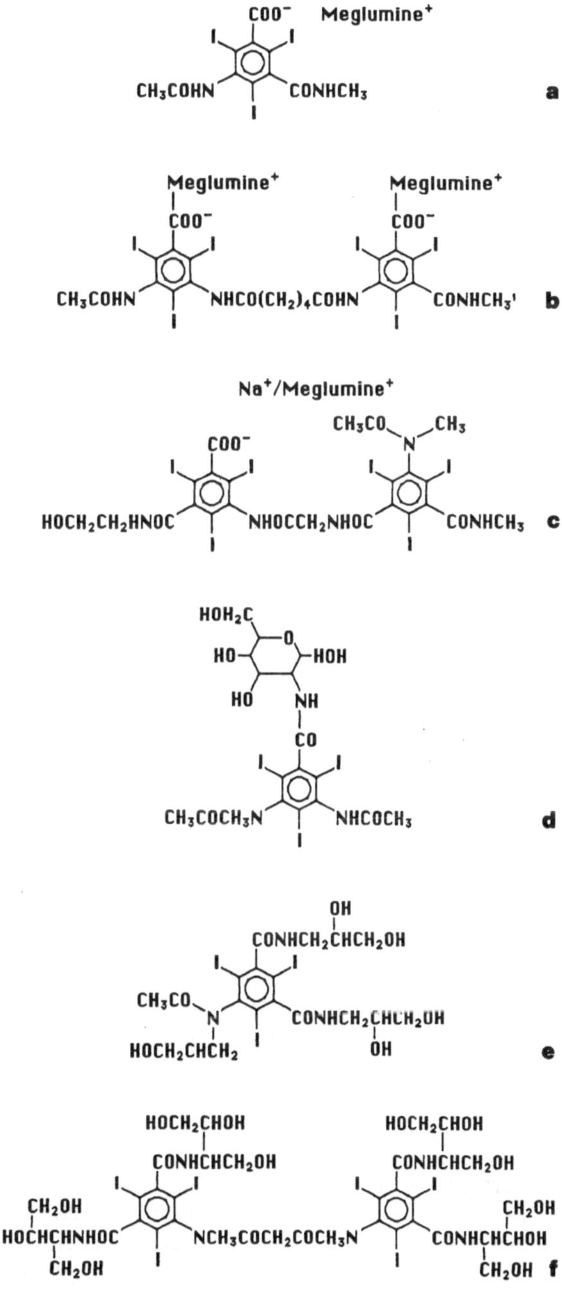

The osmolality of a solution is proportional to the number of particles in the solution and the contrast provided by the contrast agent depends on the number of iodine atoms in the solution (Grainger 1980; Dawson and Howell 1986). Conse-

Fig. 12.1. Water-soluble contrast agents. **a** Meglumine iothalamate; **b** meglumine iocarmate (dimer X); **c** meglumine sodium ioxaglate (Hexabrix); **d** metrizamide; **e** typical representative of second generation non-ionic monomeric agents; **f** a typical non-ionic dimer.

quently, the ratio of contrast provided by any particular solution to the osmolality yielded by that solution may be represented as a ratio of number of iodines on the molecule to the number of particles provided by that molecule. If it does not ionise, only one particle, the whole molecule, is yielded.

These ratios for the compounds illustrated in Fig. 12.1 are, respectively, 3/2, 6/3; 3/1; 6/2; 6/1 or simplifying, 3/2; 2/1; 3/1; 3/1; 6/1. This represents a progressive increase in the ratio or a decrease in the osmolality of the solutions for any given iodine concentration. High osmolality is certainly a significant contributor to several aspects of contrast agent toxicity and compounds with high ratios would be expected to have somewhat lower toxicities than the compounds with lower ratios (Grainger 1980; Dawson and Howell 1986). This is, broadly, found to be the case but there are other factors. Contrast agent toxicity in its many forms is dependent not only on the osmolality of the solutions but also on chemical structures and ionicity (Dawson 1985, 1987). In neurotoxicity the part played by osmolality is not a great one and the chemistry of the molecules and the ionicity are of greater interest. Uncharged non-ionic agents are much to be preferred because of their lower neurotoxicity. The intrinsic or chemotoxicity of contrast agent molecules is a function of their hydrophilicity (Dawson 1985, 1987). This may be expressed as the partition co-efficient (Dawson 1987). Iodine is a highly hydrophobic entity and iodinated molecules are therefore intrinsically toxic, a fact which no doubt explains why experiments with iodinated "natural" chemicals such as amino acids were unsuccessful (Left and Maclean 1942; Schober 1964). As can be seen from their structures, the non-ionic agents have many hydrophilic hydroxyl groups to maintain their water solubility and to some extent these shield these the iodines in a steric hindrance phenomenon thereby reducing their toxicity (Dawson 1987). (For this reason the non-ionic agents have the best systemic and neurotoxicity profile.) Their low osmolality may be advantageous but it is their lack of charge and their hydrophilic nature which lies at the heart of their low toxicity to neural tissue. It is interesting that metrizamide, the first generation non-ionic medium, should be inferior to the second generation agents such as iohexol. The reason for this is that its hydrophilic groups are all carried on a sugar moiety at one corner of the molecule leaving iodines elsewhere unmasked and rendering the molecule, overall, relatively hydophobic and toxic (Dawson 1987).

Pharmacodynamics of Water-Soluble Agents

Following intravascular injection the water-soluble agents are rapidly distributed in the intravascular and extracellular extravascular spaces (McChesney and Hoppe 1957; Dean and Kormano 1977; Newhouse 1977; Gardeur et al. 1980; Muetzel and Speck 1980). After this early distribution phase the extra-cellular contrast filled space may be viewed as a single compartment obeying first order kinetics with virtually exclusive renal excretion by passive glomerular filtration. The serum half-life is of the order of two hours.

Blood–Brain Interface

The water-soluble agents, especially the non-ionic agents with their high hydrophilicity, penetrate the central nervous system very poorly because of the existence of the blood–brain barrier (Sage et al. 1982a, b). It is for this reason that normal brain enhances poorly on contrast administration. However, there are regions such as the pituitary gland where the blood–brain barrier is absent and radiocontrast media may enter freely (Lalli 1980) and, when they are injected in high concentrations directly into the cerebral vessels, the agents themselves may cause significant disruption of the blood–brain barrier thereby effecting an entry (Hoppe 1959; Jeppson and Olin 1970; Murphy 1973; Rapoport and Levitan 1974; Rapoport et al. 1974; Waldron et al. 1974; Raninko 1979; Lulli 1980; Sage et al. 1982b). High osmolality plays a role (Hoppe 1959; Raininko 1979) but neurotoxicity does not correlate well with the osmolality of the agent (Rapoport and Levitan 1974; Sage et al. 1982a). Other factors such as chemotoxocity play a significant role both in disruption of the blood–brain barrier and in subsequent neurotoxic events (Rapoport and Levitan 1974; Rapoport et al. 1974; Waldron et al. 1974).

The penetration is dose-dependent (McClennan and Becker 1971) and appears to be a function of the plasma/CSF concentration gradient. The degree of penetration correlates with toxic manifestations. McClennan and Becker (1971) found that the CSF concentration of an ionic contrast agent one hour after IV injection was approximately 1.5% of initial blood concentration. Given the great sensitivity of neural tissues it seems reasonable to consider a role for the CNS in the toxic "systemic" adverse reactions to iodinated contrast agents (Hoppe 1959; Lalli 1980).

Possible protective measures against neurotoxic effects have been explored. Pretreatment with steroids and low-molecular-weight dextran, alone and in combination, has proved efficacious in reducing CNS toxicity (Crocker et al. 1976). Steroid pretreatment apparently reduces penetration of contrast agents into the CNS even after injury to the blood–brain barrier (Crocker et al. 1976; Neuwelt et al. 1982). It is known that neurotoxic effects are greater in patients with defects of the blood–brain barrier and in patients with high plasma levels of contrast (Kendall and Pullicino 1980). The neuro-protective effects of steroids may be postulated to form the basis for their claimed protective effects against major adverse reactions. However, the use of intrathecal corticosteroids to reduce arach-noiditis paradoxically potentiates its development (Harvey et al. 1961; Eldevik et al. 1978b).

Cerebrospinal Fluid–Brain Interface

The CSF–brain interface is at the pia mater over-lying the brain and cord and at the ependyma lining the ventricular system. These form an ineffective barrier between CSF and extracellular fluid of the brain and cord as far as the passage of relatively small radiocontrast media molecules is concerned. These appear to enter neural tissue from the CSF by simple diffusion after injection into the sub-arachnoid space. The depth of penetration into neural tissue appears to be much the same for ionic and non-ionic agents in dog experiments. The differences in neurotoxicity between various agents do not, therefore, obviously relate to any differences in penetration but rather to differences in toxicity.

It is believed that the central nervous system distribution of the agents is overwhelmingly extra-cellular. The blood–brain barrier prevents their reabsorption into capillaries and this appears to be maintained even when high concentrations of contrast are present in the neural tissues. It has been suggested that metrizamide with its deoxyglucose moiety may compete with glucose for transport into neurones but this remains speculation (Bertoni et al. 1980; Northington et al. 1982).

CSF Circulation and the Elimination of Contrast Agents

In an adult male, the total CSF volume is approxi-mately 150 ml, of which 30 ml is in the cerebral ven-tricles and a similar volume in the lumbar sac. The production rate is approximately 0.35 ml per minute or approximately 500 ml per 24 hour period. It is secreted by the choroid plexus and to a small extent by the ependyma. Reabsorption is by the arachnoid villi and spinal granulations into the venous sinuses and epidural veins respectively. Circulation of CSF is driven by hydrostatic pressures resulting from the production process, body movement, coughing, arterial pulsations and venous pressure changes resulting from respiration. Circulation in the spinal subarachnoid space is poor and inconsistent. The drive for CSF reabsorption is the 6 cm H_2O or so pressure difference between the CSF and venous sinuses. It is worth noting that this pressure differ-ence can easily be lost as a result of the lumbar

puncture itself if more CSF leaks out than the amount of contrast injected. The reabsorption process may of course also be inhibited after men-ingitis. Clearance of contrast agents from the sub-arachnoid space depends on mixing within the CSF and the rate of CSF resorption. Contrast in the spinal subarachnoid space has to move slowly up and down the spinal column rather than to circulate and is predominantly reabsorbed by the spinal arachnoid villi. Horizontal posture produces rapid reabsorption because of greater contact with the whole length of spinal granulations. The whole process depends in a complicated physical way on the volume injected, the posture of the patient, and the viscosity of the material, which determines its rate of movement and distribution. Keeping the patient in a head up position is only useful in the first few hours in preventing a significant bolus of contrast agent entering the intracranial subarachnoid space. Computed tomography (CT) studies show that contrast medium is routinely found in the brain for up to three days after myel-ography (Ahlgren 1972). Eldevik and Haughton (1978) showed that in repeat myelography, reab-sorption of contrast was diminished, presumably because of an element of arachnoiditis caused by the earlier procedure. Paradoxically, Hammer and Lackner (1980) found in a comparison of metri-zamide with iopamidol that the higher the rate of elimination of contrast the higher the incidence of headache.

The production of CSF, it should be noted, is diminished in several situations including the con-comitant administration of diuretics, acetazolamide (Rubin et al. 1969), various cardiac drugs and radio-contrast agents themselves (Ingvar 1957; Lindgren 1959; Reed 1968a, b; Domer 1966; Harnish and di Stefano 1984, 1985).

CSF–Blood Interface

The CSF–blood interface is principally at the choroid plexi which, as discussed, are responsible for some 85% of CSF production and filtration of some small molecules. The capillaries of these plexi, unlike cerebral capillaries in general, are fenestrated and therefore allow ultrafiltration of plasma with contrast molecules into the choroid interstitium. This accounts for the enhancement on CT scans of the plexi after administration of contrast. This interstitium, however, is enclosed by a cuboidal epithelial layer of cells linked by tight junctions. This considerably restricts the passage of small mol-ecules such as contrast agents.

Another CSF–blood interface is the arachnoid membrane. The capillaries of the dura are also fenestrated and allow passage of contrast media into the dural extracellular space. This explains dural enhancement on CT head scans after contrast administration. However, the outer layers of the arachnoid have capillaries with tight junctions so that contrast agent molecules cannot pass into the CSF. Any contrast agent in the cerebral or cord extracellular fluid, having entered through areas of disrupted blood–brain barrier, may exchange freely with the CSF.

Neurotoxicity of Contrast Agents

Clinical Phenomena

Angiography

Contrast agents are intended only to provide contrast and any effects on physiology, biochemistry or haematology must be viewed, no matter how apparently clinically unimportant some of them may be, as toxic effects. It should be realised that contrast media exert a number of systemic effects which may play a part in CNS effects. Thus the marked peripheral vasodilatation and cardioinhibitory effects associated with their systemic administration may engender a marked decrease in systemic blood pressure leading to secondary cerebral ischaemic events, particularly if the cerebral circulation is already impaired by disease. Furthermore, contrast agents have adverse effects on blood rheology (Dawson et al. 1983a) and, on selective injection, replace blood temporarily in the cerebral circulation.

In cerebral angiography the effects of contrast agents on the cerebral circulation itself are similar to those found in other vascular beds with vasodilatation particularly of the external carotid bed. However, there are some important reflexes resulting in bradycardia and, on occasion, asystole and hypotension (Fischer et al. 1962; Hilal 1966a, b; Lynch et al. 1969; Hilal 1974; Howieson 1974; Higgins and Schmidt 1979; Morris et al. 1979). The agents appear to act on cerebral vasomotor centres and on baro- and chemoreceptors in the extracranial cerebral vasculature (Lindgren 1958, 1959; Higgins and Schmidt 1979). Both osmolality and chemotoxicity appear to play a part (Hilal 1966a, b; Lynch et al. 1969). All these phenomena are less marked with the non-ionic contrast media (Fischer et al. 1962; Gonsette 1978; Kido et al. 1985).

Changes in blood rheology, systemic hypotension and replacement of blood by contrast media acutely on injection also contribute to adverse effects on the cord in spinal arteriography.

Clinical phenomena in cerebral angiography range from minor feelings of warmth and discomfort and head and face pain or numbness at one end of the scale, through dizziness and confusion, and transient amnesia (Suzuki et al. 1976b), to muscle twitching, leg cramps (Boijsen and Lindholmer 1971), minor and major convulsions, hemiparesis, transient and permanent hemiplegia (Brendler and Hayes 1959; Kendall 1964), temporary or permanent blindness (Labauger et al. 1968), decerebrate state and death at the other extreme end of the spectrum (Abbott et al. 1952; Studdard et al. 1981). The incidence of severe clinical adverse effects is low (Howieson 1974; Mani and Eisenberg 1978; Reisner et al. 1980). An analysis of more than 4000 cerebral angiograms performed with conventional ionic agents showed an incidence of some 13% of transient complications of which 3% were of the neurological/psychiatric type. They occurred mostly in younger patients and in patients in whom cerebral vascular disease was already present (Kachel et al. 1980). The relatively minor symptoms are all significantly reduced when the newer agents are used, pain in particular being apparently predominantly osmolality-related since metrizamide, in spite of its relatively high chemotoxicity, is associated with less pain than iohexol, presumably because of its lower osmolality. A variety of electrocardiographic and electroencephalographic changes have also been noted in cerebral angiography (Lundervold and Engeset 1969).

Adverse effects in spinal angiography and, incidentally, on occasion in aortography and other angiography (Feigelson and Ravin 1965; Epsen 1966; Henson and Parsons 1967) range from sensory and motor loss, commonly associated with a sensory level and extensor spasm lasting for 1–3 hours resolving without specific therapy (Cornell 1969) through medullary epilepsy, manifest as intermittent clonic jerking of the legs and to disastrous cord infarction (Margolis et al. 1959).

Intravenous digital subtraction angiography utilises large amounts of contrast medium. The concentrations to which neural tissues are exposed are not high but McClennan and Becker (1971) have shown that significant amounts of contrast injected intravenously may be found in the CSF.

Subarachnoid Administration

Common toxic manifestations (Baker et al. 1978) include headache, nausea and vomiting, all of which are related, at least in part, to the lumbar puncture itself and loss of CSF. The incidence of headache is unaccountably higher in females (Rolfe and Maguise 1980) and may be less marked in well hydrated (Eldevik and Haughton 1987; Eldevik et al. 1978a) and ambulant patients (Gulati et al. 1981). It is likely that the early headache is largely mechanical and related to lumbar puncture and that the late headache is due to direct toxic effects of the contrast media. One study (McClennan 1973) has shown that headache may be reduced or abolished in Pantopaque myelography by administration of intrathecal corticosteroids. Unfortunately the incidence of late arachnoiditis may thereby be increased (Ahlgren 1972, 1980; Dullerud and Morland 1976).

Seizures are uncommon with metrizamide and even less common with the second generation non-ionic agents (Kaada 1973; Hindmarch et al. 1975; Nielsen 1975; Oftedal 1977; Oftedal and Kayed 1983; Ropper et al. 1978). They may be spinal or cortical in origin and associated with electroencephalographic changes. Early entry of contrast agents into the intracerebral CSF increases their incidence. This makes the case for keeping the patient as far as possible in a head up position during, and for some hours following the examination. At least with metrizamide, if not with the second generation non-ionic agents, phenothiazines and neuroleptic drugs lower the seizure threshold and should be avoided (Hindmarch et al. 1975). Those with a high alcohol intake also appear to be at greater risk for seizures. The intrathecal administration of dextrose with metrizamide, on the belief that metrizamide may produce some of its toxic effects by competing with glucose for hexokinase, has been shown to produce no significant reduction in the seizure incidence in dogs (Northington et al. 1982).

Aseptic meningitis is an uncommon but well recognised complication and presents with all the symptomatic and CSF changes of septic meningitis but with no organism being present (Oftedal 1982; White 1984). A variety of encephalopathic disorders are common in mild degree and for short periods but occasionally are seen in more dramatic form and may be prolonged for up to two weeks (Bertoni et al. 1981). There may be changes in mood and affect, delirium, hallucination, confusion and manic disorder (Gelmers 1979; Koppejan et al. 1981; France and McCraken 1984; Galle et al. 1984; Kwentus et al. 1984). Occasionally neurological deficits including cortical blindness, aphasia, hemiplegia, quadriplegia and ophthalmoplegias may occur (Angiari 1974; Occhiogrosso et al. 1979; Smith and Laguna 1980; Wales and Nov 1981; Peroutka et al. 1982; Masdeu et al. 1983; Perlman and Barry 1984).

The whole spectrum of common and less common adverse effects may be reduced in incidence and severity by good hydration and elevation of the head for a few hours after the procedure to minimise entry of contrast agent into the intracranial subarachnoid space.

Pathological Effects

Pathological specimens are, naturally, only available from the laboratory, from animal studies and in the most severe and fatal cases of clinical neurotoxic adverse effects. Evidence of injury to the blood–brain barrier is seen in cerebral angiography with high dose and high concentrations of contrast media, particularly of ionic type (Rapoport and Levitan 1974; Rapoport et al. 1974; Waldron et al. 1974; Raninko 1979). There is swelling of cells and disruption of tight junctions. This is largely osmolality mediated but chemotoxocity plays a part (Rapoport and Levitan 1974; Rapoport et al. 1974; Waldron et al. 1974). Non-ionic contrast agents, both monomeric and dimeric, are less injurious than the ionic agents (Sovak et al. 1980, 1982a, b; Muetzel et al. 1984). Once through the blood–brain barrier, intravascular contrast agents can exert their effects directly on neural tissues. In pathological cases which have been studied, petechial cerebral and cord haemorrhages and/or areas of infarction are seen (Henson and Parsons 1967).

Mechanisms of Neurotoxicity

Blood–Brain Barrier Injury

Injury to the blood–brain barrier is the initial phenomenon in the chain of events leading to neurotoxicity of intravascular contrast agents. Rapoport and Levitan (1974), Rapoport et al. (1974) and Waldron et al. (1974) suggested that contrast agents in high concentrations caused shrinkage of vascular endothelial cells with disruption of tight junctions. The disruption appears to be reversible and of a severity related to osmolality and chemical factors (Rapoport and Levitan 1974; Rapoport et al. 1974; Waldron et al. 1974; Raninko 1979) with sodium salts being more injurious than meglumine salts of ionic agents and diatrizoates being more injurious than the iothalamates (Melartin et al. 1970). Several studies (Hammer and Lackner 1980; Sage et al. 1982a; Cronquist 1983; Dahlstrom 1984; Haughton 1985) show that non-ionic contrast agents are associated with less injury than conventional agents and that this is not simply a function of osmolality.

Direct Toxicity

In spite of a considerable amount of investigation and speculation, the detailed mechanisms of direct contrast agent neurotoxicity remain obscure. When contrast agents come into contact with neural tissues they are known to have direct cytotoxic effects, as on other cells, which are mediated by a combination of osmolality and chemotoxicity (Sovak et al. 1980; Dawson et al. 1983a), an effect exacerbated by the photoelectric phenomenon when the tissues are also exposed to X-rays (Dawson et al. 1987). Once again the lower chemotoxicity of non-ionic contrast agents is manifest in a lower cytotoxicity (Sovak et al. 1980). It is believed, though not rigorously proved, that contrast agents do not significantly enter neurones. This is a reasonable assumption in view of their chemical structures and hydrophilicity. It has, however, been postulated that metrizamide with its deoxyglucose moiety might compete with glucose for transport mechanisms in neurones (Bertoni et al. 1980; Caillé et al. 1980; Ekholm et al. 1983; Ekholm 1985). Sodium salts of ionic agents are more toxic than meglumine salts (Melartin et al. 1970). Addition of calcium or magnesium ions reduces toxicity (Golman 1979). These ions, it has been suggested, may limit penetration of anions whereas sodium may allow the anionic particle to enter the cell by interfering with normal cell metabolism and transport processes.

Charge certainly appears to play a significant part in the neurotoxic phenomena. Changes in electrical activity of isolated laboratory nervous tissue, in experimental animal models, and in man monitored by invasive techniques or external EEG recordings appear much greater with the ionic materials than the non-ionic materials (Lundervold and Engeset 1969; Kaada 1973; Gonsette and Brucher 1980; Sovak et al. 1980; Bryan and Hershkowitz 1982; Lamb 1984).

Contrast agents are known to inhibit enzyme systems on a dose/concentration dependent basis (Dawson and Edgerton 1983; Dawson 1985; Howell and Dawson 1985) and it has been suggested that they may exert some of their toxic effect in this manner or by similar inerference with neurotransmitters. Metrizamide, in particular, with its deoxyglucose moiety competes with glucose for the enzyme hexokinase and this has been postulated to be a mechanism of neurotoxocity (Bertoni et al. 1980; Callé et al. 1980; Ekholm et al. 1983). The second generation non-ionic agents and non-ionic dimers with no such glucose moieties have no significant effect on hexokinase (Ekholm 1985). This could go some way to explaining their lower neurotoxicities. Intrathecal injection of dextrose with metrizamide has been found, however, to be of no benefit in reducing the seizure rate in animal studies (Northington et al. 1982).

Another phenomenon which may play a part in neurotoxic phenomena is the reduction of CSF production by contrast agents (Harnish and di Stefano 1984, 1985; Harnish et al. 1986, 1988). CSF production is an important factor, as discussed earlier, in the excretion and clearance of toxic materials from the CNS. It has been shown, for example, that brain concentrations of methotrexate are increased, retention time prolonged and brain tissue penetration enhanced if CSF turnover is decreased. Reed (1968) found that pentobarbital sleep time in rats increased in proportion to the acetazolamide-induced decrease in CSF production (Rubin et al. 1966). The basis for this phenomenon may be inhibition of the enzyme adenylate cyclase which plays a role in CSF production (Harnish et al. 1986).

A great number of studies of EEG changes in which neural tissue is exposed to radiocontrast medium have been carried out in isolated tissue, experimental animals and in man (Lundervold and Engeset 1969; Sovak et al. 1980; Bryan and Hershkowitz 1982; Hershkowitz and Bryan 1982; Lamb 1984). These monitor the disruptive influence on normal neural activity of contrast agents, particularly the ionic variety.

Future Developments

Non-ionic Dimers

The osmolalities of the non-ionic dimers in solution in iodine concentrations of 300–700 mg I/ml are less than that of plasma. Addition of a little saline adjusts the osmolalities of all the clinical preparations to exactly that of plasma. They appear to offer significant advantages over previous agents and early studies have indeed revealed low neurotoxicity. Their high viscosities may make them less than ideal for angiography but this property and their large molecular size, by reducing the reabsorption rate, may actually make them ideal for myelography (Dawson and Howell 1986). Initial clinical studies appear to bear out this prediction (Sovak et al. 1982b).

Magnetic Resonance Imaging

Magnetic resonance imaging (MRI) has firmly established itself as a powerful tool for imaging the CNS. Historically, all imaging modalities have ultimately benefited from the development of image contrast enhancing agents and MRI has proved no exception. MR proton imaging is based on quite different physicochemical properties of tissues from

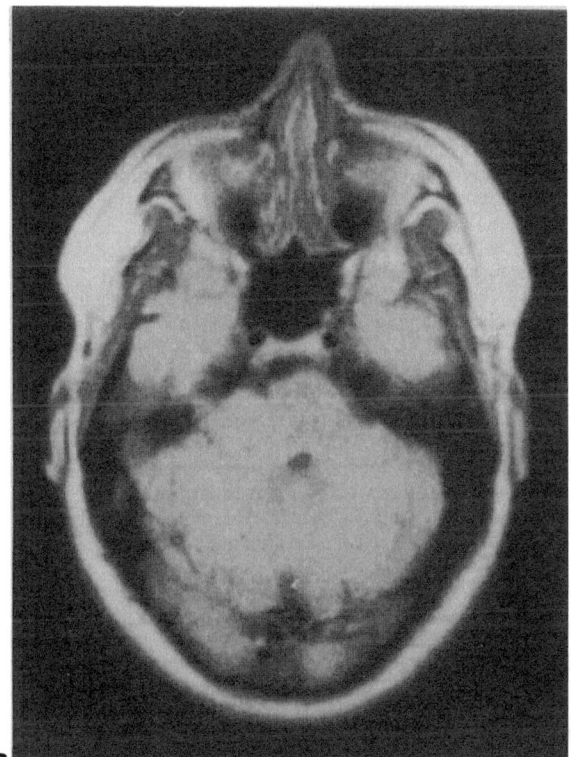

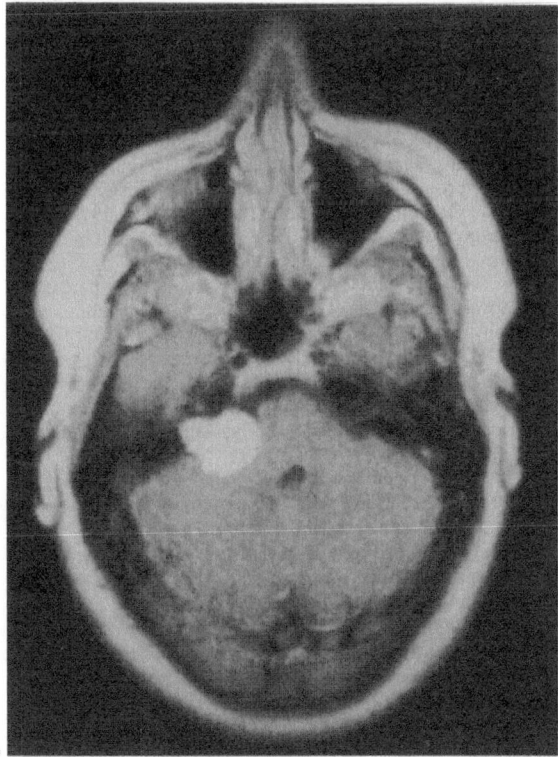

Fig. 12.2. Cranial MRI (axial T1 weighted images). Acoustic neurinoma before (**a**) and after (**b**) gadolinium DTPA. (By courtesy of I. Isherwood, Manchester.)

X-ray absorption or ultrasound reflection and practical MR agents exercise indirect effects by enhancing T1 and/or T2 relaxation times. To achieve this the molecules of the agents must closely approach the proton. Agents enhancing T1 relaxation times are usually particulate. This is a broad generalisation and most agents have some effect on both T1 and T2 relaxation times (Wolf and Popp 1984).

Paramagnetic materials are made up of atoms with unpaired electron spins. The best known and most successful MRI enhancing agent is the paramagnetic gadolinium. To render toxic gadolinium biologically acceptable it is powerfully bound to the chelating carrier molecule diethylenetriamine penta-acetic acid (DTPA). Inevitably this adversely affects its paramagnetic influence but is essential. Theoretically the nature of the carrier molecule can be changed in order to obtain different pharmacodynamics and excretion or to dictate specific tissue or organ uptake.

The pharmacokinetics of gadolinium DTPA closely parallel those of the water-soluble iodinated compounds. The agent is exceptionally safe with a lethal dose/effective dose ratio some 15 times higher than that for the ionic iodinated agents (Wolf and Popp, 1984). It has been used successfully as an enhancing agent in MRI of the CNS and exhibits no significant neurotoxicity. The nasal and paranasal sinus mucosa enhances normally with gadolinium as does the pituitary gland. Delayed scanning is therefore recommended for the study of pathology in these regions. T1 weighted pulse sequences are ideally used since the enhancement of gadolinium is exerted through a shortening of the T1 relaxation time (Stack et al. 1988) (Fig. 12.2).

As with the iodinated contrast media, gadolinium DTPA detects the abnormal blood–brain barrier but there can be no enhancement of arteries since rapidly flowing blood returns no signal. The recommended dose of gadolinium DTPA is 0.1 mmol/kg.

References

Abbott KH, Gray JR, Goodall RJ (1952) Clinical complications of cerebral angiography. J Neurosurg 9:258–274

Ahlgren P (1972) Dimer-X. A new contrast medium for lumbar myelography without spinal anaesthesia. Acta Radiol [Diagn] (Stockh) 13:753–761

Ahlgren P (1980) Early and late side-effects of water soluble contrast media for myelography and cisternography: a short review. Invest Radiol 15:S264–S266

Albertson K, Doppman JL (1974) Meglumine diatrizoate v iothalamate: comparison of seizure-inducing potential, Br J Radiol 47:265–267

Angiari P, Crisi G, Merli GA (1974) Aphasia and right hemiplegia after cervical myelography with Amipaque. A case report. Neuroradiology 26:61–63

Ansell G, Tweedie MCK, West CR, Evans P, Couch L (1986) The current status of reactions to intravenous contrast media. Invest Radiol 15:S32–S39

Arnell S, Lidstrom F (1931) Myelography with Skiodan (Abrodil). Acta Radiol 12:287–291

Baker RA, Hillman BJ, McLennan JE, Strand RD, Kaufman SM (1978) Sequelae of metrizamide myelography in 200 examinations. AJR 130:499–502

Bertoni JM, Alexander GM, Schwartzman RJ (1980) Metrizamide competitively inhibits hexokinase. In: Duvoisin RC (ed) Transactions of the American Neurological Association, vol 105. Springer, Berlin, Heidelberg, New York, pp 218–220

Bertoni JM, Schwartzman RJ, Van Horn G, Partin J (1981) Asterixis and encephalopathy following metrizamide myelography: Investigation into possible mechanisms and review of the literature. Ann Neurol 9:366–370

Boijsen E, Lindholmer E (1971) Serious complications from myelography with meglumine iothalamate. An account of 324 lumbar myelographies together with a description of 2 cases of severe leg cramp. Nord Med 85:520–522

Boyd JT, Langlands AO, MacCabe JJ (1968) Long-term hazards of Thorotrast. Br Med J ii:517–521

Brendler SJ, Hayes GJ (1959) Hypaque in cerebral angiography: report of complications in 617 angiograms. J Neurosurg 16:454–460

Broman T, Olsson O (1984) The tolerance of cerebral blood vessels to a contrast medium of the diodrast group. Acta Radiol 30:326–342

Bryan RN, Hershkowitz N (1982) Intracellular effects of radiographic contrast agents on the rat hippocampus (abstr). AJNR 3:93

Bull JWD (1961) History of neuroradiology. The presidential address delivered at the British Institute of Radiology, 20 Oct 1960. Br J Radiol 34:69–84

Caille JM, Guibert-Tranier F, Howa, JM, Billerey J, Calabet A, Piton J (1980) Cerebral penetration following metrizamide myelography, J Neuroradiol 7:3–12

Camp JD (1950) Contrast myelography: past and present. Radiology 54:477–505

Cornell SH (1969) Spasticity of the lower extremities following abdominal aortography. Radiology 93:377–379

Cristi G, Scialfa G, Di Pierro G, Tassoni A (1974) Visual loss: a rare complication following oil myelography. Case report and review of the literature. Neuroradiology 7:287–290

Crocker EF, Zimmerman RA, Phelps ME, Kuhl DE (1976) The effects of steroids on the extravascular distribution of radiographic contrast material and technetium pertechnetate in brain tumours as determined by computer tomography. Radiology 119:471–475

Cronquist S (1983) Iohexol in cerebral angiography. Survey and present state. Acta Radiol [Suppl] (Stockh) 36:135–139

Dahlstrom K (1984) Summary of US and European intra-vascular experience with iohexol. Presented at "A worldwide clinical assessment of a new contrast medium, iohexol", Boca Raton, Fla, May 1984, pp S117–S120

Dandy WE (1919) Roentgenography of the brain after the injection of air into the spinal canal. Ann Surg 70:397–403

Dandy WE (1925) The diagnosis and localisation of spinal cord tumours. Ann Surg 81:223–227

Dawson P (1985) Chemotoxicity of contrast media and clinical adverse effects; a review. Invest Radiol 20:S84–S91

Dawson P (1987) Iodinated intravascular contrast agents; a review. J Intervent Radiol 2:51–58

Dawson P, Edgerton D (1983) Contrast media and enzyme inhibition–1 cholinesterase. Br J Radiol 56:653–656

Dawson P, Howell M (1986) The non-ionic dimers; a new class of contrast agents. Br J Radiol 59:987–991

Dawson P, Harrison MJG, Weisblat E (1983a) Effect of contrast media on red cell filtrability and morphology. Br J Radiol 56:707–710

Dawson P, Grainger RG, Pitfield J (1983b) The new low osmolar contrast media – a simple guide. Clin Radiol 34:221–226

Dawson P, Penhaligon M, Smith E, Saunders J (1987) Iodinated contrast agents as radio-sensitisers. Br J Radiol 60:201–203

Dean PB, Kormano M (1977) Intra-arterial bolus of ^{125}I labelled meglumine diatrizoate. Early extravascular distribution. Acta Radiol [Diagn] (Stokh) 18:425–432

Djindjian R (1969) Arteriography of the spinal cord. Am J Roentgenol Rad Ther Nucl Med 197:461–478

Dormer FR (1969) Effects of diuretics on cerebrospinal fluid formation and potassium movement. Exp Neurol 24:54–64

Drayer B, Ross M, Allen S, France R, Bates M (1984) Iotrol myelography: initial clinical trial. Invest Radiol 19:S141

Dullerud R, Morland TJ (1976) Adhesive arachnoiditis after lumbar radiculography with Dimer-X and Depo-Medrol. Radiology 119:153–155

Ekholm SE (1985) Iohexol versus metrizamide in studies of glucose metabolism. A survey. Invest Radiol 20:S18–21

Ekholm SE, Reece K, Coleman, DK Jr, Fischer H (1983) Metrizamide – a potential in vivo inhibitor of glucose metabolism. Radiology 147:119–121

Eldevik OP, Haughton VM (1978) The effect of hydration of the acute and chronic complications of aqueous myelography. An experimental study. Radiology 129:713–714

Eldevik OP, Nakken KO, Haughton VM (1978a). The effect of dehydration on the side effects of metrizamide myelography. Radiology 129:715–716

Eldevik OP, Haughton VM, Ho KC, Williams AL, Unger GF, Larson SJ (1978b) Ineffectiveness of prophylactic intrathecal methylprednisolone in myelography with aqueous media. Radiology 129:99–101

Epsen F (1966) Spinal cord lesion as a complication of abdominal aortography. Acta Radiol [Diagn] (Stockh) 4:47–61

Erickson TC, Van Baaren HH (1953) Late meningeal reaction to ethyl iodophenyl undecylate used in myelography: report of a case that terminated fatally. JAMA 153:636–639

Feigelson HH, Ravin HA (1965) Transverse myelitis following selective bronchial arteriography. Radiology 85:663–665

Feny DW, Gooding R, Standefer JC, Weise GM (1973) Effect of Pantopaque myelography on cerebrospinal fluid reactions. J Neurosurg 38:167–171

Fischer HW, Eckstein JW, Perret G (1962) Comparison of cardiovascular effect of contrast media in cerebral angiography in man. J Neurosurg 19: 943–946

France RD, McCracken J (1984) Delirium following metrizamide myelography. Psychosomatics 25:338–339

French L, Blake PS (1950) Complications following the use of neo-iopax in cerebral angiography. Am J Roentgenol Rad Ther Nucl Med 64: 816–818

Gabrielson TO, Geparski SS, Knake JE, Latack JT, Yang PJ, Hoff JT (1984) Iohexol versus metrizamide for lumbar myelography: double-blind trial. AJR 142:1047–1049

Galle G, Huk W, Arnold K (1984) Psychopathometric demonstration and quantification of mental disturbances following myelography with metrizamide and iopamidol. Neuroradiology 26:229–233

Gardeur D, Lautrou J, Millard JC, Berger N, Matzger J (1980) Pharmacokinetics of contrast media: experimental results in dogs and man with CT implications. J Comput Assist Tomogr 4:178–185

Gelmers HJ (1979) Adverse side effect of metrizamide in myelography. Neuroradiology 18: 118–123

Golman K (1979) The blood–brain barrier effects of non-ionic contrast media with and without addition of Ca^{2+} and Mg^{2+}. Invest Radiol 14:305–308

Gonsette R (1971) An experimental and clinical assessment of water soluble contrast medium in neuroradiology. A new medium: Dimer-X. Clin Radiol 22:44–56

Gonsette R (1973) Biologic tolerance of the central nervous system to metrizamide. Acta Radiol [Suppl] (Stockh) 335:25–44

Gonsette R (1978) Animal experiments and clinical experiences in cerebral angiography with a new contrast agent (ioxaglic acid) with a low hyperosmolality. Ann Radiol 21:271–273

Gonsette R, Brucher JM (1980) Neurotoxicity of novel water soluble contrast media for intra-thecal application. Invest Radiol 15:S254–S259

Grainger RG (1980) Osmolality of intravascular radiological contrast media. Br J Radiol 53:739–746

Grainger RG (1982) Intravascular contrast media – the past, the present and the future. Br J Radiol 55:1–18

Greenberg MK, Vance SC (1980) Focal seizure disorder complication of iodophendylate myelography (letter). Lancet i:312–313

Gulati AN, Guadagnoil DA, Quigley JM (1981) Relationship of side effects to patient position during and after metrizamide lumber myelography. Radiology 141:113–116

Hammer B, Lackner W (1980) Iopamidol, a new non-ionic hydrosoluble contrast medium for neuroradiology. Neuroradiology 19:119–121

Harnish PP, Di Stefano V (1984) Decreased CSF production by Intravenous sodium diatrizoate. Invest Radiol 19:318–323

Harnish PP, Di Stefano V (1985) Pharmacological action of radiographic contrast media reduced CSF production in the dog. J Pharmacol Exp Ther 232:88–93

Harnish PP, Northington RK, Di Stefano V, Banarjee SP (1986) Mechanisms of decreased cerebrospinal fluid production by radiographic contrast media: role of adenylate cyclase activation. J Pharmacol Exp Ther 236:464–469

Harnish PP, Northington FK, Samuel KA (1988) Iohexol Inhibits adenylate cyclase. Invest Radiol 23:139–142

Harvey JP, Freiberger RF, Werner G (1961) Clinical and experimental observations with methiodal, an absorbable myelographic contrast agent. Clin Pharmacol Ther 2:610–614

Haughton VM (1976) Changes of arachnoiditis after metrizamide myelography: experimental work in monkeys. Myelography and the water soluble contrast medium. University of Wisconsin, Madison, 26 March

Haughton VM (1985) Intrathecal toxicity of iohexol versus metrizamide. Survey and current state. Invest Radiol 20:S14–S17

Haughton VM, Ho KC (1980) Arachnoiditis from myelography with iopamidol, metrizamide and iocarmate compared in the animal model. Invest Radiol 15:S267–S269

Haughton VM, Ho KC, Larson S et al. (1977) Arachnoiditis following intrathecal injection of blood and aqueous contrast media. Acta Radiol [Suppl] (Stockh) 355:373–378

Haughton VM, Ho KC, Larsen SJ, Unger GF, Correa-Pax F (1978) Comparison of arachnoiditis produced by meglumine iocarmate and metrizamide myelography in an animal model. AJR 131:129–132

Henson RA, Parsons M (1967) Ischaemic lesions of the spinal cord: an illustrated review. QJ Med 36:205–222

Hershkowitz N, Bryan RN (1982) Neurotoxic effects of water-soluble contrast agents on rat hippocampus extracellular recordings. Invest Radiol 17:271–275

Higgins CB, Schmidt WS (1979) Identification and evaluation of the contribution of the chemoreflex in the hemodynamic response to intracarotid administration of contrast materials in the conscious dog: comparison with the response to nicotine. Invest Radiol 14:438–446

Hilal SK (1966a) Haemodynamic responses in the cerebral vessels to angiographic contrast media. Acta Radiol [Diagn] (Stockh) 5:211–231

Hilal SK (1966b) Haemodynamic changes associated with intra-

arterial injection of contrast media. Radiology 86:615–633

Hilal SK (1974) Cerebral hemodynamics assessed by angiography. In: Newton TH, Potts DG (eds) Radiology of the skull and brain. CV Mosby, St Louis, pp 1067–1085

Hindmarch T, Grepe A, Widen L (1975) Metrizamide–phenothiazine interaction: report of a case with seizures following myelography. Acta Radiol [Diagn] (Stockh) 16:129–134

Hoppe JO (1959) Some pharmalogical aspects of radiopaque compounds. Ann NY Acad Sci 78:727–739

Howell MJ, Dawson P (1985) Contrast media and enzyme inhibition. II Mechanisms. Br J Radiol 58:845–848

Howieson J (1974) Complications of cerebral angiography. In: Newton TH, Potts DG (eds) Radiology of skull and brain: Angiography, CV Mosby, St Louis, Chap. 53

Hughes R (1953) Chronic changes in the central nervous system following Thorotrast ventriculography. Proc R Soc Med 46:191–195

Ingvar DH (1957) EEG during cerebral angiography. Acta Radiol 47:181–184

Irastam L, Sellden U (1976) Adverse effects of lumbar myelography with Amipaque and Dimer-S. Acta Radiol [Diagn] (Stockh) 17:145–159

Irastam L, Sundstrom R, Sigstedt B (1974) Lumbar myelography and adhesive arachnoiditis. Acta Radiol [Diagn] (Stockh) 15:356–368

Jacobaeus HG (1921) On insufflation of air into the spinal canal for diagnostic purposes in cases of tumors in the spinal canal. Acta Med Scand 55:555–564

Jaeger R (1950) Irritating effect of iodized vegetable oils on the brain and spinal cord when divided into small particles. Arch Neurol Psychiatry 64:715–719

Jeppson PG, Olin T (1970) Neurotoxicity of Roentgen contrast media. Study in the blood–brain barrier in the rabbit following selective injection of contrast media into the internal cerebral artery. Acta Radiol [Diagn] (Stockh) 10:17–34

Jones DF (1980) Postoperative convulsions due to iophendylate (Myodil). Report of a case and review of the causes of postoperative convulsions. Anaesthesia 35:50–56

Kaada B (1973) Transient EEG abnormalities following lumbar myelography with metrizamide. Acta Radiol [Suppl] 33:380–386

Kachel R, Ritter H, Schiffmann R, Schumann E (1980) Complication following cerebral angiography: Report on 4,181 cerebral angiographies. Zentralbl Chir 105:504–512

Kendall BE (1964) Cerebral angiography using Conray. Br J Radiol 37:581–589

Kendall BE, Pullicino P (1980) Intravascular contrast injection in ischaemic lesions. Neuroradiology 19:241–243

Kendall B, Schneidau A, Stevens J, Harrison M (1983) Clinical trial of Iohexol for lumbar myelography. Br J Radiol 56:539–542

Kido DK, Gordon-Potts D, Bryan NR et al. (1985) Iohexol cerebral angiography. Multicentre clinical trial. Invest Radiol 30:S55–S57

Koppejan EH, Bejeer N, Bosch DA, Vencken LM (1981) Organic psychosyndrome correlated with high density of grey matter on CT following metrizamide cervical myelography. Clin Neurol Neurosurg 83:63–66

Kun M, Alwaskiak J, Gronska J (1978) Morphological changes in the CNS after Dimer-X ventriculography. Neuroradiology 15:99–106

Kwentus JA, Silverman JJ, Sprague M (1984) Manic syndrome after metrizamide myelography. Am J Psychiatry 14: 700–702

Labauger R, Cailar J, Xhardex M et al. (1968) Cortical blindness after cerebral angiography; reversibility under hyperbaric oxygen therapy. Rev Neurol (Paris) 118:283–289

Lalli AF (1980) Contrast media reactions: Data analysis and hypothesis. Radiology 134:1–16

Lalli AF, Greenstreet R (1981) Reactions to contrast media:

testing the CNS hypothesis. Radiology 138:47–49

Lamb JT (1984) A comparison of Iopamidol and Iohexol for myelography. Neuroradiology 26:157

Lefft HH, Maclean JA Jr (1942) Visualization of the brain and spinal cord with diodothyrosine-gelatin contrast medium, including observation on the fate of this material. Arch Neurol Psychiatry 48:343–347

Lindblom K (1947) Complications of myelography by Abrodil. Acta Radiol 28:69–73

Lindgren P (1958) Blood pressure and heart rate responses in carotid angiography with sodium actrizoat. Acta Radiol 50:160–174

Lindgren P (1959) Carotid angiography with tri-iodobenzoic acid derivatives: A comparative experimental study of the effects on the systemic circulation in cats. Acta Radiol 51:353–362

Luce JC, Leith W, Burrage WC (1951) Pantopaque meningitis due to hypersensitivity. Radiology 57:878–881

Lundervold A, Engeset A (1969) Electroencephalographic and electrocardiographic studies of complications in cerebral angiography. Acta Radiol [Diagn] (Stockh) 9:399–406

Lynch PR, Harrington GJ, Michie C (1969) Cardiovascular reflexes associated with cerebral angiography. Invest Radiol 4:156–160

Mani RL, Eisenberg RL (1978) Complication of catheter cerebral arteriography: analysis of 5,000 procedures. III. Assessment of arteries injected, contrast medium used, duration of procedure and age of patient. AJR 131:871–874

Margolis G, Griffin AT, Kenan PD et al. (1959) Contrast medium injury to the spinal cord: the role of altered circulatory dynamics. J Neurosurg 16:390–406

Masdeu JC, Glista GG, Rubino FA, Martinex-Lage JM, Marani E (1983) Transient motor aphasia following metrizamide myelography. AJNR 4:200–202

Mason MS, Raof J (1962) Complications of Pantopaque myelography: case report and review. J Neurosurg 19:302–311

McChesney EW, Hoppe JO (1957) Studies of the tissue distribution and execretion of sodium diatrizoate in laboratory animals. Am J Roentgenol Rad Ther 78:137–144

McClennan BL, Becker JA (1971) Cerebrospinal fluid transfer of contrast material at urography. AJR 113:427–432

McLennan JE (1973) Prevention of post-myelographic post-pneumoencephalographic headache by single dose intrathecal methyl-prednisolone acetate. Headache 13:39–48

Melartin E, Tuohimaa PJ, Dabb R (1970) Neurotoxicity of iothalamate and diatrizoates. I. Significance of concentration and cation. Invest Radiol 5:13–21

Moniz E (1927) L'encephalographie arterielle, son importance dans la localisation des tumeurs cerebrales. Rev Neurol 2:72–90

Morris TW, Francis M, Fisher HW (1979) A comparison of the cardiovascular responses to carotid injections of ionic and nonionic contrast media. Invest Radiol 14:217–223

Muetzel W, Speck U (1980) Pharmacokinetics and biotransformation of iohexol in the rat and the dog. Acta Radiol [Suppl] 362:87–92

Muetzel W, Press W-R, Weinmann HJ (1984) Preclinical experience with iotrol. Invest Radiol 19:S140–S141

Murphy DJ (1973) Cerebrovascular permeability after meglumine iothalamate administration. Neurology 23:926–936

Neuwelt EA, Barnett PA, Bigner DD, Frenkel EP (1982) Effects of adrenal cortical steroids and osmotic blood–brain barrier opening on methotrexate delivery to gliomas in the rodent: the factor of the blood–brain barrier. Proc Natl Acad Sci USA 79:4420–4423

Newhouse JH (1977) Fluid compartment distribution of intravenous iothalamate in the dog. Invest Radiol 12:364–367

Nielsen H (1975) Case reports: epileptic seizures following cervical myelography, Neuroradiology 10:59–60

Nishikawa M, Yonekawa Y (1976) Intracisternal dimer X: toxicity and prophylaxis. Neuroradiology 11: 61–65

Northington JW, Biery DN, Lawrence TG (1982) Intrathecal Dextrose to prevent seizures after metrizamide myelography in dogs. Invest Radiol 17:282–283

Occhiogrosso M, Troccoli V, Vailati G (1979) A rare complication following iodized myelography: Late blindness. Case report. Acta Neurol (Napoli) 34:76–78

Oftedal SI (1977) Toxicity of water soluble contrast media injected suboccipitally in cats. Acta Radiol [Suppl] 335:84–92

Oftedal SI (1982) Meningeal reactions to water soluble contrast media: a comparison of iophendylate and metrizamide in experimental animals. Radiology 143:699–702

Oftedal SI, Kayed K (1983) Epileptogenic effects of water soluble contrast media: an experimental investigation in rabbits. Acta Radiol [Suppl] 335:45–56

Perlman EM, Barry D (1984) Bilateral sixth nerve palsy after water soluble contrast myelography. Letter. Arch. Ophthalmol 102:986

Peroutka SJ, Ullrich CG, Fisher RS, Suss RA, Brooks BR (1982) Transient areflexia and quadriplegia following metrizamide myelography (Letter). Ann Neurol 12:406–407

Petrovitch M (1981) Radiological evaluation of the spinal cord. CRC Press, Boca Raton

Raininko R (1979) Role of hypertonicity in the endothelial injury caused by angiographic contrast media. Acta Radiol [Diagn] (Stockh) 20:410–416

Ramsey GH, French JD, Strain WH (1944) Iodinated organic compounds as contrast media for radiographic diagnosis. IV. Pantopaque myelography. Radiology 43:236–241

Rapoport SI, Levitan H (1974) Neurotoxicity of X-ray contrast media. Relation to lipid solubility and blood brain barrier permeability, AJR 122:186–193

Rapoport SI, Thompson HK, Bidinger JM (1974) Equiosmolal opening of the blood–brain barrier in the rabbit by different contrast media. Acta Radiol [Diagn] (Stockh) 15:21–32

Reed DJ (1968) The effects of actazolamide on pentobarbitol sleep-time and cerebrospinal fluid flow of rats. Arch Int Pharmacodyn 171:206–215

Reed DJ (1969) The effect of furosemide on cerebrospinal fluid flow in rabbits. Arch Int Pharmacodyn 178:324–330

Reisner H, Samec P, Zeiler K (1980) On the complication rate of cerebral angiography. Neurosurg Rev 3:23–29

Rolfe EB, Maguise PD (1980) The incidence of headache following various techniques of metrizamide myelography. Br J Radiol 53:840–844

Ropper AH, Chiappa K, Young RR (1978) The effect of metrizamide on the EEG: A prospective study in 62 cases. Trans Am Neurol Assoc 103:159–162

Rosenbaum AE, Baker RA (1984) Pneumomyelography. In: Shapiro R (ed) Myelography, Yearbook Medical Publishers, Chicago

Rubin RC, Henderson ES, Ommaya AK, Walker MD, Rall DP (1966) The production of cerebrospinal fluid in man and its modification by actazolamide. J Neurosurg 25:430–436

Sage MR, Wilcox J, Evill CA, Benness GT (1982a) Brain parenchyma penetration by intrathecal ionics and non-ionic contrast media. AJNR 3:481–483

Sage MR, Wilcox, J, Evill CA, Benness GT (1982b) Comparison and evaluation of osmotic blood brain barrier disruption following intracarotid mannitol and methylglucamine iothalamate. Invest Radiol 17:276–281

Schober R (1964) Roentgen-Kontrastmittel und Liquor-Raum. Springer, Berlin, Heidelberg, New York

Shaw DD, Gansmo TB, Dahlstrom K (1985) Iohexol. Summary of North American and European clinical trials in adult lumbar, thoracic and cervical myelography with a new non-ionic contrast medium. Invest Radiol 20:S44–S50

Shehadi WH, Toniolo G (1980a) Adverse reactions to intravascularly administered contrast media. AJR 124:145–152

Shehadi WH, Toniolo G (1980b) Adverse reactions to contrast media. Radiology 137:229–302

Sicard JA, Forestier JE (1922) Methode generale d'exploration radiologique par l'huile iodie (lipidoil). Bull Soc Med Hop Paris 46:463–469

Skalpe IO (1976) Adhesive arachnoiditis following lumbar radiculography with water soluble contrast agents. Radiology 121:647–651

Smith MA, Laguna JF (1980) Confusion, dysphasia, and asterixis following metrizamide myelography. Can J Neurol Sci 7:309–311

Sovak M, Siefert HM, Ranganathan R (1980) Combined methods for assessment of neurotoxicity. Testing of new nonionic radiographic media. Invest Radiol 15:S248–S253

Sovak M, Ranganathan R, Speck U (1982a) Nonionic dimer: Development and initial testing of an intrathecal contrast agent. Radiology 142:115–118

Sovak M, Siefert HM, Ranganathan R (1982b) Combined methods for assessment of neurotoxicity: Testing of new nonionic radiographic media. Invest Radiol 15:6

Stack JP, Antoun NM, Jenkins JPR, Metcalfe RA, Isherwood I (1988) Gadolinium DTPA as a contrast agent in magnetic resonance imaging of the brain. Neuroradiology 30: 145–154

Steinhausen TB, Dungan CE, Furst JB et al. (1944) Iodinated organic compounds as contrast media for radiographic diagnosis. III. Experimental and clinical myelography with ethyl iodophenylundecylate (Pantopaque). Radiology 43:230

Strain WH (1971) Radiocontrast agents for neuroradiology. In: Knoefel PK (ed) Encyclopaedia of contrast media, vol 11. Pergamon Press, Oxford, p 369

Strain WH, French JD, Jones GE (1946) Iodinated organic compounds as contrast media for diagnosis. Escape of Pantopaque from intracranial subarachnoid space of dogs. Radiology 47:47–50

Studdard WE, Davis DO, Young SW (1981) Cortical blindness after cerebral angiography. A case report. J Neurosurg 54:240–244

Suzuki S, Kawaguchi S, Mita R, Ito K, Iwabuchi T (1976a) Ventriculography with methylglucamine iocarmate (Dimer-X). Experimental and clinical study. Neurol Surg (Tokyo) 3:849–858

Suzuki S, Kawaguchi S, Mita R, Iwabuchi T (1976b) Ventriculography with methylglucamine iocarmate (Dimer-X). Experimental and clinical study. Acta Neurochir (Wien) 33:219–223

Taren JA (1960) Unusual complication following Pantopaque myelography. J Neurosurg 17:323–326

Thomas SF, Heary GW, Kaplan HS (1951) Hepatolienography: Past, present and future. Radiology 57:669–683

Usbeck W, Assmann H (1977) value of Dimer-S myelography in the diagnosis of lumbar intravertebral disk lesions. Zentralbl Neurochir 38:165–174

Waldron RL, Bridenbaugh RB, Dampsey EW (1974) Effect of angiographic contrast media at cellular level in the brain: hypertonic vs chemical action. AJR 122:469–476

Wales LR, Nov AA (1981) Transient global amnesia: Complication of cerebral angiography. AJNR 2:275–277

Wallingford VH (1953) The development of organic iodide compounds as X-ray contrast media. J Am Pharmacol Assoc 42:721–728

White WB (1984) Metrizamide meningitis. South Med J 77:88–89

Wolf GL, Popp C (1984) NMR. A primer for medical imaging. Slack Incorporated, New Jersey

Subject Index